Safety Education

Safety Education

Fourth Edition

A. E. Florio, E.D.
Professor Emeritus of Safety Education
and Program Director of
Safety and Driver Education
University of Illinois

W. F. Alles, Ph.D.
Professor of Health and Safety
Pennsylvania State University

G. T. Stafford, E.D.
Deceased, Professor Emeritus
of Health and Safety Education
University of Illinois

HV
676
A 2
F 55
1979

McGraw-Hill Book Company
New York   St. Louis   San Francisco   Auckland   Bogotá   Düsseldorf
Johannesburg   London   Madrid   Mexico   Montreal   New Delhi
Panama   Paris   São Paulo   Singapore   Sydney   Tokyo   Toronto

SAFETY EDUCATION

Copyright © 1979, 1969, 1962, 1956 by McGraw-Hill, Inc. All rights reserved.
Printed in the United States of America. No part of this publication may be
reproduced, stored in a retrieval system, or transmitted, in any form or by any
means, electronic, mechanical, photocopying, recording, or otherwise, without
the prior written permission of the publisher.

1 2 3 4 5 6 7 8 9 0   F G F G   7 8 3 2 1 0 9

This book was set in Helvetica Light by University Graphics, Inc.
The editors were Richard R. Wright and Barry Benjamin;
the designer was Charles A. Carson;
the production supervisor was Dominick Petrellese.
New drawings were done by Allyn-Mason, Inc.
Fairfield Graphics was printer and binder.

Library of Congress Cataloging in Publication Data

Florio, A. E
    Safety education.

    Includes bibliographies and index.
    1. Safety education—United States.
I. Alles, W. F., joint author. II. Stafford,
George Thomas, joint author.
HV676.A2F55 1979   614.8'07   78-21902
ISBN 0-07-021371-2

Contents

Preface

Great advances have been made in this country toward preventing untimely deaths and crippling injuries. The results of the past have brought the American death rate to an all-time low. But the task is far from complete. In spite of the great advances that have been made, much more needs to be done to help solve this great social problem.

Accidents on the road, at work, at play, and in the home are still the leading cause of death among Americans aged 1 to 38, and, among persons of all ages, accidents are the fourth leading cause of all deaths. For youths aged 15 to 24 years, accidents claim more lives than all other leading causes combined and about four times more than the next leading cause of death. This epidemic still kills over 100,000 Americans annually, disables over 10 million, and causes injuries requiring treatment of over 63 million. The cost in a recent year was close to $53 billion.

There is no question that safe living is still an important and complicated problem. Living safely is a challenge that must be accepted by everyone if we are to continue to move forward in an ever-changing society. Although much progress has been made, the general public still must be strongly motivated to action. The complexity of modern living demands not only greater knowledge of the growing hazards that surround us but effective ways of coping with them.

We must realize that orderly living is a prerequisite to staying alive. We must learn how to remove all unnecessary dangers and to compensate for those which cannot be removed. All this points clearly to the need for increased emphasis on education in safe living. We must know more, care more, and act more prudently if we are to survive.

As this fourth edition is published, our society is beginning to become concerned with the urgent need for conservation of our human, financial, and natural resources. More and more, people are becoming aware of the many deaths and the destruction that occur daily on our streets and highways. The nation's National Highway Safety Administrator has said that "highway accidents are by far the leading form of violence in American life."

Although society has been faced with this problem for many years, only recently has the public started to show much interest in it. The specific area of traffic safety has drawn the greatest attention. The topic has been front-page news across the country, as we read of the thousands of motor vehicles recalled because they are considered unsafe. Increased attention has also been given to consumer product safety and safer conditions for the industrial worker. On three different occasions more than 40 million television viewers took traffic and disaster safety knowledge tests.

Many new laws have been passed by local and federal governmental bodies, and while these laws will help combat the problem, accidents will continue to take their gruesome toll until we teach everyone how to live safely in a changing world.

Safety education has made considerable progress since it was first introduced five decades ago. Its value has been most vividly demonstrated in the marked reduction of traffic accidents among elementary school children and in the lower incidence of motor-vehicle accidents and violations among those who have participated in traffic-safety education programs.

Accidents, however, remain the foremost cause of death among school-aged children, accounting for many more fatalities than are attributed to any single disease. Home and traffic accidents claim most lives, but drownings and fire casualties also help keep the death toll high. Technological advancement, while unquestionably adding to the enjoyment of life, has also multiplied its dangers, and individuals have not yet learned how to function safely in an increasingly hazardous environment. Although welcoming these new developments, they fail to adopt the careful procedures that alone can protect them from the risks inherent in using the powerful equipment now at their disposal. The mechanical safety devices designed to counteract these risks have therefore been unable to lower the accident rate to the extent that antibiotic drugs and other scientific advances have reduced the number of disease fatalities.

Preventing accidents is not a simple matter, for so many variables affect the accident rate that it is difficult to determine the most effective remedial action. But since human error is probably the outstanding cause of 85 percent of all accidents, education for safe living seems the best approach to the problem of minimizing them. Excellent results have already been reported in those areas that have received primary emphasis. This book holds that the scope of safety education must be enlarged to embrace all the times and places of ordinary life—the home, the factory, the farm, the school, and the community—working hours and hours of leisure.

No safety program can have any appreciable effect on the overall accident rate if it concentrates on only one or two activities. Although the intensive efforts of industry have reduced the workers' death rate by 60 percent, off-the-job accidents occur as frequently as ever, outnumbering on-the-job accidents by a ratio of three to one. The precautions observed in one occupation are not necessarily carried over into others, but if safety education is provided in all areas, the principles and procedures taught in one will tend to complement the instruction given in others. Thus education may contribute to the development of a general preoccupation with the subject that will enable people to safeguard their contact with the physical world.

American educators recognize that education for safe living is an integral part of the school's responsibility to society, and today the challenge of preventing accidents is greater than ever. Although safety education in public schools is required by law in many states, all too often the subject suffers because of inadequate time allotment, complacency of administrators, and incompetent instructors. Education can be the cure for this epidemic and, through the use of the content of this book, accidents can be prevented and consequences of accidents can be lessened.

This volume provides readers with concepts that will vividly alert them to the magnitude of the accident problem, the competencies needed to cope with the problem, and possible solutions.

The text presents fifteen major areas of safety and accident prevention that are related to today's major accident problems. The reader is given not only a broad coverage of each area but extensive specifics needed to be knowledgeable in the discipline of safety.

The fourth edition is expanded, updated, and rewritten. It is aimed at students in all curricula interested in improving the quality of life for all members of our society. The content is up to date and reflects the philosophy of the writers as well as a modern philosophy of accident prevention. Threading the text is the concept that accident prevention is the responsibility of every individual; and, through appropriate knowledge, skill, attitude, and behavior, accidents can be prevented.

The chapters have been reorganized to present a more orderly progression of material. A list of instructional objectives has been provided at the outset of each chapter, and extensive learning activities appear at the conclusion of each chapter to aid readers in achieving their objectives. Two chapters are entirely new ("Highway Safety" and "Community Safety"). The remaining twelve chapters have been rewritten and, in many instances, the thrust has been redirected. The content areas have been selected and presented in detail as they affect our society according to studies of the accident problem by national and local organizations dealing exclusively with accident prevention.

The authors wish to express their appreciation to the reviewers for their critical analysis, suggestions, and high support of this new edition. Expression of appreciation is also extended to the many federal, state, and private agencies, professional organizations, insurance companies, industries, and publishers who generously contributed material and assistance and granted permission to use quotations and illustrations. Also mentioned with gratitude are the many pioneers in the field of safety education, whose efforts have been an inspiration to the authors. Special mention should be made of George T. Stafford, who was an original coauthor prior to his death in 1968. His imagination, creativity, and foresight led to many early successes in the professional preparation of safety educators. We also wish to express our appreciation to our wives Marana and Barbara for their forbearance during this revision.

A. E. "Joe" Florio
W. F. "Wes" Alles

The Need for Safety Education

OVERALL OBJECTIVE:

The student of safety should understand the magnitude of the accident problem and the need for a comprehensive prevention program.

INSTRUCTIONAL OBJECTIVES:

After completing this chapter the student will be able to:

1 List the four principal classes and the nine types of accidents.
2 State in round numbers the death and injury toll for the four principal classes of accidents.
3 Cite the cost of accidents and the various elements that make up that cost.
4 Define certain terms that are used in *Accident Facts*.
5 List the major causes of accidents.
6 Define an *accident* and a *disabling injury*.
7 Describe the trends for traffic, home, public, and work accidents.
8 Compare the various causes of accidental injury and death with the other leading causes of injury and death.
9 Explain the various forces that were behind the safety movement, and show how they brought about a decline in accidents and injuries.
10 List the professional organizations that are major forces behind today's safety programs, and indicate the role of each organization.

THE SCOPE OF SAFETY EDUCATION

As we enter the last quarter of the twentieth century, we can look back with some satisfaction that progress in safety has been made during the previous decades (see Figure 1–1). It is also encouraging to note that in the last decade there has been a decline in the death rate for all age groups and a dramatic decline for

1

Between 1912 and 1976 accidental deaths per 100,000 population were reduced 43 percent from 82 to 47. The 68 percent reduction from 79 to 25 in the nonmotor-vehicle death rate was offset in part by the sevenfold increase in the motor-vehicle death rate from 3 to 22. The reduction in the overall rate during a period when the nation's population more than doubled has resulted in 1,850,000 fewer people being killed accidentally than would have been killed if the rate had not been reduced.

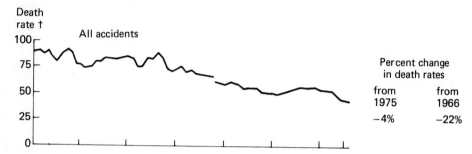

Death rate †

All accidents

Percent change in death rates

from 1975	from 1966
−4%	−22%

All rates on this page are adjusted to the age distribution of the population in 1940 to remove the influence of changes in the average age of the population through the years.

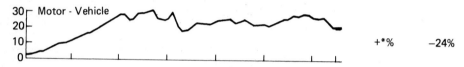

Motor - Vehicle

+*%   −24%

In 1976, there were 24 times as many deaths as in 1910, but about 300 times as many vehicles on the highways.

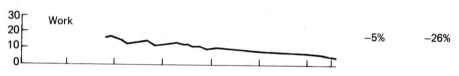

Work

−5%   −26%

These rates are based on total population, not worker population.

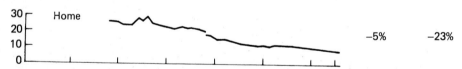

Home

−5%   −23%

For persons under 65, the 1976 standardized death rate was 10 percent below the 1966 rate; for persons 65 and over, the rate decreased 43 percent.

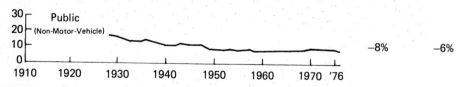

Public (Non-Motor-Vehicle)

−8%   −6%

1910   1920   1930   1940   1950   1960   1970 '76

The recent rise in the rate is partly due to an increase in recreational activity.

†Deaths per 100,000 population, adjusted to 1940 age distribution.   *Less than 0.5 percent.

Figure 1-1 Trends in accidental and nonmotor-vehicle death rates. (Source: Accident Facts, 1977, p. 10, National Safety Council, Chicago, Ill.)

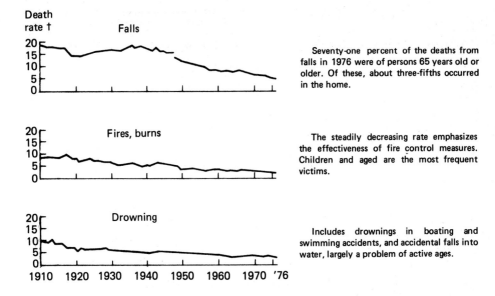

Death rate †

Falls

Seventy-one percent of the deaths from falls in 1976 were of persons 65 years old or older. Of these, about three-fifths occurred in the home.

Fires, burns

The steadily decreasing rate emphasizes the effectiveness of fire control measures. Children and aged are the most frequent victims.

Drowning

Includes drownings in boating and swimming accidents, and accidental falls into water, largely a problem of active ages.

†Deaths per 100,000 population, adjusted to 1940 age distribution.

Figure 1-1 *(Continued)*

the very young and for older people (see Table 1–1). Many fatalities have been prevented and billions of dollars have been saved. The efforts of many organizations, along with improved school codes and laws, improved and increased legislation, new and expanded accident-prevention agencies [Occupational Safety and Health Administration (O.S.H.A.) and Consumer Product Safety Commission (C.P.S.C.)], greater public awareness, and consciousness of the consequences of accidents, have combined to bring about these positive changes.

TABLE 1–1
Decline in the Death Rate
from 1966 to 1976

Age, yr	Decline, %
All ages	20
Under 5	30
5–14	16
15–24	12
25–44	19
45–64	28
65–74	31
75 and over	34

Source: *Accident Facts,* National Safety
Council, Chicago, 1977.

Although progress has been made in the first three-quarters of this century, we must not relax our efforts in behalf of accident prevention. We still have a long way to go in establishing comprehensive safety education programs in our schools. As we move toward the twenty-first century, we are still faced with many challenging problems. The complexity of life in the modern world requires greater knowledge of the hazards which surround us. Albert Wurts Whitney, a pioneer of the safety movement, said: "We must conserve our most valued resources—our people—especially from accidental life loss, crippling and injury." Whitney has made us aware of the extent of the material and property losses that result from accidents. Analysis of the facts clearly demonstrates that the accident toll continues to be intolerably high.

If an epidemic killed over 100,000 people, disabled, permanently or temporarily, close to 11 million others, and injured over 61 million others,[1] it would evoke an immediate and dramatic emotional response from our citizens. These figures represent the exact annual losses to this country from accidents. Yet we still tolerate this waste of human lives and resources that constitutes a serious threat to the national economy and social structure. It is essential that our citizens become familiar with the hazards of modern living.

Safety results from the effective adaptation of people to their environment. It is attained by concentrated individual effort and group cooperation. It can be achieved only by informed, alert, skillful people who respect themselves and have a regard for the welfare of others.

Accidents rank fourth on the list of the main causes of death among persons of all ages in this country. Responsible for an injury every 3 seconds and a fatality every 5 minutes, they account for six times more casualties than were attributed to World War II and for more deaths among children aged one to fourteen than the next four most common causes of death *combined.* In the age group of one to forty-four years, accidents rank as the number-one killer. Yet many people who can be terrorized by the threat of war remain relatively undisturbed by the announcement of accident statistics, and millions of parents were more alarmed by an epidemic of infantile paralysis than by the fact that accidents claim the lives of more than 12,000 children[2] every year (see Figure 1–2).

Unlike epidemics, which usually occur in one area, accidents are scattered throughout the country. Unlike either a war or a plague, they cannot be attributed to a single dramatic cause that suddenly disrupts normal conditions. Also, it is commonly believed that accidents happen to the other person. After all, they are not contagious, and it is easy to feel that one will be careful enough or lucky enough to avoid them. For these reasons, most people remain indifferent to the country's consistently high accident rate, although it should be a matter of grave concern to all citizens and a stimulus to preventive action (see Figure 1-3).

[1]*Accident Facts,* National Safety Council, Chicago, 1977. Unless otherwise noted, all statistics cited in this chapter are drawn from this source.
[2]Adding figures for the ages from birth to one year would raise the total to almost 14,000.

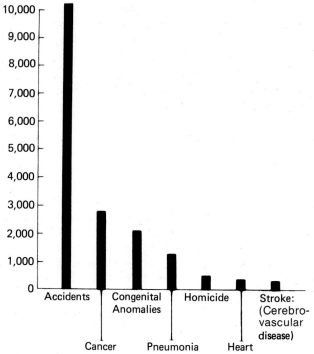

Figure 1-2   Chief causes of death among children aged 1-14 years. Chief causes of death among persons from age 5 to 75 and over are illustrated in Figure 1-3 by age groups.

ACCIDENT FACTS AND FIGURES

Varying only slightly from year to year, the annual accident toll amounts to over 100,000 fatalities and over 10 million disabling injuries, 380,000 of which result in permanent impairments. Although the previous all-time high of 110,052 accidental deaths was reported in 1936, the figures for the last decade have averaged over 112,000. Tragic as these figures are, they represent a decline of about 30 percent in the accident death rate in the last 50 years.

In 1960 accidents cost $13 billion, almost twice the amount spent on education during that year. The annual cost rose to $27 billion in the next 10 years and to $47 billion by the middle of the 1970s. Of this figure, more than $15 billion represented the cost of wages lost from temporary inability to work, lower wages caused by permanent impairment, and the current value of the calculated future earnings of those totally incapacitated or killed in accidents. Medical and hospital expenses totaled approximately $6 billion. The administrative and claim-settlement costs of insurance totaled more than $6 billion. (The amounts paid in actual claims are included in the figures given for medical expenses and wage losses.) The property damage by motor-vehicle accidents alone exceeded $8 billion, and property valued at over $4 billion was

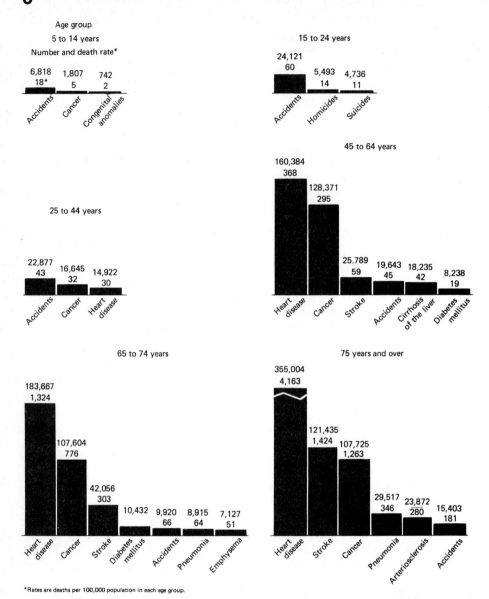

Age group

5 to 14 years

Number and death rate*

6,818	1,807	742
18*	5	2
Accidents	Cancer	Congenital anomalies

15 to 24 years

24,121		
60	5,493	4,736
	14	11
Accidents	Homicides	Suicides

25 to 44 years

22,877	16,645	14,922
43	32	30
Accidents	Cancer	Heart disease

45 to 64 years

160,384	128,371				
368	295	25.789	19,643	18,235	8,238
		59	45	42	19
Heart disease	Cancer	Stroke	Accidents	Cirrhosis of the liver	Diabetes mellitus

65 to 74 years

183,667	107,604	42,056	10,432	9,920	8,915	7,127
1,324	776	303		66	64	51
Heart disease	Cancer	Stroke	Diabetes mellitus	Accidents	Pneumonia	Emphysema

75 years and over

355,004	121,435	107,725	29,517	23,872	15,403
4,163	1,424	1,263	346	280	181
Heart disease	Stroke	Cancer	Pneumonia	Arteriosclerosis	Accidents

*Rates are deaths per 100,000 population in each age group.

Figure 1-3 Leading causes of all deaths. (Source: National Center for Health Statistics, U.S. Department of Health, Education and Welfare. Accident Facts, 1977, National Safety Council, Chicago, Ill.)

destroyed by fires. Property damage and production curtailed through occupational accidents represented a loss of $7 billion.

The cost of accidents is enormous, (Table 1–2), and we mourn for those whose lives have been snuffed out by accidents. But what about the grief and suffering of those who have survived *seemingly* less tragic, nonfatal accidents, persons who must live with a permanent disability? Lost eyesight, unsightly scars, artificial arms or legs, and the frustrations of thwarted plans for the

TABLE 1-2

1976 Accident Costs by Class of Accident

Type of Accident	Cost, Billions of Dollars
Motor-vehicle accidents	$24.7
This cost figure includes $7.6 billion in wage loss, $2.1 billion in medical expense, $6.1 billion in insurance administration cost, and $8.9 billion in property damage from moving motor-vehicle accidents. Not included are the cost of public agencies such as police, fire departments, and courts, indirect losses to employers, the value of cargo losses in commercial vehicles, and damages awarded in excess of direct losses. Fire damage to parked motor-vehicles is not included here but is distributed to the other classes.	
Work accidents	17.8
This cost figure includes $3.6 billion in wage loss, $1.9 billion in medical expense, $2.4 billion in insurance administration cost, $2.0 billion in fire losses ($1.7 billion from building fires and $0.3 billion from nonbuilding fires), and $7.9 billion in the other, indirect costs arising out of work accidents. Not included is the value of property damage other than fire losses and the indirect losses from fires.	
Home accidents	6.3
This cost figure includes $2.9 billion in wage loss, $1.8 billion in medical expense, $0.1 billion in health insurance administration cost, and $1.5 billion in fire losses ($1.4 billion in building fires and $0.1 billion in nonbuilding fires, primarily parked motor-vehicles). Not included are the costs of property damage other than fire losses and the indirect costs to employers.	
Public accidents	5.0
This cost figure includes $2.9 billion in wage loss, $1.2 billion in medical expense, $0.1 billion in health insurance administration cost, and $0.8 billion in fire losses ($0.5 billion in building fires and $0.3 billion in nonbuilding fires). Not included are the costs of property damage other than fire losses and the indirect costs to employers.	
Total, all accidents	$53.8

Source: *Accident Facts*, National Safety Council, Chicago, 1977, p.5.

future—all these must be considered as a part of the cost of accidents. They become grim reminders that for every person killed there may be five or six people who must face life under varying degrees of permanent disability.

TRAFFIC ACCIDENTS

More than 38 million miles of public highways serve the nation's 129 million motorists, who drive over 1,332 billion motor-vehicle miles annually on these facilities.

Since approximately 4 million young people reach driving age each year, the number of motorists will probably continue to grow (Figure 1-4). In addition, there are approximately 100 million bicycle riders, 50 percent of whom are children under fourteen years of age. In recent years the traffic situation has been complicated by increases in motorcycles, and more recently by the introduction of the Moped or motorized bicycle.

In 1960 there were slightly more than 500,000 motorcycles registered in this country. In 15 years this number has increased to 5,494,000. At the present rate of growth we can predict that close to 8½ million cycles will be traveling on our streets and highways by 1980.

Motor-vehicle accidents receive more publicity than any other type except major disasters. From 1900 through 1975, motor-vehicle deaths in the United States totaled about 2,100,000. Fatalities from the Revolutionary War through the Vietnam war totaled 1,156,000 (See Table 1–3). One can readily see that our streets and highways constitute more hazardous environment than existed in

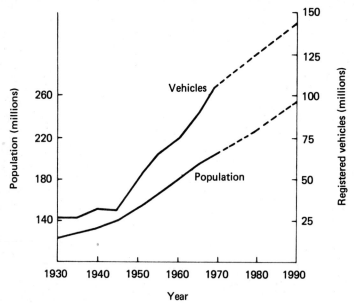

Figure 1-4 Population and vehicle growth in the United States. (Source: Transportation and Traffic Engineering Handbook, Institute of Traffic Engineers, p. 2, 1976, Prentice Hall, Inc., Englewood Cliffs, New Jersey.)

TABLE 1–3
United States Military Casualties in Principal Wars

War	Deaths			Nonfatal Wounds
	Total	Battle	Others*	
Total	1,156,000†	649,534	506,400†	1,580,000‡
Revolutionary War (1775–83)	4,435	4,435	N.A.	6,188
War of 1812 (1812–15)	2,260	2,260	N.A.	4,505
Mexican War (1846–48)	13,283	1,733	11,550	4,152
Civil War (1861–65)				
Union Forces	364,511	140,414	224,097	281,881
Confederate Forces	133,821	74,524	59,297	N.A.
Spanish-American War (1898)	2,446	385	2,061	1,662
World War I (1917–18)	116,708	53,513	63,195	204,002
World War II (1941–45)	407,316	292,131	115,185	670,846
Korean War (1950–53)	54,246	33,629	20,617	103,284
Viet Nam War (1961–75)	56,897	46,510	10,387	303,569

*Includes deaths from disease, accidents, etc.
†Rounded.
‡Incomplete and rounded.
N.A. Not available.
Source: Office of Secretary of Defense, as reported in *Accident Facts,* National Safety Council, Chicago, 1977, p. 49.

our principal wars. It must also be kept in mind that nearly everyone is exposed to motor-vehicle accidents whereas a much smaller number are exposed to war.

In one recent year (1972) alone, over 56,000 deaths and 1,800,000 disabiling injuries occurred (see Table 1–4). Statistics pertaining to the nation's number-one killer warrant all the attention they have received. Bicycle acci-

TABLE 1–4
Motor-Vehicle Deaths

Period	Average Yearly Deaths
1913–1917	6,800
1918–1922	12,700
1923–1927	21,800
1928–1932	31,050
1933–1937	36,315
1938–1941	34,859
1942–1945 (war years)	26,125
1946–1950	32,906
1951–1955	37,359
1956–1959	38,311
1960–1965	42,882
1966–1970	54,250
1971–1975	51,714
1976–	46,700

Source: *Accident Facts,* National Safety Council, Chicago, 1977, p. 58.

dents claim 1,000 lives and result in approximately 40,000 disabling injuries annually, but considering the 100 million bicycles in use, these figures are relatively low.

There has been a noticeable change in the proportion of bicycle-related deaths by age group in recent years. In the early 1950s the majority of bicycle fatalities were suffered by the zero to fourteen age group (see Table 1–5). Today 28 percent of fatalities occur in the fifteen to twenty-four age group and 23 percent in the twenty-five and over age group. From present trends we can anticipate a further increase in adult bicycle useage because the bicycle provides one of the most economical forms of transportation and recreation, and promotes physical fitness. With the increasing use of bicycles come increasing problems in the highway aspects of bicycling safety. These problems must receive immediate attention from appropriate federal, state, and local governments, and private agencies, with special emphasis in our elementary and secondary schools, since formal training usually produces positive results.

A recent study of motor-driven cycle accidents, by the National Safety Council, reveals that 3,160 cyclists lost their lives in one year, and thousands were injured. The majority of these victims were youthful operators. In a ten-year period (1966 to 1976) the number of motorcycles increased from 1,752,801 to 5,110,000. Although there are no accurate mileage figures for motorcycles and motor scooters available, it is estimated that the mileage death rate would be around 13 deaths per 100 million vehicle miles of travel. This compares with a death rate between 3 and 4 for all motor vehicles.

TABLE 1–5
Pedalcycle Rates and Deaths by Age, 1935–1976

Year	Pedalcycles* (millions)	Deaths	Death Rate†	Percent of Deaths by Age			
				All Ages	0–14	15–24	25 & Over
1935	3.5	450	12.80	100%	57	29	14
1940	7.8	750	9.59	100%	48	39	13
1945	9.0	500	5.55	100%	56	22	22
1950	13.8	440	3.18	100%	82	9	9
1955	23.1	410	1.78	100%	71	12	17
1960	28.2	460	1.63	100%	78	9	13
1965	38.8	680	1.75	100%	64	18	18
1970	56.5	780	1.38	100%	66	15	19
1972	71.4	1,000	1.40	100%	50	27	23
1973	80.0	1,000	1.25	100%	49	30	21
1974	90.0	1,000	1.11	100%	47	31	22
1975	95.0	1,000	1.05	100%	49	28	23
1976	95.0	900	0.94	100%	48	33	19

*Pedalcycles in use for a given year is the ten-year total (that year and the previous nine years) of domestic production plus imports less exports.
†Deaths per 100,000 pedalcycles in use.
Source: Data from National Center for Health Statistics, state traffic authorities and NSC estimates. Reported in *Accident Facts*, National Safety Council, Chicago, 1977.

A more recent addition to the traffic scene has been the Moped—a vehicle that is a cross between a bicycle and a motorcycle. Although the Moped is not as popular as either the motorcycle or the bicycle, it has been estimated that by 1980 several million will be using our streets and highways. As Mopeds get 120 to 200 miles per gallon of fuel, with low exhaust emissions, there is little doubt as to their future popularity. Who can predict the accident toll if motorcycles, motor scooters, and Mopeds become as numerous as bicycles?

PEDESTRIANS

For the past decade, pedestrian fatalities have averaged around 10,000 a year. Recently there has been a slight decline in this average; nevertheless pedestrians still constitute a serious traffic problem. In the various traffic safety programs that have been instituted in the past decade, the pedestrian problem has probably received the least amount of attention. Tables 1–6 and 1–7 analyze pedestrian accidents by comparing age-group involvement and pedestrian action, and pedestrian and vehicle action, respectively.

Six out of ten pedestrian deaths and injuries happen when persons cross or enter streets. Two-fifths of all actions occur between intersections, but the proportion varies for persons of different ages.

PEDESTRIAN AND VEHICLE ACTIONS. According to 1974 data from Alabama and Arizona, in pedestrian accidents involving turning vehicles, two-thirds of the pedestrians were struck while crossing intersections and crosswalks. For all pedestrian-vehicle accidents, more than two-fifths of the pedestrians were involved while crossing *not* at an intersection or crosswalk. Table 1-7 illustrates the proportional relationship of pedestrian actions and selected vehicle actions.

HOME ACCIDENTS

Traditionally people's homes are their castles, places of security, but this concept seems to have little basis in fact. There seems to be a lack of understanding as to what is and what is not safe in and around the home. Today the home is a major source of accidental death and injury. There may be some consolation in the fact that since the end of World War II accidental home deaths per 100,000 population have dropped 50 percent, from 25.3 in 1945 to 10.0 in 1976. Nevertheless, there are still close to 25,000 deaths and 4 million disabling injuries each year. The National Health Survey reports an additional 17,500,000 less serious injuries annually.

Home accidents usually occur to the very young, children under five, and people over sixty-five. The causes of home accidents fall under two headings: (1) mechanical causes, such as disorder, improper equipment, improper use of equipment, neglect of needed repairs, slippery surfaces, and insufficient light; and (2) personal causes, such as poor judgment, adult negligence in the

TABLE 1–6

Deaths and Injuries of Pedestrians by Age and Action, Statewide, 1976*

Actions	All Ages		Age of Persons Killed and Injured							
	No.	%	0–4	5–9	10–14	15–19	20–24	25–44	45–64	65 and Over
Total Pedestrians	**108,300**	**100.0%**	**100.0%**	**100.0%**	**100.0%**	**100.0%**	**100.0%**	**100.0%**	**100.0%**	**100.0%**
Crossing or entering	67,000	61.9	71.2	77.8	63.5	47.2	45.3	48.2	61.8	75.0
—at intersection	24,700	22.8	8.0	19.2	23.4	20.4	20.1	21.7	30.1	41.5
—between intersections	42,300	39.1	63.2	58.6	40.1	26.8	25.2	26.5	31.7	33.5
Walking in roadway	8,600	7.9	2.2	2.4	8.6	15.0	12.2	9.5	8.7	6.7
—with traffic	6,200	5.7	1.3	1.3	6.0	11.1	10.2	7.5	5.6	4.2
—against traffic	2,400	2.2	0.9	1.1	2.6	3.9	2.0	2.0	3.1	2.5
Standing in roadway	4,600	4.2	1.2	0.4	2.1	7.1	8.9	7.6	5.7	2.1
Pushing or working on vehicle in roadway	2,300	2.1	†	0.1	0.5	3.3	4.5	4.9	2.5	1.3
Other working in roadway	1,500	1.4	1.3	0.8	0.5	0.8	2.4	3.3	1.5	0.4
Playing in roadway	4,200	3.9	11.3	8.6	6.2	1.6	0.2	0.3	0.2	0.5
Other in roadway	9,400	8.7	6.3	6.4	10.9	11.5	11.8	10.5	7.7	4.7
Not in roadway	10,700	9.9	6.5	3.5	7.7	13.5	14.7	15.7	11.9	9.3

*Totals not comparable to previous years due to classification changes.
†Less than 0.05%.
Source: Based on reports of deaths and injuries from 18 state traffic authorities. Reported in *Accident Facts*, National Safety Council, Chicago, 1977.

TABLE 1–7
Pedestrian Action by Vehicle Action, 1974

Pedestrian Action	Vehicle Action					
	Total	Straight	Overtaking	Right Turn	Left Turn	Backing
Total	**100.0%**	**100.0%**	**100.0%**	**100.0%**	**100.0%**	**100.0%**
Crossing at intersection or crosswalk	25.3	21.0	24.9	69.7	68.8	5.3
Crossing not at intersection or crosswalk	41.3	45.2	12.5	9.3	15.2	13.2
Walking in roadway with traffic	5.7	6.0	12.5	5.8	1.6	0.0
Same against traffic	2.7	2.8	6.3	3.5	0.0	0.0
Standing in roadway	4.1	4.1	6.3	3.5	1.6	15.7
Pushing or working on vehicle in roadway	1.2	1.2	0.0	0.0	0.8	5.3
Other working in roadway	2.7	2.9	0.0	0.0	2.4	0.0
Playing in roadway	1.9	1.8	18.7	1.2	0.0	7.9
Other in roadway	5.8	5.6	6.3	2.3	4.0	26.3
Not in roadway	9.3	9.4	12.5	4.7	5.6	26.3

Source: 1974 reports from Alabama Department of Public Safety and Arizona Department of Transportation. Reported in *Accident Facts,* National Safety Council, Chicago, 1977.

supervision of children, personal frailty, hurry, intoxication, and physical handicaps.

OCCUPATIONAL ACCIDENTS

Between 1912 and 1976, work accidents have had a dramatic decline of 71 percent. The rate per 100,000 workers went from 21 to 5.8. In 1912, an estimated 18,000 to 21,000 workers' lives were lost. At present, with a work force more than twice as large and producing more than seven times as much, there were only 12,500 work deaths.

In comparing work accidents with the other major classes—motor-vehicle, home, and public—work accidents involved the lowest number of fatalities and disabling injuries. Although we are still faced with over 12,000 fatalities and over 2 million disabling injuries annually, the progress that has been made in reducing accidents and fatalities has been significant (See Figure 1–5). Because of poor working conditions and high accident rates during the Industrial Revolution and after, a great deal of emphasis has been placed on industrial safety since the turn of the century. Early inspections and regulations, workmen's compensation laws, and more recently the Occupational Safety and Health Act have all contributed to today's organized safety movement. Today, industries that have an organized safety program can illustrate lower injury-frequency and injury-severity rates.

Apparently, many workers who have been trained to observe safety principles and practices while they are at work have not been motivated to apply these same procedures to their off-time activities. Fatalities are three times

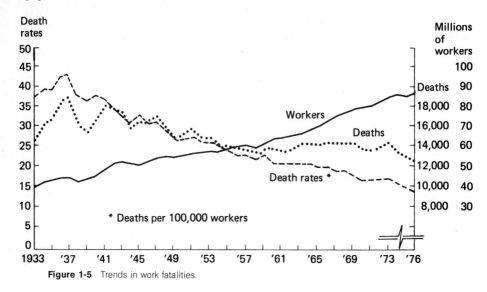

Figure 1-5 Trends in work fatalities.

greater off the job than at work, and over a million more disabling injuries occur. In one year, production time lost because of off-job accidents totaled nearly 70 million man-days, compared with 45 million man-days lost by workers being injured on the job. As a result, employers have been making an all-out effort to promote safety. One company, for example, has a record of more than 61,979,-357 man-hours of work without a disabling injury.[3]

HISTORY AND DEVELOPMENT OF THE SAFETY MOVEMENT[4]

The accident-prevention movement is a product of the twentieth century. It was born in the field of industry, and today there is cooperation between government, industry, private and public organizations, and education, with virtually hundreds of organizations providing specialized safety services.

Although factory workers of today may not find working conditions all they desire, they do not have to undergo the harrowing experiences suffered by factory hands in England in the early days of mechanized industry.

The appalling number of workers killed or injured at their jobs began to register in the public consciousness in the middle of the nineteenth century. Workers began to leave farms and small shops in ever-increasing numbers to work in larger plants. New machinery created new hazards and led to new injuries. Labor was plentiful and disabled workers could be easily displaced.

[3]E. I. DuPont De Nemours and Co., Kinston Plant, Kinston, N.C. For other no-injury records, see the current edition of *Accident Facts*.

[4]For a detailed account of the history of the safety movement, see: H. W. Heinrich, *Industrial Accident Prevention*, 4th ed., McGraw-Hill Book Company, New York, appendix 1; Herbert James Stock and J. Duke Elkow, *Education for Safe Living*, 4th ed., Prentice-Hall, Inc., Englewood Cliffs, N.J., 1966, chap. 1; and U.S. Department of Labor, *The Development of the Safety Movement*, Washington, 20402.

Despite a growing concern for safety, there was a lack of unity among labor, industry, and government. At first, employers assumed a limited degree of liability for injuries. In defense against damage suits, the company lawyer had many ways of proving that the worker or a coworker had contributed to the cause of the accident. In many cases the principle of assumption of risk relieved the employer of any responsibility.

The continuously rising rate of deaths and injuries finally led to some action, and stricter legislation to protect the worker began to evolve. In 1867 Massachusetts passed a law providing for the services of factory inspectors, and two years later created the first bureau of labor statistics to study the accident problem. In 1877, the Massachusetts Legislature voted to compel employers to protect workers from hazardous machinery. The stimulus for initiating these early programs arose from the humanitarian and social arguments voiced by the clergy and the press. Although some of the early laws enacted in this country in the late 1880s helped effect accident prevention, the financial burden on the employers was still not sufficient to spur them to establish programs to protect workers from death and crippling injuries.

It was not until adequate records were kept as a result of workmen's compensation laws and increased accident experiences that industry began to realize the seriousness of occupational accidents. Although a limited act was passed in 1908 at the demand of President Theodore Roosevelt, it was not until 1910–1911 that comprehensive employers' liability laws were enacted. The acts caused employers to secure insurance coverage against workers' injuries and to remove many hazards from factories. These laws also compelled industries to use mechanical safeguards to give workers greater protection from accidents, because the employer was now required to remunerate the injured employee *whether or not negligence could be proved.* Between 1911 and 1915, thirty states enacted workmen's compensation laws, and today all states have them. The requirements of these laws impressed both employee and employer with the high cost of accidents. This led to increased interest in safety on the part of employers and industry and to the implementation of their own safety programs.

Probably the greatest stimulus to safety programs occurred in 1912, when a group of engineers representing insurance companies, industry, and government met in Milwaukee, Wisconsin, to exchange data on accident prevention. The organization formed at this meeting was to become the National Safety Council, which today carries on major programs and campaigns in practically all areas of safety. Its annual safety congress draws thousands of representatives of industry, government, and education from all over the United States and many foreign countries. From 35,000 in 1912, the yearly average of industrial deaths has dropped to slightly more than 13,000.

However, for the long-range program, to impart the knowledge of safe behavior and to effect its immediate and continuing practice has been the task of education. Such educators as E. George Payne and Albert W. Whitney developed philosophies of safety in the early 1920s that have been instrumental in strengthening the place of safety instruction in the field of education. Whitney's philosophy of "safety for more and better adventure" captured the imagination of educators and others interested in the safety movement.

The early efforts of Detroit and Kansas City to establish training in safety measures as an integral part of their educational programs were instrumental in guiding other cities in similar directions. Early publications such as *The Present Status of Safety Education,* twenty-fifth yearbook of the National Society for the Study of Education; *Safety Education,* eighteenth yearbook of the American Association of School Administrators; and the magazine *Safety Education* (no longer published) were of inestimable value in gaining recognition for safety education.

Grateful recognition should be given to Herbert J. Stack for his early work as educational director of the National Bureau of Casualty and Surety Underwriters and later as director of the New York University Center for Safety Education. Recognition should also be given to Amos E. Neyhart of Pennsylvania State University, who pioneered some of the early developments in high school driver education. Both these men represented organizations that formulated the first high school driver education textbooks. *Man and the Motor Car* was published first by the National Bureau of Casualty and Surety Underwriters and later by the Safety Center. *Sportsmanlike Driving,* first in booklet form and later as a text, was published by the American Automobile Association, whose consultant was Amos Neyhart. These two early texts were instrumental in promoting driver education in high schools. Later, many other excellent textbooks and publications furthered the cause. Although further progress must still be made, education has made great contributions to the safety movement.

Today, many professional organizations contribute to our safety programs.[5] The United States American Standards Association, along with various societies and associations, has helped develop safety standards. The unions have been major forces in the safety movement. They have campaigned vigorously for safe working conditions, have established safety education programs, and have worked with management in formulating safety regulations. Various insurance associations, state and federal governments, and virtually hundreds of other organizations have provided specialized services for accident prevention.

There have been many forces behind the safety movement, and these forces have given the movement great impetus. The forces that have assisted most in the evolution of the accident-prevention movement are

1 *Legislation.* Standards for improved health conditions in factories, fire protection, licensing of drivers, driver education in secondary schools, and workmen's compensation have all emerged from legislative acts.

2 *Disasters.* [see Table 1–8] Concern is always present after a major disaster strikes the nation. Legislation, improved standards, and control pro-

---

[5]Some of the prominent safety organizations are listed in the source note for Table 1-8.

TABLE 1–8

Largest United States Disasters by Category

Type and Location	No. of Deaths	Date of Disaster
Floods		
Galveston tidal wave	6,000	Sept. 8, 1900
Johnstown, Pa.	2,209	May 31, 1889
Ohio and Indiana	732	Mar. 28, 1913
St. Francis, Calif. dam burst	450	Mar. 13, 1928
Ohio and Mississippi River valleys	380	Jan. 22, 1937
Hurricanes		
Florida	1,833	Sept. 16–17, 1928
New England	657	Sept. 21, 1938
Louisiana	500	Sept. 29, 1915
Florida	409	Sept. 1–2, 1935
Louisiana and Texas	395	June 27–28, 1957
Tornadoes		
Illinois	606	Mar. 18, 1925
Mississippi, Alabama, Georgia	402	Apr. 2–7, 1936
Southern and Midwestern states	318	Apr. 3, 1974
Ind., Ohio, Mich., Ill. and Wisc.	272	Apr. 11, 1965
Ark., Tenn., Mo., Miss. and Ala.	229	Mar. 21–22, 1952
Earthquakes		
San Francisco earthquake and fire	452	Apr. 18, 1906
Alaskan earthquake-tsunami hit Hawaii, Calif.	173	Apr. 1, 1946
Long Beach, Calif. earthquake	120	Mar. 10, 1933
Alaskan earthquake and tsunami	117	Mar. 27, 1964
San Fernando-Los Angeles, Calif. earthquake	65	Feb. 9, 1971
Marine		
"Sultana" exploded—Mississippi River	1,547	Apr. 27, 1865
"Titanic" struck iceberg—Atlantic Ocean	1,517	Apr. 15, 1912
"Empress of Ireland" ship collision—St. Lawrence River	1,024	May 29, 1914
"General Slocum" burned—East River	1,021	June 15, 1904
"Eastland" capsized—Chicago River	812	July 24, 1915
Aircraft		
Two-plane collision over New York City	134	Dec. 16, 1960
Two-plane collision over Grand Canyon, Ariz.	128	June 30, 1956
Scheduled jetliner crash in New York City	113	June 24, 1975
Jetliner crash into mountainside near Juneau, Alaska	111	Sept. 4, 1971
Scheduled plane crash near Miami, Fla.	101	Dec. 29, 1972
Railroad		
Two-train collision near Nashville, Tenn.	101	July 9, 1918
Two-train collision, Eden, Colo.	96	Aug. 7, 1904
Avalanche hit two trains near Wellington, Wash.	96	Mar. 1, 1910
Bridge collapse under train, Ashtabula, Ohio	92	Dec. 29, 1876
Rapid transit train derailment, Brooklyn, N.Y.	92	Nov. 1, 1918
Fires		
Peshtigo, Wisc. and surrounding area forest fire	1,152	Oct. 9, 1871
Iroquois Theatre, Chicago	575	Dec. 30, 1903
Cocoanut Grove nightclub, Boston	492	Nov. 28, 1942
North German Lloyd Steamships, Hoboken, N.J.	326	June 30, 1900
Ohio penitentiary, Columbus	320	Apr. 21, 1930

TABLE 1-8 (*continued*)
Largest United States Disasters by Category

Type and Location	No. of Deaths	Date of Disaster
Explosions		
Texas City, Texas ship explosion	561	Apr. 16, 1947
Port Chicago, Calif. ship explosion	322	July 18, 1944
New London, Texas school explosion	294	Mar. 18, 1937
Eddystone, Pa. munitions plant explosion	133	Apr. 10, 1917
Cleveland, Ohio gas tank explosion	130	Oct. 20, 1944
Mines		
Monongha, West Va. coal mine explosion	361	Dec. 6, 1907
Dawson, New Mexico coal mine fire	263	Oct. 22, 1913
Cherry, Ill. coal mine fire	259	Nov. 13, 1909
Jacobs Creek, Pa. coal mine explosion	239	Dec. 19, 1907
Scofield, Utah coal mine explosion	200	May 1, 1900

Source: National Almanac, World Almanac, Official Associated Press Almanac, National Fire Protection Association, Chicago Historical Society, Texas Inspection Bureau, American Red Cross, U.S. Bureau of Mines, National Oceanic and Atmospheric Administration, city and state Boards of Health, and the Metropolitan Life Insurance Company. Quoted in *Accident Facts,* National Safety Council, Chicago, 1977.

grams usually are implemented while public attention is high and focused upon the disaster.

3 *Economic Measures.* Accidents cost money; therefore industries, states, and business concerns welcome the implementation of loss prevention programs. Such measures have been very influential in the advancement of accident prevention programs.

4 *Social Mores.* People from all avenues of life have joined together from time to time in the betterment of mankind. Conferences, public forums, and workshops have been conducted to influence the development of the safety movement.

5 *Protective Equipment.* Equipment such as seat belts, hard hats, radar, safety glass, and guards for industrial machinery have contributed significantly to the safety of people engaged in all types of activities.[6]

INGREDIENTS THAT CAUSE ACCIDENTS

Before suitable remedies can be prescribed that will lead to an effective accident-prevention program, the causes of the problem must be diagnosed. At this point it may be advisable to define the term *accident*. The National Safety Council defines an accident as that occurrence in a sequence of events which usually produces unintended injury, death, or property damage.[7] It can be broadly stated that all accidents are the result of environmental hazards and/or

[6]James E. Aaron, Frank A. Bridges, and Dale O. Ritzel, *First Aid and Emergency Care. Prevention and Protection of Injuries.* The Macmillan Company, New York, 1972, p. 30.
[7]The National Safety Council definitions of the four major classes of accident, as well as the major types of accident, are listed later in this chapter.

unsafe behavior, but any thoroughgoing attempt to explain why accidents happen involves the study of many variables—not only the innumerable objects and forces in the outer world that can injure people, but also the variety of attitudes and emotions that motivate their actions.

An understanding of the ingredients that cause accidents will be helpful in establishing corrective and remedial controls.

INADEQUATE KNOWLEDGE

Today's technological advances and those of the past decade almost defy one's imagination. The electron microscope makes it possible to actually see viruses so small that almost a million of them cover only 1 square inch. "Breaking the sound barrier," "space ships," and "rockets, and even men, to the moon" are commonplace terms today. And people must have the knowledge of safe practices that will enable them to make the necessary adjustments to their technological environment, in order to live a safe and satisfying life.

Knowledge of common safety rules is not as widespread as might be imagined. Partial information often serves merely to give people an unwarranted sense of security, which may blunt their alertness to danger. Some drivers realize that speeding is responsible for many accidents but fail to understand that a rate of 35 miles an hour in city traffic can be more hazardous than twice that speed on the newer interstate roads. Although most people are aware in a general way that drinking alcoholic beverages is dangerous, many do not realize that it can have an effect on vision, judgment, the brain, and motor skills, and that just two beers can affect their driving ability.

IMPROPER ATTITUDES AND HABITS

Accidents are usually attributed to the attitude and behavior of individuals, involving common faults, such as carelessness, foolhardiness, procrastination, and irresponsible and selfish conduct. The expressions "Take a chance," "Nothing ventured, nothing gained," and "Safety is for the other person" suggest some of the attitudes that are inconsistent with safe living. This kind of thinking often leads people to drive too fast, to pass red lights when a police officer is not in sight, to pile up oily rags in a corner of the attic, to smoke in bed, or to assume that a few drinks will not impair their driving skill.

The willingness to take a chance is sometimes reflected in the habit of procrastinating. A motorist may realize that his or her brakes are not holding properly and intend to have them adjusted at the first opportunity, but until then the motorist is likely to assume that the car will be able to stop in time to prevent a collision. Too often a motorist is involved in an accident before getting around to having the necessary repairs made. A housewife may notice some dangerous condition in the house and even comment repeatedly on the necessity of correcting it before someone is hurt. But her family will probably go on living with the hazard until an injury occurs. *After* a fall on the stairs, she may decide to remove the throw rug on the landing, or install a handrail, or remove the children's toys from the steps.

UNSAFE BEHAVIOR

People have not learned to live safely with the powerful forces now at their disposal. Although their environment has changed, they have not changed with it; they persist in careless actions, once relatively harmless, that now endanger their lives. The still-prevalent habit of crossing streets at will did not involve much risk in the horse-and-buggy days, but in the light of present traffic conditions it has become potentially suicidal. If in 1900 a carriage driver drowsed on the way home from an evening party, the chances were good that the horse would proceed safely to their destination. Today's motorist who falls asleep at the wheel is lucky to survive. The housewife of 50 years ago could mix a cake batter without fear of losing a finger in an electric beater, and if her child did not look in both directions before chasing a ball into the street, the consequences were not likely to be disastrous.

The customs and traditions that prevailed for generations permitted relaxed, carefree behavior, but circumstances now demand alertness and control, for the complexities of a mechanized civilization make order a necessity. With our increased dominion over the natural world, accidents rarely "just happen"; they are caused by undisciplined conduct that violates the order essential to safety in the modern world. Of all accidents in recent years, 85 percent could have been prevented if the victims had reacted properly to their environment.

Howard Pyle, emeritus president of the National Safety Council, stated, "We can only get as much safety as people want to have." Better ways of motivating people must be found. Research shows that underlying causes of accidents are deep-seated in human personality; therefore, continuous attention should be focused on human behavior. Legislating safety in and for the use of motor vehicles and other kinds of mechanical equipment may be of some help, but the human factor will continue to be the major agent in accident prevention and control. Therefore, safety education is a worthy and effective approach.

INSUFFICIENT SKILL

Accidents sometimes occur because people, especially children, attempt to perform feats beyond their abilities. A child is permitted to ride a new bicycle in the street before really knowing how to operate it or understanding traffic rules. Victims of drowning are frequently inexperienced swimmers who have overestimated their endurance and have set themselves goals that they are unable to reach. The novice skier may break a leg in attempting a maneuver that he or she has seen a professional perform with ease.

Sometimes psychophysical characteristics, such as faulty vision, faulty reaction time, fatigue, muscular weakness, senility, intoxication, or overwrought emotions, decrease people's skills so that they cannot safely accomplish tasks that are ordinarily well within their abilities. Emotional pressures and intoxication can also influence attitudes. Individuals under the influence of liquor or extremely upset may disregard all the safety precautions they would otherwise observe. Some people, for example, give vent to their pent-up anger through daredevil, aggressive driving. The various sections of this book provide information that encourages training in developing skills for accident prevention.

ENVIRONMENTAL HAZARDS

Life today is undeniably more convenient and comfortable than it was in 1900, but in many respects it is potentially far more dangerous. In making possible a world of ease and plenty, automobiles, high-powered industrial equipment, electrical household appliances, and the countless other achievements of modern technology have created many hazards that were unknown 60 years ago.

Despite the risks inherent in present-day conditions, only about 15 percent of all accidents are caused by forces external to man. Most modern machinery is not necessarily dangerous, for the development of safety apparatus has kept pace with the invention of equipment, and today there are probably more protective devices than people willing to use them. When greater power is offered to people, they are usually given the means of controlling it. As car speeds have been increased, for example, such improvements as smoother roads, brighter headlights, and more effective brakes have made safe travel possible at a faster rate. Since all the mechanisms and gadgets and special features designed to protect us from environmental hazards have not appreciably lowered the accident rate, it can only be concluded that most accidents occur primarily because people fail to take the precautions necessary to protect themselves.

Accidents are to be expected in an uncontrolled environment; but people have the ability to control the conditions of their lives to a certain extent and thus reduce their accident threshold. Engineering science can anticipate strains in structures and can supply the means to withstand the known tensions. However, our rapidly advancing, complex social order often outstrips the individual's ability to acquire and use the knowledge and skill necessary to cope with the changing patterns of the world we live in. People must learn not only to avoid the hazards of their environment, but also to use their new-found way of living for a worthwhile purpose.

THE VARIETY OF POSSIBLE CAUSES

Since human motivation is a complex study, it is often difficult to understand why the victim of a preventable accident failed to take the necessary precautions. Many explanations are usually possible. Although the following news story may be dated, as there are few wringer-type clothes washers today, it does illustrate the interplay of conditions that can cause a tragedy.

> Mrs. Paul Jones, twenty-eight, was going to have her waist-long hair cut any day, but just didn't get around to it. Monday, she bent over her washing machine in her apartment at 4445 Main Street. Her hair was caught in the wringer and pulled through the rollers. A fuse blew—but too late. Mrs. Jones had died of head injuries and loss of blood. The body was discovered by her husband, a barber, when he came home from work. "She was meaning to get her hair cut," Mr. Jones told the police. The couple have two children, John, aged four, and Ann, aged two.

Although this accident could have been prevented if Mrs. Jones had not put off having her hair cut, procrastination cannot necessarily be considered the "cause" of her death. Her survival did not depend on her having a haircut—which, in any case, was probably dictated by considerations of style rather than of safety—for she could have avoided injury merely by carefully tying back her loose hair. If she did not realize that she was risking her life by failing to do so, the accident can be attributed to inadequate knowledge. But perhaps she recognized the danger, at least remotely, and nevertheless decided to take a chance, since she had often done so safely. It is also possible that she was emotionally upset on the fatal Monday and therefore did not give any thought to safety. The superficial explanations suggested here indicate only a few of the possibilities.

Lack of supervision is a common cause of many childhood accidents, although education of the child should gradually lessen the amount of supervision needed. Surely the deaths from suffocation in plastic bags and discarded refrigerators and from driving bicycles in traffic must be charged to adult negligence and failure to foresee what young, adventurous, curious children will do when they are "on their own."

Failure to assume personal responsibility for one's own behavior may be the result of too much supervision. Many people have become overly dependent upon others for many things which they could and should do for themselves. Drowning accidents rarely occur where swimming places are supervised, but many drownings do occur when victims have no one to prevent their unsafe behavior. The success of any program of accident prevention is dependent upon the individual responsibility assumed by everyone who participates in it.

Inadequacy of attitudes, skill, or knowledge may be ultimately responsible for an accident, but more often several accident-producing factors operate together. Without the habit of taking a chance, for example, people are less likely to attempt feats beyond their ability; and with sufficient knowledge of the degree of danger in a situation, they may not be willing to assume the inherent risk. It has been found, in fact, that there is a high correlation between faulty attitudes and lack of knowledge. Often the careless driver is one who has never properly learned or understood the rules of the road. Careless drivers take chances because they do not realize the extent to which they are jeopardizing themselves and others.

It may not always be possible to isolate the particular faulty attitude or other characteristic responsible for a specific accident, but every possibility should be considered in order to identify all the traits that tend to increase human vulnerability to accidents. Remedial efforts can then be directed toward helping people recognize and overcome the failings that endanger them.

THE CHALLENGE OF SAFETY EDUCATION

Even a superficial analysis of the causes of accidents suggests the approach to be used in attempting to prevent accidents. Prevention does not consist primarily of devising more and more safety devices, however important these may be, but in improving a person's knowledge, skill, attitudes, and habits. However, knowledge, skill, and habits are not adequate without the all-important attitude of social responsibility. Safe living, fortunately, does not require freedom from all potentially hazardous conditions, for this is neither possible nor desirable. Rather, it requires the ability to function at an optimum level in the presence of necessary hazards. To develop this ability in American citizens, and thereby to reduce the country's accident rate, is the challenge that safety education must accept. If it is to achieve this goal, ample time must be provided in an already "overcrowded" school curriculum from preschool through high school.

RELATIONSHIP TO SCIENTIFIC PROGRESS

Safety education must help us to adjust to our changing environment, to utilize effectively and safely the forces which science has placed at our disposal, and thus to enjoy to the full all the opportunities for a richer life that these forces represent.

Technology continues to advance. Journeys that once required days of arduous travel now take only a few hours, and the speeds attainable in the future may reduce the traveling time to a matter of minutes. It is quite possible that the wonders wrought through the peaceful use of atomic power will far surpass all preceding accomplishments. But as greater forces are harnessed to serve society, we may face increasingly greater dangers.

If society cannot learn to recognize the hazards in our ever-changing world, to remove needless hazards, to compensate for those that cannot be removed and certainly to avoid creating unnecessary hazards, the only way to ensure its welfare may be to curtail scientific progress, to deprive people of opportunities that involve greater risk than they can safely face. Education in accident prevention must help society acquire the sense of responsibility, the skill, and the knowledge that will entitle it to all the advantages available through technological advance. The challenge education faces will require a herculean effort in all areas. New methods will have to be discovered and implemented if we are to meet the challenge.

With technological advances comes a greater need for knowing how to use one's leisure time safely. There will be greater need for emphasis on accident prevention and injury control in recreational activities such as camping, boating, and hunting, and in the traveling and proper use of vehicles they involve.

CONTRIBUTION TO NATIONAL STRENGTH

Unsafe behavior weakens the country by squandering the human and material resources that form its economic base. The early American settlers found a land of abundance, but the country's natural wealth has been consumed at such an alarming rate during the last 150 years that we are now living beyond our geographical income and devouring our principal. The government's conservation program cannot be wholly effective without the voluntary support of every citizen. Valuable forests are sometimes destroyed by carelessly discarded cigarettes or half-extinguished picnic fires, and the nation's labor supply is diminished and its productive power curtailed whenever employees are seriously injured. By helping prevent accidents, safety education can help preserve America's economic strength.

Safety education can make another important contribution by fostering democratic ideals. A democracy offers its members both freedom and responsibility. It sets up laws to guarantee personal rights and securities, but requires citizens to organize and govern themselves under these laws so that the nation's basic social and economic processes will be carried on in harmony with society's commonly held beliefs and aspirations. Unsupported by public opinion, laws cannot be enforced, and the order essential to the welfare of all cannot be maintained. Gaining public support for that order is one of the important functions of safety education, for accident prevention, like democracy, depends on order, self-discipline, and consideration for others. In many respects, education for safety *is* education for democracy; it is preparation for effective citizenship.

A democracy holds out to every citizen, for example, the right and the opportunity to earn a living in an occupation of one's own choosing. But a disabled worker may have to forfeit this privilege. By attempting to overcome the careless habits and the ignorance that are responsible for many crippling accidents, a safety program helps protect and enrich the equality of opportunity that is the birthright of every American.

Despite the regulations enacted in this country to protect citizens, the number of lives that will be lost over any holiday weekend—and most accidents occur during leisure time—can be predicted with fair assurance. It is not the law, but its enforcement, that is inadequate. A traffic officer cannot be stationed at every intersection, but perhaps people can learn to abide by the law voluntarily if they can be made to understand that their own security, the security of others, and ultimately the good of society as a whole depend upon their doing so. The good citizen and the safe driver choose to drive at posted speed limits even when a policeman is not in the vicinity. They assume individual responsibility for their own safe behavior; this is the key to safe living.

Safety programs provide countless opportunities for learning democratic principles. Student patrols, for example, enable members to gain experience as leaders and other students to discover the responsibilities of intelligent follow-ers. Students learn to respect the patrol's authority, to recognize the value of safety regulations, and to regard the rights of others. They come to understand that order is necessary to protect individual liberties, that the private good and the public good are often allied. The school's accident-prevention program, by promoting democratic as well as safe practices, serves as an ideal laboratory for training in good citizenship.

The basic function of safety education is to educate people to prevent accidents. Although safety education is probably gaining greater acceptance and growth at a time when accidents have become one of the nation's most serious problems, there will be still greater emphasis as our population grows. There has been a significant change in population characteristics. In the United States between 1930 and 1970, the urban population increased from 56 percent of the total to 73 percent. The U.S. Department of Transportation has estimated that the urban population will reach 81 percent by 1990. The resulting increased congestion will have implications for the kinds of accident-prevention programs offered. An abundance of people, increased personal income and leisure time, and resulting demands for better standards of living have created an unrelent-ing pressure that increases the potential for accidents.

EVALUATION

Some may doubt that safety education is equal to the difficult challenge it faces. It may be argued that the various human characteristics responsible for acci-dents are such fundamental parts of people's nature that we cannot learn to overcome them, that education cannot effectively change attitudes, and that people will be safe only insofar as they can avoid potentially dangerous situations. Although safety education has not received the emphasis it needs, the promising results it has thus far achieved support a belief in its value. One example that illustrates gratifying results is the school safety-patrol program. Evidence of its success, however, must be cautiously interpreted, for so many different considerations affect the accident rate that the influence of any single factor cannot be easily determined.

THE RESULTS ACHIEVED

The death rate for children between the ages of five and fourteen has shown a reduction since safety education was introduced into school programs in 1922. Although the death rate for young people between the ages of fifteen and twenty-four showed little change in the two decades prior to 1962 (see Table 1–9), there has been a dramatic increase (almost double) each year since then. Approximately 80 percent of all fatalities in this group are due to motor-vehicle accidents, with drowning, poisons, and firearms accidents responsible for most of the rest. If quality driver education courses become more widespread,

TABLE 1–9
Accidental Deaths and Death Rates by Age, 1903–1976*

Year	All Ages	Under 5 Years	5–14 Years	15–24 Years	25–44 Years	45–64 Years	65–74 Years	75 Years and Over†
				Deaths				
1903–1912 avg	73,700	9,800	7,700	11,200	21,200	13,200	10,600	
1913–1922 avg	78,600	10,200	9,200	10,800	20,400	14,800	13,200	
1923–1932 avg	92,100	8,600	9,500	12,800	22,300	19,900	19,100	
1933–1942 avg	98,765	6,983	7,232	13,171	22,257	22,739	26,383	
1943–1952 avg	95,420	8,270	6,157	13,040	20,529	19,584	27,840	
1953–1962 avg	93,447	8,557	6,427	13,136	20,250	19,156	9,794	16,127
1964	105,000	8,670	7,400	17,420	22,080	22,100	10,400	16,930
1965	108,004	8,586	7,391	18,688	22,228	22,900	10,430	17,781
1966	113,563	8,507	7,958	21,030	23,134	24,022	10,706	18,206
1967	113,169	7,825	7,874	21,645	23,255	23,826	10,645	18,099
1968	114,864	7,263	8,369	23,012	23,684	23,896	10,961	17,679
1969	116,385	6,973	8,186	24,668	24,410	24,192	10,643	17,313
1970	114,638	6,594	8,203	24,336	23,979	24,164	10,644	16,718
1971	113,439	6,496	8,143	24,733	23,535	23,240	10,494	16,798
1972	115,448	6,142	8,242	25,762	23,852	23,658	10,446	17,346
1973	115,821	6,037	8,102	26,550	24,750	23,059	10,243	17,080
1974	104,622	5,335	7,037	24,200	22,547	20,334	9,323	15,846
1975	103,030	4,948	6,818	24,121	22,877	19,643	9,220	15,403
1976	100,000	4,800	6,200	24,000	22,000	19,100	8,800	15,100

Year	Index			Death Rates†				
1903–1912 avg	85.9	100.0	95.0	41.8	64.6	83.2	104.1	272.4
1913–1922 avg	76.8	89.9	89.5	42.5	57.6	67.0	91.3	268.4
1923–1932 avg	77.4	90.5	75.0	39.4	59.0	63.4	97.0	299.4
1933–1942 avg	76.2	85.2	66.8	29.9	56.4	57.2	90.9	312.9
1943–1952 avg	66.3	70.6	56.7	25.6	60.7	47.8	66.4	242.5
1953–1962 avg	54.3	58.0	44.3	19.6	57.6	43.3	55.2	93.9	312.4
1964	54.9	59.0	43.1	19.1	59.9	47.3	57.6	88.9	264.0
1965	55.8	59.9	43.4	18.7	61.6	47.7	58.8	88.5	268.7
1966	58.1	62.3	44.4	19.9	66.9	49.6	60.7	89.9	267.4
1967	57.3	61.6	42.2	19.4	66.9	49.7	59.2	88.5	257.4
1968	57.6	61.8	40.6	20.5	69.2	50.1	58.5	90.2	244.0
1969	57.8	62.1	40.2	20.0	71.8	51.2	58.4	86.6	232.0
1970	56.2	60.1	38.5	20.1	68.0	49.8	57.6	85.2	220.0
1971	55.0	58.5	37.8	20.2	66.3	48.5	54.8	82.8	214.9
1972	55.4	58.6	36.2	20.8	68.1	47.7	55.3	80.9	217.1
1973	55.2	58.3	36.2	20.8	68.8	48.4	53.5	77.5	210.2
1974	49.5	51.9	32.7	18.4	61.6	43.1	46.9	68.9	191.3
1975	48.4	50.6	31.2	18.1	60.3	42.8	45.1	66.5	180.6
1976	46.6	48.5	31.3	16.7	59.1	40.1	43.7	62.0	172.7

Year				Changes in Rates				
1966 to 1976	−20%	−22%	−30%	−16%	−12%	−19%	−28%	−31%	−35%
1975 to 1976	−4%	−4%	+*%	−8%	−2%	−6%	−3%	−7%	−4%

TABLE 1-9 (*continued*)
Accidental Deaths and Death Rates by Age, 1903–1976*

Year	All Ages	Under 5 Years	5–14 Years	15–24 Years	25–44 Years	45–64 Years	65–74 Years	75 Years and Over†
			1976 Population (millions)					
Total	214.65	15.34	37.17	40.61	54.90	43.70	14.19	8.74
Male	104.47	7.84	18.95	20.43	26.97	20.92	6.16	3.20
Female	110.18	7.50	18.22	20.18	27.93	22.78	8.03	5.54

*Rates are deaths per 100,000 resident population in each age group. The All Ages crude rates are based on U.S. Census Bureau figures. The index numbers are based on rates standardized for age (base 1940) to remove the influence of changes in age distribution between 1903 and 1976.
†Includes "age unknown". In 1975 these deaths numbered 74.
Source: 1903 to 1932 based on National Center for Health Statistics data for registration states; other figures are NCHS totals except 1964 and 1976 which are NSC estimates. *Accident Facts,* National Safety Council, Chicago, 1977.

*Less than 0.5 per cent.

however, the death rate for adolescents and young adults should also be reduced. At present, more than 2½ million students are enrolled in these courses, which are offered by over 15,000 high schools. Many studies show that both the accident rate and the incidence of traffic violations are lower among alumni of these courses than among other drivers of the same age.[8] Actuarial calculations of insurance companies have also demonstrated the effectiveness of traffic safety education programs.

An Illinois study, which included several hundred thousand youthful drivers, showed that the trained group was 2 to 1 better in avoiding accidents and almost 4 to 1 better in avoiding traffic violations. Some of the studies showing the effectiveness of driver education may be questioned as to their accuracy. However, there is no proof that there is any better way to teach young people how to handle a motor vehicle in modern traffic, and to give them the necessary sense of their social responsibilities.

AREAS FOR IMPROVEMENT

Despite encouraging evidence that safety education can be an effective means of dealing with the accident problem, much remains to be done, especially in areas where accident statistics are most alarming. The number of home accidents has not been appreciably reduced, even though schools, industry, public health organizations, and some safety councils have made an attempt to promote household safety. Students have been guided in devising checklists of avoidable home hazards, and excellent safety training has been offered in homemaking classes, which, unfortunately, have small enrollments and are attended almost exclusively by girls. Home safety instruction, like all training in

[8]Leon Brody and Herbert J. Stack, *Highway Safety and Driver Education,* Prentice-Hall, Inc., Englewood Cliffs, N.J., 1966, pp 344–345.

TABLE 1-10
Accidental Deaths by Age, Sex, and Type, 1975

Age and Sex	All Types	Motor-Vehicle	Falls	Drowning	Fires, Burns	Ingest. of Food, Object	Firearms	Poison (Solid, Liquid)	Poison by Gas	% Male All Types
All Ages	103,030	45,853	14,896	8,000	6,071	3,106	2,380	4,694	1,577	70%
Under 5	4,948	1,576	197	800	752	504	71	114	38	58%
5 to 14	6,818	3,286	137	1,300	580	77	424	49	81	70%
15 to 24	24,121	15,672	497	2,520	502	223	758	1,332	357	81%
25 to 34	13,823	7,680	428	1,080	500	218	359	1,215	263	81%
35 to 44	9,054	4,289	530	660	461	241	249	638	208	77%
45 to 54	9,993	4,089	1,057	630	757	369	215	545	216	74%
55 to 64	9,650	3,574	1,392	490	845	429	143	381	176	71%
65 to 74	9,220	3,047	2,148	310	795	451	115	233	139	63%
75 & over	15,403	2,640	8,510	210	879	594	46	187	99	47%
Male	72,376	33,597	7,696	6,782	3,733	1,829	2,042	3,147	1,165	
Female	30,654	12,256	7,200	1,218	2,338	1,277	338	1,547	412	
Per cent male	70%	73%	52%	85%	61%	59%	86%	67%	74%	

Source: *Accident Facts*, National Safety Council, Chicago, 1977.

accident prevention, must be extended to everyone. As safety education gains its proper place in the school curriculum and as better teaching techniques continue to be discovered through experience and study, increasingly gratifying results should be achieved.

RELATIONSHIP TO THE COMMUNITY.   If safety education is to meet its challenge, it must be extended not only to more students but to their parents as well, and to all members of the community. The school's program functions best when it is supported by outside agencies. The public must get involved. In this way people will be made conscious of the social and economic purpose of safety. The effectiveness of classroom instruction in bicycle safety, for example, is weakened when parents permit a child to ride in the street before acquiring sufficient skill and knowledge. When a student brings home a checklist of home hazards, it is important that the student's parents pay attention, for any indifference or opposition on their part may negate the value of what he or she has learned. The training which students receive at school must be strengthened by their outside experiences; otherwise they may take the proper precautions only when they are closely supervised. It is far easier to induce children to behave safely at all times if adults set a good example.

RELATIONSHIP TO STUDENTS' NEEDS.   Accident prevention is related to all phases of the school curriculum. It is not an incidental, isolated subject, but vital to all phases of democratic living. Wherever possible, the materials and learning experiences used in teaching safety should be related to students values and attitudes.

A program based exclusively on expressed interests and needs, however, may be unduly restricted. People do not always recognize their own needs. Attention should also be given to important personal and community problems of which the students may be unaware. The use of atomic energy and the related considerations of health and safety should concern everyone, even though their importance has not yet been fully recognized. Education cannot neglect the problems of living in the atomic age until there is greater public interest; by that time considerable damage may already have been done. Safety instruction must give students a better understanding of the world in which they live so that they will know how to escape injury and how to make the life saved more satisfying.

SAFETY AND PSYCHOLOGY.   The far-reaching importance of safety education and its potential contribution to society have not always been fully appreciated, and instruction in this subject has too often been superficial. At times the "teaching" of accident prevention has consisted merely in imparting information. Unless children are *motivated* to develop and practice protective skills, unless they acquire the *habit* of conscientiously observing general as well as specific safety principles, they will not have learned to live safely even though they have been taught the rules of safety and have been given protective devices. Conformity to safe behavior is often challenged by the desire to be "different." Our standards of safe living have little or no appeal to too many youths of today. Education should engender in all children the desire and the ability to shield themselves from potential danger in all circumstances, including those that are new and that involve hazards which have not previously been encountered. This can be accomplished without reducing the pleasures of living.

The attempt to foster proper attitudes is sometimes blocked by the persistence of improper habits. Such habits may be so firmly entrenched that they cannot be easily uprooted, especially when they are a manifestation of deep-seated emotional needs. A motorist's habit of speeding, for example, may be traced to a sense of inferiority that makes him or her resent being outdistanced. At such times the motivation to "get even" may be so strong that the motorist will try to overtake the other car regardless of the danger to himself and others. Since many accidents are ultimately caused by such unhealthy psychological traits, safety education must be concerned with developing well-adjusted personalities, adequate to the world in which they live—personalities in which aggressive tendencies are held in check and in which the inevitable compensatory mechanisms of life are constructive.

Teachers can do much to achieve this goal by helping students arrive at self-understanding. They can give students opportunities to express themselves in socially desirable ways and to receive recognition for their achievements from the other members of their group. It is particularly important that safety education use a group approach. In an age when the approval of others is often essential to personal adjustment, individuals should be made to feel that careful, orderly behavior is sanctioned, not ridiculed, by their peers.

School-age children usually derive greater satisfaction from the respect of their classmates than from the commendation of their parents and teachers. Too often the daredevil is praised by other students while the child who refuses to take needless risks is ostracized as a sissy. The "sissy" of grade-school days may develop a sense of inferiority that manifests itself during adult life in aggressive driving and other dangerous tendencies. This might be counteracted if more commendation was given to safe behavior. The reckless student whose daring exploits delight his or her friends may go on taking a chance as a means of winning their admiration. An important function of the school's safety program is to prevent the formation of such undesirable personality traits. Prevention, however difficult it may be, is far easier than overcoming such traits once they are formed. When unsafe behavior patterns result from serious maladjustments, a psychiatric problem is involved, and safety education can do little to change it.

In the light of present knowledge, for example, it is unlikely that safety education can cure "accident-proneness." Studies have shown that certain persons have accidents repeatedly, no matter how much safety apparatus is placed at their disposal. Although there is some indication that this characteristic is neurotically induced, further research is necessary before its causes and symptoms can be fully understood. With further study, safety education can at least help those who are accident-prone to recognize their particular vulnerability to injury. Through understanding, they may be consciously motivated to develop safe habits. Through patient teaching and continued practice, they may learn to protect themselves and to compensate for their condition until proper treatment removes its cause.

If safety education is to consist merely in exposure to the rules of accident prevention, it obviously cannot fulfill all its potentialities. Rightly conceived, however, it should be equal to the challenge it faces. It is properly concerned with individuals in relationship to their environment, with their motivations as well as their behavior, with the hazards that confront them, and with their ability to protect themselves from those hazards. So comprehensive and important a subject cannot be confined to the classroom. Safety education must not only pervade the entire school program as the responsibility of all personnel, but extend its influence throughout the community.

NATIONAL SAFETY COUNCIL DEFINITIONS OF THE FOUR MAJOR CLASSES OF ACCIDENTS[9]

- **Motor Vehicle** Includes deaths involving mechanically or electrically powered highway-transport vehicles in motion (except those on rails) both on and off the highway or street.
- **Work** Includes those accidents which arise out of and in the course of gainful work, except that (1) work injuries to domestic servants, and (2) injuries occurring in connection with farm chores, are classified as home injuries.
- **Home** Includes those accidents in the home and on home premises to occupants, guests, and trespassers. Also includes domestic servants but excluding other persons working on home premises.
- **Public** Includes those accidents in public places or places used in a public way, not involving motor vehicles. Most sports and recreation deaths are included. Excludes accidents in the course of employment.

NATIONAL SAFETY COUNCIL DEFINITIONS OF TYPES OF ACCIDENTS

- **All Accidents** The term "accident" covers most deaths from violence; excluded are homicides, suicides, deaths for which none of these categories can be determined, and deaths in war operations.
- **Motor Vehicle** Includes those accidents involving mechanically or electrically powered highway-transport vehicles in motion (except those on rails) both on and off the highway or street.
- **Falls** Includes deaths from falls from one level to another or on the same level. Excludes falls in or from transport vehicles, or while boarding or alighting from them.
- **Drowning** Includes all drownings (work and nonwork) in boat accidents

---

[9] *Accident Facts*, National Safety Council, Chicago 1977, pp. 6, 72, 80, 97.

and those resulting from swimming, playing in the water, or falling in. Excludes drownings in floods and other cataclysms.

- **Fires, burns, and accidents associated with fires** Includes those accidents from fires, burns, and from injuries in conflagrations—such as asphyxiation, falls, and being struck by falling objects. Excludes burns from hot objects or liquids.
- **Poisoning by solids and liquids** Includes deaths from drugs, medicines, mushrooms and shellfish, as well as commonly recognized poisons. Excludes poisonings from spoiled foods, salmonella, etc.—which are classified as disease deaths.
- **Suffocation-ingested object** Includes deaths from accidental ingestion or inhalation of objects or food resulting in the obstruction of respiratory passages.
- **Firearms** Includes deaths in firearms accidents principally in recreational activities or on home premises. Excludes deaths from explosive material or in war operations.
- **Poisoning by gases and vapors** Mostly carbon monoxide due to incomplete combustion, involving cooking and heating equipment and standing motor vehicles. Excludes deaths in conflagrations, or associated with transport vehicles in motion.
- **All other types** Most important types included are: mechanical suffocation, struck by falling object, electric current, air and rail transport, and medical complications.

LEARNING EXPERIENCES

The following assignments are recommended for anyone concerned with planning and conducting a safety education program. They are intended to facilitate recognition of the seriousness of the accident problem in one's own community, its causes, and some of the preventive measures that could prove effective.

1 Bring available accident figures and tables up to date, and discuss the possible causes of changes.

2 Deaths caused by diseases have been reduced by immunization and other health measures. Compare the almost static figures of accident fatalities with those of nonaccident deaths. Discuss possible ways of using methods which have been successful in reducing nonaccident deaths to reduce accident deaths.

3 Secure from police and hospital files a record of the accidents in your community during the current year. Arrange them in groups according to the ages of the victims. Discuss the need for safety education in your community.

4 Prepare a chart showing the number of accidents that have occurred in the home, at the school, in industrial plants, during recreational activities, etc.

5 Keep a record of all accidents reported in your local newspaper during a single month, and report your findings to the class.

6 Compare the accident record of your community with that of (a) a nearby community of similar type and size and (b) the national figures as stated in the publication *Accident Facts*.

7 Observe an intersection for a half-hour at a time when traffic is comparatively heavy, and record the number and variety of unsafe actions by (a) pedestrians, (b) motorists, (c) bicyclists, and (d) Moped operators.

8 Interview an individual in your community who has had a serious accident, and report the facts of the case to the class (how the accident happened, how it might have been prevented, how much expense it entailed, etc.).

9 Secure current copies of a number of popular magazines, such as *Ladies Home Journal, Time, Life, Newsweek, Vogue, Good Housekeeping,* and *Better Homes and Gardens,* and write a review of articles dealing with the need for safety education. Note especially the *practical safe behavior* emphasized in the articles.

10 Select a frequent cause of accidents in your community, and plan suitable means of eliminating it. (This assignment may be treated as a class project.)

11 Discuss the implications of the cost of accidents to our national economy.

SELECTED REFERENCES

Accident Facts, National Safety Council, Chicago. Yearly.
Automobile Facts and Figures, Automobile Manufacturers Association, Detroit. Yearly.
Haddon, William, Jr.: *Accident Research: Methods and Approaches,* Harper & Row, Publishers, Incorporated, New York, 1964.
Metropolitan Life Insurance Company Statistical Bulletin, vol. 57, January, May, June, November, December, 1976, vol. 58, April, January 1977.
National Safety Council, Chicago:
    Accident Facts, yearly
    Public Safety Report to the Nation, yearly
    Transactions of the National Safety Congress, yearly
Safety Education, Eighteenth Yearbook of the American Association of School Administrators, National Education Association, Washington, 1940.
Stack, Herbert James (ed.): "Safety for Greater Adventure," *The Contributions of Albert Wurts Whitney,* New York University Center for Safety Education, New York, 1953.
————, and J. Duke Elkow: *Education for Safe Living,* 4th ed., Prentice-Hall, Inc., Englewood Cliffs, N.J., 1966.
Statistical Abstracts, Bureau of Vital Statistics, U.S. Department of Commerce. Monthly.
Strasser, Marland K., et al.: *Fundamentals of Safety Education,* The Macmillan Company, New York, 1973.
Thygerson, Alton L.: *Accidents and Disasters,* Prentice-Hall, Inc., Englewood Cliffs, N.J., 1977.
————: *Safety, Concepts and Instruction,* 2d ed., Prentice-Hall, Inc., Englewood Cliffs, N.J., 1976.
Vital Statistics of the United States, National Office of Vital Statistics. Yearly.

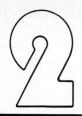

Psychological Considerations

OVERALL OBJECTIVE:

The student should begin to develop a philosphy of safety that positively influences his or her behavior and promotes a safer way of life.

INSTRUCTIONAL OBJECTIVES:

After completing this chapter the student will be able to:

1 Describe how the science of epidemiology is applied to the study of accident prevention.
2 Discuss the relationship between safety education and accident prevention.
3 Explain the *social pathology* theory of accident causation.
4 List the personality characteristics commonly associated with accident-prone and non-accident-prone individuals.
5 Explain the *ecologic model* of accident causation.
6 Discuss the *health belief model* as it relates to accident-preventive behavior.
7 Describe how teachers can use self-preservation and self-enhancement to motivate students toward safe behavior.

In view of the statistical data presented in Chapter 1, it is curious to note that many people still behave as if accidental injury and death represent only a minor problem. It is extremely important to recognize that *safety is no accident*. Responsibility for safety lies with the individual. Nevertheless, many people have a complacent attitude toward self-preservation. The purpose of this chapter is to offer a perspective on the relationship between human behavior and the occurrence of accidents.

Accidents are not the result of chance. Since accidents are not distributed randomly among the population, it must be assumed that certain factors contribute to the causation of accidents. If this is true, the concept of "accidental" as understood by the general public is entirely inappropriate. When an individual believes that accidents are unforeseen events of chance, his or her behavior response becomes one of helplessness: accidents, which are neither foreseeable nor preventable, defy personal action that will reduce the likelihood of injury or property damage.

EPIDEMIOLOGY AND ACCIDENT PREVENTION

The study of epidemiology in this country began as a scientific approach to the investigation of infectious disease. In recent years, the epidemiologic techniques which were used successfully in analyzing diseases such as plague, yellow fever, and polio have been applied to the study of chronic diseases and accidents. Epidemiology is the study of the distribution and determinants of disease and injury in human populations.

The ultimate goal of medical investigation is the prevention of disease. The first step toward achievement of that goal is accurate identification of the causes of disease. Then it is up to the individual to take appropriate action to minimize the risk of becoming ill. The specific causes of most diseases have already been determined, yet the incidence of some of these diseases continues to rise. To benefit from the knowledge of cause, the individual must be willing to take appropriate action directed toward prevention. To the extent that risk factors can be minimized or avoided, the frequency of disease can be reduced or eliminated. For example, an individual may develop clinical heart disease after years of being overweight and having high blood pressure, high serum cholesterol, atherosclerosis, and taxing levels of stress. By eliminating one or more of these risk factors a person can reduce the probability of suffering a fatal heart attack.

Accidents and chronic disease share certain unique characteristics. Both elicit such a strong sense of fear that many people repress their feelings with rationalizations like "When you time is up, it's up" or "There's nothing you can do about it anyway, so why worry?" Accidents and chronic disease allow risk factors to accumulate over a long period of time so that their consequences are not readily apparent. The effects of both are often expensive and permanent, leaving their victims with residual disability. Fortunately, both are largely preventable through a modification of individual behavior aimed at limiting the known risk factors.

Accidents do not occur evenly throughout the population. It is possible to study subgroups of people who experience frequent accidents in an attempt to find common elements among these groups. Similarly, subgroups with low accident rates could be studied for common factors which contribute to that phenomenon. The ultimate goal of epidemiologic investigation in this area is the prevention of the injurious occurrences known as accidents. Safety researchers have identified the contributing causes of accidents, but the frequency of accidents continues to rise because, as individuals, we have not fully accepted responsibility for accident prevention. We need to seriously address the question, "What actions am I willing to take in order to remain healthy, to remain safe?"

Think of prevention as taking place along a time continuum:

1 Primary prevention occurs before the accident happens.

2 Secondary prevention is the minimization of the consequences of the accident by expedient treatment of injury.

3 Tertiary prevention is the limitation of disability by long-range treatment and rehabilitation.

Obviously, the most effective results will be achieved when efforts are focused on the level of primary prevention. Unfortunately, the safety movement has often stressed the later stages of prevention. It has been said that more effort is spent on reducing the extent of injury after an accident than on preventing the accident in the first place. Primary prevention is the best alternative because it is the most effective and least expensive of the three levels. Primary prevention represents the reduction of injury through the reduction of accidents. The following poem illustrates the difference between primary and secondary levels of accident prevention.

> 'Twas a dangerous cliff, as they freely confessed,
>   Though to walk near its crest was so pleasant;
> But over its terrible edge there had slipped
>   A duke, and full many a peasant.
> The people said something would have to be done,
>   But their projects did not at all tally.
> Some said, "Put a fence 'round the edge of the cliff";
>   Some, "An ambulance down in the valley."
> The lament of the crowd was profound and was loud,
>   As their hearts overflowed with their pity;
> But the cry for the ambulance carried the day
>   As it spread through the neighboring city.
> A collection was made, to accumulate aid,
>   And the dwellers in highway and alley
> Gave dollars or cents—not to furnish a fence—
>   But an ambulance down in the valley.
> "For the cliff is all right if you're careful," they said;
>   "And if folks ever slip and are dropping,
> It isn't the slipping that hurts them so much
>   As the shock down below—when they're stopping."
> So for years (we have heard), as these mishaps occurred
>   Quick forth would the rescuers sally,
> To pick up the victims who fell from the cliff,
>   With the ambulance down in the valley.
> Said one, to his plea, "It's a marvel to me
>   That you'd give so much greater attention
> To repairing results than to curing the cause;
>   You had much better aim at prevention.
> For the mischief, of course, should be stopped at its source,
>   Come, neighbors and friends, let us rally.

It is far better sense to rely on a fence
  Than an ambulance down in the valley."
"He is wrong in his head," the majority said;
  "He would end all our earnest endeavor.
He's a man who would shirk this responsible work,
  But we will support it forever.
Aren't we picking up all, just as fast as they fall,
  And giving them care liberally?
A superfluous fence is of no consequence,
  If the ambulance works in the valley."
The story looks queer as we've written it here,
  But things often occur that are stranger.
More humane, we assert, than to succor the hurt,
  Is the plan of removing the danger.
The best possible course is to safeguard the source;
  Attend to things rationally.
Yes, build up the fence and let us dispense
  With the ambulance down in the valley.[1]

Although this poem is admittedly humorous, it represents an "after the fact" philosophy shared by many Americans. Chapter 1 presented the statistical data needed for understanding how, to whom, when, and where accidents are most likely to occur. With this information available, primary prevention becomes a plausible approach to solving the accident problem. For safety education to be effective, we need the answer to the question: *"Why do accidents occur?"*

TOWARD AN UNDERSTANDING OF ACCIDENT PREVENTION

One's concept of what is accidental can often be changed by education. The more thoroughly a person understands the specific dangers of a situation, the less likely it becomes that he or she will consider an unexplained injurious event to be accidental. Until bacteria were identified under a microscope it was impossible to define the etiologic agent (cause) of tuberculosis. The sickness was attributed to bad luck or explained by one of a multitude of the supersitions which often surround the unknown. Today, the etiology of accidental occurrences is subject to the same scrutiny as the etiology of diseases. We no longer need to attribute accidents to bad luck or explain them in terms of superstition. To a large degree they are preventable. Avoidance of risk factors will provide significant protection against the many consequences of accidents.

The safety-educated person is more likely to regard an accident as being predictable, preventable, and nonaccidental. Rather than rationalize the event as an "act of God," such a person would be more likely to identify an accident as the result of an irresponsible "act of man." This viewpoint encourages a shift in attitude away from the fatalistic acceptance of dangerous circumstances and toward a philosophic idealism that considers virtually all accidents pre-

[1]Author unknown, but it is believed the poem first appeared in a newsletter from the National Safety Council in 1957.

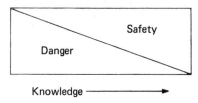

Figure 2-1 Relationship between knowledge and safety.

ventable. Understanding and intelligent application create a diminishing danger potential in the life of the safety-educated individual.

Words like unexpected, unavoidable, and unintentional have become elements of the accident concept held by the general public. For many people:

1 The less an event can be anticipated, the more likely it will be considered an accident.

2 The less an event results from deliberate action, the more likely it will be considered an accident.

3 The less an event can be avoided, the more likely it will be considered an accident.[2]

Safety education plays an important role in the preventive process. As knowledge increases, one's behavior becomes more intentional, so that unanticipated events are less likely to result in injury.

Assume that you are unfamiliar with the operation of a corn harvester. While you are working this piece of machinery it suddenly jams, causing the tractor to stop. In an attempt to locate the source of the problem you begin pushing buttons and levers; eventually one button releases the jam and sets the tractor into motion. Not expecting this sudden forward lunge, you are thrown off balance and cannot stop yourself from falling out of the seat. Thus, the potential for personal injury became actual because of lack of knowledge. Part of the role of safety education is to increase knowledge, thereby decreasing the proportion of unintended behavior and increasing the level of anticipation and the possibility of avoiding danger. It is important to repeat that increased understanding diminishes the potential for accidents.

THEORIES OF ACCIDENT CAUSATION

SOCIAL PATHOLOGY

Some social scientists believe that accidents may reflect a person's attitude toward life. They reason that frequent accidents are symptomatic of inadequate social adjustment. They state that as one's sense of social responsibility increases, the potential for accidents decreases correspondingly. The assumption is that one lives by an internalized set of rules which govern one's behavior

[2]Edward A. Suchman, "A Conceptual Analysis of the Accident Phenomenon," in William Haddon, Edward Suchman, and David Klein (eds.), *Accident Research Methods and Approaches,* Harper & Row, Publishers, Incorporated, New York, 1964, p. 276.

in all activities. The more these rules reflect social irresponsibility, the more likely it is that the individual will suffer an accident. It has been suggested that drivers' licensing examinations include not only written and skills tests but also personality inventories to screen out people who are psychologically unfit to operate a motor vehicle.

Suchman theorized that rejection of social constraints leads to a higher incidence of accidental injuries. He studied more than 1,500 high school and college students through personal interviews and written questionnaires. A significant relationship was found between accidents and characteristics commonly associated with social deviance.

He reasoned that behavioral activities such as fighting and cheating on tests represented an attitude of social irresponsibility and could cause a person to be a high-risk candidate for accidental occurrences. Students with attitudes such as "It is all right to get around the law as long as you don't break it" and "I get a kick out of taking chances, even if it means getting hurt" were found to have significantly more accidental injuries than students who didn't display such attitudes. Students displaying the most extreme levels of deviance were three to five times more likely to incur accidental injuries than students whose attitudes were closer to the conforming end of the scale. He concluded: "A hostile, aggressive, impulsive individual placed in a situation that requires constant attention, self control, consideration of others and respect for laws and regulations . . . is more susceptible to having an accident."[3]

ACCIDENT-PRONENESS

Accident-proneness is generally understood to refer to those personality characteristics which predispose an individual toward having accidents. The concept was formulated as early as 1919. It was based on the observation that some people seem to experience more than their share of accidents. This kind of thinking represented an important change in the study of accident causation, which had previously centered on environmental hazards. For the first time, scientists began to study the human element as a contributing cause of accidents.

Type X (Non-Accident-Prone)	Type Y (Accident-Prone)
Conventional values	Unconventional values
Goal-oriented	No clearly defined goals
Satisfied with everyday life	Dissatisfied with everyday life
Respects the rights and opinions of others	Insensitive to the rights and opinions of others
Nondomineering	Doesn't relate easily or warmly
Noncombative	Difficulty controlling hostility
Concern for others	Self-oriented

[3]Edward A. Suchman, "Accidents and Social Deviance," *Journal of Health and Social Behavior,* vol. 11, p. 6, 1970.

Shaw and Sichel recently compiled a comprehensive list of characteristics associated with accident-prone and non-accident-prone personalities.[4] By applying their data we can classify individuals as good or bad accident risks.

THE BAD ACCIDENT RISK

- The mental defective or psychotic.
- The person who is extremely unintelligent, unobservant, and unadaptable.
- The disorganized, disoriented, or badly disturbed person.
- The badly integrated or maladjusted person.
- The person with a distorted apperception of life and a distorted sense of values.
- The person who is emotionally unstable and extremistic.
- The person who lacks control, and particularly the person who exhibits uncontrolled aggression.
- The person with pronounced antisocial attitudes or criminal tendencies.
- The selfish, self-centered, or id-directed person.
- The highly competitive person.
- The overconfident, self-assertive person.
- The irritable and cantankerous person.
- The person who harbours grudges, grievances, and resentments.
- The blame-avoidant person who is always ready with excuses.
- The intolerant and impatient person.
- The person with a marked antagonism to and resistance against authority.
- The frustrated and discontented person.
- The inadequate person with a driving need to prove him or herself.
- The extremely anxious, tension-ridden, and panicky person.
- The person who is unduly sensitive to criticism.
- The helpless and inadequate person who is constantly in need of guidance and support.
- The chronically indecisive person.
- The person who has difficulty in concentrating.
- The person who is easily influenced or intimidated.
- The careless and frivolous person.
- The person who is lacking in personal insight and an appreciation of personal limitations.
- The fatalistic person who makes no attempt to control his or her destiny; the person who is prone to mysticism, superstition, or primitive, unreasoning beliefs.
- The person who already gives evidence of addiction to alcohol or drugs.
- The person who has the sort of personality pattern that predisposes him or her to drink or drugs.

[4]Lynette Shaw and Herbert S. Sichel, *Accident Proneness*, Pergamon Press, Oxford, 1971, pp. 335–338.

- The person who has suicidal tendencies or who indulges in suicide fantasies.
- The person who exhibits undue signs of aging.
- The person who exhibits the personality characteristics commonly associated with immaturity: foolhardy impetuosity, irresponsibility, exhibitionism, inability to appreciate the consequences of one's actions, hypersensitivity, easily aroused emotionalism, unrealistic goals, and a general lack of self-discipline, personal insight, worldly wisdom, and common sense.

THE GOOD ACCIDENT RISK

- The balanced, mature, and well-controlled person with a healthy and realistic outlook, satisfactory interpersonal relations, a kindly and tolerant attitude to others, a well-developed social and civic conscience, and an ingrained sense of responsibility.
- The person who is essentially a moderate individual, able to exercise adequate control over his or her impulses and emotions.
- The positive person who is able to assess a situation as a whole and make decisions—provided the person is not too aggressive. (This is what one might call the "executive" class of good accident risk: people who, though they may be dominant and forceful in their business lives, are realistic enough to minimize their aggressive drives in a traffic situation.)
- The person who is not yet quite mature but whose motivations are sound and who demonstrates an ability to learn quickly by experience and profit from mistakes. (This sort of person will undoubtedly have a learning period before his or her record stabilizes at a good level.)
- The contented person who is in no way outstanding but who is friendly, cheerful, adaptable, and accepting—provided the person is reasonably intelligent, realistic, and mature.
- The person who has weaknesses and limitations but is realistically aware of them, one who is careful and cautious and moderates behavior according to personal limitations.
- The introverted person—provided the person is not too maladjusted.
- The person who, though reasonably well integrated, is nevertheless unimpressively negative; the passive, somewhat compliant and subservient person who is anxious to conform and does not wish to be in any way conspicuous; the person with a strong need for acceptance and security.

Apparently, certain personality characteristics predispose individuals to greater risk of accidental injury. However, accident-proneness is a matter of degree rather than of having it or not having it. Changes in a person's behavior will make the person more accident-prone at different times of his or her life. It is also important to differentiate between accident-proneness and accident-repetitiveness. Some people are placed at great risk by occupational hazards or their chosen life-style. Taxi drivers might be expected to have a high accident rate because of the many miles they drive in high-density traffic. Finally, it must be stated that accident repeaters do not incur the overall majority of accidents. Having a type X personality does not ensure immunity from accidental injury.

THE ECOLOGIC MODEL

Ecology may be defined as the study of the relationship of organisms to each other and to their environment. The essence of the ecologic model is that accidents cannot be attributed to the operation of any *one* factor. It is more appropriate to consider an unsafe situation as the result of an ecology of danger (see Figure 2–2). This concept of multiple causation is also known as multifactorial (more than one cause) etiology.

Accidents are often attributed to a single act or condition, such as speeding, intoxication, or wet, slippery pavements. Although all of these can be contributory factors in highway accidents, it cannot be accurately stated that they are "the" cause. Many people speed, drive while under the influence of alcohol, and negotiate wet, slippery pavements without experiencing an accident. Accidents result from a dynamic interaction between human and environmental factors. The end result is the product of the total combination of forces through which it was created. Human factors are sometimes called intrinsic, and environmental factors are sometimes referred to as extrinsic.

Intrinsic Factors Contributing to Accidents	Extrinsic Factors Contributing to Accidents
Physical incapability	Imperfect weather conditions
Poor visual acuity	Overcrowding
Stress	Defective equipment
Fatigue	Inadequate law enforcement
Distractibility	Nonsupportive social environment
Lack of knowledge	Inadequate legislation
Poor attitudes	Lack of safety education
Bad habits	programs beginning at the
False sense of security	preschool age and continuing
	throughout life

Ecological relationships are complex. Intervention will not succeed so long as attempts at remediation are narrowly focused upon one "best" solution. Efforts toward accident prevention are often simplistic and directed exclusively toward the control of extrinsic factors. Modification of human factors must also occur if accident-prevention programs are to be truly effective. The only rational approach to multiple causation is a carefully designed program which is oriented toward a multiple solution.

An individual enters into each new situation with an established behavior pattern that is uniquely his or her own. This pattern is based upon an accumulation of knowledge, skills, habits, and attitudes that intermingle to form a repertoire of behavior. People who have acquired adequate knowledge, and

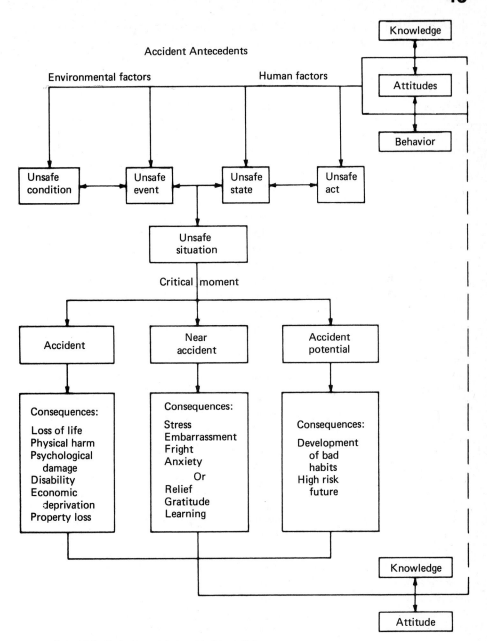

Figure 2-2 Ecologic model of accident causation.

more importantly, have developed attitudes that facilitate accident prevention, are in a safer position throughout a potential accident encounter. Because their actions are for the most part intentional, such people can reduce the possibility of an accident by controlling the unexpected and the unavoidable.

Antecedents are those events which, when combined, lead to an unsafe situation.

1 *Unsafe conditions* are the environmental circumstances in which the event is occurring, for example, rainy weather or crowded highways.

2 *Unsafe events* are unanticipated extrinsic occurrences. Examples include a blowout, or an irresponsible driver suddenly pulling in front of your vehicle.

3 *Unsafe state* is the sum total of the human's physical, emotional, and psychological distress. Examples include poor depth perception, anger, stress, and neurotic tendencies.

4 *Unsafe acts* are the behavioral responses of individuals to relevant goal-directed stimuli. This might be illustrated by driving at an excessive speed or weaving from lane to lane in order to arrive on time for an appointment.

As the model indicates, all the unsafe antecedents interact to create an unsafe situation.[5] Thus, on a rainy evening after a stressful day at the office, you are driving at an excessive rate of speed on a wet and slippery highway in order to arrive on time for an important appointment. An irresponsible driver suddenly violates your path of travel. You recognize the danger too late because you are not wearing your glasses and the windshield wipers have not worked in a month. The unsafe situation is the result of its combined antecedents. The ensuing collision is not the result of any one of the human or environmental hazards.

In every unsafe situation there is a critical moment of decision that ultimately determines the consequences of the situation. In some instances this critical moment occurs well after the unsafe situation has been recognized. The safety of a person walking along the edge of a steep cliff is guaranteed only so long as the center of gravity remains inside solid boundaries. In this situation, where the interval between initiation of the unsafe activity and the critical moment is great, the potential for avoidability is great. Conversely, when another driver suddenly pulls in front of your vehicle, the time available for interpretation, prediction of the consequences, selection of an alternative, and execution of avoidance behavior may not be adequate. In fact, avoidability is a function of the amount of time available between recognition of a dangerous situation and the conclusion of the event.

When a person is fortunate enough to escape an accident situation without incurring injury or property damage, a number of favorable results may occur. Knowledge of a dangerous situation is established or reinforced. Attitudes may

[5]This ecologic model was adapted from Alan D. Swain, *The Human Element in Systems Safety,* In Com Tec House, Surrey, England, 1974, p. 6.

shift toward an appreciation of health and well-being. Future behavior may reflect the experience of the near miss. On the other hand, some people would attribute their safety to the "luck was with me" myth. Such people would leave the situation unaware of its antecedents, and without knowing how to predict unsafe situations or take preventive measures for future encounters. They would leave the situation free to "try their luck" again, having learned nothing from the near-miss event.

The non-safety-educated person who experiences an "accident potential" may not perceive its operative factors or know that the situation is dangerous. The unsafe conditions, unsafe events, unsafe state, and unsafe acts are not recognized. The deceptive feeling of safety permits bad habits to develop. A person may experience hundreds of accident-potential situations without ever recognizing the danger. This concept is demonstrated by the individual who has committed numerous traffic violations without receiving a citation. Eventually, the individual comes to believe that speeding, tailgating, etc., are not dangerous.

Accident victims have much to lose. It is frightening to think of the physical, mental, and social consequences of a serious accident. The consequences are even more difficult to accept when one realizes that most accidents are preventable.

Safety education is an effective technique for primary prevention of accidents. The safety-educated person has learned to recognize, and where possible to eliminate, important risk factors. Such a person can anticipate unsafe environmental and human forces, thereby avoiding many unsafe situations. Knowledge, adequate skill, and favorable attitudes allow behavior that is planned, deliberate, and intentional, so that unavoidable circumstances rarely occur. Vicarious learning through safety education demonstrates that experience is not always the best teacher.

THE HEALTH BELIEF MODEL AND ACCIDENT PREVENTION

During the 1950s the U.S. Public Health Service wanted to know why more people did not take advantage of the preventive health services that were available. Research was conducted to determine why some people protected themselves and others did not. The health belief model shown in Figure 2-3 is an outgrowth of this research. The model is based upon the premise that preventive health behavior is an attempt to avoid negatively valued outcomes (disease). It is therefore appropriate to apply the model to the prevention of accidents.

The essence of the model is that preventive behavior depends on the world view of the perceiving individual. For an individual to take action to avoid disease or injury, the individual would need to believe:[6]

[6]Irwin M. Rosenstock, "Historical Origins of the Health Belief Model," *Health Education Monographs,* vol. 2, p. 330, Winter, 1974.

46

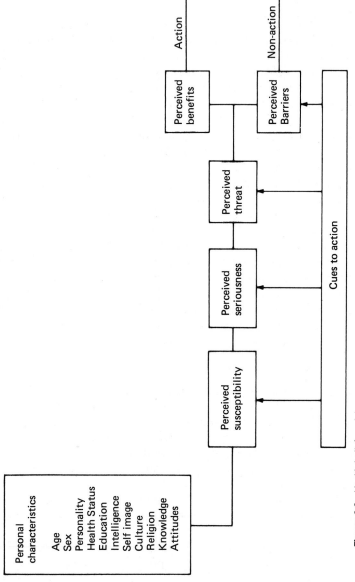

Figure 2-3 Health belief model.

1 That he or she was personally susceptible

2 That the occurrence would have at least moderate severity on some aspect of the individual's life

3 That taking a particular action would be beneficial by reducing susceptibility or severity

Perception of susceptibility varies along a continuum. At one extreme are people who deny any possibility of danger to themselves. A more moderate perception, and one which is perhaps representative of the majority of people, is that a statistical possibility of accidents exists, but that such an event is improbable (the "other guy" syndrome). Finally, some people understand that a real danger exists for them personally.

Perceived seriousness is the degree to which an individual feels threatened by an accident situation. One person might perceive only the medical consequences of an accident, whereas another person might see the consequences in medical, psychological, and economic terms. The intensity of fear may vary according to the nature of the specific threat. A person who is paranoid about cancer may be only slightly affected by the prospect of accidental injury. Generally, a more thorough understanding of the facts enhances perception of both susceptibility and seriousness.

The individual's subjective estimate of the probabilities and consequences of a situation, rather than the actual facts, determines the individual's behavior. Thus, information alone will not help a person develop accident-preventive behavior. Many people "know" that seat belts save lives, that one should always cut away from one's body when using a knife, and that smoking in bed is dangerous. Without proper perception of susceptibility and seriousness, such information will probably not lead to accident-preventive behavior[7] (see Figure 2–3).

"Passive" cues serve to make a person consciously aware of danger. They can raise the levels of perceived susceptibility and perceived seriousness. "Active" cues can tip a person's perception of the benefit-to-barrier ratio in favor of action. For the cues to be effective, they must be relevant to the learner. A clever slogan, a detailed pamphlet, or a safety lecture will be ineffective cues unless they are meaningful to the recipient of the message.

The following statements about cues are also generally true:

1 The more frequently they occur, the more likely it is that action will result.

2 The more varied the source of the cue, the more likely that action will result.

3 The more recent the cue, the more likely that action will result.

4 The more emotional the cue (to a point), the more likely that action will result.

5 The more the cue represents an existing belief, the more likely that action will result.

[7]Irwin M. Rosenstock, "Historical Origins of the Health Belief Model," *Health Education Monographs*, vol. 2, p. 334, Winter, 1974.

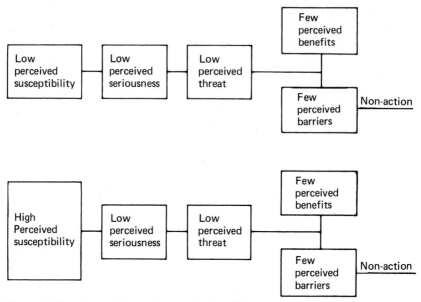

Figure 2-4 Nonaction variations of the health belief model.

Variations of the model which depict circumstances leading to nonaction are presented in Figure 2–4.

One nonaction variation of the health belief model needs explanation. Perceived threat leads to preventive action only when a "reasonable" amount of fear is produced. When the threat becomes overwhelming, the fear can actually inhibit safe behavior. The individual compensates for the stressful emotions by denying or rationalizing the potential harm. Fear may also stimulate a person to magnify existing barriers and to create artificial barriers so that nonaction is assured. This supports the widely held belief that scare techniques in safety education are usually ineffective (see Figure 2–5).

For safety education to encourage preventive behavior, one's perception of susceptibility, seriousness, and threat must be raised to a sufficient level, and

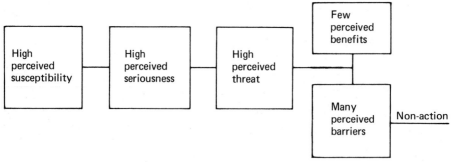

Figure 2-5 The health belief model and fear.

the benefits must clearly outweigh the barriers. Since people's beliefs about accidents are subjective, the mere exchange of information will not alter their behavior. There is a need to create positive attitudes and a sense of motivation that encourages people to protect themselves against accidental harm. The belief system must be changed so that people will no longer be willing to accept accidents as events of chance.

IMPLICATIONS FOR SAFETY EDUCATION

If *learning* is defined as the progressive organization of knowledge, motivation, and behavior, the process of learning to live safely involves (1) understanding the many hazards that a person must encounter in his or her various daily activities, (2) developing attitudes that predispose one to adjust properly to one's environment, and (3) mastering skills that enable one to cope with potentially dangerous situations. Through this process, students should acquire not only specific habits that will protect them against particular hazards, but general habits that will protect them under an infinite variety of circumstances.

The teacher faces the difficult but essential task of convincing students not only that safety has advantages but that these advantages are more desirable than any possible gain from recklessness. It is imperative that the strongest motivating forces, which too often lead to dangerous actions, be cultivated as inducements to careful, orderly behavior. Students need guidance in directing their energy toward satisfying experiences that are socially acceptable. There is no point in stressing the connection between proper conduct and the good of society if students have considerably less interest in contributing to the general welfare than in achieving their own immediate goals. The driver speeding down the highway may want to be a good citizen but would rather set the record for the fastest trip to town. If the teacher understands the satisfactions derived from dangerous behavior, he or she may be able to plan safe activities that offer similar satisfactions as well as other rewards.

SELF-PRESERVATION

Emphasizing the self-preservation drive as an incentive to proper conduct is of questionable value, for focusing attention on the accident that has not yet happened may foster timidity rather than respect for safe behavior. Fear-ridden individuals are more likely to avoid all potentially dangerous situations than to face them with prudence and courage. They may refuse to participate in sports, travel by airplane, or avail themselves of many other valuable opportunities that involve unusual risk.

When safety is taught primarily as protection against injury it conflicts with some of the ideals that people have held since childhood. Their heroes are those who dared; their desire to avoid physical harm is often weaker than their need to live adventurously and to win respect and admiration by facing risks bravely. Football fields would be deserted if exemption from injury were a primary goal. Even young children take chances despite parental warnings, for safety per se is a pallid condition of life.

People can learn to recognize the need for caution. Safety education must convince students that true adventure, which requires skill and sound judgment, is not only safer but more worthwhile than recklessness, and that really courageous adventurers do not needlessly endanger themselves and others. The teacher should point out that airplane pilots, mountain climbers, astronauts, and explorers need long periods of study and training before they are considered ready for their vocations. Students must be made to realize that taking chances is a characteristic not of the hero but of the immature person who is trying to compensate for deficiencies. Young people are more likely to accept these facts if educators can provide them with meaningful, constructive experiences that fulfill their desire for thrills and excitement and lessen their need to participate in the dangerous activities that now attract them. The task is not easy, for adolescents seem to find destructive behavior more appealing than experiences that build character.

It is important that students learn to avoid foolish risks, but it is at least as important that they recognize the value of expert performance as a means of living courageously and safely in the face of necessary hazards. If the self-preservation urge is to serve as an inducement to safe behavior, the emphasis should not be on preserving oneself *from* injury but on preserving oneself *for* a full, adventurous life of greater personal enjoyment and greater service to others. "Survival of the fittest" may be interpreted as the survival or self-preservation of the person who adheres to the basic pattern of safe and orderly behavior. Safety should be taught as a dynamic, positive expression of the moral aspirations of the individual, not as a method of escaping danger and thus satisfying only the desire to stay alive, the basic drive shared by all animals. The well-known slogan, "Be careful—the life you save may be your own," although undoubtedly a deterrent to reckless driving, appeals exclusively to selfish motivation. Ideally it should include a reminder of one's responsibility to others.

SELF-ENHANCEMENT

Although safety teachers should encourage the development of altruistic feelings, they must recognize that the desire for personal gain is often a stronger motive. One who wonders why he or she should comply with a request is likely to ask, "What's in it for me?" Students must be convinced that they, as well as others, profit from careful behavior and that they gain nothing from courting accidents. Our problem is to help them appreciate their responsibility for acquiring a status that is consistent with safe living.

THE IMPORTANCE OF THE GROUP. The need for self-enhancement usually manifests itself as a desire to win the respect and admiration of others.

Most people today want to "belong"; they must have status and security as approved members of a group in order to adjust to society and to function effectively. The desire for group recognition is one of the strongest motives in contemporary American life. To avoid disapproval and gain prestige, individuals often subordinate themselves to the interests of the group, conform to its standards, adopt its values, and pattern their actions after its model; they do what the crowd does. Mothers need to understand the nine-year-old child's desire to avoid group ridicule by not wearing a hat—even though it might be to his or her health advantage to wear one.

Safety education, therefore, must foster *group* approval of its aims, lest social pressure hinder rather than support the development of proper habits and attitudes. Where there is general admiration of recklessness, efforts to promote careful, orderly behavior make little headway. Most people prefer the praise of their own group, or of the group to which they wish to belong, to the respect of outsiders; a student is not likely to risk the ridicule of classmates in order to please the teacher. As long as reckless driving brings students not only excitement and adventure but popularity among their classmates, safety instruction will not seem important to them; they would rather risk injury than be known as a "mama's boy" or a "teacher's pet."

INCONSISTENT SOCIAL VALUES. Cooperation and interdependent activity are generally utilized to satisfy basic needs. To some extent, most groups value cooperation, helpfulness, courtesy, responsibility, self-control, and other characteristics of the good citizen that are conducive to safe behavior. Those who customarily display these qualities are usually accepted and admired, whereas the impolite, selfish, or uncooperative person may be excluded from the group. Teachers should therefore help students understand that such attributes as self-restraint and consideration for others indicate maturity and enhance social status.

Social standards are not always consistent; in many cases they militate against safe behavior. For example, although democratic ideals are generally endorsed, contrary practices are also sanctioned. The very high school group that ordinarily values thoughtful, considerate behavior may also idolize the daredevil with the fastest hot rod and disparage the boy or girl who obeys all the traffic laws.

Such inconsistent attitudes are not restricted to adolescents. Adults often set a poor example. Children are raised in an atmosphere where "influence" is powerful, where, all too often, the leading members of society are permitted to violate safety regulations. Speeding tickets are sometimes "fixed" if the offender has enough money or power. A wealthy theater owner may not be forced to shut down his or her building for repairs even though it is a firetrap, but the owner of a small grocery store may be fined for a minor violation.

It is difficult to teach young people to respect the law when there are people in high office whose interests and purposes seem unsuited to their positions and whose actions are sometimes downright dishonest. Individuals who get away with infractions are often not condemned, but admired and envied. It is therefore not surprising that many adolescents strive to emulate the privileged few who seem able to serve their own selfish interests unhindered by rules and regulations.

SOCIETY AND THE INDIVIDUAL.   To prevent the development of asocial attitudes, safety education—along with all other phases of the school program—must be concerned with imparting a thorough understanding of what democracy means. When this goal has been achieved, students will recognize and disapprove of the unsafe practices that violate democratic principles. Beyond concern for their own safety, they must develop a feeling of responsibility for the welfare of other group members. Only as they acquire this sense of social obligation will they be free to act as they please. Students must be made to see that each member of the community has a place and function, and that progress is measured by the degree to which this place and function become increasingly significant, both for the self and for the community. With the development of this common purpose of society, students should have less difficulty in realizing that their prestige is enhanced by sharing in activities that promote the general welfare, and that personal goals and altruistic ideals are not in conflict one with the other.

Adolescent groups should be guided in selecting standards that uphold the social processes by which the benefits, safeguards, and moral responsibilities that belong by right to every member of a democracy will actually be extended to all citizens. Young people must be taught the value of citizenship in a free society, the necessity of fulfilling the obligations accompanying citizenship, and the importance of upholding its ideals and principles. Teachers can best accomplish these objectives by giving students opportunities to practice democracy in their daily activities. Although pupils must be given tasks commensurate with their varying abilities, each should be expected to contribute his or her share to projects designed to benefit the entire group.

RESPONSIBILITY.   One is most likely to do a job well if it is within one's capacity and if successful performance will bring personal recognition. Often children who are careless about household chores become thorough and willing workers when stimulating tasks outside the home give them a chance to prove their maturity and to show that they deserve to be treated as adults. Since an employer usually takes it for granted that the adolescent employee is capable of assuming responsibility, the youth is eager to show that this trust is not misplaced and that he or she is entitled to respect as a working member of the community.

Early participatory experiences in adult society promote a feeling of individual worth. If a girl has to make a contribution to the life of a family or other group as early as her level of maturity will permit, she will become more conscious that the policies and goals of her group are her concern and that their fulfillment depends upon her. Even the best-organized program of accident prevention is ineffectual without individual responsibility.

Parents who expect their child to show adult judgment often fail to give the child any indication that they consider him or her sufficiently grown up to assume a reasonable degree of responsibility. This contradictory attitude is confusing and frustrating to a youth. When a youth is expected to do only simple, routine jobs that younger children could easily perform, he or she has little incentive to work well, however necessary the task. Surely young drivers whose parents express faith in their dependability by allowing them to use the family car are more likely to behave safely than those whose parents treat them as if they were hopelessly irresponsible and reckless.

The knowledge that one has been entrusted with responsibility can be a strong incentive to proper behavior, and experience in handling challenging assignments can help to develop safe habits. Young people should be given ample opportunity both at home and at school to display their competence and reliability, provided that they are adequately trained for the work they are to do. An alert teacher can often bring out the best in students by showing confidence in their ability and trustworthiness, and by praising their achievements. The safety teacher has many opportunities to assign character-building duties that students will enjoy performing, such as making surveys of home hazards, planning and conducting safety programs, organizing bicycle clubs, and serving on school patrols.

SELF-GOVERNMENT.   The popularity of reckless conduct among some adolescent groups stems partially from a need to rebel against the authority of parents and teachers, who—they feel—neither consider their interests nor respect their opinions. Young people may decide that they have had enough of adult-imposed restrictions, including safety rules and regulations, and that it is time to show they are on their own. Failing to gain status in socially approved ways, they may seek to assert themselves through destructive behavior.

Safety education must help students recognize that our vulnerability to injury makes certain laws necessary for our survival. Observing these laws is not a matter of submitting to arbitrary authority but of playing the game of life according to tested rules. Students should be made to understand that safety regulations are actually for their own protection. In exchange for this protection they must give up the right to do exactly as they please.

Adherence to the rules of games may help young people accept rules in other activities. For example, the batter in baseball must attempt to hit a ball thrown in the "strike zone," or be charged with one strike. If the batter commits this delaying tactic three times, he is "out" and his team is penalized. The pitcher must deliver the ball into some part of the strike zone. If he or she fails to do so four times, the batter becomes a base runner. Such rules are recognized as necessary for the orderly progression of the game.

It is easy enough for students to recognize the necessity of conforming to the inevitable laws of nature. They realize, for example, that they must swim with their heads above water—or at least come up for air at frequent intervals—if they are to avoid drowning. Through proper counseling, students may learn to accept society's laws in the same spirit; to acknowledge the fact that a swimmer's safety may depend not only on keeping her head above water but on obeying all accepted rules for aquatic safety.

Adolescents are more likely to obey safety rules that they have helped formulate. They should be given an opportunity to evaluate the regulations they are expected to obey. They will feel that they have an approved status in society if they are consulted about the laws that govern them. The chance to verbalize their objections and resentments about existing rules may act as a catharsis that frees them to consider alternative procedures for ensuring safety. The result will often be essentially the same set of rules, but because the rules have been worked over by the students themselves and stated in a slightly different manner, the "new" code will seem more acceptable.

Teachers should encourage group discussions of incidents that indicate a need for new safety rules or for better enforcement of existing rules. If the students themselves recognize the necessity of taking corrective action, they will work out a solution that seems reasonable to them. Wherever possible, offenders should be brought into line by group pressure and not by faculty or parental authority. The group will then be clearly on record as supporting *its own rules.*

EVALUATION

A school can judge the overall effectiveness of its accident-prevention efforts by studying the postgraduation records of its graduates to see how well they have adjusted to their environment. Since external conditions are not static, the safety program may have to be modified from time to time to meet changing needs. The answers to the following questions should indicate the areas of strength and weakness in the program.

- Are students given opportunities to gain actual experience in democratic living?
- Does the school sponsor civic and social education that deals frankly, rationally, and sympathetically with significant issues of the contemporary world?
- Is there adequate provision for integrating safety education with social science courses and other subject areas?
- Are activities planned to suit the varying interests and capacities of individual students?
- Is the system flexible enough to utilize new resources without sacrificing the best in traditional education?
- Are teachers adequately prepared to teach safety? If not, are they learning through in-service training?

- Do students fully understand and sanction the objectives of education, or are they simply attending school because of habit, legal requirements, and social pressure?
- Does the safety program foster the development of personal responsibility? Has the school a functioning safety council with student representation?
- Are students acquiring the wholesome critical attitude necessary for effective problem solving?
- Are accidents reported? Are the data studied regularly in an attempt to plan ways of preventing similar accidents?
- Is the vocational education program concerned with inculcating basic economic understandings as well as with developing trade skills?
- Is there provision for meeting students' avocational and recreational needs? Are pupils given opportunities for worthwhile adventure? What trips are taken? Are these trips used to demonstrate some phase of safety?
- Do students receive intelligent and adequate guidance to aid them in developing mature, well-adjusted personalities?
- Does the school sponsor a program emphasizing good physical, social, and mental health as a means of leading a fuller, richer, and safer life?
- Has there been any evidence of (1) reduction in the student accident rate, (2) improvement in the students' attitudes towards safety, (3) community support for safety patrols and other school-initiated measures, and (4) parewntal and faculty interest and participation in safety efforts?

If these questions can be answered affirmatively, graduating students will have acquired certain personal characteristics that tend to promote safe, democratic practices. Perhaps safety education can best achieve its objectives by fostering development of the following personal characteristics:

1 *Commitment to the common purposes of society.* Participating in student-government associations and other school organizations that promote self-rule, personal responsibility, and respect for delegated authority will help students understand through actual experience that contributing to the social good is ultimately more satisfying than pursuing one's own selfish interests without regard for others. Membership in religious groups that stress broad ethical principles and the common goals of all mankind rather than denominational differences can also stimulate the development of altruistic attitudes.

2 *Emotional maturity.* Appropriate activities can help students develop mature attitudes toward sportsmanship, teamwork, cooperation, and the rights of others—to acquire a sense of responsibility for their own welfare and safety and for the welfare and safety of others. Students should be helped to realize that attaining maturity is not like reaching one's destination at the end of a journey, but more like covering the allotted distance on each successive stage of a journey. Fourteen-year-olds for example, are considered immature if they neglect their schoolwork and chores, continually whine and complain when they cannot have their way, and need to have most of their activities planned for them.

3 *Knowledge of important contemporary problems.*

4 *A sound philosophy of life.* Sympathetic counseling should help students develop a strong and wholesome personal philosophy.

5 *Dependence upon rational, not emotional, thinking to control behavior.*

LEARNING EXPERIENCES

The following activities are designed to supplement the study of this chapter.

1 Gather statistical information from sources such as the National Center for Health Statistics, the National Safety Council, the United States Census, and your state department of public health.

    a Compare the accident data with figures for specific chronic and communicable diseases.

    b Identify cyclic and long-term trends and make predictions about the future priorities of safety education.

    c Analyze the accidental occurrences in terms of age, sex, occupation, educational level, ethnic background, and place of residence (urban versus rural). Prepare a list of possible reasons which account for differences in the accident rate according to these factors.

2 Write a position paper on "The responsibility of a humanistic society for the provision of safety education to enhance the quality of life."

3 Discuss the various levels of accident and disease prevention.

    a Why has our health-care delivery system focused so much effort on the tertiary level of prevention?

    b Why does the general public fail to use primary-prevention techniques in protecting themselves against the hazards of accidental injury or death?

    c What steps can be taken to encourage a change of philosophy so that prevention occurs at the primary level?

4 Debate the following issue: "The use of personality inventories as a criterion for drivers' licensing examinations would significantly affect the incidence of highway accidents."

5 Develop a creative model to explain the concept of accident causation.

6 Brainstorm a list of health superstitions which exist as the result of an unknown cause-and-effect relationship.

7 Create an artificial accident story using as many antecedents as possible leading to the unsafe situation. This might be done as a contest among students to see who can provide the most antecedents for a single accident.

8 Develop a new safety slogan which uses self-preservation or self-enhancement as its focus.

9 Write a position paper on the topic, "Safety is important to me because . . .

SELECTED REFERENCES

Allport, Gordon W.: "Values and Our Youth," in Robert E. Grinder (ed.), *Studies in Adolescence,* The Macmillan Company, New York, 1963, pp. 17–27.

Brody, Leon: "Personal Characteristics of Chronic Violators and Accident Repeaters," *Highway Research Bulletin,* no. 152, National Academy of Sciences, National Research Council, Washington, 1957.

Dietrich, Harry Fredrick: "The Role of Education in Accident Prevention," *Journal of Pediatrics,* vol. 17, pp. 297–302, February, 1956.

Guilford, Joan S.: "Prediction of Accidents in a Standardized Home Environment," *Journal of Applied Psychology,* vol. 57, pp. 306–313, no. 3, 1973.

Haddon, William Jr., Edward A. Suchman, and David Klein, (eds.): *Accident Research Methods and Application,* Harper & Row, Publishers, Incorporated, New York, 1964.

Hale, A. R., and M. Hale: "Accidents in Perspective," *Occupational Psychology,* vol. 44, pp. 115–121, 1970.

Margolis, Bruce L., and William H. Kroes: *The Human Side of Accident Prevention,* Charles C Thomas, Publisher, Springfield, Ill., 1975.

Miller, Gary, and Neil Agnew: "First Aid Training and Accidents," *Occupational Psychology,* vol. 47, pp. 209–218, 1973.

Rosenstock, Irwin M.: "Historical Origins of the Health Belief Model," *Health Education Monographs,* vol. 2, pp. 328–335, Winter, 1974.

Shaw, Lynette, and Herbert S. Sichel: *Accident Proneness,* Pergamon Press, Oxford, 1971.

Stafford, G. T.: "Safety: Your Responsibility," *Journal of Health, Physical Education and Recreation,* vol. 30, p. 6, November, 1959.

Suchman, Edward A.: "Accidents and Social Deviance," *Journal of Health and Social Behavior,* vol. 11, pp. 4–15, March, 1970.

Swain, Alan D.: *The Human Element in Systems Safety,* In Com Tec House, Surrey, England, 1974.

Williams, Alan F., and Henry Weschler: "Dimensions of Preventive Behavior," *Journal of Consulting and Clinical Psychology,* vol. 40, no. 3, pp. 420–425, 1973.

3

Planning the School Safety Program

OVERALL OBJECTIVE:

The student should understand the procedures necessary for planning, implementing, and evaluating the school safety program.

INSTRUCTIONAL OBJECTIVES:

After completing this chapter the student will be able to:

1 Explain the basic concepts which lay the foundation for the school's safety program.
2 List the basic principles which serve as a guide for the development of a safety education program.
3 Discuss the major components of the *Safety Charter for Children and Youth* (home, school, and community).
4 Show how the *School Safety Council* functions as the administrative mechanism in planning a comprehensive safety program.
5 Identify the many sources of data available to a School Safety Council when conducting a *needs assessment.*
6 State, in precise terms, several major goals of a comprehensive school safety program.
7 List alternative methods for evaluation of the school safety program.
8 Discuss the objectives of adult safety education.
9 List the goals of the Campus Safety Association.

Safe living has become an important and complicated issue in our society. The home and community have not dealt adequately with this issue. Because of the availability of professional safety educators, the school must assume responsibility for preparing our young people for safe living. In many states, legislative enactments require the teaching of safety at various grade levels.

Our children and youth must learn to live safely in an increasingly complex environment where the safety hazards of everyday living are constantly changing. To develop this capacity, they must be able to recognize unsafe conditions; they must learn when and how to modify their environment, as well as their behavior, to eliminate or minimize unsafe situations. Toward this end, a well-planned school safety program is recommended.

When a new subject such as safety education takes its place in the school curriculum, confusion and misunderstanding are likely to occur. Educators and administrators frequently have conflicting interests, and areas of study are often poorly defined. Teachers of the traditional subjects often do not understand the new field and sometimes object to the innovation. But as technological advances change American living conditions, creating hazards along with improvements, safety education is gaining acceptance as an integral part of school programs, with a relationship to all aspects of the total school curriculum.

Education represents the one real hope for reducing the accident rate, for it is through education that meaning can be given to safety. A school's safety program is capable of helping students understand what safety means; it demonstrates the benefits of safe living. A well-planned school safety program can make significant contributions to accident prevention in our fast-moving society. The primary function of the school safety program is to influence the behavior of young people toward safe living for greater adventure throughout life.

BASIC CONCEPTS

Before presenting basic principles about the school's safety program, it is necessary to start with basic concepts or beliefs, and to lay the foundation for understanding the problem of accident prevention and control.[1]

    I. Almost all accidents can be avoided.
        1. Accidents are the end result of a series of circumstances, of which the elimination of any one would prevent the accident.
        2. Accidents do not just happen but are caused. They are caused by what people do or don't do.
        3. Basic to the prevention of accidents is a consideration of the rights of others.
    II. Emphasis must be placed on higher standards of safe performance with an accompanying reduction in the acceptance of foolish risks and defiance of the law of chance.
        1. It is of little value to encourage or urge people to be safe unless they understand "what is safe" and "what is unsafe."

---

[1]"Accident Prevention: Seriousness of the Problem," unpublished report of a Curriculum Commission Committee under the direction of W. K. Streit, Chairman, Cincinnati Public Schools, Sept. 23, 1965.

    2. One is more likely to comply with a safety rule or regulation if he understands its purpose and realizes that it is intended for his welfare and protection.

III. A reduction of accidents will be achieved when man accepts greater self-responsibility for his acts and when there are better environmental controls.

    1. When we accept some responsibility for the safety of others, we can reduce accidents by being "our brother's keeper."

    2. Pre-planning in the elimination of hazards in the environment and in the establishment of controlling regulations for safe movement is desirable.

    3. One of the major functions of society is to protect the individual against the hazards of his environment and to find ways in which he can protect himself.

    4. Inspection and care of equipment will help reduce accidents.

    5. Supervision of activity can play an important role in accident prevention.

IV. To be safe requires adjustment to the situation, not merely perfunctory behavior.

    1. Hence, it is important that we learn to swim in order that we may save our own life and perhaps that of others; that we learn to fall and roll in a coordinated and relaxed manner; and that we learn to drive a motor vehicle in a "defensive" manner by anticipating the actions of others in order to avoid accidents.

    2. Accidents can be avoided through thought and precaution. They are caused through imitation, failure to follow directions, carelessness, and failure to recognize hazards.

    3. Human factors which are of greater significance for the control of accidents include age, training and personal adjustments.

V. Safety is related to physical and mental health.

    1. Accidents are more likely to occur when one is physically, psychologically, or socially unfit; when one is frustrated; when one is emotionally upset; when one is fatigued; when one is taking certain medication; when one is not accepted by the peer group.

    2. The innate drive toward emotional and physical wholeness must be reinforced by and predicated upon the causal factors of accidents—mechanical and human.

    3. Antisocial behavior has a predictive value relating to accidents.

VI. Safety enables the individual to enjoy adventure without the hazards of accidents.

    1. Skill in the performance of an act helps to reduce accidents.

    2. The positive approach is an incentive for the right action based on a way to perform safely.

    3. Life is at its best when we are not robbed of adventure and worthwhile activities by stupid acts or careless mishaps.

VII. Accidents waste time, money, life.
1. Loss of life and the incapacity resulting from accidents is greater than from any known disease entity.
2. Accidents are the leading cause of death among young people, ranking first for persons up to about 34 years of age, and second for persons between 35 and 44.
3. Each year local, state and national figures reveal tremendous losses in earning power and productivity, property damage, and shortened lives resulting from unsafe acts.
4. Being put out of condition by an accident is just as serious as being ill.
VIII. In order to prevent accidents, we need to know how they occur. This can be accomplished by
1. Understanding the hazards as they relate to persons, places, and things.
2. Removing the hazards.
3. Compensating for hazards that cannot be removed.
4. Creating no unnecessary hazards by an act or failure to act.
IX. Accident prevention is not the task of a few people but the responsibility of many.
1. Teachers and administrators should develop some familiarity with its scope, purposes, methods and objectives.
2. Parents should lay the foundation for safe living from birth to maturity. Boys and girls need love, security and self-esteem. Lack of these basic human needs results in accident-prone people who are characteristically impulsive, resentful, and self-absorbed in their relations with their surroundings.
3. Community education in safe practices is pursued constantly in a variety of ways and through many individuals, groups and organizations, voluntary and official.
4. Each community has the responsibility for determining its own requirements for safety by identifying the problems.

BASIC PRINCIPLES FOR SAFETY EDUCATION[2]

Our democratic way of life operates in accordance with certain basic principles which have been derived from past experiences in an ever changing society. It emphasizes self-realization and encourages a critical evaluation of living, to the end that a better way of life may be achieved for all.

The school is an agency of society and is responsible for designing and guiding the development of an educational program which will meet the needs of the individual in an era of cultural change. The needs of human beings living in a particular environment give direction to the total educational process. This considers our democratic ideals and values, the needs and interests of the individuals, and the needs of society.

[2]"Basic Principles for Safety Education," *Safety Education*, vol. 36, pp. 12–13, December, 1955.

Therefore, the following principles may serve as a guide for the development of a safety education program.

Safety education should be a responsibility of society and should be consistent with our best understanding of human growth and the development of society.

The machine age has redesigned our pattern of living. It has introduced hazards into all phases of human activity with the result that accidents in our age are a major problem which can be met with the help of an effective educational program.

The school should provide leadership in promoting safe living.

The rapid scientific strides of our time make it imperative that education focus specific attention on the persistent problems of accidents. Educational leadership has the responsibility of providing effective guidance and direction toward cooperative participation in a democratic society for safety conditions.

Safety instruction should be an integral part of the school program and should further develop understandings, attitudes, values, skills, habits and appreciations which will assist the learner in meeting the responsibilities of safe living in today's world.

Safety instruction should seek to develop fully the potentialities of the "whole child" as a happy, well-integrated personality, who can contribute to a better way of life for all. The school should carefully select and plan safety experiences, the method of instruction, and the use of instructional materials to meet the needs of each individual. The learning environment, therefore, should provide experiences that continuously challenge the individual to think clearly and to act wisely in terms of safe living for himself and others.

The school should utilize community resources to implement its program and to further supplement its efforts in safety education.

Safety education should be a vital part of community life. It requires cooperative planning, selecting, and utilizing of community resources to the extent that they will contribute to and enrich the quality of safety education. It must be developed with an awareness of the pattern and characteristics of child growth and development. Educating each child for safe living must take into consideration all factors that influence his attitude toward life.

Safety education should develop a continuous awareness of the value of human life and the physical well-being of individuals, and at the same time recognize the achievement of others in meeting these requirements.

Life and human well-being are priceless and can be conserved only to the extent that we are aware of and can appreciate their value.

Safety education should be continuous and contribute to the enrichment of all areas of living.

Education is the ongoing process of life, and safety education is the continuous process of conserving it. The safety experiences in school should be continuous and consistent with those out of school. Safety education should help each individual not only to avoid accidents, but also to free him to live "life more abundantly."

These principles suggest the function of a safety education program but offer no easy solution to the persistent problems involved, not merely in transmitting information, but in fostering safe behavior. The schools must face these responsibilities, however, for no day passes without widely publicized reports of tragic accidents that remind us of the imperative need for effective safety education.

In planning the school safety program, careful study must be made of the *Safety Charter for Children and Youth*. The charter was developed by a joint committee representing seven departments of the National Education Association, the Society of State Directors for Health, Physical Education and Recreation, and the National Safety Council. The American Academy of Pediatrics, the American Medical Association, and the Boy Scouts of America also endorsed the charter. The major components of the charter include the home, the school, and the community.

A SAFETY CHARTER FOR CHILDREN AND YOUTH

Children and youth are the nation's most valuable asset. They are wholesome and eager; they possess great vigor; they are adventurous. At the same time they are ingenious and mischievous. Most of all, they have faith and trust in adults whenever and wherever their safety is involved. This fact places a tremendous responsibility upon us all to provide:

I. For every child a dwelling-place safe, . . .
A home that assures freedom to live, work and play safely; an environment with progressively reduced physical hazards; and a family program of continuous guidance that develops confidence and ability to protect one's self and others.
All children and youth need:
1. A home built, equipped, and maintained for safe living.
2. A home where there is an atmosphere of acceptance of each individual—where sympathy, understanding, love and affection promote the mental and emotional health essential to the development of desirable attitudes and practices of safe living.
3. A home where parents and children alike assume their individual responsibilities for safe behavior in all situations.
4. A home where the family practices safe living at all times.
II. For every child education for safety and protection against accidents to which modern conditions subject him . . .
A school that recognizes ever-changing needs; progressively reduces physical hazards; and educates for safe living through instruction, example, and participation.
All children and youth need:
1. A school that provides and maintains a safe environment—buildings, grounds, equipment, supplies, machinery, heating, and lighting.
2. A school that bases its education for safe living on continuous research, local and national.
3. A school that uses a 24-hour a day accident-reporting system as one factor in planning and evaluating its instruction in safe living.
4. A school where guidance, supervision, and instruction are geared to personal responsibility for one's safety and that of others, and where due emphasis is given to proper knowledge, skills, attitudes, and habits.
5. A school that provides, in all its activities, opportunities for pupils to develop the ability to make adjustments for safe living, both present and future.
6. A school that permits democratic participation of children and adults in planning and enforcing rules and regulations designed for safe living.
7. A school that reflects a philosophy which emphasizes educational experiences for youthful participants and which substitutes an increasing sense of personal responsibility for restrictive and supervisory measures imposed by others.
8. A school that facilitates interaction with the community for better safety.
III. For every child a community which recognizes and plans for his needs, protects him against physical dangers—provides him with safe and wholesome places for play and recreation. A community where all agencies and organizations, through individual and cooperative effort, develop a program of action that meets conditions affecting the safety of youth.

All children and youth need:

1. A community that provides for the safety of its citizens.
2. A community, rural or urban, that provides for and encourages safe living on the streets and highways, on the job, in recreation, and at home.
3. A community that considers the safe route to and from school, church, playground, and other youth centers in its planning.
4. A community with adequate regulations and enforcement for traffic, transportation, building, and fire safety.
5. A community that accepts its responsibility for appropriate leadership and supervision of group functions.
6. A community wherein safe and reasonable recreation programs are provided for children and youth, under adult guidance and supervision competent to assist children and youth in making appropriate social adjustments.

We, as educational leaders, recognizing that conservation of life depends upon the safety education of our children and recognizing that every individual has the right to contribute to safe living for all Americans, do hereby pledge ourselves to do all that is within our power to meet these needs of children and youth.

PROGRAM PLANNING FOR SAFETY EDUCATION

The success of the school safety program largely depends on the quality of the planning which precedes the teaching and learning process. Although the components of program planning may vary, depending on circumstances, the following elements are absolutely essential:

1 An administrative mechanism for the planning, development, promotion, implementation, and evaluation of the program
2 A formal and detailed needs assessment
3 Planned strategies for implementing safety education
4 Adequate techniques for evaluation of program effectiveness
5 Techniques for stimulating public support

SCHOOL SAFETY COUNCIL

The administrative vehicle recommended for a comprehensive safety education program is known as a school safety council. The organization consists primarily of teachers and students, but it is often desirable to solicit membership among parents, safety professionals, and community leaders who are interested in promoting a safer way of life. The building principal need not belong to the council, but it is imperative that the council receive administrative recognition and support.

To be truly effective in its efforts to establish a comprehensive safety program, the council must be willing to work with community resources. People are more likely to support a program when they have had an opportunity to participate in its formulation. Therefore, a wide variety of input is recommended. The responsibilities of the council include, but are not limited to, needs assessment, implementation, and evaluation.

The council should function as a clearinghouse for all safety matters brought to its attention. It should coordinate the various school activities concerned with accident prevention, and establish safety regulations governing such matters as the use of bicycles and motor vehicles and the conduct of students in halls, stairways, and play areas. Although a faculty member may initiate a council, it is usually organized and operated largely by the students themselves as a phase of student government.

The importance of having a safety specialist on the council must be stressed. No teacher can be expected to provide all the guidance, learning experiences, and safety activities for students who may range from elementary school to high school and college age. The specialist, whether from the school or from an outside agency, can give teachers and students a broad view of and deep insight into the problems of safety education.

In organizing the safety program, the council should observe the general objectives and principles of curriculum planning. The resulting plan should permit continuous growth, research, evaluation, and revision. The program should not remain static once it has been developed but adjust to fit changing conditions and to meet student needs. The basic objectives formulated in this chapter should always be kept in mind. The program should have continuity; it should include the cooperative efforts of teachers and students, and utilize the students' experiences both outside and within the school.

Like other permanent organizations, the council should develop and adopt a constitution that meets the needs and interests of the students, the school administration, and the community. Since large groups cannot operate efficiently, an elementary school council should probably be restricted to two members from each grade, and a junior or senior high school council to one representative from each home room. Officers are usually chosen by popular vote to serve for the entire school year. It is advisable to schedule the election shortly before the summer vacation so that the new council can begin functioning as soon as school reconvenes in the fall.

The various committees usually organized by the council are responsible for the following functions:

1 The program committee organizes assemblies and other special programs dealing with safety, secures speakers and movies, plans skits, etc.

2 The publicity committee informs local newspapers and radio and television stations of school safety work, arranges bulletin-board displays, and prepares materials for the school paper.

3 The accident-reporting committee collects information pertaining to school accidents and assists in making accident reports.

4 The inspection committee regularly examines play areas, locker rooms, stairs, etc., and reports its findings to the responsible person, usually the school principal or the committee adviser.

In addition to its regular duties, the council may plan special activities such as excursions to police and fire stations, traffic courts, radio and television studios that are presenting safety programs, and industrial plants. It may also arrange a series of safety exhibits to illustrate a safe home, a safe play area, and safe routes to and from school. It may display maps that indicate hazardous areas. The council may also set up a safety suggestion box to encourage student recommendations on accident prevention. A council can do much to help ensure a school safety program. Principals and teachers who are willing to devote time and energy to organizing and guiding a council will find that their efforts pay off in a better school safety record.

NEEDS ASSESSMENT

A needs assessment can be thought of in much the same way as a visit to the doctor for diagnosis of an illness. Positive action can be taken only after it has been understood that a problem exists. Upon thorough and scientific analysis of the problem, an accurate diagnosis can be rendered. When the nature of the disability is understood, plans can be developed to improve the unsatisfactory state of being by application of corrective and remedial controls.

A needs assessment for program planning is somewhat more complicated than this and requires additional steps. It is important to determine the needs and interests of the target population. This necessitates a vast amount of research. Data may be obtained from:

1 Student, staff, and teacher accident records
2 State and national accident figures
3 Legal requirements and mandates from the state board of education
4 Interviews with police, ambulance, fire, hospital, and public health personnel
5 Safety inspector forms that identify potential or existing hazards
6 Observation of student behavior
7 Knowledge tests
8 Skills tests
9 Attitude inventories
10 Community surveys and questionnaires
11 State-provided curriculum guides
12 Safety consultants

The content of a safety education program should be based primarily upon a careful analysis of these data and upon:

1 The students' interests
2 Their level of maturity
3 Their knowledge
4 Their readiness to learn

5 Their desire for improvement, as indicated by tests and classroom discussion

6 Their previous preparation in safety education.

7 Legal requirements

STATEMENT OF GOALS AND OBJECTIVES

The next step in the planning process is to identify goals and objectives. Goals are long-range statements of expectation. Objectives are short-term, measurable statements that provide some degree of accountability for the program. Goals and objectives provide a framework for the total safety program. They generate program policies, curriculum content, learning activities, and supportive safety programs. Program policies must be stated clearly, accurately, and precisely.

Once the safety needs of a group are understood, it is not difficult to set goals for the school program. The following are suggested:

1 To develop attitudes, habits, knowledge, and skill for one's self-protection and the protection of others

2 To cultivate an attitude of social responsibility that pertains to law and order, courtesy, and respect for others

3 To develop respect and regard for national and local resources

4 To develop an appreciation of democratic living and the highest respect for the worth of the individual

5 To develop an understanding of responsibility and cooperation in local, state, and national endeavors for accident prevention and control

6 To develop an understanding of the difference between a foolhardy, rash, devil-may-care attitude and alertness, foresight, conscientiousness, forethought, and probity

7 To develop the perception that the absence of accidents and injury provides opportunities for greater and better adventure

The teacher will be more likely to achieve these fundamental goals if more specific objectives are formulated in accordance with the particular subject matter and the students' level of maturity. The aims applicable to the various areas of safety education are discussed in later chapters, but it is well to indicate here how the objectives of safety education for elementary school children differ from those for high school students.

Children in the *elementary grades* should be trained to recognize hazardous situations and to develop skill and knowledge in meeting those situations. They must be taught to perceive, understand, and obey the various rules and regulations that apply to their safety and to the safety of others. If the teacher fosters appreciation and respect for the law and for law-enforcement officers, pupils are more likely to cooperate in accident-prevention efforts. Children should be taught to practice safe habits of conduct in the home, at school, and in the community. Activities should provide actual experiences in safe behavior, and should help develop neuromuscular skill, strength, coordination, and agility, for physical fitness helps children avoid injuries.

In safety education at the *secondary school level,* the teacher should help students understand why accidents happen and how adequate knowledge, proper attitudes, and sufficient skill can help prevent accidents. In this way, students will learn to appreciate and observe safety rules and regulations. Attention should be focused on subjects such as fire prevention; safeguards against vocational and traffic hazards; proper pedestrian, motorcycle, and bicycle-riding habits; and the safe handling of automobiles (taught in a driver and traffic-safety education course). Throughout the program, the teacher should try to instill a sense of group and community responsibility for the prevention of accidents and the preservation of property.

The goals and objectives suggested here illustrate some commonly accepted aims of safety education at the elementary and secondary school levels, but the list could be extended. The teacher will find many helpful suggestions for preparing objectives in various textbooks, teachers' guides, state courses of study, and materials prepared by such organizations as the National Education Association and the National Safety Council, as well as by state departments of education and city school systems.

PLANS FOR IMPLEMENTATION

Implementation is the phase of planning that makes a program operational. A needs assessment and a statement of goals and objectives must be completed prior to implementation, but this alone will not guarantee program success. It is important to be able to predict potential problems and to plan strategies which will alleviate their occurrence. To achieve its goals and objectives, the council must:

1 Identify steps necessary for implementation
2 Develop a time line to ensure adequate progress
3 Allocate responsibilities (to committees)
4 Establish effective communication with the principal, school board, and community
5 Identify strategies for public relations
6 Solicit input from a variety of sources
7 Specify and prioritize objectives
8 Predict problems and identify solutions
9 Recruit qualified personnel who are supportive of the program
10 Develop written policies
11 Evaluate the program throughout its course

SELECTING THE UNITS OF WORK

Once the overall curriculum has been planned, a committee should organize the instructional units. Suggestions for these units may arise from group discussion or from new interests that develop as the students pursue their work. For this reason, specific units of safety education will not be recommended here. All too often the teacher, or prospective teacher, employs a prearranged program that does not fit the particular needs and interests of the students. As has been previously stated, the program should be prepared by those who will teach it for the particular groups of students who will use it. In planning the unit of work, the following steps are suggested:

1 Prepare a statement of the desired results in terms of students' attitudes, knowledge, and skills. The objectives of a particular unit can be more specific than the objectives of the entire program.

2 Select an approach that will be interesting and meaningful to the students

3 Select the type of learning activities that will create the proper attitudes and develop the necessary skills and practices. These learning experiences should include out-of-school activities in the home and community.

4 Select culminating activities that will not only summarize the unit but measure, objectively and subjectively, the degree to which its purposes have been achieved.

5 Select and list specific and easily obtainable references that will help the student. These may include textbooks, pamphlets, magazine articles, and audiovisual materials.

6 Allow time for students to evaluate their accomplishments as the work progresses.

The instructional program should cover the following areas: pedestrian safety; bicycle safety; motorcycle safety; traffic safety, including driver and traffic-safety education; home safety; fire prevention; civil defense; vocational safety; safety in and around the school, and on the way to and from the school; and safety in play, sport, and other recreational activities. Although it can be difficult to plan units in safety education, it is well within the combined abilities of teachers, administrators, and students, especially when assisted by a safety expert. Organizing an effective program presents a challenge to everyone in the school, a challenge which must be accepted by all.

EVALUATION

Evaluation is a continuous process. It begins with the needs assessment and continues as long as the program remains in operation. The primary purpose is to determine whether and to what extent the program objectives are being achieved. Evaluation is useful in recommending program changes to fit the varying needs and interests of the target population. Methods of evaluation include:

1 Student test scores
2 Attitude inventories
3 Skills testing
4 Observation of student behavior
5 Analysis of accident report records
6 Inspections of buildings and grounds
7 Student evaluation of program activities

PLANNING AN ADULT SAFETY EDUCATION PROGRAM

An area of safety education that has not been developed sufficiently is education for adults. Although this chapter is primarily concerned with safety instruction in elementary and secondary schools, the adult program is so closely related that it should be mentioned here. The success of a school safety program is largely dependent on the knowledge, interests, and efforts of the adults within the community. The school can help influence the behavior of children, but unless safe practices prevail in the home and community, the learned knowledge, skills, and attitudes may not be used outside the school. Since adults determine local safety practices and set the community standard for accident prevention, their influence on the effectiveness of the school program should not be underestimated. It is logical, therefore, for the school to organize a safety education program for adults.

A safety program for adults includes essentially the same subject matter as programs for school-age students. Many of the principles that apply to education at any level can be utilized in planning and conducting a safety program for adults. The curriculum must be geared to the needs, interests, and problems of the group, and educational leaders must be carefully selected.

Organizations other than the school may sponsor or conduct adult education programs, and the schools have an excellent opportunity to work with these groups. The schools can furnish leadership, assist in formulating the program, and act as the coordinating agency.

Among the objectives of an adult program are:

1 To develop an appreciation and an understanding of what the schools are doing, through safety education, to prevent accidents to children
2 To help adults recognize the contributions of legislation, law enforcement, engineering, and education to public safety
3 To develop a spirit of community responsibility and cooperation in preventing accidents and promoting the welfare of the group
4 To encourage self-enforcement of rules and regulations and to stimulate enthusiasm for encouraging others to obey safety laws voluntarily

5 To develop interest in promoting and supporting local, state, and national legislation concerned with safety and accident prevention

6 To develop an interest in safety education throughout the adult's life

COORDINATING LOCAL SAFETY EFFORTS

The *school, home,* and *community* share responsibility for safety education, and the success of the school program requires the cooperation of outside agencies. For example, if the home provided children with early training in safety, accidents to preschool children would be reduced and fewer children would enter school with careless habits already established. Parents can teach children not only to develop behavior patterns that contribute to their own safety, but to consider the rights of others, to wait their turn, and to observe the courtesies that contribute to the general welfare. Children should be given ample opportunity at home and at school to learn how to do things on their own. If they make mistakes, these can be easily corrected. Many of the great tragedies of life occur because an individual has not developed judgment and cannot master social situations.

Once enrolled in school, children learn best when they can relate the safety instruction they receive to actual situations in the home and community. They should be given opportunities to do fieldwork in safety—to investigate real accidents and hazardous conditions and report their findings before the entire class, so that causes and possible preventive measures can be discussed. The cooperation of parents and various outside agencies is obviously necessary. Home safety, for example, can be illustrated by having a small committee of students, with the cooperation of the parent-teacher association, prepare two homes for a safety-inspection check—one to represent a variety of possible hazards and the other to illustrate the safest living conditions possible. The class can then inspect each home. The final report should provide sufficient problem material of a meaningful type to cover a number of class meetings. The many hazards found in the "fixed" home should provide excellent subject matter. Students, rather than being lectured on these hazards, should be encouraged to discuss what they would do about them.

Whether or not instruction can be supplemented by actual experience, safety measures should always be taught in the school with a view to their wider application in the community. First-aid methods can be explained in terms of home accidents. Participation in the school's physical education and athletic medical insurance plan can lead to better understanding of the need for prompt diagnosis and treatment of all injuries, and for financial protection in case of accident or illness. The school is rich in laboratory resources for teaching safety. Safety education is most effective, however, when the entire community participates in accident-prevention efforts.

A communitywide safety program offers an opportunity to demonstrate democracy in action. Students learn how to work and play together harmoniously, to develop a genuine concern for one another's safety, and to refrain voluntarily from actions that might injure others. A community safety program in which teachers and parents set and follow a pattern of friendly cooperation makes a more lasting contribution to the student's understanding of democracy than anything he or she might read on the subject.

SAFETY IN HIGHER EDUCATION. In recent years greater attention has been given to teaching safety at the college and university level. The traditional functions of education have been expanded and several hundred institutions have developed teacher education programs in safety education. These programs will continue to grow and expand as our schools give greater emphasis to accident prevention.

Our institutions of higher education have recently been offering safety courses to individuals who are not majoring in education. The meaningful nature of such courses has made them extremely popular. Safety information and attitude development have widespread applications to daily living.

In 1974, the American Academy of Safety Education was created to recognize individuals who have made outstanding contributions to safety education. This prestigious organization meets annually for its National Safety Congress. It provides an opportunity for exchange of ideas among academy members working toward the solution of problems related to safety.

The College and University Safety Educators Association was also founded in 1974. It is part of the School and College Division of the Higher Education Section of the National Safety Council. Members are drawn from athletics, physical education, recreation, driver and traffic safety education, elementary and school safety education, and other professional organizations concerned with safety in higher education. The organization sponsors an annual convention for safety educators and publishes a monograph of the conference proceedings.

SAFETY CENTER. Although the first Center for Safety Education was established in 1938 at New York University, only in recent years has this movement been expanded. The best way to describe these centers is the description adopted by the Safety Center Division of the Higher Education Section of the National Safety Council:[3]

> A safety center is an organization formed by a college or university dedicated to accident prevention and related fields. It functions as a focal point for the institution's resources, providing a liaison unit that serves college and university personnel, state or local officials, business, industrial and professional interests and the public at large. It makes use of a staff of professional safety specialists and the services of other disciplines and units on or off the campus to provide leadership for and assistance in coordinating and improving accident prevention efforts. Activities related to a safety center may include safety courses, conferences, research projects, production of materials and publications, and public information on safety matters, and make available consultation services on accident prevention problems.

[3]"Definitions of a Safety Center," in *Transactions, School and College Conference,* National Safety Council, Chicago, 1960.

CAMPUS SAFETY ASSOCIATION. After World War II, the sudden increase of enrollment in colleges and universities brought increases in accidents among students, faculty, and staff. Some institutions developed committees for accident prevention and fire control. As increased enrollment continued to bring more construction, activity, and congestion, many institutions began employing full-time safety coordinators. In 1949 a group of coordinators and other members of university staffs dealing with housing, intramural activities, and traffic met at the University of Illinois and formed the Campus Safety Association. Later it became a division of the Higher Education Section of the National Safety Council. Today it has a membership of more than one thousand. The safety coordinators' functions have been developed by their own association. They deal with the following:[4]

1 A basic safety policy
2 Safety leadership
3 Safety organization
4 Maintenance of a safe environment
5 Fire prevention and protection
6 Reporting and follow-up of accidents
7 Training
8 Promotion of interest
9 Education for safe living
10 Off-campus activities
11 Implementing O.S.H.A. standards as they pertain to the campus environment

LEARNING EXPERIENCES

The following activities are designed to supplement the study of this chapter:

1 Prepare a detailed charter for a school safety council.
2 Conduct a detailed needs assessment to be used in planning safety education for grades K through 12. On the basis of these findings, develop specific long-range goals and instructional objectives for the program.
3 Discuss the procedures necessary for implementing a comprehensive safety program. Prepare a time line to facilitate progress.
4 Obtain from your state department of education a copy of:
a. the school code—and examine it for mandates related to safety and health
b. the state syllabus or curriculum guide for safety education—and critique the document according to the findings of the needs assessment previously completed.
5 Interview a variety of community residents (bankers, insurance brokers,

[4]*National Conference on Campus Safety Report,* National Safety Council, Chicago.

police and fire officials, school board members, etc.), and determine their feelings about the role of safety education in the public schools.

6 Role-play a group of concerned citizens who are speaking before the board of education in support of the development of a safety education program. The board should ask critical questions of the group, which should.have satisfactory answers prepared.

7 Prepare a unit plan for a specific content area. Teach the unit to a class of elementary or secondary-level students. Develop and administer an objective test for measuring student knowledge. Develop and administer a teacher-evaluation form.

8 Write to the many agencies concerned with safety and request that free materials be sent to you. Begin a file of such materials and evaluate their quality.

9 Ask the campus safety coordinator to discuss efforts to make your campus a safer place to live.

10 Conduct a safety-needs assessment on campus by interviewing the safety coordinator, the director of housing, the security police, the director of health services, and others in a position to provide valuable information about campus accidents.

11 Plan, implement, and evaluate a safety training seminar for all dormitory counselors.

SELECTED REFERENCES

Beauchamp, George A.: *Curriculum Theory,* 2d ed., The Kaag Press, Wilmette, Ill., 1968.

Gronlund, Norman E.: *Stating Behavioral Objectives for Classroom Instruction,* The Macmillan Company, London, 1970.

Haas, Glen: *Curriculum Planning: A New Approach,* 2d ed., Allyn & Bacon, Inc., Boston, 1977.

Mager, Robert F.: *Preparing Instructional Objectives,* Fearon Publishers, Belmont, Cal., 1962.

Manning, Duanne, *Toward a Humanistic Curriculum,* Harper & Row, Publishers, Incorporated, New York, 1971.

Morley, Franklin P.: *A Modern Guide to Effective K-12 Curriculum Planning,* Parker Publishing Company, Inc., West Nyack, N.Y., 1973.

National Conference on Safety Education, *Policies and Guidelines for a School Safety Program,* American Driver and Traffic Safety Education Association, Washington, 1974.

Oberteuffer, Delbert, Orvis A. Harrelson, and Marion B. Pollock: *School Health Education,* Harper & Row, Publishers, Incorporated, New York, 1972.

Payne, David A.: *Curriculum Evaluation,* D.C. Heath & Company, Lexington, Mass., 1974.

Popham, W. James, and Eva I. Bailer: *Establishing Instructional Goals,* Prentice Hall, Inc., Englewood Cliffs, N.J., 1970.

Tyler, Louise L.: *A Selected Guide to Curriculum Literature: An Annotated Bibliography,* National Education Association, Washington, 1970.

4

The School Safety Program

OVERALL OBJECTIVE:

The student should understand the complex nature of the school safety program. As a teacher, parent, or concerned citizen, the student should support its existence as an integral part of the total school curriculum.

INSTRUCTIONAL OBJECTIVES:

After completing this chapter the student will be able to:

1 Discuss the interrelated nature of the components of the school safety program.
2 List the administrative concerns of the school safety program.
3 Describe how a safe-school inspection form can be used to develop appropriate administrative policy.
4 List school-sponsored services which encourage safe behavior among students.
5 Discuss the specific responsibilites of teachers for the provision of safety services.
6 Describe the functions of school safety patrols.
7 Compare basic patterns of instruction by analyzing the organization, advantages, and disadvantages of each pattern.
8 List and compare the advantages of a variety of instructional techniques commonly used in safety education.
9 Describe the various types of audiovisual materials that are effective in teaching safety.

The term *school safety program* is used to describe all school activities which promote the safety of school-age youth. The overall purpose of the

75

program is to favorably influence knowledge, attitudes, and behavior for the benefit of the individual and the community. Safety education, therefore, is more than just an instructional program of formalized classroom learning. It involves a safe school environment, safety and protective services provided by the school, and administrative guidelines which promote all phases of the school safety program. A school which offers safety instruction in a safe and healthful environment is contributing to the attainment of the goals and objectives of this chapter. Similarly, a school with excellent safety services offers these services largely as a result of sound, written administrative policy.

Fire drills illustrate the interrelation of these components of the school safety program. Administrative policy is necessary to ensure that fire drills will be held frequently enough to be effective. Specific provisions for conducting the drill also depend on the quality of written policy statements. Fire drills are a service that the school provides to ensure safe behavior in the event of an actual emergency. Teachers serve as role models of appropriate attitudes and behavior. The drill provides students with an opportunity to assume responsible attitudes toward the protection of themselves and others. Students learn that it is prudent to plan for emergencies. The safety of the environment is tested by a drill. The effectiveness of the warning system and the planned evacuation procedures are evaluated before an actual emergency, so that changes can be implemented to prevent a future malfunction. Formal classroom instruction on fire drills, planning for emergencies, responsible and courteous behavior, etc., provides factual information for future reference. Knowing why fire drills occur makes the experience more relevant and meaningful to the students. The learning experience may carry over throughout adult life.

The interrelated nature of the various school safety components is illustrated in Figure 4–1.

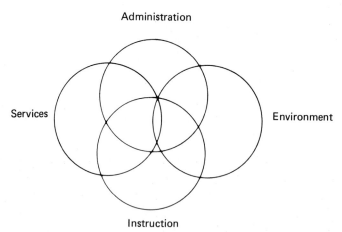

Figure 4-1 Comprehensive school safety program.

ADMINISTRATIVE CONCERNS

Every educational program requires strong administrative support and encouragement. Established administrative policy enables the school safety program to function so that each part supports the efforts of the other components. This coordination fosters the attainment of the important goals of the school safety program. Some of the administrative concerns and responsibilities are to:

1 Formulate safety policy and procedures

2 Arrange for emergency health care, including parental approval for transportation to a hospital (see Figure 4–2)

3 Provide for the needs of exceptional children

4 Maintain a variety of records, especially health-related information about students

5 Systematize accident reporting (see Figure 4–3)

6 Investigate and analyze accident occurrence so that future accidents may be prevented

7 Acquire adequate funding to support the program

8 Arrange for safe student transportation, and student mobility within the school building and grounds

9 Maintain an appropriate level of discipline and morale

10 Provide for supervision of all activities, especially when large numbers of people congregate

11 Maintain an adequate level of security to protect students, teachers, staff, buildings, and equipment

12 Develop policies for use of the school after hours by nonschool groups

13 Provide student accident and teacher liability insurance

Parent's or Guardian's Authorization for Emergency Medical Aid

Name of Child _____ School _____

In the event of illness or accident to a child or children of mine attending school, which in the judgment of the principal of the school, would seem to demand medical attention, I hereby authorize the said principal to summon medical help at my expense if I cannot be promptly reached by phone. I further authorize the principal to cause the child's transportation to a place where appropriate medical aid can be rendered, if in the principal's judgment such transportation is necessary. I would prefer that the principal call:

Dr. _____ Phone _____, or

Dr. _____ Phone _____, if

available, but otherwise he shall use his own judgment as to the doctor to be called.

In my absence the following persons are authorized to act for me in the above respect in behalf of my child:

Name _____ Phone _____ Address _____

Name _____ Phone _____ Address _____

Signed _____ Date _____

Home Address _____ Home Phone _____

Father's Business Address _____ Phone _____

Mother's Business Address _____ Phone _____

Figure 4-2 Emergency medical aid authorization form.

(check one)		RECOMMENDED		(check one)

<table>
<tr><td colspan="2">(check one)
☐ School Jurisdictional
☐ Non-School Jurisdictional</td><td colspan="2" align="center">RECOMMENDED
STANDARD STUDENT ACCIDENT REPORT
(See instructions on reverse side)</td><td>(check one)
Recordable ☐
Reportable Only ☐</td></tr>
</table>

School District:

City, State:

General

1. Name		2. Address		
3. School	4. Sex Male ☐ Female ☐	5. Age	6. Grade/Special Program	
7. Time Accident Occurred Date: Day of Week: Exact Time:				AM ☐ PM ☐

Injury

8. Nature of Injury

9. Part of Body Injured

10. Degree of Injury (check one)
    Death ☐   Permanent ☐   Temporary (lost time) ☐   Non-Disabling (no lost time) ☐

11. Days Lost
        From School: From Activities Other Than School: Total:

12. Cause of Injury

Accident

13. Accident Jurisdiction (check one)
    School: Grounds ☐   Building ☐   To and From ☐   Other Activities Not on School Property ☐
    Non-School: Home ☐   Other ☐

14. Location of Accident (be specific)	15. Activity of Person (be specific)

16. Status of Activity	17. Supervision (if yes, give title & name of supervisor)
	   Yes ☐
	   No ☐

18. Agency Involved	19. Unsafe Act
20. Unsafe Mechanical/Physical Condition	21. Unsafe Personal Factor

22. Corrective Action Taken or Recommended

23. Property Damage
    School $ Non-School $ Total $

24. Description (Give a word picture of the accident, explaining who, what, when, why and how)

Signature

25. Date of Report	26. Report Prepared by (signature & title)
27. Principal's Signature	

This form is recommended for securing data for accident prevention and safety education. School districts may reproduce this form adding space for optional data. Reference: *Student Accident Reporting Guidebook*, National Safety Council, 425 N. Michigan Avenue, Chicago, Illinois 60611. 1966. 34 pages.

(over)

Figure 4-3 Recommended standard student accident report.

14 Be familiar with state laws, local ordinances, and sections of the school code pertaining to safety and health

15 Receive parental approval for nonroutine school activities

16 Require appropriate professional preparation for teachers of safety education

INSTRUCTIONS
Please read carefully — Fill out form completely

Use the form on the reverse side to report each school and each non-school jurisdictional accident. In the upper left corner, check appropriate box:

School Jurisdictional. Any accident which results in any injury to a pupil and/or property damage which occurs in a school building, on school grounds, on the way to or from school, or in connection with any other school-sponsored activity even though not on school property.

Non-School Jurisdictional. An accident which causes restriction of activity to the pupil, occurring anywhere not definitely specified above.

In the upper right corner, check appropriate box:

Recordable. If the accident results in

a. Pupil injuries severe enough to cause the loss of one-half day or more of school time, or

b. Pupil injuries severe enough to cause the loss of one-half day or more of pupil activity during non-school time, or

c. Any property damage as a result of a school jurisdictional accident.

Reportable Only. If the accident does *not* cause a *lost time* injury or property damage.

NOTE: Only those forms checked **Recordable** are to be included in the *Annual Student Accident Summary* forms which are submitted to the National Safety Council.

1. **Name.** Name of injured student.

2. **Address.** Home address.

3. **School.** School attended.

4. **Sex.** Check box.

5. **Age.** Age of student at last birthday.

6. **Grade/Special Program.** Grade level such as K—for kindergarten, 1—for first grade, 2—for second grade, etc.; Special Education, Adult Education, Junior College, etc. If a special program, such as Head Start, Student Work Program, Adult Re-Training or Pre-Primary, so indicate.

7. **Time Accident Occurred.** Indicate the time the accident occurred as follows: Date (month, day of the month, and year); day of the week; the exact time and check AM or PM.

8. **Nature of Injury.** Indicate, *to the best of your knowledge,* what the injury was, such as burn, fracture, abrasion, etc. If multiple injuries, so indicate and list each.

9. **Part of Body Injured.** Indicate part of body injured, such as lower left arm, right ankle, scalp, etc. If more than one part of body is injured, indicate as "multiple" and list each part.

10. **Degree of Injury.** Check one box. If the degree of injury is not immediately known, estimate or use a follow-up system. Reports should not be held up for lack of this information.

Death. If fatal.

Permanent. If injury results in a complete loss of, or loss of use of, a body part or parts, such as the loss of an eye, the loss of use of a limb, amputation of a part of the body, etc.

Temporary (lost time). If the injury does not cause permanent disability, but causes the child to lose one-half day or more of school, or one-half day or more of normal activity, during a non-school period.

Non-Disabling (no lost time). If the injury did not cause permanent disability and/or lost time, or loss of activity.

11. **Days Lost.** Indicate from one-half or more, the number of days that the student was absent from school; and/or the number of days from one-half day or more, the student was restricted from normal activities if during a non-school period. One-half day's lost time in school is defined as one-half of the normal school day for that particular student. The time charge for death is 1,200 days. See *Guidebook,* page 24, for permanent disability charges. If lost time is not immediately known, estimate or use a follow-up system. Reports should not be held up for lack of this information.

12. **Cause of Injury.** Identify the event which resulted in the injury, such as "struck against moving object," "fall from elevation," "rubbed or abraided," "over-exertion," etc.

13. **Accident Jurisdiction.** Check one box to indicate where the accident occurred.

14. **Location of Accident.** Indicate exact location of the accident. Example: Second floor corridor near room 210, girls' gymnasium, sidewalk at northeast corner of 12th and Locust, inside stairway at home, etc.

15. **Activity of Person.** Indicate what person was doing at time of the accident. Example: Conducting a science experiment, playing second base in soft ball, riding as a passenger in parents' car, driving a bicycle, etc.

16. **Status of Activity.** Indicate status of activity at time of the accident. Example: Regular classroom period, physical education class, intramural athletic practice, interscholastic athletics, recess, lunch period, supervised before or after school activities, at a friend's home, in the kitchen, at a supermarket, etc.

17. **Supervision.** Check box to indicate whether an adult was present at the scene of the accident; if "yes," indicate by name and title whether this adult was the teacher, another school employee, the parent, another adult, etc.

18. **Agency Involved.** Indicate the equipment, substance, material, or the thing most closely related to the accident. Example: Glass test tube, motorcycle, ground surface, other person, dog, etc.

19. **Unsafe Act.** Indicate any act on the part of the person or persons involved which may have caused or contributed to the accident. Example: Using equipment unsafely, feet in aisle, body contact in sports or other action in excess of intent of rule, not following established rules, etc.

20. **Unsafe Mechanical/Physical Condition.** Indicate any unsafe mechanical or physical conditions such as deep ruts in play area, ice on sidewalk, improperly guarded machine, improperly stored material, poor lighting, porch railing in need of repair, etc.

21. **Unsafe Personal Factor.** Indicate any unsafe personal factors that may have contributed to the accident. Example: Bodily defects such as defective hearing; lack of knowledge, skill or experience, such as failure to recognize hazards; emotional upsets such as death in the family, new sibling, parental separation or school failure.

22. **Corrective Action Taken or Recommended.** Indicate what action was taken locally and/or what further action is recommended, if needed action cannot be taken by local school personnel. Example: Maintenance action such as play area holes were filled and leveled; procedural action such as a study is being made to improve the flow of students into the auditorium; engineering recommendation such as the ventilating system should be studied to determine if sufficient for the area involved; curriculum recommendation such as the present course of study for woodworking shop should be reviewed to insure that safe procedures are included; counseling action such as referred child to guidance department.

23. **Property Damage.** Estimate in dollars the amount of damage, if any, to school property and/or other property as the result of the accident. Do not hold up report for this information. If there was no property damage write "none."

24. **Description.** Give a *word* picture of the accident, explaining who, what, where, when, why and how of the accident. Include such items as weather, equipment, unsafe conditions, unsafe acts, personal factors, and whether other persons may have contributed to the accident, and how.

25. **Date of Report.** Date report was completed.

26. **Report Prepared by.** Signature and title of person preparing report.

27. **Principal's Signature.**

(National Safety Council—Form School 1)
Rev. 100M86701

Printed in U.S.A.
(over)

Stock No. 429.21

Figure 4-3 *(continued)*

17 Provide for in-service education of teachers, custodians, cafeteria workers, bus drivers, nurses, and secretaries

18 Keep personnel informed of school dangers, student accident records, and individual student health needs

19 Insist on standards of safe behavior among faculty and staff to serve as a model for students

20 Coordinate efforts of school personnel and the community
21 Develop a safe-school inspection form.

SAFETY INSPECTION FORM

The specific details obtained from these forms can help guide and improve a school's entire safety program. Such data can provide the school superintendent with information upon which to base:[1]

1 Curriculum guidance to educate the child for safe living.
2 A realistic evaluation of safety program efforts on a regular basis.
3 Changes in building structures and facilities, or procedures, to improve the environment of the school system.
4 Organizational and administrative improvements to strengthen the management aspects of the safety program.
5 A strong public relations program, thus lessening public demands for crash programs of little value if an unusual incident occurs.
6 A strong leadership role in community safety efforts.
7 An assessment of the costs of accidents and injuries and their relationship to operating expenses of the school system.

The principal may use the reports to:

1 Check on what is happening in his school.
2 Spot an unsafe condition or hazardous procedure which can be corrected locally by the custodian or by the principal himself; or, the report can provide the basis for a work order for repair and maintenance of facilities.
3 Initiate special safety studies with the school.
4 Strengthen staff interest in accident prevention activities by having members of the staff, such as the faculty safety coordinator, nurse, or custodian, review the report and make recommendations.
5 Establish a repeater file, or to note the accident in the pupil's personnel folder for reference throughout the child's school years.

The school system safety supervisor may use the reports to:

1 Spot unsafe conditions or deficiencies not recognized at the school level, and which can be corrected at his level.
2 Initiate special studies when unusual accidents appear, such as when skate boards came into use.
3 Watch for trends in normal activities so that immediate analytic and preventive action can be taken in cases of rising trends.
4 Initiate procedural studies and changes.
5 Emphasize a particular subject area in regular or special bulletins.
6 Alert supervisors in other departments, such as physical education, elementary, industrial arts, science, and medical departments, to incidents relative to their specialty, and to ask for their recommendations or suggestions.
7 Spot weaknesses inthe reporting procedures, which can be corrected or minimized.

[1]*Student Accident Reporting Guidebook,* National Safety Council, Chicago, 1966, pp. 1–2.

8 Screen out unusual occurrences which will provide a little levity or change of pace for bulletin material.

9 Keep the superintendent fully informed of serious or unusual incidents in case of question by the board or other local officials.

10 Keep the business or law office informed of reports which may have legal implications.

11 Establish a repeater file at the school system level for purposes of special studies.

These functions can be fulfilled only if all faculty members cooperate in filling out and recording reports, in collecting and tabulating data from the entire school system, and in formulating specific plans for using this material. When these tasks have been accomplished, the various school departments will have sufficient information on which to base their particular attack on the accident problem. The teacher responsible for physical education and the intramural athletic program, the director of vocational education, the head of the home economics department, the supervisor of playgrounds, the teachers in charge of science laboratories, and the physical-plant personnel can then analyze the accidents that have occurred within their areas of supervision, and work out means of preventing similar accidents.

To establish uniformity in accident reporting it is desirable to have an understanding of terms and definitions. The terms suggested in the National Safety Council's *Student Accident Reporting Guidebook* are recommended. They are as follows:

1 A reportable accident.
   a Any school-jurisdictional* accident which results in any injury to a pupil and/or property damage:†
   b Any nonschool-jurisdictional‡ accident which results in injury causing restriction of activity§ to the pupil.
2 A recordable accident. Is any accident which results in:
   a Pupil injury severe enough to cause the loss of one half day¶ or more of school time;
   b Pupil injury severe enough to cause the loss of one half day or more of pupil activity during nonschool time;
   c Any property damage as a result of a school-jurisdictional accident.

*School jurisdiction includes school building, grounds, route to and from school, and school-sponsored activities away from school property.
†The concept of property damage includes damage to the school's own equipment, material, or structures; or damage to nonschool property as a result of a school jurisdictional accident.
‡Nonschool jurisdiction includes all other areas and activities not under the jurisdiction or sponsorship of the school, such as home, public buildings, and the like.
§Restriction of activity infers a loss of one half day or more of school time, or loss of one half day or more of normal activity if during a nonschool period.
¶For standardization, one half day loss of school time is defined as one half day of the normal school day for the particular student involved.

The reports should be tabulated and summarized every month if possible, but compilation every semester or year should be a minimum. In most situations hand tabulation is adequate, but in large school systems machine tabulation and data processing can be used. The summaries should be made available to everyone in the school system so that all may evaluate their particular phases of the safety program. At the conclusion of the spring term, the accident record for the entire academic year should be reviewed and used as a basis for planning future efforts.

Although accident data are gathered primarily for local use, a school may sometimes wish to compare its figures with those of other schools. The National Safety Council facilitates comparison by tabulating all monthly accident reports received from schools and making the statistics available in its annual publication, *Accident Facts*. Standard accident-reporting sheets and summary forms can be obtained from the council. Schools wishing to participate in this program should write for detailed information to the School and College Division of the council.

EMERGENCY POLICY

Every school administrator should develop a systematic procedure for handling any accident or emergency illness that occurs while children are under the school's jurisdiction. Although no one policy or set of rules can fit all situations, whatever plan is devised should include clear and definite answers to the following questions:

1 What immediate action should be taken when a student is injured in an accident?
2 Who should be permitted to administer first aid?
3 When should the parents or family physician be notified?
4 Who should assume responsibility when parents cannot be reached?
5 What are the provisions for transporting the injured student home or to a hospital?

When the administrator has settled these issues, he or she must make sure that the entire staff understands the regulations that have been formulated for them. The accident policy should be explained at the beginning of every school term so that if an accident should occur, even new personnel will know what procedures to follow. The school accident policy should be printed on the inside back cover of the student roll book. In this manner it will be available for the teacher to follow in case of of an accident. This procedure is of significant value to the new teacher in a school system.

SAFETY SERVICES

Safety services and the protection of students, faculty, staff, and visitors represent another aspect of the school safety program. Some of the activities, such as teacher observation of student behavior, are informal and require little or no written administrative policy. Other activities, such as fire drills, emergency care, and safety patrols, require substantial planning and specific policy statements. The primary purposes of this school-safety component are the detection, prevention, and correction of circumstances which represent a potential danger to human well-being. Safety services include:

1 Planned emergency drills
2 Provisions for exceptional children, notably the handicapped
3 Maintenance of health and accident records
4 Availability of student counseling
5 Cooperative efforts among staff and faculty
6 Health screening of students, faculty, and staff
7 Referral of health and safety needs to parents and appropriate community agencies
8 Special safety events and assemblies
9 School safety-patrol organizations
10 Crossing guards
11 Utilization of safety inspection forms
12 Accident-reporting systems
13 In-service education of faculty and staff
14 Provision of accident and liability insurance
15 Enforced safety standards for cafeteria, pool, shop, gymnasium, locker rooms, play areas, home-economics suites, laboratories, stairs, etc.
16 Replacement of broken or defective equipment
17 Employment of qualified personnel who minimize danger because of professional knowledge and capability.

Teachers are especially important to the safety effort. Among their other duties, teachers should:

1 Set a good example
2 Provide a safe environment
3 Provide opportunities for safe behavior
4 Insist on the proper use of protective equipment and provide guidance in the safe use of all equipment
5 Help develop a positive self-image in their students
6 Provide adequate supervision and leadership
7 Identify and report accident hazards
8 Report cases of possible child abuse
9 Fulfill the legal duties and policy expectations of their jobs
10 Ask the nurse to help them understand the health and safety files of their students, and seek advice about how to deal with potential problems
11 Carry out emergency drills with an appropriate attitude toward safety
12 Stay knowledgeable about safety and accident prevention
13 Know first aid and teach it to their students
14 Evaluate the safety curriculum and the effectiveness of school safety services on a continuing basis
15 Interpret the school safety program to the community

A SAFE SCHOOL ENVIRONMENT

Safe living is dependent upon our physical environment and the social environment in which we live. A safety program must establish and maintain an environment that is free of hazards. The concerns central to establishing a safe environment are the physical, social, and emotional situations which are potentially dangerous to students and staff.

Too often those concerned with safety education for young people become so involved in classroom safety instruction that they ignore or fail to emphasize the total school environment. They should teach students not only how to make wise choices with regard to safe behavior, but how to create an environment which encourages safe behavior. The school is a laboratory for learning and living. Efforts to create a safe school environment have considerable educational value and can effectively supplement classroom instruction. Although accident fatalities at school are relatively low, the proportion of the total accidents to young people which occur in school is surprisingly high. It is obvious that educators cannot ignore the safety of the students' environment.

THE SCHOOL BUILDING

The school building and surrounding grounds are two important areas to consider in effecting a safe school environment. The School Plant Planning Commission of the National Safety Council has developed a statement of principles, endorsed by the National Council of School House Construction and the Association of School Business Officials, defining our responsibility for environmental safety. New building codes usually provide for a high degree of safety, but modification of older structures is a major problem facing many boards of education. High costs sometimes affect the construction of school buildings, but a safe environment must be provided.

> Safety is one of the prime requisites of any school building. No one will disagree with the statement that a school building should be a safe place for children. In the controversy that arises in many communities over construction costs, little thought is given to the possibility that lives of children may be endangered through the false economy of cheap construction or the continued use of old and obsolete buildings.[2]

A safe school environment requires that accident records be consulted for evidence of particualr danger spots. Both the building and the surrounding grounds must be thoroughly examined for possible hazards. Special attention should be given to the condition of corridors and stairways; they should be free of obstacles and sharp projections, and firm handrails should be located on both sides of all stairways. Although the stairways in most new school buildings have been constructed with rough surfaces, old stairways have often been worn smooth and slippery, and may have to be equipped with safety treads. Floor

---

[2]William H. Roe, School Business Management, McGraw-Hill Book Company, New York, 1961, p. 192.

surfaces should be tested to see that they provide a sure footing; nonslip waxes and preservatives should be used to keep them in good condition. Exit doors should be well lighted, designed to open outward, and furnished with panic bolts. Exits to the auditorium and to other areas where large groups assemble should be inspected before a program or meeting is held.

School-building patrols, although they are not concerned exclusively with accident prevention, can be used effectively in the safety program. In most schools the patrol serves primarily to monitor the building while classes are in session and while students are in transit. In addition to guiding students and visitors, patrol members are usually authorized by the principal to control conduct in the halls and on the stairway. The prankster who wants to tamper with fire-fighting equipment, the boys and girls who would like to race each other down the stairs, and the child who might slide down the banister if no one was looking—children like these can be prevented from pursuing such dangerous activities by an alert building patrol.

Patrol members may be selected by popular vote or by the principal, the faculty adviser, or the student-government organization; girls as well as boys should be considered as candidates. One patrol member is usually chosen from every thirty-five to forty-five pupils in an elementary school, and from every twenty-five to thirty students in a junior or senior high school. It may be desirable to provide members with some type of insignia—such as badges, arm bands, belts, or distinctive caps—so that other students may identify them easily. A school-building patrol requires some adult guidance and supervision, but members derive the greatest educational benefit from their position if they are allowed as much self-direction as possible.

THE PLAYGROUND

The school grounds require constant attention if they are to be kept clear of hazards. Besides supervising play areas and furnishing adequate instruction in all activities, school personnel should inspect the playground thoroughly every day to see that it is free of holes, sharp objects, and rubbish, and that all equipment is in good operating condition. The area should be as level as possible, well drained, and large enough to accommodate all students who are likely to use it at one time. If it is located near a busy street, it should be enclosed by a fence. Permanent play equipment should be set up around the sides of the area rather than in the center, so that the swings, slides, seesaws, etc., will not interfere with one another, and adequate space will be left for other activities. Such equipment should be held to a minimum, for the children using it must be supervised constantly if accidents are to be avoided. Whatever equipment is provided should be kept in excellent repair. It should never be used if there is any question about whether it can be operated safely.

Student playground patrols, which are useful in elementary schools, can assist teachers in supervising students during recess and lunch periods. Each member, after being assigned a definite section of the play area to observe, should stop dangerous behavior, report any damaged or broken equipment to the responsible person, and help custodians keep the grounds clear of debris. The principal or faculty adviser who supervises the patrol usually appoints one member for every thirty-five to fifty students.

STUDENT BEHAVIOR

No school environment can be considered safe unless students are willing to cooperate in preventing accidents. If a school's safety-instruction program is effective, however, students should develop the proper attitudes; they should be safety-conscious, and concerned not only about their own welfare but about the welfare of others. They must also be taught:

1 To walk safely through halls, on stairways, and around chairs, desks, and other objects

2 To carry chairs, working materials, and other equipment safely in the classroom, in halls, and on stairs

3 To handle scissors, knives, glass objects, and tools properly

4 To avoid pushing, crowding, and running in the building

5 To refrain from interfering with anyone who is using the drinking fountain

6 To avoid using the toilet rooms as play areas

7 To observe clean and orderly habits

8 To observe safety procedures, rules, and regulations in play areas and in going to and from play areas

9 To play only in areas designated for their age group

10 To help keep play areas clean and safe by removing glass, sticks, stones, and rubbish

11 To develop a safety sportsmanship code applicable to the play areas

12 To participate in organizing playground and school-building patrols and to obey such patrols

13 To recognize hazards in and around the school, such as broken and cracked windows, rough surfaces, and loose and worn electrical equipment

14 To observe the proper procedure if an accident should occur

The solution to the problem of accidents in the school environment lies largely within the scope of the adminstration and other school staff members. Keeping the school hazard-free, sanitary, properly equipped, well ventilated, well lighted, and adequately supervised can do much to prevent accidents. It can also help students develop safe habits that will carry over into their homes, neighborhoods, and places of employment.

FIRE EXIT DRILLS

Although fire prevention is discussed in Chapter 13, fire-exit drills are such an important part of the school safety program that they deserve special mention here. As a result of the recent large and rapid increase in enrollments, many schools have become overcrowded, and old buildings that are not fireproof are still in use. Under these circumstances, the need for the exit drills cannot be questioned.

It has been estimated that over 9,300 fires occur annually in our schools and colleges. Despite these alarming figures, some school officials, believing that their own buildings are not susceptible to fire, menace the lives of their students by failing to conduct drills in accordance with well-established practices. Since it does not seem possible to eliminate all school fires, administrators must make sure that everyone knows how to leave the building as quickly as possible in case of fire. Adequate exits, unobstructed doors equipped with panic bolts, and efficient drills are the best insurance against fire casualties.

GENERAL CONSIDERATIONS. School administrators must make sure that fire-exit drills are well planned, efficiently taught and supervised, and conducted so frequently that everyone will react without doubt or hesitation when he or she hears the fire alarm. Each principal, assisted by teachers, custodians, and student leaders, must develop an evacuation plan suited to the particular building. The local fire chief, who is usually well acquainted with the latest safety measures, can often help officials formulate drill procedures. Police officers may also be able to offer suggestions. Those planning the drill must consider the number and the age of the persons to be evacuated, and must make special provisions for the disabled and physically handicapped. Once the procedure has been established it should be explained to everyone, preferably with the aid of diagrams, charts, and blueprints, and thereafter modified as little as possible.

In organizing the drill, every school administrator must personally decide whether or not students should be allowed to serve as monitors. In some schools, members of the building patrol or of a special fire-drill patrol are assigned certain functions during a drill. Many principals hesitate to follow this practice since these students have greater responsibility and face far more potential danger than do members of other patrols.

There is no doubt, of course, that fire-drill patrols can help supervise the evacuation of the building by keeping students alert and helping them follow directions. If student monitors are to be used, they should be selected by the principal and the faculty. The patrol should include members of both sexes. Usually one patrol member is adequate for each classroom of students.

Fire-exit-drill regulations should be taught at the beginning of every school term for the benefit of new students and staff members. If drills are conducted frequently in the fall, everyone should be so well acquainted with the procedure by winter that fewer drills will be necessary at that time. Some drills should be held during cold weather since fires are more likely to occur then. The short time in which children are outside for a fire drill will not ordinarily endanger their health, and winter drills can be conducted as students are entering or leaving the building and are dressed for the outdoors.

Regular drills tend to remove the sense of panic that often develops at the sound of the fire alarm. They should be conducted as many times as necessary to teach students to leave the building as quickly as possible in a natural, unhurried manner. Ordinarily, this process should take no longer than 2 minutes; the school principal who always insists upon good order and discipline should have little difficulty in training students to carry out the drill properly in the minimum time recommended. Usually, fewer drills are required in high schools than in elementary schools.

All drills should be conducted on the assumption that an actual fire exists. They should be held at varying times of the day, and neither teachers nor students should be notified of a drill in advance. Sometimes the building should be evacuated through alternate exits that have been designated for use when the usual route is blocked by fire, smoke, or some other obstacle.

THE SAFEST ROUTE TO SCHOOL PROJECT. A program known as the *Safest Route to School Project* has recently been prepared by the Traffic Engineering and Safety Department of the American Automobile Association. The program is based on the belief that it is possible to reduce traffic hazards for children by careful selection of the walking routes to and from school. The program fosters cooperation between the home and school in helping children develop safe walking skills. Although the program is designed for school safety education, there is ample opportunity for transfer of learning to nonschool pedestrian travel situations.

In deciding the best walking route, consider the basic principles of the *Safest Route to School Project:*[3]

1 *Directness.* Sacrifices in directness are permissible only when such sacrifices enhance safety.

2 *Minimum use of roadway.* The number and length of street crossings must be examined.

3 *Complicated intersections.* Complicated intersections should be avoided unlesss police officers or crossing guards are present.

4 *Converging routes.* Make efficient use of adult-supervised routes so that children converge at one place before crossing a hazardous street.

5 *Police supervision.* Because of their complete authority to control traffic, police officers provide the best protection. This protection is only effective if police are *always* on duty when children are going to and from school.

6 *Adult crossing guards.* Having been trained by the police department, they are usually granted the authority to regulate the flow of traffic.

7 *School safety patrols.* The function of the patrol is to instruct, direct, and control children in crossing streets. Students should take advantage of safety-patrol protection.

8 *Traffic signals.* Although they afford an appreciable level of protection, traffic signals should not be regarded as a guarantee of safety.

[3]The American Automobile Association has published a *Teachers Guide for the Safest Route to School Project* and a film called "The Safest Way." Readers who have children are encouraged to write to the AAA for additional information about this project.

9 *School crossings.* Some areas, adjacent to school grounds, provide warnings of potential student pedestrian traffic by flashing yellow lights that are clearly visible to motorists.

10 *Vehicular volume at crosswalks.* Vehicular volume should be analyzed before selecting a walking route. Preference should be given to crosswalks which are crossed by: (a) the fewest number of vehicles turning right; (b) the fewest number of vehicles turning left; and (c) the fewest number of total vehicles.

11 *One-way streets.* Generally, one-way street intersections offer greater safety than intersections of two-way streets. However, vehicular volume must be analyzed before reaching a decision.

12 *Stop signs.* Although not as good as traffic signals, stop signs provide some protection by forcing vehicles to come to a complete stop even if only momentarily.

13 *Pedestrian accident experience.* Consider factors such as the number and types of pedestrian accidents that have occured at various intersections.

14 *Other factors.* Numerous other factors need to be considered for individual communities. Steep grades, sharp curves, the availability of sidewalks, etc., are matters for careful analysis.

SCHOOL SAFETY PATROLS

In the early 1920s, schools began to employ older students to protect younger children from the hazards of crossing streets en route to or from school. In 1930 the American Automobile Association, the National Congress of Parents and Teachers, and the National Safety Council established standard rules for the operation of school safety patrols. The original policies have been revised several times. Several other organizations have since become affiliated with the nationwide program: the National Education Association, the United States Office of Education, and the International Association of Chiefs of Police.

There is no doubt that school patrols have saved many students from injury and death during the last decade. They have become an indispensable national institution, offering protection to millions of youngsters on their way to and from school, in the school building, on the school bus, and on the playground. They fulfill an important educational function by training students to become good leaders and good followers. The value of learning through direct experience is nowhere better illustrated than in the operation of these groups.

The success of a school patrol will depend upon the combined efforts of the principal, who is responsible for organizing it, the faculty adviser, the students, their parents, and the outside agencies that are interested in this work. All too often the patrol is used only as a means of enforcing safe behavior, and its potential educational services are ignored. Some of these potentialities are the encouragement and development of (1) leadership, (2) a desire to serve, (3) respect for authority, (4) self discipline and self-control, (5) self-reliance and self-confidence, and (6) courtesy. If the full value of the patrol is to be realized, both its members and its adviser must be carefully selected, with full consideration given to those qualities that enable any group to operate smoothly and efficiently.

The teacher chosen as sponsor should be a good teacher, enthusiastic about his work or her work, and fully aware of the safety needs of the school and community. The teacher can acquire the needed specific technical information through in-serivce training and participation in the 1-day workshops conducted and sponsored by teacher education institutions or by local and state departments of education. By studying existing school-patrol programs and reading prepared materials on the subject, he or she can gain firsthand knowledge of the problems involved and develop skill in handling them. The various patrols, their specific functions, and the special considerations that apply to them are discussed individually in relation to their particular areas of school safety.

POLICIES AND PRACTICES FOR SCHOOL SAFETY PATROLS[5]

1 Functions

The functions of school safety patrols are to instruct, direct, and control the members of the student body in crossing the streets and highways at or near schools and to assist teachers and parents in the instruction of school children in safe pedestrian practices at all times and places.

Patrols should not be charged with the responsibility of directing vehicular traffic, nor should they be allowed to do so through the use of flags, hand signs or other signaling devices. They need not, therefore, be recognized by city ordinance or state law dealing with the control of vehicular traffic.

2 Establishment and support

The approval, understanding, support, and encouragement of all school authorities, administrators, and teachers, are essential to the effective functioning of the school safety patrol.

a Authorization—The governing board or other directing authority is the appropriate group to authorize the organization and operation of school safety patrols.*

b Administration—The school superintendent should assume the leadership in determining the overall school safety patrol policy.

The principal of each school should provide leadership in developing good relationship among teachers, student body, and members of patrols in matters of selecting, instructing, and giving immediate supervision to patrol members, and carrying out administrative details. Administrative responsibility for actual operation of the patrol may be delegated to an individual teacher or a committee.

c Community Support—Every community has civic and service organizations which will work cooperatively with schools upon invitation. The local automobile club, safety council, parent-teacher-association, and others may cooperate by offering assistance to school administrators for the successful operation of school safety patrols. Assistance may include the

*Because of varying state laws, each school administrator should review liability responsibilities in his own state relating to school safety patrol programs.

[5]American Automobile Association, *Policies and Practices for School Safety Patrols*, rev., Washington, 1972.

provision of equipment. Such community participation fosters the development of community understanding and support of the school safety patrol program.

3 Selection and appointment

The school safety patrol members should be selected from the upper grade levels—preferably not below the fifth grade. Qualities such as leadership and reliability should determine selection. Patrol service should be voluntary and open to all who qualify. Written approval of parent or guardian [see Figure 4-4] should be secured. After selection, patrol members may be formally appointed by the principal.

Removal or suspension from duty for any cause should immediately result in notification of the member's parent or guardian. An explanation should be made to the pupil and to the parent or guardian through a letter or personal interview.

4 Size of patrol and officers needed

The number of members of a school safety patrol should be determined by local factors, such as street and highway conditions, number of intersections, volume of vehicular traffic, school enrollment, and number of school dismissal times. Schools may wish to consult with police or other qualified individuals in determining the number of patrol members and the most strategic locations for them. Every patrol should have such officers (captain, lieutenant, sergeant) as are necessary for effective operation. It is desirable that officers and members serve for at least one school year. Members may be changed periodically to minimize the time required of one pupil and permit a maximum number of pupils an opportunity to serve.

5 Instructions and supervision

School safety patrols offer a way of extending traffic safety education beyond the classroom. Careful instruction and supervision of patrol members are essential if the patrol is to be efficient and continuous. The best results are obtained by delegating the continuous guidance to a teacher, supervisor, or other professional person within the school system who is interested in safety education. This person should work cooperatively with the police department and other civic and service organizations.

New patrol members, after initial instruction, should serve with and under the guidance of experienced members until qualified to assume their duties.

PARENT'S CERTIFICATE

Date _____ 19 _____

Understanding the aims and accomplishments of the School Safety Patrol as printed on the reverse side, I hereby give my consent for _____

_____

a student in _____ school to act as a Patrol Member during this school year.

Submitted by   Signed

_____   _____
Patrol Supervisor or Principal   Parent or Guardian

Figure 4-4 Patrol member's approval form. Front of card. (Source: Chicago Motor Club.)

6 Insignia

A standard insigne is desirable for school safety patrols and bus-patrol members. Such insigne should be readily identifiable, and worn in plain view at all times while patrol members are on duty. The standard insigne for patrols is the white or fluorescent orange Sam Browne belt of two-inch-wide material. Any auxiliary equipment (such as badge or arm band) used in patrol operation should be uniform throughout the community. Other patrols, such as hall, playground, etc., should not wear the Sam Browne belt, but may use another type of identification.

7 Adequate advance warning of school crossing

The white Sam Browne belt is usually adequate to attract the attention of drivers approaching school crossings under normal conditions. However, hilltops, curves, foliage, or other conditions may make it difficult for the driver to see the patrol member in time to ensure a safe stop or whatever other driving adjustments should be made.

Where conditions are such that the patrol member cannot be seen at least as far away as the safe stopping distance for the legal speed at that location, one of the following procedures is recommended:

a Select a safer location for the crossing at which the patrol is to serve.

b When it is not possible to select another crossing, the matter should be taken up with appropriate traffic authorities for a solution.

8 Positions and procedures

The patrol member should stand back of the curb—*not in the street*—and remind the children to wait behind him until he sees an adequate gap in traffic. When the gap occurs, he should step aside and motion for the children to cross the street in a group.

When the patrol member's view of traffic is obstructed, it may be necessary for the patrol member to step into the street. In this event, the patrol member should go no further than the outer edge of the obstruction (usually a parked vehicle). Children should remain on the sidewalk near the curb until motioned to cross. After the children have crossed, the patrol member should return to his station back of the curb.

School authorities should confer with traffic authorities in arranging for appropriate parking restrictions on streets adjacent to or near schools and school crossings. If possible, off-street parking areas should be provided to minimize congestion and safety hazards caused by parked cars.

A school crossing traversing a one-way street should be located, if possible, on the approach side where traffic enters the intersection. Most complications arise from turning cars, whether turning from a one-way street into a two-way street, or where two one-way streets intersect. Patrol members should be cautioned frequently to be alert for vehicle turning movements.

When vehicular traffic is such that adequate safe gaps do not occur at school crossings at reasonably frequent intervals to allow pupils to cross the street or highway safely, the traffic problem is not a safety patrol responsibility. It is the function of appropriate traffic authorities to create the necessary interruption of vehicular traffic. A survey (preferably a cooperative survey by school officials, traffic engineers, and other qualified individuals) should be made to determine the additional measures to be provided at times when children are going to and from school.

9 Relation to traffic signals, police orders, and adult crossing guards

When the vehicular traffic is such that control by a police officer, authorized adult crossing guard, or traffic signal is required, the safety patrol member should assist by directing children to cross in conformance with the direction given by the police officer or authorized adult assigned to the crossing, or in conformance with the time cycle of the signal.

10 Hours on duty

The hours that patrol members are on duty should be determined by the needs of the school area from an accident prevention standpoint and the time schedule of the school being served. The schedule of each patrol member should be so planned as to make it unnecessary for him to miss regular school work for lengthy periods. Parents should be informed of the amount of time pupils are scheduled to serve on patrols.

Patrols should be on duty at all times while children are crossing streets or highways in going to and from school. Members should be at their posts at least 10 to 15 minutes before the opening of classes in the morning and in the afternoon. At dismissal times, arrangements should be made for them to leave their classes two or three minutes before the dismissal bell. They should remain on duty until all pupils who are not stragglers have passed their posts.

SCHOOL-BUS PATROLS

A student patrol may be organized to assist children entering and leaving the bus, to supervise them during the trip to and from school, and to direct the driver when the bus must be maneuvered in close quarters or at dangerous intersections. The general principles observed in selecting school-traffic patrols also apply to school-bus patrols. Two members, a front and rear guard—one of whom lives near the end of the route—should be assigned to every bus. Each team should:

1 See that all students are properly seated in their assigned places before the bus starts

2 Assist the driver in checking attendance

3 See that aisles are free of obstacles such as books, lunch kits, and protruding feet

4 Make students understand the rules of safe conduct on buses and help enforce those rules

5 Prevent children from leaning out of the window or extending their hands or arms outside the window

6 Direct the driver at railroad crossings and dangerous intersections

7 Help the driver make children leave the bus in a quiet, orderly manner. Patrol members should get out first so that, if necessary, they can assist the other students.

8 Prevent children from crossing streets or highways when approaching or leaving the bus, until the driver signals that the road is clear[6]

9 Know when and how to use the emergency door

10 Gain the respect and cooperation of fellow pupils by setting an example of good conduct

---

[6]Instruction in highway crossings merits emphasis. The usual practice of crossing in front of a stopped passenger vehicle is a procedure unique to travel on school buses. Current laws should be carefully reviewed and appropriate uniform instructions given. Where instruction will deal with definite needs and specific locations, such as crossing a multilane highway, a procedure should be worked out and made familiar to everyone concerned, including parents. All states have laws requiring motorists to stop for school buses taking on or discharging passengers. However, the laws and practices are not uniform throughout the United States. All possible consideration should be given to the routing of buses so that passengers are picked up and discharged at stops that do not require crossing of streets or highways.

THE SCHOOL-BUS DRIVER. The selection of qualified drivers is an essential part of the school-bus safety program, but not enough attention is devoted to this matter. The character and habits of a school-bus driver should be considered as carefully as those of a teacher. The driver should be selected for dependability, good habits, unquestionable character, and complete willingness to follow the instructions and requirements of the superintendent and school board. A parent is usually best qualified for the position. A driver should not be too old or too young for the job, or inexperienced in working with children. A candidate for the position should be evaluated according to the following criteria:

1 *Age.* Is he or she old enough to assume responsibility but young enough to fulfill the special requirements of the job?
2 *Health.* Is he or she in good condition, emotionally as well as physically?
3 *Experience.* Has he or she had the necessary background? Does he or she have sufficient driving skill and mechanical knowledge to be able to handle the bus properly?
4 *Attitude.* Is he or she willing to cooperate fully with local and state authorities?
5 *Driver Record.* Is the driving record evidence of safe behavior?

A person who has qualified as a licensed bus driver by passing state and local tests and satisfying various other legal requirements is not prepared to handle the problems of operating a school bus until he or she has received specialized training. In addition to keeping drivers informed of new legislation and improved safety procedures, the school administrator should see that they have an opportunity to take short refresher courses and to attend conferences which offer new approaches to their work.

LEGALITY AND LIABILITY

The question of liability for accidents to patrol members or students under the supervision of the school safety patrol is important to school officials. The regulations governing accident liability are not uniform throughout the country. Some states specifically authorize school safety patrols, and others have no laws which apply directly to them.

According to the latest information available, most legal advisers believe that (1) school boards may organize traffic patrols to guide students in crossing streets, provided that members are not allowed to direct motorists, and (2) school boards may not be liable if a patrol member is injured while performing his or her approved duty, but individuals and the board may be liable if a patrol member is injured while directing vehicular traffic.[7]

[7]The reader is encouraged to obtain the most recent edition of *School Safety Patrol Supervisor's Manual* from the Safety and Traffic Engineering Department of the Chicago Motor Club, 66 South Water Street, Chicago, Ill. 60601. This resource may also be available through affiliated AAA clubs throughout the nation.

All school administrators should become thoroughly familiar with the pertinent legislation in their own state by consulting the state department of education and the legal adviser to the local board of education. They may gain a better understanding of the issues involved if they ask the adviser to answer the following specific questions:[8]

1 Are pupils engaged in patrol activities in potentially more hazardous positions than other students?

2 Is the school district liable for damages if a school patrol member is injured?

3 In the few states where legislation has done away with the common-law immunity of school districts, does this legislation include injuries sustained by reason of school patrol activities?

4 Can the school board buy insurance to cover pupil injuries sustained through patrol activities?

5 Is the classroom teacher or principal in charge of patrols liable for negligence, if inadequate instructions or warnings are given to students who undertake these activities?

6 Does permission of parents relieve the school personnel of liability if the pupil is injured in a sanctioned activity?

7 To what extent, if any, are school personnel relieved of liability in cases where the patrol activity is sponsored or supported jointly by the school and a nonschool agency in the community?

8 Can a patrol member who is injured while at his post of duty be charged with contributory negligence? Does the answer depend wholly on whether or not he was following instructions?

9 In an injury caused by the patrol member's own negligence, does this fact relieve the insuror from paying a claim on the injury?

10 How can school patrol activities best be conducted to avoid injuries to the patrol members and at the same time allow patrols to serve as a protective influence for other pupils?

ADULT CROSSING GUARDS

It is becoming increasingly difficult for student patrols to function effectively without assistance, for many schools are located near streets and highways where the flow of traffic is rarely interrupted. Under these circumstances, adult crossing guards are frequently employed to direct motorists.

The adult-guard program began more than 30 years ago when mothers took it upon themselves to stop cars and guide children across the street. Thereafter, various cities became interested in their efforts and began authorizing women to control traffic at school crossings. This practice gradually spread throughout the country, expanding rapidly immediately after World War II, when police departments could not fulfill all the requests by school administrators and parents to station officers at busy intersections. As school enrollments and highway traffic continue to increase, more communities are relying on the services of adult crossing guards to lessen demands on the police force and to supplement the work of student patrols.

The following criteria should be considered when utilizing adult crossing

---

[8] *The Expanding Role of School Safety Patrols,* pp. 31–32; also *Who is Liable for Pupil Injuries?* National Education Association, Washington, February, 1963, pp. 50–61.

guards after it has been determined that a particular location needs control by an adult.[9]

1 An adult crossing guard is more feasible and economical than either a pedestrian grade separation structure or a traffic-control signal specially installed to handle the crossing problem.

2 The traffic conditions at the location do not meet the specific warrants set forth for the installation of traffic-control signals.

3 Special hazards exist at either signalized or nonsignalized locations that can be properly handled only by adult supervision. Such hazards would include unusual conditions such as extreme fog, complicated intersections, heavy vehicular turning movements and high vehicular approach speeds.

4 A change in school routes or school districts is imminent, thus requiring protection at a location for only a limited time.

The following information, adapted from the American Automobile Association booklet *Adult Crossing Guards,* describes the procedures for the administration and operation of adult crossing guard programs. These suggestions should be adapted for local use in the light of community needs, resources, and particular problems concerned with protection by school crossing guards.[10]

Organization and administration

Most adult crossing-guard programs are organized and administered by local police departments. Usually a member of the department's traffic division is assigned to supervise the operation of crossing guards as well as conduct necessary training programs. While close cooperation and communication is carried out with school authorities, it has proved more effective to have one single agency completely responsible for the operation and administration of adult crossing-guard programs.

a Scope of Authority. Adult crossing guards should not generally be given regulatory and enforcement powers. The scope of their responsibilities and duties should be clearly spelled out and understood by both police and crossing guards alike. A local ordinance should be enacted to outline responsibilities and authorization for the operation and administration of a crossing-guard program.

b Liability. Crossing guards should be included under the state's workmen's compensation laws. Their insurance protection should be effective only during hours of duty and not include protection for walking back and forth to work.

c Pay. The average city pays an adult guard about $4 a day—one dollar for each period (morning, noon, afternoon dismissal), of duty. It has proved more efficient to pay guards on the basis of periods of duty worked rather than trying to pay by an hourly rate, since the duty does not fall into hourly segments. With duty time cards mailed in at the end of each week, guards could be paid at two-week intervals,

d Uniforms. It is important that crossing guards be uniformly and distinctively outfitted with belts, badges, caps and insignia so that motorists and pedestrians can recognize them and respond to their signals. Some areas also specify the use of uniform blouses or jackets and lowheel shoes. Adult guards should not wear regular police uniforms unless they have full police authority. Elaborate uniforms not only add unnecessary costs to the program, they give the public an erroneous impression of the extent of authority vested in crossing guards.

e Duty Period. Generally, crossing guards are on duty four periods a day—morning, noon dismissal, noon starting, and afternoon dismissal time. Sometimes the number of work

[9]*A Program for School Crossing Protection*, Institute of Traffic Engineers, Washington, 1971.
[10]*Adult Crossing Guards: A Guide to Selection, Training, and Warrants for Operation*, American Automobile Association, Washington, 1964, pp. 11–19.

periods may vary depending upon a school's particular needs. Guards report for duty one half hour before the tardy bell and remain on duty until at least five minutes after classes begin.

It is important that crossing guards be instructed to call in at least one half hour before duty time to report inability to be on duty. This obviates the need for calling in daily unless the guard cannot make it for some reason. In some areas, more than two unexcused absences is cause for dismissal.

Recruitment and selection

Recruitment and selection of adult crossing guards is generally the responsibility of the police department. Women are most frequently hired as guards because they are more readily available at the times needed. Selection of crossing guards should be based on the following:

- Character. Good character references should be obtained on every individual who is being considered for an adult crossing-guard position. An interest in and an understanding of children are essential for adult crossing guards. They must also know how to work effectively with adults.
- Physical Fitness. Physical examinations for candidates should give particular attention to the important areas of vision, hearing, and reflexes, which are vital for adult crossing guards in adequately performing their duties.
- Dependability. Areas deemed hazardous enough to warrant adult crossing guards require continuous supervision. It is paramount that guards assigned these duty posts be persons who can be relied upon for prompt, consistent, and efficient service.
- Availability. Whenever possible, adult guards should live within walking distance of the post to which they are assigned. This not only assures their steady availability and accessibility at all times and under all conditions, it also avoids increasing operation costs for transportation to duty posts.

Training program

As is true for all professions, a training program is also essential for smooth and effective operation of adult crossing guards. It is important that before crossing guards are assigned to actual duty, they be given instruction and training so that they will know what is expected of them. In such an in-service training program, these areas should be covered:

Classroom Instruction.

1. Purpose and goals of an adult crossing-guard program.
   a. Discussion of school child accident problem
   b. Warrants for use of adult crossing guards
   c. Relationship of adult crossing guard to other traffic-control aids, particularly school safety patrols
2. Extent of responsibilities of adult guards.
3. Orientation on the Police Department.
4. Personal conduct.
5. Knowledge of local traffic regulations.
6. Traffic-control devices.
7. Vehicle identification.
8. Filing reports.
9. Emergency procedures.
   a. How to get help
   b. First aid instruction

In-The-Field Training. The control and direction of motor vehicle and pedestrian traffic in helping children to safely cross the street is the major function of adult school crossing guards.

Therefore, considerable attention should be given to proper instruction for crossing guard procedures in carrying out this responsibility. A school crossing guard's actions must be crisp and clearly informative so that both pedestrians and drivers will know what is required of them.

SAFETY INSTRUCTION

For many people, the primary function of the school safety program is the planned exchange of information in the classroom. The establishment of an adequate plan for organizing the teaching-learning process will help achieve the objectives of the program efficiently. It is appropriate to plan the learning experiences only after identifying the needs, interests, and comprehension ability of the students. The design of the program should provide an effective means of achieving the stated goals and objectives.

Recently, the curriculum of public education has been criticized in two ways. Some people regard the learning material as irrelevant to the needs of youth in our modern society. Other people state that education needs to return to the "basics" so that young adults will be able to demonstrate essential skills and competencies upon graduation from high school. Instruction in safety education has a justifiable place in the school curriculum on the basis of relevance and utilitarian application.

It has been estimated that several quadrillion pieces of nonredundant information are known to humankind. Knowledge doubles approximately every 9 years. The junior high school adolescent of today probably possesses more factual knowledge than the scientists of the Middle Ages. Therefore, it is important for safety education to help students acquire concepts to which precise facts can be attached. When students have conceptualized and internalized relevant material, practical application becomes more likely. The goal of instruction is not the accumulation of specific facts but the formulation of concepts which have practical applications and which are useful in arriving at meaningful decisions.

Concepts are broad, generalized ideas which furnish a frame of reference for subsequent learning. They help to organize information and systematize facts into larger constructs that have extensive applications. It is rather pointless to memorize that in 1 year (1975) accidents cost the American public $47.1 billion and caused an estimated 102,500 deaths. It is more useful for students to realize that accidents represent a major cause of death, disability, and loss to the economy. The learning processes of inquiry, analysis, comparison, interpretation, and synthesis are more effective than the memorization of data.

PATTERNS OF INSTRUCTION

DIRECT TEACHING

The curriculum pattern of direct instruction provides the most effective teaching and learning process. In this pattern, safety education is offered as a separate course, with curricular time allocated specifically for the accomplishment of the stated goals and objectives of the school safety program. The teacher, after appropriate academic preparation and with enthusiasm toward the content and mission of safety education, meets with the students on a regularly scheduled basis.

An important benefit of the direct teaching pattern is that learning activities can be planned to encourage the development of concepts, positive attitudes, and safe behavior. After long-range goals and specific objectives are identified, the content and learning activities are carefully selected to achieve these goals. Students begin to perceive the interrelated network of information as a whole. Generalizations are established. The possibilities for useful application are multiplied. An appropriate analogy is to the weaver who blends the separate strands of fabric into a useful piece of cloth. At the end of the process, the whole is greater than the sum of its parts.

Direct teaching is efficient. It offers an opportunity for comprehensive planning. In a kindergarten-through-twelfth-grade sequence the learning is based upon previous understanding. Although some material might be repeated at a higher level, the repetition provides reinforcement, and unnecessary repetition can be avoided. Similarly, this pattern of instruction ensures that all the material needed for concept development will be available to the student.

Many secondary schools do not employ full-time safety educators, but it is possible to offer instruction on a block-of-time basis with another subject. For example, safety education can be offered as part of health education, with a 6-week unit devoted to safety. Obviously, the teacher in this situation needs adequate preparation in both areas of study. Safety education should never become an addendum to another subject merely for the sake of convenience. The time appropriated for safety must be used exclusively for the attainment of the goals and objectives of the school safety program.

There is one inherent danger in this pattern of instruction: teachers who tend to compartmentalize learning according to subject area may conclude that safety instruction is the responsibility of the safety educator alone. They may feel no need to correlate safety information with their subjects because "the students learn that in Safety." Since learning is essentially an integrative process, correlation should be encouraged.

CORRELATION

A correlated pattern of instruction is the *planned* inclusion of safety education into another subject. It involves more than an incidental, "opportune moment" type of coverage. The purpose is to blend safety education into the total school curriculum so that it does not become isolated content. However, correlation is supplementary to direct instruction and should never occur in place of it.

Virtually all school subjects have important relationships to safety. An issue discussed in safety education may be reinforced and brought to life in the home-economics classroom. Similarly, safety education can make the content of many other curricular areas more meaningful.

The following conditions, as stated by Oberteuffer and Beyrer, are necessary in developing and administering an effective correlated safety program:[11]

1 An individual or small committee must become sufficiently familiar with all areas of study and with the wide area of safety education to recognize where each could enrich the other, and be prepared to make recommendations for the inclusion of health [safety] material in the other areas.

2 The faculty must be receptive to the idea of correlation and ready to receive and use such recommendations as appear reasonable.

3 A program of in-service training should be provided for the teachers involved, to improve their ability to handle the acceptable health [safety] material.

4 Conferences should be held during the year as necessary for the exchange of ideas between teachers in the different areas, for example, between the social science teachers and the health [safety] group. Such conferences would be useful in checking facts, exchanging teaching materials and ideas, agreeing on purpose, and setting direction.

The following list indicates curricular areas that may be correlated with specific aspects of safety instruction:

- **Health education**

Poison prevention and proper use of medicine
First aid
Fitness and health
Prevention against infectious disease
Air, water, and noise pollution, and envrionmental health
Relationship between stress and illness
Adequate maintenance of health records
Selection and proper utilization of the family physician
Mental health and personality as factors in safety
The Food and Drug Administration

- **Science**

Use of electricity
Plants and animals
Nuclear power and radioactivity
Starting and controlling fires
Traffic safety and engineering
Smoke detectors

- **Social studies**

Transportation safety
Industrial safety
Control of public health
Government and safety
Communications and safety
Citizenship and safety

[11]Delbert Oberteuffer and Mary K. Beyrer, *School Health Education*, 4th ed., Harper & Row, Publishers, Incorporated, New York, 1966, p. 219.

- **Home economics**

Proper storage, preparation, and serving of foods
Interior design and accident prevention
Kitchen safety
Flammable fabrics
The Consumer Product Safety Commission
Child growth and development

- **Language arts**

Writing letters for safety education materials
Talks and panel discussions
Safety column in school paper or letter to the editor of city newspaper
Reports on special topics such as fire prevention
Creative work: art, safety posters, etc.
Spelling exercises using safety terminology

- **Arithmetic** (quantitative thinking)

Tables and graphs of accidents by cause, type, age of person injured, place of accident, etc.
Percentage of increase and/or decrease in accident figures
Calculating loss of time and money caused by accidents

- **Art, music**

Creative drawing, coloring, and painting
Illustrating safety booklets
Posters
Suitable songs, original or popular
Bulletin boards and collages

- **Shops**

Use and care of tools and equipment
Safety practices in shop activities
Safety in industry
Good housekeeping
Safety consciousness

- **Problems of democracy**

Student government
Trips and excursions
Surveys and inspections
Safety patrols and committees, safety council
Assemblies and radio programs
Citizenship and safety

- **Physical education**

Proper use of recreational equipment
Lead-up activities
Responsible leadership and supervision
Development of self-reliance and self-image
Aquatic safety and swimming
Training and conditioning

INTEGRATION

An integrated curriculum is not arranged according to subject matter. Therefore it represents a noticeable departure from the traditional organization of curriculum. It is also known as a "core" curriculum, in which relationships across content areas are sought. The curriculum is not compartmentalized into narrowly defined subjects. The premise is that all areas of instruction contribute to the acquisition of common goals and objectives.

The word integrate means to relate the parts of something to a unified whole. The identified core concept is ordinarily too broad to be the exclusive concern of any one subject. The statement "community responsibility enhances the quality of living" has implications for virtually all subjects in the school curriculum. Every teacher within the core can provide information that relates to the concept. To facilitate integration, schools would no longer be organized by subject area or department. Instead, a team composed of teachers from each discipline would cooperatively plan the learning experiences for all students assigned to their team. Although the system of teaching safety by integration has tremendous possibilities, it requires imagination, planning, experimentation, and skill on the part of the teacher.

A core program, as described by Grace Wright, is characterized by broad preplanned problem areas. Within each problem area there should be provisions for dealing with (1) the interests, concerns, and needs common to all youths in our society, (2) the major areas of everyday life (social functions and living safely), (3) problems of major significance to all members of our society (societal problems), and (4) persistent life situations. The core program should help youth acquire basic citizenship education to deal with significant personal and social problems, to understand their own behavior and that of others, and to live democratically.[12] There are a multitude of concepts which could serve as appropriate topics for an integrated curriculum. Each area of instruction must contribute to the acquistion of knowledge. An important outcome of this type of learning is the discovery of meaningful relationships that have practical application. Listed below are a few concepts which could be used in a core curriculum.

1 Independence demands responsibility as well as freedom.

2 Productivity is enhanced whenever people work together toward a common goal.

3 There are many forms of communication.

4 Transportation is important to our national economy.

5 Peer pressure often helps to influence decision making.

6 Government seeks to protect us in many ways.

7 Helping others in time of need provides an opportunity to practice human kindness.

8 Selecting a career requires one to consider many factors.

[12]"The Core Program: Unpublished Research, 1956–63," prepared by Grace S. Wright, U.S. Department of Health, Education, and Welfare, 1963, p. 2.

INSTRUCTIONAL TECHNIQUES

Many different instructional techniques, ranging from lectures to puppet shows to student participation in solving actual problems, are used in safety education courses. Some techniques are more commonly used than others, but to varying degrees all recognize the value of providing students with direct experiences that enable them to learn by doing.

The method selected should take into account the educational maturity of the group, with allowances made for individual differences, and should provide challenging experiences for all grade levels. Subject matter should be integrated with real-life situations, and the activities provided should stimulate student motivation. Teaching should proceed from psychological appeals to logical reasoning. The instructional technique must be a suitable means of achieving the stated objectives of the safety education program. Its aims should be made clear to the students so that they can participate in evaluating results. The final criterion of any method is its effectiveness in increasing the students' knowledge of safety and in improving their habits, skills, attitudes, and behavior patterns.

Insofar as possible, any method of teaching should have the objective of leading students to make discoveries independently. The primary goal of safety education—to ensure correct behavior—cannot be achieved by merely teaching students and then testing them. Nor is it sufficient only to impart information and develop habits and skills. Learning rules and regulations, slogans and warnings, does not necessarily produce discretion. Assigning appropriate readings and transmitting essential facts to students does not always constitute good teaching.

The essence of the problem is to motivate the student to accept beliefs, since motivation is essential to learning. Without proper motivation a person will not pay attention, practice, or make a real effort to comprehend. A teacher's choice of instructional methods will depend upon the:

1 Objectives to be attained
2 Age of the group
3 Skills and abilities of the class
4 Intellectual capacity of the students
5 Experience of the group
6 Group and individual differences
7 Space, time, and equipment available
8 Competence, interest, and ability of the teacher
9 Personality of the teacher

The instructional techniques used in many other academic disciplines can be utilized in the teaching of safety. A resourceful teacher will use a variety of techniques to achieve the objective. The following annotated list of successfully used methods is quoted from R. K. Means. The list is not intended to be all-inclusive, and does not specifically state what grade level each method may be applied to. The purpose is to provide the prospective teacher with a wide variety of techniques, with the hope that several will be tried in various classroom situations. The listing is alphabetized, and the order in no way reflects degree of importance.[13]

1. Audiovisual Aids. The supplementation of learning through the senses of seeing hearing, and/or feeling and often used simultaneously with verbal presentation by the health education teachers, such as bulletin boards, charts, collections, exhibits, filmstrips, flannel boards, maps, mock-ups, models, motion pictures, puppets, recordings, slides, television and others.

Examples

a. Make a bulletin board display of the kinds and incidences of local traffic accidents.
b. Prepare a flannel or magnetic traffic board depicting traffic situations.

2. *Brainstorming.* The division of the class into groups to present possible solutions to a problem. No negative statement may be made, only positive answers, and the recorder writes down all that is said. No moderation is deemed necessary. An intriguing method that stimulates thinking and individual expression.

Examples

a. List all the possible dangers in the home and solutions for overcoming them.
b. List positive suggestions for learning how to swim safely.

3. *Buzz Sessions.* A technique whereby the class is divided into groups of from four to eight members for the discussion of a specific health (safety) problem or controversial issue for a limited time. The chairman of each section presents the group viewpoints following individual group discussion. Works well with large groups to give individuality to presentation of material. Promotes understanding by group and organizational ability and leadership on the part of the chairman.

Examples

a. Conduct a buzz session on the effects of alcohol and drugs on driving.
b. Discuss smoking as related to home fires.

4. *Committee Work.* The segmentation of class members into designated groups to accomplish concentrated group study or research on a particular health (safety) topic or unit of work. Stimulates group action and improves relations among students.

Examples

a. Prepare an oral report on safety practices for skin and scuba diving.
b. Develop a safe code for bicycle and motorcycle operators.

5. *Conference.* An individual or group meeting of student, teacher, parent, and/or other school personnel to discuss, plan, interpret, and evaluate school experiences and student health (safety) problems. Provides an excellent opportunity for personal expression and interpersonal relations between teacher and student.

[13]R. K. Means, "Practical Instructional Methods in Health Education," *Journal of School Health,* vol. 28, pp. 223–227, September, 1958, as quoted in Jack Smolensky and L. Richard Bonvechio, *Principles of School Health,* D. C. Heath Company, Boston, 1966, pp. 259–269. The examples have been supplied.

Examples

a. Plan a youth traffic-safety conference for the schools in your county.

b. Invite various safety agencies to discuss local, state, and national accident problems.

6. *Creative Activities.* Individual or group composition of stories, posters, music, film-strips, charts, models, dramatizations, and other materials concerning a particular health (safety) problem or area. Promotes understanding through practical application with realistic outcomes.

Examples

a. Write a story for your school paper concerning the hazards in and around the school building.

b. Plan a radio or TV program on what the school is doing in driver education.

7. *Debate.* The division of the class into equal groups of from four to eight members, each representing opposite viewpoints regarding a health (safety) question. Each participant is allowed an individual presentation and rebuttal following a limited preparation period. Stimu-lates thinking, organization and expression in a structural experience.

Examples

a. Have a debate on the argument that teen-agers are too young to drive.

b. Debate the question that civil defense is a waste of time, for we shall all be affected by radioactivity.

8. *Demonstration.* The process of presentation by the health (safety) education teacher in front of the class in order to illustrate a principle, show a technique, or establish certain facts. Usually used to supplement a presentation and facilitate learning and understanding.

Examples

a. Demonstrate the three elements needed for starting a fire.

b. Illustrate how hair sprays can act like a blow torch.

9. *Discussion.* Student oral participation toward the resolution of a health (safety) prob-lem or question. Discussion may proceed with or without active teacher direction but ordinarily employs some degree of moderation to guide the thinking of the group. Allows clarification of certain aspects of a presentation and stimulates thinking and expression.

Examples

a. What are the findings of research as to the effectiveness of seat belts?

b. How can better attitudes be developed by the general public for accident prevention?

10. *Drill.* The repetitive practice of fundamental health (safety) knowledge or skill intended to bring about automatic response or performance in a subject. Not necessarily mechanical and uninteresting. Can be functionally used in conjunction with other procedures for subject matter or behavioral understanding.

Examples

a. Practice fire drills from unusual locations within the school building, gymnasium, swimming pool, and auditorium.

b. Illustrate how to protect yourself in the classroom when a tornado warning is given.

11. *Exploration.* The process of obtaining health (safety) knowledge and understanding through studious inquiry and contact with many sources and a wide range of experiences. Excellent technique to facilitate the learning of concepts and understanding relative to scientific research.

Examples

   a. Analyze research articles on current traffic-accident problems.
   b. Find out why your local community does not have a safety council.

12. *Field Trips.* An excursion planned by the student, teacher and/or school and undertaken for educational purposes in order to observe and study health (safety) materials and processes in their functional setting. Provides by observation an understanding of social or personal needs and problems in a distinctly functional manner.

Examples

   a. Visit a local traffic court and observe its operation.
   b. Visit a police or fire department and observe how calls are handled.

13. *Games.* The participation by class members in health (safety) activities, which counstitute and establish a conducive learning situation through creation of favorable emotional appeal. Promotes desirable outcomes by creating an atmosphere conducive to participation.

Examples

   a. Conduct a hazard hunt at home, at school, on the farm, in your fraternity, sorority, or dormitory, and then analyze it in class.
   b. Conduct a "spell down" on safety terminology.

14. *Interview.* A face-to-face consultation of student and teacher or other school personnel often conducted as an important aspect of health (safety) guidance and counseling. It is also used as related to a guest speaker when he is asked specific questions.

This is a practical manner of discovering problems, asking and answering questions, and improving student-teacher relations.

Examples

   a. Interview the school safety coodinator about his role in accident prevention.
   b. Interview a local pediatrician to determine how many and what type of accidents he handles weekly.

15. *Laboratory Experimentation.* The process of conducting a scientific health (safety) experiment to test various hypotheses or to demonstrate certain processes. Practical and functional approach toward problem-solving and the influence of attitude toward scientific endeavor.

Examples

   a. Have the chemistry teacher explain the effects of various poisons found in the home when taken accidentally.
   b. In a driver education laboratory, test the various physical characteristics of a person as they may relate to driving a motor vehicle.

16. *Lecture.* An attempt to impart knowledge, create interest, influence opinion, stimulate activity, or promote critical thinking by the use of verbal language with little student participation. Unexcelled in comprehensive presentation of material. Becomes functional when used to furnish information in order to proceed or complete a particular study.

Sample topics

a. Today's traffic problem.
b. How to combat accidental deaths.
c. The economic waste caused by accidents.
d. What causes carbon monoxide poisoning?
e. How to prepare for an atomic bomb attack.
f. The federal government's Highway Safety Act and its implications for state and local government.

17. *Lecture-Discussion.* A composite presentation utilizing both the lecture and discussion techniques. Incorporate desirable qualities of lecture and discussion when functionally utilized.

Sample topics

a. What are the effects of drugs on driving a motor vehicle?
b. What are the effects of alcohol on driving a motor vehicle?
c. Why are teen-agers considered poor drivers?
d. Are college student motorcycle operators inconsiderate of pedestrians and other motor-vehicle operators?
e. Should high school students be allowed to drive motor vehicles to school?
f. How should a youngster walk to and from school safely?

18. *Oral Report.* The verbal presentation before the class or an audience of the results of a health (safely) study or problem, conducted by the student or group of students. Promotes initial study with opportunities for organization, original thinking and expression. Particularly effective when used with other techniques to encourage informality.

Examples

a. Have a student report on his findings after making an inspection of fire extinguishers in the school building.
b. Have a student report on backyard swimming pool drownings and how they occurred.
c. Have a student report on the school administrator's legal responsibilities for providing a safe school environment.

19. *Outside Speaker.* The utilization of a well-informed specialist from the community to talk to or discuss with the students some relevant health (safety) issue or subject about which he is an expert. Excellent method of obtaining information and insuring understanding from a practical viewpoint.

Examples

a. Invite an insurance agent to describe various types of automobile insurance.
b. Invite a police officer to speak on local accident problems.
c. Invite a fireman to speak on fire safety.

20. *Panel Discussion.* An oral presentation or discussion by selected class participants of a health (safety) problem, topic, question, or controversial issue. Class or audience participation is sometimes invited following the panel presentation by an impartial moderator. Provides for diversity of views and reactions, stimulates research, study and expression.

Sample topics

a. What are the pros and cons of raising the legal driving age to twenty-one years?
b. What is the function of a local or state safety council, and what is its effect on accident reduction?
c. High school youths should be better drivers than they are. Why aren't they?

21. *Problem-Solving.* The technique of arriving at a desired goal by means of selecting, defining, collecting data, interpreting, finding, and testing the best soulution to a problem having more than one possible response and evaluating the results. Stimulates deeper values, understanding, judgment, and decision making. Promotes group discussion and provides for practice of democratic procedure.

Examples

a. Observe pedestrians and count how many use good pedestrian practices.
b. Analyze campus pedestrian, bicycle, motorcycle and motorist problems, and formulate plans for solving them.

22. *Project.* The planning, investigation and written solution to a health (safety) topic or problem by the student, accomplished in a real-life situation. Functional and active opportunities with objective outcome. Usually correlated with other techniques.

Examples

a. Inspect all school fire extinguishers to determine when they were last serviced.
b. Keep a monthly local spot map to determine where there were pedestrian, bicycle, motorcycle, and automobile accidents. Write a story for your local paper describing your findings.

23. *Reading Assignments.* The delegation of supplemental health (safety) education reading materials to the student to further understanding of a particular topic or unit of work promotes and stimulates thinking or understanding by exposure to other views and opinions when properly utilized.

Examples

a. Read research reviews in safety magazines.
b. Read various magazines to supplement textbook reading on a variety of accident problems—sports, fire, school, pedestrian, traffic, home, etc.

24. *Review.* A re-examination of health (safety) material or a health activity previously presented and studied or a critical review of a literary work, motion picture, television program, play, or musical event concerning health or safe living. Encourages critical thinking, constructive analysis and general comprehension.

Examples

a. Critically analyze various films on traffic safety.
b. Review safety advertisements in popular magazines for their effectiveness.

25. *Role-Playing.* A spontaneous, unrehearsed and on-the-spot acting-out of a health (safety) problem or situation by selected students and presented before the group to stimulate interest, thinking, and interpretation or to provide a common basis for discussion. Excellent functional approach to reflect knowledge, attitude or behavior concerning a problem.

Examples

a. Plan a home fire drill and act it out in your home.
b. You smell smoke in your home. Act out your procedure.

26. *Skit.* A rehearsed and planned dramatization of a health (safety) problem or situation by students and presented before the group to stimulate interest, discussion or interpretation. Provides information in a unique manner and is particularly effective in influencing attitudes concerning a situation or problem.

Examples

a. Write a play for presentation to the PTA on home safety.
b. Dramatize safety practices when riding and getting off and on a school bus.

27. *Story-telling.* A device utilized by the health (safety) education teacher to supplement oral presentation by illustration or to enliven class discussion. Also may be undertaken by the student. Adds humor, realism or feeling to a presentation or subject. Can be used spontaneously and is feasible for any age level.

Examples

a. Have the captain of the school traffic-safety patrol tell a story to primary grade pupils on how the patrol helps them.
b. Have students tell a story concerning a safety incident in order to illustrate a safety concept.

28. *Survey.* The scientific gathering and compilation of information concerning a particular health (safety) problem or area by an individual or group in order to emphasize an existing circumstance. Facilitates group action experiences and understanding of specific health problems.

Examples

a. Do a community survey with the help of local police to determine how many drivers are using seat belts.
b. Have students make a survey of their home, dormitory, fraternity, or sorority to find unsafe conditions.

29. *Test.* A device or procedure utilized to measure health (safety) knowledge, attitude, interest, ability, achievement or behavior, constructed by the teacher or pupil. Self-tests help to stimulate interest, motivate and cement teacher-student understanding.

Examples

a. Take a pretest of general safety knowledge followed by a culminating test at the end of the course or unit.
b. Give a variety of tests such as short quizzes, essay, true-false, matching, multiple-choice, fill-in, or completion.

30. *Verbal Explanation.* An informal, brief, concise and to-the-point oral description of a health (safety) situation or activity by the teacher or pupil. Usually a phase of another procedure. Should be functionally correlated to further a concept or understanding.

Examples

a. Briefly explain a serious school safety problem such as a news reporter might have to do.

b. Explain the reasons for having a compulsory motor-vehicle inspection lane.

31. *Workshop.* A group session of a designated time devoted to the production, preparation or accomplishment of a specific health (safety) project or topic. Provides unlimited opportunities for leadership, group organization and exploration. Often a combination of many other procedures.

Examples

a. Sponsor a countywide youth farm-safety project, including: farm machinery, traffic, bicycles, fire, hunting, etc.

b. Plan a safety program for a university, high school, community, church, etc.

VALUES CLARIFICATION

Although it is not a new teaching technique, *values clarification* has only recently gained popular acceptance. This approach attempts to help young people build a value system. Planned "values activities" enable students to better understand the relationship between beliefs and behavior. When encouraged to consider alternatives, students learn to examine the benefits and consequences of their actions as compared with other types of behavior. This teaching method offers significant opportunities for safety education. (The Selected References at the end of this chapter provide several excellent sources of information on values clarification.)

AUDIOVISUAL AIDS

Some of the instructional techniques listed above explicitly require the use of audiovisual materials, but such materials can enhance the value of most other teaching methods. A lecture can often be clarified by illustrative materials, and class discussion can be stimulated by educational films.

One of the important jobs of the teacher of safety education is to make students see clearly the causes and results of accidents and the methods of avoiding them. Children in the primary grades especially need graphic impressions of environmental dangers and protective safety measures. It is with this group that audiovisual materials are most effective. Children cannot be made to understand easily all phases of safety in the time allotted to the subject within the school day. It is not always possible to provide them with the direct, firsthand experiences that are most valuable in dramatizing problems. Audiovisual materials are the next best way of making the subject matter vivid and of giving students realistic concepts of safe behavior.

The various types of audiovisual materials effective in teaching safety have been classified by Kinder as follows:[14]

I. Repetitive Materials
   A. Blackboards
   B. Bulletin boards
   C. Duplicating devices
II. Pictorial and Graphical Representation
   A. Photographs
   B. Textbook illustrations
   C. Prints and etchings
   D. Cutouts
   E. Post cards
   F. Newspaper clippings
   G. Drawings and sketches
   H. Charts, graphs, and tables
   I. Cartoons
   J. Pictorial statistics
   K. Posters
   L. Maps and globes
   M. Diagrams and schematics
III. Still Projected Pictures
   A. Stereographs
   B. Lantern slides
   C. Filmstrips
   D. Opaque projections
   E. Positive transparencies
   F. Microslide projections
   G. Tachistoscopes
IV. Projected Motion Pictures
   A. Silent
   B. Sound-on-film motion pictures
V. Auditory Materials
   A. Phonograph records
   B. Electrical transcriptions
   C. Radio broadcasts
      1. Amplitude modulation
      2. Frequency modulation
   D. Centralized sound system
VI. Audiovisual Aids in Combination
   A. Sound motion pictures
   B. Television
   C. Sound filmstrips
VII. The School Journey (Field Trip)
VIII. The Museum
IX. Representation and Relief Displays
   A. Models
   B. Objects
   C. Specimens, collections, samples

[14]James S. Kinder, *Audio-visual Materials and Techniques,* 2nd ed., American Book Company, New York, 1959, pp. 10–11.

       D. Relics
       E. Dioramas
       F. Sand tables, miniature sets, floor representation
       G. Mock-ups
       H. Miniatures, dolls, etc.
   X. Dramatization
  XI. Demonstrations
 XII. Miscellaneous
       A. Flash cards
       B. Albums
       C. Illustrated booklets, scrapbooks

Insufficient in themselves, audiovisual materials should supplement rather than supplant the textbook, the teacher, and other media. No single type of audiovisual material can be effective in all situations. The teacher should preview materials before using them in the classroom and should plan ahead to have the proper materials available at the appropriate time. The success achieved in using particular aids should be evaluated, and a record should be kept of the results. When handled properly, audiovisual materials should give the student a richer, fuller learning experience, and can assist the teacher in vitalizing safety education.

LEARNING EXPERIENCES

The following activities are designed to supplement the study of this chapter.

1 Interview a school principal and discuss the components of a comprehensive school safety program.

2 Develop a safe-school inspection form with major headings covering administrative policy, safety services, safe environment, and safety instruction. Secure permission from the principal to make recommendations which would strengthen the school's safety program.

3 Identify an administrative concern of the school safety program. Determine the ways in which adequate policy can positively affect the safety services, environment, and instruction. Conversely, determine how a poor administrative policy, or a lack of policy, would negatively affect each of these major safety components.

4 Make appropriate arrangements to visit a class on safety education at an elementary or a secondary school. Discuss your observations with the class.

5 Carefully examine a school district or state curriculum guide and critically evaluate issues such as:

   a. philosophy of the safety program
   b. identified goals and objectives
   c. content
   d. selected learning activities

    e. techniques of evaluation

    f. progression from grade level to grade level

    6 Brainstorm the special needs of the handicapped on campus. What kinds of architectural changes are needed to make buildings accessible to this special population?

    7 Prepare a comprehensive school emergency plan. Consider the following:

    a. What plans exist for locating and contacting parents of injured students?

    b. Who shall render first aid, and under what circumstances?

    c. What is the line of authority for making decisions relevant to emergencies?

    d. What provisions should be made for transporting injured children to the hospital?

    e. What procedures govern emergency evacuation of the building?

    f. Should trained personnel be available after school for all intramural and interscholastic events?

    8 Select an elementary school and determine the attendance boundaries. Prepare a street map and identify potentially dangerous areas. Select the Safest Route to School for several areas of the map. Where would you locate members of the school safety patrol?

    9 Visit with a school nurse and review the school's accident records. Analyze the data according to type of injury, location of the accident, probable cause, and time of the day when the accident occurred. What recommendations could you make to reduce the accident rate at this school?

    10 Develop a list of safety topics which can be correlated with other curricular areas. How can the content of other studies be correlated with safety education?

    11 Develop a values-clarification activity for use in the instructional part of the school safety program. Prepare a short teaching demonstration using this activity.

    12 Preview safety materials available to you from various local, state, and national sources. Compile a list of agencies where resources are available, indicating the address of each organization.

SELECTED REFERENCES

American Automobile Association:
    Adult School Crossing Guards, Washington
    Is Liability a Factor Affecting School Safety Programs today, Traffic Engineering and Safety Department, Falls Church, Va.
    Policies and Practices for School Safety Patrols, rev. ed., Washington, 1972
    Teacher's Guide for the Safest Route to School Project, Falls Church, Va.
American Driver and Traffic Safety Education Association, National Education Association, Washington:*Personnel Functions and Preparation*
    Policies and Guidelines for a School Safety Program, 1974

Chicago Motor Club, Safety and Traffic Engineering Department: *School Safety Patrol Supervisor's Manual,* Chicago, Ill.

Institute for Traffic Engineers: *A Program for School Crossing Protection,* Washington, 1971.

National Safety Council: *Student Accident Reporting Guidebook,* Chicago, Ill., 1966.

Nemir, Alma, and Warren E. Schaller: *The School Health Program,* W. B. Saunders Company, Philadelphia, 1975.

Raths, Louis E., Merrill Harmin, and Sidney B. Simon: *Values and Teaching,* Charles E. Merrill Publishing Company, Columbus, Ohio, 1966.

Simon, Sidney B., Leland Howe, and Howard Kirschenbaum: *Values Clarification,* Hart Publishing Co., Inc., New York, 1972.

Safety in Physical Education, Athletics, and Recreational Activities

OVERALL OBJECTIVE:

The student should know that physical education, athletics, and recreational activities increase one's chance of incurring an accident. The student should be able to recognize and guard against the hazards associated with these activities, remove or compensate for potential hazards, and avoid creating new hazards by action or failure to act.

INSTRUCTIONAL OBJECTIVES:

After completing this chapter the student should be able to:

1 List ten environmental hazards and faulty practices responsible for injuries sustained in interscholastic and recreational sports and to discuss methods to minimize these dangers.
2 Select ten popular athletic, physical education, and recreational activities, and list the risks involved in the performance of each activity.
3 List and discuss preventive measures to reduce the risk of accident for each of the ten chosen activities.
4 Discuss the relation of facilities, equipment, fitness, and skills to safe athletic performance.
5 List the administrative measures that can be taken to control risks.
6 Know the various types of accident-reporting systems that pertain to athletic, recreational, and physical education activities.
7 Know the significance of the accident-reporting system and know how to apply the data to accident prevention.
8 Know the five major factors in the health supervision of athletics.
9 Know the specific hazards of popular outdoor seasonal recreational and

115

sports activities (camping, hunting, fishing, skiing, snowmobiling, aquatic activities, etc.) and know preventive measures to reduce or eliminate the risks.

TRENDS IN SPORTS SAFETY

In sports, recreational, and physical education activities, participants seek exciting, vigorous, and emotionally satisfying experiences. Today, many people participate in these activities to improve their health and physical fitness.

In recent years, significant changes that have implications for safety have occurred in these activities. The great increase in the participation of women in sports activities, particularly at the level of varsity competition; the expansion of intramural and recreational sports programs; and the overall increased participation in athletic and recreational activities have caused greater exposure to accidents. An increase in injuries and fatalities in newer activities such as skateboarding and snowmobiling has also caused concern. The increase in sports-related lawsuits has caused professional leaders to become concerned about program participation and the financial drain on individuals and on the organizations conducting recreational programs. These developments should arouse increased interest in accident prevention and injury control. If individuals are to enjoy and achieve success in sports, physical education, and recreational activities, they must (1) understand the hazards related to an activity, (2) remove the hazards, (3) compensate for hazards that cannot be removed, and (4) create no unnecessary hazards by action or failure to act.

The physical education program, which includes athletics, play, and recreational activities, obviously exposes participants to more than normal classroom risks. Thus, it is not surprising that a high percentage of all school-jurisdictional accidents involving children occur during participation in these activities[1] (Tables 5-1, and 5-2).

The element of danger makes participation in sports activities sufficiently thrilling and exciting to attract adolescents and young adults. Sports activities can direct students' energies away from the more harmful pursuits on which the students might otherwise depend for challenge and adventure.

By helping fulfill the physical, emotional, and social needs of youth, sports and related activities contribute to the development of well-adjusted personalities and strong, healthy bodies. They provide an acceptable means of release from the tension of modern living; promote good social relationships, including wholesome companionship between the sexes; foster fair play, cooperativeness, leadership, and tolerance; and offer opportunities for achievement that may compensate, at least in part, for failures and disappointments elsewhere.

Despite the many benefits of recreational activities, some parents and teachers point to the high accident rate in this area. They recommend that the program be curtailed, on the fallacious assumption that the only way to prevent

---

[1]*Accident Facts,* National Safety Council, Chicago, 1977, pp. 90–91.

TABLE 5–1

Boys—Student Accident Rates by School Grade

Location and Type	Total	Kgn.	1–3 Gr.	4–6 Gr.	7–9 Gr.	10–12 Gr.	Days Lost per Inj.
Enrollment Reported (000)	1,157†	77	249	268	295	243	
Total School Jurisdiction	9.94	5.73	6.39	8.95	13.63	12.29	1.03
Shops and labs	0.73	0	0.01	0.05	1.31	1.70	0.63
Homemaking	0.01	0	‡	‡	0.02	0.01	1.09
Science	0.06	0	‡	0.01	0.16	0.09	0.50
Driving (practice)	‡	0	0	0	0.01	‡	1.20
Vocational and arts	0.51	0	0	0.01	0.93	1.16	0.59
Agricultural	0.01	0	0	0	0.01	0.01	0.58
Other labs	0.03	0	‡	0.01	0.06	0.06	0.73
Other shops	0.11	0	0.01	0.02	0.12	0.37	1.04
Building—general	2.01	1.82	1.53	1.85	3.18	1.53	0.88
Auditoriums and classrooms	0.88	1.24	0.79	0.93	1.24	0.51	0.69
Lunchrooms	0.10	0.04	0.09	0.12	0.15	0.07	0.87
Corridors	0.50	0.26	0.25	0.34	0.95	0.48	1.03
Lockers (room and corridor)	0.07	0	0.01	0.02	0.16	0.10	1.02
Stairs and stairways (inside)	0.20	0.07	0.09	0.15	0.40	0.18	1.23
Toilets and washrooms	0.10	0.12	0.16	0.13	0.06	0.05	0.96
Grounds—unorganized activities	1.98	2.48	3.39	3.76	0.73	0.21	1.00
Apparatus	0.40	1.04	0.95	0.55	0.07	0.02	1.13
Ball playing	0.44	0.06	0.37	1.20	0.22	0.07	0.84
Running	0.55	0.61	1.12	0.94	0.17	0.04	1.02
Grounds—miscellaneous	0.36	0.48	0.40	0.49	0.29	0.28	1.20
Fences and walls	0.04	0.06	0.06	0.07	0.03	0.01	1.61
Steps and walks (outside)	0.12	0.25	0.13	0.13	0.11	0.10	1.01
Physical education	3.27	0.35	0.69	2.29	6.09	4.64	1.04
Apparatus	0.30	0.04	0.12	0.22	0.52	0.38	1.05
Class games	0.35	0.07	0.21	0.42	0.55	0.29	0.90
Baseball—hard ball	0.03	0	‡	0.01	0.08	0.06	0.96
Baseball—soft ball	0.16	0	0.02	0.17	0.31	0.16	1.39
Football—regular	0.11	0	‡	0.04	0.20	0.25	1.59
Football—touch	0.24	0	0	0.09	0.49	0.43	1.14
Basketball	0.52	0	0.01	0.19	0.99	1.02	1.06
Hockey	0.03	0	‡	0.01	0.04	0.05	0.65
Soccer	0.19	0	0.03	0.16	0.32	0.31	1.18
Track and field events	0.12	0	0.01	0.08	0.26	0.13	1.27
Volleyball and similar games	0.14	0.02	0.01	0.08	0.21	0.31	0.72
Other organized games	0.43	0.04	0.11	0.40	0.82	0.45	0.90
Swimming	0.07	0	0	0.02	0.12	0.17	0.62
Showers and dressing rooms	0.07	0	0.01	0.02	0.19	0.06	0.60
Intra-mural sports	0.16	0	0	0.04	0.32	0.31	1.50
Baseball—hard ball	‡	0	0	0	‡	0.01	1.83
Baseball—soft ball	0.01	0	0	0	0.02	0.01	6.81
Football—regular	0.07	0	0	0	0.13	0.15	1.42
Football—touch	0.02	0	0	0.01	0.04	0.02	0.68
Basketball	0.03	0	0	0.01	0.05	0.08	1.27
Inter-scholastic sports	1.04	0	‡	0.05	1.23	3.36	0.86
Baseball—hard ball	0.02	0	0	0	0.01	0.09	0.81
Baseball—soft ball	0.01	0	0	‡	0.01	0.02	0.61
Football—regular	0.66	0	0	0.01	0.74	2.17	90

117

TABLE 5–1 *(continued)*
Boys—Student Accident Rates by School Grade

Location and Type	Total	Kgn.	1–3 Gr.	4–6 Gr.	7–9 Gr.	10–12 Gr.	Days Lost per Inj.
Basketball	0.15	0	0	0.01	0.23	0.42	0.70
Track and field events	0.07	0	‡	0.02	0.10	0.18	0.81
Special activities	0.06	0.03	0.04	0.10	0.06	0.06	1.84
Trips or excursions	0.03	0.03	0.03	0.05	0.04	0.02	1.53
Student dramatics	‡	0	‡	0	‡	0.01	0.13
Student concerts	0	0	0	0	0	0	0
Going to and from school (MV)	0.16	0.34	0.18	0.14	0.18	0.12	3.95
School bus	0.07	0.07	0.06	0.06	0.09	0.04	0.92
Public carrier (incl. bus)	0.01	0.09	0.02	0.01	0.01	0	7.30
Motor scooter	0.01	0.01	0	0	‡	0.02	6.50
Other mot. veh.—pedestrian	0.04	0.12	0.09	0.04	0.04	0.01	6.71
Other mot. veh.—bicycle	0.01	0.02	0	0.02	0.02	‡	8.24
Other mot. veh.—other type	0.02	0.03	0.01	0.01	0.02	0.05	2.45
Going to, from school (not MV)	0.17	0.23	0.15	0.18	0.24	0.08	1.63
Bicycle—not mot. veh.	0.03	0	0.01	0.03	0.05	0.01	1.38
Other street and sidewalk	0.09	0.20	0.10	0.09	0.10	0.06	1.16

*This table and Table 5-2 summarize about 32,000 school-jurisdictional accidents reported to the National Safety Council for the 1974–75 school year. The rates are accidents per 100,000 student days. A rate of 10 in the total column is equivalent to about 4,500 accidents. *Accidents* cause the loss of one-half day or more of (1) school time or (2) activity during nonschool time, and/or any property damage as a result of a school-jurisdictional accident. Kindergarten rates are adjusted for half-day.
†Some totals include data not shown separately.
‡Less than 0.005.
Source: *Accident Facts*, National Safety Council, Chicago, 1977.

TABLE 5–2
Girls—Student Accident Rates by School Grade

Location and Type	Total	Kgn.	1–3 Gr.	4–6 Gr.	7–9 Gr.	10–12 Gr.	Days Lost per Inj.
Enrollment Reported (000)	1,105†	72	235	258	286	238	
Total School Jurisdiction	5.72	4.01	4.35	6.24	7.99	4.73	0.98
Shops and labs	0.17	0	0.01	0.03	0.39	0.28	0.45
Homemaking	0.06	0	0	0.01	0.17	0.08	0.35
Science	0.05	0	0	0.01	0.13	0.06	0.43
Driving (practice)	‡	0	0	‡	0	0.01	0
Vocational, ind. arts	0.03	0	0	0.01	0.05	0.06	0.45
Agricultural	‡	0	0	0	‡	0	0
Other labs	0.02	0	‡	‡	0.02	0.05	0.61
Other shops	0.01	0	0.01	‡	0.02	0.02	1.04
Building—general	1.36	1.02	0.88	1.28	2.25	1.04	0.87
Auditoriums and classrooms	0.58	0.67	0.50	0.63	0.85	0.31	0.73
Lunchrooms	0.05	0.02	0.06	0.05	0.07	0.04	1.03
Corridors	0.31	0.12	0.11	0.25	0.65	0.23	0.76
Lockers (room and corridor)	0.04	0.01	0.01	0.02	0.10	0.05	0.44
Stairs and stairways (inside)	0.23	0.05	0.05	0.16	0.44	0.28	1.38
Toilets and washrooms	0.07	0.12	0.08	0.09	0.06	0.05	0.80
Grounds—unorganized activities	1.25	1.68	2.37	2.46	0.26	0.08	0.94
Apparatus	0.38	0.99	0.93	0.57	0.04	0.01	1.20

118

TABLE 5–2   (continued)
Girls—Student Accident Rates by School Grade

Location and Type	Total	Kgn.	1–3 Gr.	4–6 Gr.	7–9 Gr.	10–12 Gr.	Days Lost per Inj.
Ball playing	0.21	0.02	0.15	0.66	0.06	0.01	0.63
Running	0.34	0.31	0.76	0.57	0.07	0.02	0.84
Grounds—miscellaneous	0.21	0.22	0.28	0.28	0.17	0.14	1.17
Fences and walls	0.02	0.03	0.04	0.04	0.01	0	1.38
Steps and walks (outside)	0.08	0.09	0.09	0.11	0.08	0.06	1.07
Physical education	2.16	0.40	0.51	1.80	4.26	2.25	0.94
Apparatus	0.37	0.11	0.11	0.27	0.69	0.44	1.01
Class games	0.25	0.09	0.13	0.39	0.36	0.14	0.80
Baseball—hard ball	0.01	0	0	‡	0.01	0.01	0.63
Baseball—soft ball	0.10	0	0.01	0.09	0.20	0.12	0.75
Football—regular	0.01	0	0	0.01	0.01	0.01	0.83
Football—touch	0.03	0	0	0.02	0.06	0.04	0.50
Basketball	0.22	0	0.01	0.08	0.52	0.30	0.88
Hockey	0.04	0	0	0.01	0.07	0.08	0.81
Soccer	0.08	0	0.01	0.11	0.14	0.07	0.91
Track and field events	0.10	0	0.01	0.08	0.24	0.07	1.37
Volleyball and similar games	0.18	0	0.01	0.11	0.34	0.29	0.98
Other organized games	0.32	0.09	0.10	0.32	0.65	0.25	0.93
Swimming	0.04	0	0	0.01	0.09	0.07	0.71
Showers and dressing rooms	0.05	0	0	0.01	0.14	0.04	0.81
Intra-mural sports	0.04	0	‡	0.05	0.07	0.05	0.84
Baseball—hard ball	‡	0	0	0	‡	‡	0
Baseball—soft ball	‡	0	0	0	0.01	0	1.00
Football—regular	‡	0	0	‡	0	0	0.50
Football—touch	‡	0	0	0	0	0.01	0.75
Basketball	0.01	0	‡	0.01	0.01	0.02	0.98
Inter-scholastic sports	0.18	0	0	0.02	0.19	0.56	0.74
Baseball—hard ball	0	0	0	0	0	0	0
Baseball—soft ball	0.01	0	0	‡	0.01	0.04	0.69
Football—regular	‡	0	0	0	‡	0.01	0
Basketball	0.07	0	0	0.01	0.08	0.22	0.62
Track and field events	0.04	0	0	0.01	0.05	0.09	1.10
Special activities	0.07	0.11	0.03	0.07	0.08	0.10	1.32
Trips or excursions	0.04	0.11	0.03	0.04	0.04	0.04	1.11
Student dramatics	‡	0	0	‡	0	‡	0.25
Student concerts	‡	0	0	0	‡	‡	0
Going to and from school (MV)	0.17	0.36	0.16	0.11	0.22	0.14	1.91
School bus	0.08	0.09	0.05	0.05	0.13	0.05	1.00
Public carrier (incl. bus)	0.01	0.08	0.01	0.01	0.02	‡	2.75
Motor scooter	‡	0	‡	0	‡	0	0.33
Other mot. veh.—pedestrian	0.05	0.14	0.07	0.03	0.05	0.02	3.85
Other mot. veh.—bicycle	‡	0	0	0	‡	‡	1.75
Other mot. veh.—other type	0.03	0.05	0.03	0.02	0.02	0.07	1.54
Going to, from school (not MV)	0.11	0.22	0.11	0.14	0.10	0.09	2.42
Bicycle—not mot. veh.	0.01	0	‡	0.02	0.01	0	1.14
Other street and sidewalk	0.07	0.17	0.07	0.09	0.06	0.07	1.32

*See footnote for Table 5-1.
†Some totals include data not shown separately.
‡Less than 0.005.
Source: *Accident Facts*, National Safety Council, Chicago, 1977.

119

injuries is to prohibit the activities in which they are likely to occur. To ensure students' safety by depriving them of valuable recreation is obviously an undesirable solution to the accident problem. Unless supervisory personnel take the necessary steps to prove that there is a satisfactory alternative, and that proper attention to safety can minimize sports casualties without restricting participation, such a solution is inevitable.

ANALYZING CAUSES AND SETTING OBJECTIVES

To plan an effective accident-prevention program, physical education teachers, coaches, and recreation leaders must thoroughly understand the environmental hazards and faulty practices responsible for injuries sustained in interscholastic and recreational sports. *Accident Facts,* as well as other sources, indicates that most of these casualties can be attributed to one or more of the following causes: inadequate leadership, faulty equipment, inadequate community recreational facilities, irresponsible student behavior, insufficient skill, poor physical condition, and risks inherent in the activity itself.

Further analysis reveals that poor leadership and supervision, at least in the past, has been *directly* responsible for fully one-third of the accidents arising from athletic participation and has been partly responsible for nearly all such accidents.[2] In other words, a thoroughly competent instructor can eliminate most of the conditions that are likely to lead to injuries.

Conscientious teachers do not attempt to minimize their own responsibility for students' safety by assuming a fatalistic attitude toward injuries resulting from voluntary participation in sports known to be hazardous. Realizing that most of the risks associated with athletic activities can be countered by precautionary measures, they try to determine all the potential dangers in the program, remove or compensate for every conceivable hazard, and help students acquire the knowledge, skills, and attitudes required for safe participation. Relatively few casualties result from the unavoidable risks inherent in an activity. As the following statistics illustrate, the number of injuries sustained in the various sports does not necessarily correlate with the degree of danger in those sports.[3]

Sport	Percentage of Injuries per 1,000 Participants
Touch football	17.11
Heavy apparatus	13.68
Football	8.75
Wrestling	5.76
Tumbling	5.10

[2]Frank Lloyd et al., *Safety in Athletics,* W. B. Saunders Company, Philadelphia, 1936, pp. 36 ff. See also current edition of *Accident Facts.*
[3]Frank Lloyd, *Safety in Physical Education,* Recreation Bulletin Service, no. 2821, 1933.

It is particularly remarkable that touch football occasions almost twice as many injuries as does football, which is a far more dangerous sport. However, this discrepancy can be readily explained. Most high school football players have competent coaches and officials, use properly fitted, up-to-date equipment, understand and respect the rules of the game, and possess strength, endurance, and skill. Touch-football players must cope with inadequate leadership and poor officiating, second-rate equipment, and unimproved playing fields. The players generally lack essential skills, assume little responsibility for their own safety, and tend to be physically inferior to members of the varsity team.[4] Although instructors recognize that football is hazardous and make a determined effort to prevent injuries in that sport, they apparently underestimate the degree of risk involved in touch football and thus fail to institute the necessary safety measures. There can be no doubt, therefore, that the teacher who fully understands the potential dangers in the activities he or she supervises can effectively compensate for most of the risks involved.

The primary aim of the safety program must be to minimize the number of injuries in sports and related activities while extending the benefits of participation to as many students as possible. The following specific objectives are implicit in this major purpose:

1 To help students accept responsibility for their own safety and that of fellow participants

2 To provide safe equipment and facilities

3 To help students develop a degree of physical fitness and skill commensurate with safe participation in athletic activities

4 To institute the administrative controls necessary to ensure optimum protection for participants in the physical education program

5 To recognize and guard against the particular hazards associated with each activity included in the physical education program

ACHIEVING THE OBJECTIVES—GENERAL PROCEDURES

The teacher must analyze each activity he or she supervises to determine the particular hazards involved and the specific steps that should be taken to remove or compensate for them. However, nearly all accidents in the physical education program spring from the same basic causes and call for essentially the same preventive measures. If instructors thoroughly understand the general safety procedures that should be instituted, they should have very little difficulty in applying them to particular activities. Competence in accident prevention necessitates a more careful reporting and study of accidents, as is done in industry. All accidents should be carefully analyzed to prevent recurrence.

[4]*Ibid.*

ACCIDENT-REPORTING SYSTEMS FOR SPORTS

In recent years a great deal of emphasis has been placed on developing an effective accident-reporting system for sports.

"Such a system will lead to the systematic collection of valid and reliable data and material evidence which, if utilized properly, can eliminate most potential accident hazards, and minimize the consequences of mishaps which do occur. Unfortunately there is no one system that is available, on a national basis, that would provide the kind of information needed for supervisory and administrative personnel to implement accident-prevention programs. This is particularly true in sport activities where certain inherent features exist, such as:

1 Certain unique risks and potential hazards which are associated with each sport activity.
2 Competitive behaviors common to all sports in varying degrees of aggressiveness.
3 The dynamics of risk-taking desires or needs possessed to some extent by all sports participants.
4 Personal variables of participants such as their interest, motivation, skill, maturity, and knowledge.
5 Societal influences which affect participants' (and their leaders) behavior and performances in sport activities.
6 Inadequate and overcrowded sport areas and facilities.
7 Discrepancies and failures of sports products and especially personal protective supplies, devices and clothing, and
8 Laxity of officials in enforcing the rules and regulations designed to safeguard participants."[5]

Until an effective sports accident-reporting system is developed, it is reassuring to know that several systems exist that can help the professional sports safety practitioner attack the accident problem. A brief description of each system follows.

THE NATIONAL SAFETY COUNCIL SYSTEM

This system has provided guidelines and materials to educational institutions for many years. It publishes guidelines specifically designated for the elementary and secondary school levels, including sections on sports accidents. (See Chapter 4 for a sample of the accident report form.) For a detailed description of this system see the National Safety Council's *Student Accident Reporting Guide Book* and *Accident Surveillance System For Sports,* p. 62.

THE NATIONAL ELECTRONIC INJURY SURVEILLANCE SYSTEM (NEISS)

The U.S. Consumer Product Safety Commission was activated in May 1973. The commission was called upon to create an Injury Information Clearinghouse to provide clear and accurate information about product-related injuries. The

---

[5]Frazier C. Damron, *Accident Surveillance System for Sports,* Sports Safety Series, Monograph no. 2, American School and Community Safety Association, and Association of the American Alliance For Health, Physical Education, and Recreation, Washington, D.C. 1977, p. 22.

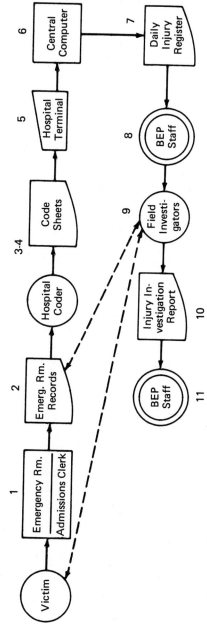

Figure 5-1 The path of an injury through the NEISS system.

123

TABLE 5–3
Injuries Associated with Selected Consumer Products Treated in Hospital Emergency Departments for March and for the 12 Months Ending June 31, 1978

Report Period   March   1978

| Product Codes | Description | Number of Cases | | Estimated Number of Cases | | Estimated Number of Product-Related Injuries per 100,000 Population* within the Contiguous United States which Were Treated in Hospital Emergency Rooms During the Last 12 Months Ending with This Report Period | | | | | | | | Estimated Mean Severity 12 Mos to Date |
| | | | | | | By Age | | | | | | By Sex | | |
		Report Period	12 Mos to Date	Report Period	12 Mos to Date	All Ages	00–04	05–14	15–24	25–64	65+	Male	Female	12 Mos to Date
12	Sports and recreational equipment													
04	Baseball, activity, related equip. and apparel	531	15,874	14,226	390,747	163.3	30.0	303.8	375.5	123.9	3.0	275.9	94.7	21
05	Basketball, activity and related equipment	2,045	16,115	47,559	354,560	166.4	4.2	223.7	513.3	65.7	.5	279.6	58.7	16
02	Bicycles and bicycle equipment	882	20,519	21,478	477,207	223.9	261.3	840.5	189.2	41.6	9.5	303.5	148.1	40
10	Fishing equipment	60	1,582	1,816	58,183	27.3	12.1	64.2	26.6	20.1	7.7	46.4	9.2	28
11	Football, activity, related equip. and apparel	252	17,622	4,624	402,541	188.9	5.4	412.2	539.1	31.0	—	370.2	16.6	22
12,13	Golf equipment (incl. golf carts)	32	701	592	18,543	8.7	8.5	20.1	4.5	6.9	4.6	12.3	5.3	36
37	Guns, gas, air and spring-operated, incl. BB guns	42	525	844	11,839	5.6	6.1	19.4	6.8	.8	—	9.4	1.9	36

TABLE 5–3 *(continued)*

33,72	Gymnastics, activity and related equipment	337	2,606	8,398	67,299	31.6	10.2	111.3	52.4	2.3	1.9	27.4	35.5	19
79,95,96	Hockey equipment and apparel	291	2,287	5,949	38,453	18.0	.6	31.5	52.9	5.4	—	31.9	4.8	24
45	Ice skates	110	1,291	3,468	35,087	16.5	3.7	35.7	21.0	12.5	2.3	16.9	15.6	29
3204	Motor scooters, minibikes. and other such vehicles	47	771	1,130	19,530	9.2	3.2	28.4	13.8	2.7	.6	14.9	3.8	56
1333	Skateboards	348	5,739	7,378	133,958	62.9	15.1	241.0	73.8	11.3	.3	86.5	40.4	32
16,98	Snow skiing and related equipment	538	3,037	19,141	107,480	50.4	2.4	77.0	122.3	29.9	.4	65.1	36.3	24
67	Soccer	146	2,843	3,539	64,370	30.2	.4	72.3	68.0	10.1	—	46.7	14.5	18
78	Swimming pool diving boards	7	339	190	8,290	3.9	1.3	10.4	6.9	1.4	—	5.3	2.5	26
77	Swimming pool water slides	1	28	9	842	.4	.4	1.0	.3	.3	—	.6	.2	20
84	Swimming pool, not otherwise specified	24	1,337	703	35,574	16.7	15.7	42.7	22.2	7.7	2.8	20.8	12.7	101
31	Swimming pools and associated equip.	13	847	188	18,337	8.6	5.4	22.2	15.6	2.8	.5	11.3	6.0	71
62	Swimming pools, above ground	1	85	14	1,614	.8	.7	2.4	.5	.4	.1	.8	.7	22
41–44,89	Swings, slides, seesaws, and climbing apparatus	309	5,008	7,830	145,310	68.2	263.1	250.9	13.8	3.3	1.2	69.1	67.3	28
17,73,74, 99	Toboggans, sleds, snow discs, and snow tubing	105	1,993	3,061	57,522	27.0	12.2	72.1	45.4	10.2	1.2	34.9	19.4	42
46	Wading pools	—	11	—	700	.3	.5	1.6	—	—	—	.6	.1	86

Source: *NEISS Data Highlights*, vol. 2, no. 3, March, 1978.

125

commission now operates the National Electronic Injury Surveillance System, which monitors 119 hospital emergency rooms nationwide for injuries associated with consumer products. Figure 5-1 provides a schematic diagram showing how the NEISS system relates to sports safety.[6]

For a detailed description of how the system operates, see U.S. Consumer Product Safety Commission, National Electronic Injury Surveillance System. *NEISS News,* vol. 1, June, 1973, Washington. In addition to published monthly reports and annual reports (Table 5-3), (the commission also provides a summary report listing injury-related products, and activities, according to satistical frequency (Table 5-4).

NATIONAL CENTER FOR HEALTH STATISTICS

This agency, a division of the U.S. Public Health Service of the Department of Health, Education, and Welfare, deals with national accident statistics but does not provide or collect information on accidents in sports or physical education activities. The agency does record some recreational accidents.

OCCUPATIONAL SAFETY AND HEALTH SYSTEM

This system was established by the Occupational Safety Health Act of 1970. It provides information pertaining to professional sports accidents, which are classified as work-related injuries.

NATIONAL ATHLETIC INJURY REPORTING SYSTEM (NAIRS)

The National Athletic Injury/Illness Reporting System was established at Pennsylvania State University in 1973. It represents the most comprehensive system in the world for the analysis of data about high school and college athletics. More than 793 sports teams participate in the system, which has been patterned after the National Electronic Injury Surveillance System (NEISS) developed by the U.S. Consumer Product Safety Commission. (Figures 5–2 and 5–3).

At the beginning of each athletic season, institution abstracts are sent to the Pennsylvania State University campus to record relevant data about the high school or college. A participant abstract, using a code number without a name, provides essential information on each male and female participant. Whenever an injury is incurred, a case abstract is completed by a trained recorder and immediately sent to NAIRS. All the information is edited for completeness and accuracy, and is prepared for computer analysis.

Many sophisticated computer programs have been developed specifically to analyze these data. Factors such as playing surface, type of equipment worn, precise diagnosis of the injury, experience of the athlete, time of day, etc., can

---

[6]Ibid., p. 8.

TABLE 5–4
NEISS Frequency Rank of Injuries Related to Sports and Recreational Equipment, July, 1972, through June, 1973.

Code Number		Frequency	Severity
1202	Bicycle and bicycle equipment	17,411	33
1214	Football, activity and related equipment	12,591	22
1205	Basketball, activity and related equipment	9,492	16
1204	Baseball, activity and related equipment	8,983	23
1265	Sports ball, not specified	3,207	18
1241	Swings	2,788	30
1216	Snow skiing and associated equipment	1,887	20
1214	Hockey equipment	1,640	27
1210	Fishing equipment	1,569	26
1231	Swimming pools and associated equipment, not including above-ground pools	1,415	79
1245	Ice skates	1,164	21
1266	Volleyball	1,161	15
1244	Playground climbing apparatus	1,094	30
1242	Slides	1,010	34
1263	Mini-bikes	1,003	34
1267	Soccer	1,000	22
1219	Tennis and badminton equipment	918	19
1270	Wrestling—organized activity and related equipment	756	25
1272	Gymnastics and associated equipment	749	22
1212	Golf equipment except golf carts	704	31
1200	Sports and recreational equipment	636	25
1233	Trampolines	551	20
1203	Boats, motors, and accessories for recreational use	502	48
1218	Snowmobiles	480	44
1206	Bowling, activity and related equipment	474	16
1237	Gas- Air- and Spring-operated guns	452	38
1262	Swimming pools, above-ground	432	59
1217	Sleds	424	33
1204	Playground equipment not elsewhere classified	414	26
1209	Exercise equipment	408	36
1264	Water skiing and associated equipment	359	24
1273	Toboggans	321	34
1268	Track and field activities and related equipment	300	23
1230	Camping trailers, other than mobile homes	264	28
1236	Unlicensed motor scooters and go-karts	248	23
1243	See saws	236	26

Source: *NEISS Data Highlights*, vol. 2, no. 3, March, 1978.

be analyzed simultaneously to identify the relative importance of each variable that contributed to the injury. Participating institutions receive credible information on the nature and extent of injury or illness among their athletes. The use of such a system also provides coaches, athletic trainers, league officials, rules committees, and sporting goods manufacturers with information to help make

CODE 0 OR 00 IF "UNKNOWN" CHECK OR PRINT CODES THAT APPLY

NAIRS—I

75—76

SPORT SEASON
CLOSEOUT
ABSTRACT

1. INSTITUTION ⬚⬚⬚⬚⬚⬚⬚ **2. SPORT** ⬚⬚

3. PRIMARY PHYSICIAN SUPERVISION
[1] Team Physician(s), Institution Staff
[2] Team Physician(s), Community based
[3] Clinic/Hospital
[4] Community Physicians as needed
[5] Other

Also Code:
[1] M.D. [3] D.C.
[2] D.O. [4] Other

4. PRIMARY NON-PHYSICIAN SUPERVISION
[71] Athletic Trainer, NATA Certified Member
[72] Athletic Trainer, NATA Associate Member
[73] Athletic Trainer, Other
[74] Coaching Staff [77] Emergency Care Personnel
[75] Student [78] Parent
[76] School Nurse [79] Other _____

5. COACHING STAFF SIZE ⬚⬚

6. HEAD COACH

Sex
[1] Male
[2] Female

Education
[1] Bacc. Degree, PE major or minor
[2] Bacc. Degree, other
[3] Masters Degree, PE major or minor, undergrad or grad
[4] Masters Degree, other
[5] Doctorate, PE major or minor, undergrad or grad
[6] Doctorate, other
[7] No college degree

Experience Coaching This Sport
[1] 1—2 years
[2] 3—5 years
[3] 6—10 years
[4] 10 + years

Experience Playing This Sport
[1] 1—2 years, h.s. only
[2] 1—2 years, college only
[3] 3—6 years, h.s. only
[4] 3—6 years, college only
[5] 3—6 years, h.s. and college
[6] 3—6 years, college and post college
[7] 6 + years, college and post college
[8] None

7. COACHING PREFERENCES*

1—Yes

	Pre-Season	In Season
Isometrics	⬚	⬚
Endurance Training	⬚	⬚
Weight Training	⬚	⬚
Flexibility Training	⬚	⬚
Taped Ankles	⬚	⬚
Wrapped Ankle	⬚	⬚

*Record yes if prescribed routinely for squad

8. PRESEASON MEDICAL EXAM
[1] Required only for athlete's first sport of year
[2] Required for each sport
[3] Required only for athlete's first sport in institution
[4] Not required

9. FACILITIES*

Surface
Primary Practice Arena ⬚⬚
Home Contest ⬚⬚

*See item 12 in Code Book under the respective sport.

10. EQUIPMENT*

		Type	Brand	% of Squad	Vintage
HEADGEAR:	1	⬚⬚	⬚⬚⬚	⬚⬚	⬚
	2	⬚⬚	⬚⬚⬚	⬚⬚	⬚
	3	⬚⬚	⬚⬚⬚	⬚⬚	⬚
	4	⬚⬚	⬚⬚⬚	⬚⬚	⬚
DENTAL GUARD:	1	⬚⬚	⬚⬚⬚	⬚⬚	
	2	⬚⬚	⬚⬚⬚	⬚⬚	
SHOES, Natural Surface:	1	⬚⬚	⬚⬚⬚	⬚⬚	
	2	⬚⬚	⬚⬚⬚	⬚⬚	
	3	⬚⬚	⬚⬚⬚	⬚⬚	
	4	⬚⬚	⬚⬚⬚	⬚⬚	
SHOES, Artificial Surface:	1	⬚⬚	⬚⬚⬚	⬚⬚	
	2	⬚⬚	⬚⬚⬚	⬚⬚	
	3	⬚⬚	⬚⬚⬚	⬚⬚	
	4	⬚⬚	⬚⬚⬚	⬚⬚	

Code for Vintage

1—New this season
2—New previous season
3—Used previous season
4—Reconditioned for this season
5—Reconditioned previous season(s)

*See item 15 in Code Book under the respective sport

11. PURCHASE OF PERSONAL EQUIPMENT (shoes, helmets, etc.)
[1] Institute responsibility
[2] Athlete responsibility
[3] Shared, primarily institution
[4] Shared, primarily athlete

12. WIN/LOSS RECORD
[1] Won at least two-thirds of contests
[2] Won between one-third and two-thirds of contests
[3] Won less than one-third of contests

RESEARCH (1) ⬚⬚ (2) ⬚⬚ (3) ⬚⬚ (4) ⬚⬚

Figure 5-2 Sample form of NAIRS Sports Season Closeout Abstract.

CODE 0 OR 00 IF "UNKNOWN" CHECK OR PRINT CODES THAT APPLY

1. INSTITUTION

2. PARTICIPANT

Sport Athlete Episode

NAIRS—I

75—76

CASE ABSTRACT

3. ONSET

Date Month

4. TIME

[1] AM (Before Noon)
[2] Aft (Noon-6pm)
[3] Eve (After 6pm)

5. RETURN

Date Month

6. DIAGNOSIS
Principal Other

If Extremity
[1] Rt
[2] Lt

REMARKS:

7. OCCASION

10 Not Sport-Related
  [11] Residence
  [12] Vehicle, Passenger
  [13] Vehicle, Pedestrian
  [14] School, not sport/phys ed
  [15] Job
  [16] Public, Other

2* Varsity Sports
  [20] Competition, Home
  [21] Competition, Away
  [22] Competition, Warmup
  [23] Team Travel, Vehicle
  [24] Team Travel, Other
  [25] Locker/Shower/Training Room
  [26] Between Lockerroom/Arena
  [27] Practice/Skill Training
  [28] Practice/Conditioning
  [29] Practice/Competition

3* Sub-Varsity Sports

4* Club Sports

5* Intramural Sports

6* Physical Education

7* Community Recreation

8* Other Varsity Sport

90 Other: _____

*for second digit, refer to
Varsity Sport subheadings

WHEN STRICKEN:

9. POSITION

10. ACTIVITY

11. SITUATION

12. SURFACE

**13. SURFACE
CONDITION**

[1] Normal
[2] Icy
[3] Snow-covered
[4] Wet
[5] Slippery, not wet
[6] Muddy
[7] Baked/Hard
[8] Irregular

**14. PROTECTION OF
INJURED BODY
PART**

[1] None
[2] Taped
[3] Wrapped
[4] Specially padded
[5] Customary uniform
[6] Bandaged
[7] Brace
[8] Cast

15. EQUIPMENT INVOLVED

Type Brand Vintage

Code for Vintage

1 New this season
2 New previous season
3 Used previous
  season
4 Reconditioned for
  this season
5 Reconditioned pre-
  vious season(s)

16. NATURE OF INJURY/ILLNESS

[1] New Problem, this season and last
[2] Recurrence, this sport, this season
[3] Recurrence, this sport, last season
[4] Recurrence, other sport, since last season
[5] Complication, this sport, this season:

EPISODE

[6] Complication, other sport, since last season

17. ACTION TAKEN

[1] Not hospitalized, not confined to bed
[2] Hospitalized overnight or less and released
[3] Hospitalized at least two days
[4] Confined, other, at least two days

**18. PRINCIPAL MANAGEMENT OF
INJURY/ILLNESS**

[1] Surgery
[2] Superficial debridement, minor suturing, etc.
[3] Nonsurgical immobilization
[4] Formal physical therapy
[5] Prescription drug therapy
[6] Proprietary management (aspirin, butterfly bandage)
[7] Rest
[8] Post-season surgery scheduled (returned to play)

8. SOURCE OF DIAGNOSIS

Physician OR Non-Physician

[1] Team Physician,
  Institution Staff
[2] Team Physician,
  Community based
[3] Clinic/Hospital Staff
[4] Community Physician
[5] Other: _____

Also Code:
[1] M.D. [3] D.C.
[2] D.O. [4] Other: _____

[71] Athletic Trainer,
  NATA Certified Member
[72] Athletic Trainer,
  NATA Associate Member
[73] Athletic Trainer, Other
[74] Coaching Staff
[75] Student Trainer
[76] School Nurse
[77] Emergency Care Personnel
[78] Parent
[79] Other: _____

19. RESEARCH

(1) (2) (3) (4)

Figure 5-3 NAIRS abstract form for reporting details of reportable injuries.

participation in sports as safe as possible. Additional information can be obtained by writing to: The National Athletic Injury/Illness Reporting System, White Building, The Pennsylvania State University, University Park, Pa. 16802.

THE NATIONAL COLLEGIATE ATHLETIC ASSOCIATION (NCAA)

The American Football Coaches Association: The National Federation of State High School Associations Systems

These organizations support an extensive annual survey of football fatalities. "The program was initiated in 1931 with the main objective to make the game of football a safe and more enjoyable sports activity. At the conclusion of each season an annual report is issued which provides information on the number of fatalities directly related to football, age of players, activity engaged in, part of the body involved, and specific location of the injuries.[7]

Other data on sports accidents are made available through statewide Insurance Benefit Plans. A detailed description of one such successful plan is provided in *Accident Surveillance System For Sports,* pp. 32–42.

When a good accident-reporting system is implemented, it has a positive influence on the participants, school, and community. It demonstrates a sincere interest and concern for the safety of the individual participants. In numerous cases, a good accident-reporting system has assisted in avoiding legal entanglements and adverse public criticism.

DEVELOPING INDIVIDUAL RESPONSIBILITY

Many accidents in the physical education program can be prevented by adequate supervision. In swimming very few drownings occur where there is good supervision of the sport, but many drownings occur when no one is at hand to prevent a swimmer from taking unnecessary risks. Nobody can watch every person every minute; anyone who wants to break rules will have ample opportunity to do so, despite constant vigilance on the part of the instructor. Thus, the best way to avoid needless injuries, not only in school-sponsored sports but in related leisure-time activities, is to gain students' voluntary support for all phases of the safety program. The instructor who fails to train individuals to accept responsibility for their own safety must be considered negligent, however conscientiously the instructor's other duties are fulfilled.

PROMOTING THE PROPER ATTITUDE

Individuals will voluntarily obey only those safety rules which they recognize as personally desirable. If the instructor or coach merely presents them with a list of "don'ts" proscribing dangerous behavior, without bothering to explain its

---

[7]Ibid., p. 29.

relationship to their own welfare, they are likely to rebel against what seems to be a restriction on their freedom and pleasure. The popularity of sports, however, tends to make participants amenable to safety regulations that are presented as prerequisities to continued participation. Although participants must understand that foolhardy actions, not safe practices, are the real deterrent to worthwhile adventure, primary emphasis should be placed on the value of safe performance in increasing enjoyment.

If the proper philosophy of safety is established early in the instructor-participant relationship, it will facilitate acceptance of the specific precautions taught in connection with particular sports, and help develop respect for general safety principles that can be applied to most everyday experiences. Thus, the physical education instructor, coach, or recreation leader is in an excellent position not only to minimize risks in the gymnasium and on the playing field but to contribute to all phases of the school and community safety program.

An athletic coach can do much to help students develop respect for safety by setting a good example of sportsmanlike conduct. During all interscholastic contests, the coach should treat officials and opponents with courtesy and fairness, neither abusing referees and umpires for their rulings on fouls nor encouraging any of the team's players in unnecessary roughness. The desire to win should never be allowed to take precedence over the requirements of safety, and the selfish desire of the individual must be subordinated to the best interests of the team. Rather than praise the star player who heroically stays in the game instead of reporting an injury, the coach should treat such conduct as foolish and immature. If the instructor's own competitive instinct is kept within bounds, the instructor should be able to train team members to be ruled by concern for the welfare of all participants and a sense of fair play, and to place a higher value on safe, ethical behavior than on victory.

PROMOTING SELF-GOVERNMENT

When students appreciate the various safeguards established for their protection and voluntarily obey safety rules, they will have learned to be good followers. But it is essential that they also learn to govern themselves in their own best interests, for external controls will not always be present to ensure their welfare.

Students tend to develop a sense of personal responsibility in proportion to the opportunities given them to plan, execute, and appraise their own activities. If they work out their own safety code, they will appreciate its value and the necessity of following it. With the guidance of the teacher, they can formulate regulations designed to eliminate or compensate for specific hazards that they can readily recognize, such as the danger of bumping into open locker doors or of slipping on the wet tile walk around the edge of the pool. The teacher must make sure that all standard safety measures are recommended for their consideration.

Students should be encouraged not only to formulate their own safety rules but to take an active part in enforcing them. The physical education teacher should assign carefully selected students to inspect equipment and facilities, help beginners develop basic skills, and supervise activities. Such a system provides desirable outlets for the restless energy of the most high-spirited adolescents. To ensure that all leadership duties will be adequately carried out, the instructor should assign each task to one individual, or to several, and make it clear that every student by fulfilling his or her particular duty contributes to the welfare and safety of all. Dividing responsibility helps ensure adequate coverage of all essential safety requirements and assists the teacher in carrying out his or her own duties, which might otherwise prove too demanding to be performed with sufficient care.

Students must be given every opportunity to solve their own problems so that they will assume responsibility for keeping themselves in good condition, checking equipment before using it, avoiding needless risks on the playing field, and conducting themselves with a due regard for safety at all times and under all conditions. "The ability to act in a proper and safe manner in a given situation is gained only by actually practicing in a learning situation the way of doing things which one is expected to follow in his everyday living. Therefore, activities should be planned to permit learning by doing. Pupil activities should be determined by the objectives to be achieved."[8]

PROVIDING SAFE FACILITIES AND EQUIPMENT

Faulty equipment and inadequate or improperly used facilities represent avoidable hazards that have caused many needless injuries in the physical education program. Conscientious adherence to the following practices should enable the teacher to eliminate or compensate for most environmental hazards.[9]

1 The teacher must see that sufficient funds are allotted to the physical education department to ensure purchase of the safest possible equipment and proper maintenance of all facilities and apparatus.

2 Safe, modern equipment must be provided in all areas of the physical education program. Students should be properly fitted with the personal protective equipment appropriate to the particular sport in which they are to engage—soft-soled or cleated shoes, helmets, knee guards, padded gloves, and so on. Anyone who wears glasses, unless he has unbreakable lenses or wears contact lenses, should be required to wear a guard when participating in such sports as football, basketball, and volley ball. Bows and arrows, guns, the trampoline table, the high horizontal bar, canoes, and other potentially dangerous apparatus and equipment should be used only by students who have the requisite skill and only when the teacher is present and has given his permission. Playground apparatus and all other equipment must be appropriate to the age group that is to use it.

3 Play areas should be regularly inspected and equipment and facilities kept in safe condition. Rough or splintered swing seats and slide surfaces should be immediately repaired; frayed ropes should be promptly replaced; jumping pits should be kept soft, smooth,

[8] *The Physical Education Instructor and Safety,* National Education Association, Washington, 1948, p. 26.
[9] D. C. Seaton *Safety in Sports,* Prentice-Hall, Inc., Englewood Cliffs, N.J., 1948, chap. 8.

and free of hard or sharp objects; and so on. No defective apparatus should, of course, be used until the necessary repairs have been made. All camping equipment should be carefully checked before starting for the camp site, guns must be kept in good working condition, and any personal equipment in need of repair should receive immediate attention.

All play areas should have smooth, even surfaces, and the gymnasium floor should be specially treated to minimize the danger of slipping. Any obstructions, such as pipes and radiators that protrude into the play area should be well padded, lest students injure themselves by striking against them. There should be adequate storage space, and the teacher should institute a good housekeeping system to ensure that all equipment is returned to its proper place, not left in the game areas, where it might cause falls. Good lighting must be installed in locker rooms, showers, and halls, and stable bleachers should be provided for spectators and kept in good condition. In older schools the teacher may have to compensate as well as he can for inadequate space and poor design, but if a new building is planned, he should see that the safest possible facilities are provided for physical education.

4 Adequate space should be provided for each activity. In many schools, the gymnasium and other play areas are not large enough to accommodate the student load, and activities must be restricted to those which can be safely conducted in the availabe space. When class size is a problem, the teacher should divide the group into two sections, allowing one to rest and observe while the other performs. If various activities are conducted simultaneously, sufficient room must be provided for each group in an area where its activities will not interfere with those of any other group. Playground apparatus should be concentrated in a section away from the usual flow of pedestrian traffic and away from all game areas, lest children en route to and from swings and slides risk being hit by a ball or colliding with older students. Swimming must be prohibited in the vicinity of the diving board; ample space must be allowed around jumping standards, and so on. There must be a reasonable amount of free space around tennis and basketball courts, the football field, and the baseball diamond; boundary lines should be clearly marked, and bleachers, players' benches, and other obstructions should be far enough outside the lines to meet the requirements of safety.

5 Before they are allowed to engage in a given activity, and at opportune times during such activity, students should be taught the safety rules for any apparatus they will have to use. Although primary emphasis must be placed on the positive benefits to be gained by following the proper procedures, due attention should also be paid to the injuries caused by incorrect practices and to the importance of preventive measures. Students should understand, for example, that there is some danger in falling when working on the horizontal bar or the rings and that mats must consequently be placed directly under and around such apparatus.

Participants should be encouraged to analyze all activities to determine the potential dangers represented by they various kinds of equipment and apparatus. They should recognize for themselves the precautions necessary to ensure their safety. A "break" or rest period between activities offers an ideal time for discussion of necessary safety precautions. Given an opportunity to assume responsibility, participants are much more likely to appreciate the importance of keeping away from moving swings, taking turns on gymnastic equipment, and so on, than if they are merely required to give unquestioning obedience to the teacher.

In organizing the physical education program, the instructor should allow students to help select activities and plan the safe use of available space and equipment. Students will be eager for an opportunity to participate in such enjoyable but potentially dangerous sports as canoeing and boating, archery, and hunting. If the instructor explains that these activities involve some degree of unusual risk and cannot be included in the program unless the proper precautions are faithfully observed, students should willingly help formulate and enforce the necessary safety rules.

DEVELOPING PHYSICAL FITNESS AND SKILL

Young people should need increasingly less supervision as they learn to assume responsibility for their own safety. However, it is unrealistic to hope that all students will become sufficiently self-disciplined to refrain from any activities that may be too strenuous or too difficult. Students' eagerness for adventure and excitement and their abundant energy, though desirable characteristics when properly directed, too often manifest themselves in reckless attempts to perform feats beyond their ability. Young people frequently fail to recognize the degree of strength and skill necessary for safe participation in a particular activity. They also tend to be emotionally immature, and their unrestrained feelings frequently warp their judgment and set up accident situations. High spirits following a victory by a narrow margin, for example, may show up in dangerous horseplay and daredevil stunts in the locker room unless the coach is on hand to direct the team's exuberance into desirable channels.

Students should not be allowed to engage in any activity until the instructor has made every possible effort to ensure that they are sufficiently skilled and in good enough condition, physically and emotionally, to do so without needlessly endangering themselves. To fulfill responsibility, the teacher must not only train students to participate safely in the activities he or she supervises, but discourage unorganized activities, which account for fully 20 percent of all school accidents.[10] If the physical education program is developed to meet students' interests and needs, insofar as is consistent with their natural ability and the requirements of safety, students will be less inclined to devise their own amusements.

Although eager to participate in sports, young people are often impatient with the conditioning exercises and practice sessions necessary to develop the strength, agility, and skill required for safety on the playing field. Too many students are satisfied with mediocre performance. They fail to realize, perhaps, that lack of skill in sports leads to unnecessary effort, resulting in awkwardness, a rapid onset of fatigue, and increased vulnerability to accidents.

Acquiring only a little skill too often leads to a dangerous complacency. People who manage to pass a 50-yard swimming test, for example, often develop unjustifiable faith in their proficiency and begin to take foolhardy chances. Because they fare well in supervised swimming areas, they erroneously assume that they have enough skill to risk swimming in unguarded waters. Students must learn to accept their limitations and to recognize the danger of overexerting themselves and attempting feats beyond their ability. With proper guidance, they can be made to understand that the effort required

---

[10]*Accident Facts*, National Safety Council, Chicago, 1977.

to improve skill will be amply rewarded not only by a greater assurance of safety but by the increased enjoyment that comes from doing things well.

Good physical condition, like skill, is a prerequisite for successful and safe participation in sports. Every athlete should have a thorough health examination at the beginning of the sport season. Any student who has been absent from school for even a short period because of an acute or chronic illness should be given a medical checkup before being allowed to reenter the physical education program.

Individual differences must be considered in deciding whether particular students should be permitted to engage in a given activity. Whether or not a sport should be classified as strenuous depends in largely on the individual participant. Because the physical education instructor may also be the coach, he or she is accustomed to dealing with athletically inclined youth and may underestimate the degree of stamina required for such sports as touch football and even volleyball. A trained athlete or a student who usually gets a great deal of physical exercise would not find these sports particularly strenuous, but they might be extremely taxing for one who normally leads a more sedentary life. Since physical education is usually compulsory, there are bound to be some participants who have little natural inclination to engage in sports and who must be slowly and carefully conditioned before they are required to do so.

If the instructor classifies students according to age, grade, size, and demonstrated ability, and restricts athletic competition to homogeneous groups, the less skilled will not have to overexert themselves to keep up with those who have greater natural ability, more experience, and higher performance standards. Equal competition assures each student of some success within his or her own group, thus preventing the poor athlete from developing a defeatist attitude, a sense of inferiority, and a consequent hatred of sports. In addition, it gives the potentially first-rate athlete competition as a stimulus to continued improvement. A special program, including sports as well as therapeutic exercises, should be planned to meet the interests, needs, and capacities of handicapped students.

To help students acquire the endurance, coordination, and other qualities necessary for safe participation in a given activity, the instructor should schedule a program of progressively more rigorous conditioning exercises. Special attention must be given to developing muscles and joints sufficiently strong and flexible to withstand the strain of vigorous sports. Warm-up exercises should always precede practice sessions and games to limber the muscles and prevent strains and other injuries.

Good health practices, including adequate rest, a well-balanced diet, and abstinence from nicotine, alcohol, and other harmful substances, must be stressed as an integral part of the conditioning process. High standards of hygiene must be taught in all phases of the physical education program. Athletes skilled in a particular sport should be encouraged to engage in related activities and to observe training rules throughout the year so that they will be in relatively good condition for the sport of their choice when its season arrives.

During athletic contests the coach should be alert to any signs of fatigue or injury among team members. Any player who does not seem in proper condition should be promptly taken out of the game. Although students should be instructed to report injuries immediately, love of the sport and an intensely competitive spirit will tempt many athletes to continue playing even when they are not in condition to do so safely. Coaches must therefore rely on their own observations in judging a player's condition. A sufficient number of substitutes is a necessity if team members are to be protected from overexertion; the conscientious instructor will discontinue an interscholastic sport if there are not at least twice as many qualified candidates for the team as there are positions to be filled.

ESTABLISHING ADDITIONAL CONTROLS

The following administrative controls, in addition to those governing equipment, facilities, and training, should be established to ensure that physical education injuries will be held to a minimum:

1 All activities should be supervised by a qualified teacher or a carefully trained student leader.

2 Competent officials should be secured for all contests, not merely for interscholastic games.

3 Safe transportation should be provided for all teams.

4 Games should be postponed when bad weather or other special circumstances make playing conditions particularly hazardous.

5 A definite procedure should be established for handling all accident cases and faithfully used whenever an accident occurs. Students should be urged to report all injuries without delay. First aid should be promptly administered for even minor cuts and bruises, which may lead to serious complications if neglected. A physician must be in attendance at all athletic contests and subject to call during practice sessions. Diagnosis and treatment, except for first aid, are properly the duties of a medical doctor and should never be assumed by the coach.

6 An accident-reporting system must be instituted to provide uniform, accurate records of all injuries. Reports should be studied as a basis for planning appropriate preventive measures (see Chapter 4).

7 All participants in the physical education program should be protected by health and accident insurance, which may be obtained at relatively low rates from either the state high school athletic association or a reputable commercial firm. Since a few injuries are inevitable in such sports as football, some form of insurance is an absolute necessity. Special attention should be given to the injury coverage plan for high school students, which not only finances medical care but offers such benefits as early attention to diagnosis and treatment of injuries and information on effective accident-prevention procedures.

8 Available figures show that more accidents occur in intramural sports than in varsity or physical education activities. Often lacking the safeguards of varsity sports, intramurals are participated in by students in poor physical condition, lacking adequate equipment and supervision, and with little concern about the prevention of accidents.

SAFETY GUIDELINES AND THE LAW[11]

The world of college athletics has not been able to avoid the "sue syndrome" which has permeated present day society.

In fact, the January issue of *Trial Magazine* devoted an entire article which provided guidelines for plaintiff attorneys in the preparation of a sports injury negligence case. The likelihood that a lawsuit is apt to be filed after any athletic injury of a serious nature puts an excessive amount of pressure on administrators, coaches and all involved with athletics. Sports injury litigation is a legitimate concern.

Liability

Liability—its responsibilities and ramifications—has always been a concern of responsible athletic administrators and coaches. However, in recent years, those associated with intercollegiate athletics have been exposed to a much broader interpretation of liability than ever before.

The "government immunity" concept under which educational institutions operated for many years is no longer commonly accepted. In addition, the "assumed risk" theory has been redefined. In the past, it was accepted that athletics possessed certain hazards and those who participated assumed the risk of injury.

To a certain extent, the theory is still accepted. However, if it can be proven the injured athlete was unaware of the potential dangers involved in the sport then the theory is not applicable.

The NCAA Committee on Competitive Safeguards and Medical Aspects of Sports has considered the sports injury litigation problem. The Committee assumes that those who sponsor and govern athletic programs have accepted the responsibility of attempting to keep the risk of injury reasonable.

However, lawsuits only need a complaint to exist. It is the Committee's contention the principal defense against an unwarranted complaint is documentation that adequate measures have been taken and programs have been established to minimize the risk inherent in sport. It must be noted no checklist is ever complete, but the following should serve as a review of considerations for those responsible for the administration of intercollegiate sports programs:

Preparticipation medical exam. Before an athlete accepts the rigors of organized sport, his/her health status should be evaluated. When the athlete first enters the college athletic program, a thorough exam should be required. Subsequently, an annual health history update with use of referral exams when warranted is sufficient. (A formal statement in this regard has been prepared for consideration by the membership during the annual Convention.)

Health insurance. Each student-athlete should have or secure, by parental coverage or institutional plan, access to customary hospitalization and physician benefits for defraying the costs of a significant injury or illness.

Preseason preparation. Particular practices and controls should protect the candidate from premature exposure to the full rigors of the sport. Preseason conditioning recommendations will help the candidate arrive at the first practice at optimal readiness. Attention to heat stress and cautious matching of candidates during the first weeks are additional considerations.

[11]*National Collegiate Athletic Association News,* October 15, 1977.

Acceptance of risk. "Implied consent" or "waiver of responsibility" by athletes, or their parents if of minority age, should be based on an informed awareness of the risk of injury being accepted as a result of the student-athlete's participation in the sport involved. Not only does the individual share responsibility in preventive measures, but he or she should appreciate the nature and significance of these measures.

Planning and supervision. Competent attention to a sizable group of energetic and highly motivated student-athletes can only come from appropriate planning. Such planning should ensure both general supervision and organized instruction. Instruction should include individualized attention to the refinements of skill development and conditioning. In addition, first aid evaluations should be included with the instruction. Such planning for particular health and safety concerns should take into consideration conditions which are encountered during travel for competitive purposes as well.

Equipment

Equipment. As a result of the increase in product liability litigation, purchasers of equipment should be aware of impending as well as current safety standards being recommended by authoritative groups and utilize only known reputable dealers. In addition, attention should be directed to the proper repair and fitting of equipment.

The National Operating Committee on Standards for Athletic Equipment (NOCSAE) has established a voluntary football helmet standard which has been adopted by the NCAA Football Rules Committee. By 1978, all new helmet models being worn must meet the NOCSAE Standard.

Facility. The adequacy and conditions of the facilities used for particular activities should not be overlooked, and periodic examination of the facilities should be conducted. Inspection of the facilities should include not only the competitive area, but warm-up and adjacent areas.

Emergency care. Reasonable attention to all possible preventive measures will not eliminate sports injuries. Each scheduled session, practice or contest of an institution-sponsored sport therefore should have the following:

The presence or immediate availability of a person qualified and delegated to render emergency care to a stricken participant.

Planned access to a physician by phone or nearby presence for prompt medical evaluation of the situation when warranted.

Planned access to a medical facility—including a plan for communication and transportation between the athletic site and medical facility—for prompt medical services when warranted.

A thorough understanding by all affected parties, including the leadership of visiting teams, of the personnel and procedures involved.

Records. Documentation is fundamental to administration. Authoritative sports safety regulations, standards and guidelines kept current and on file provide ready reference and understanding. Waiver forms may not prevent lawsuits but they help reflect organized attention to injury control.

ACHIEVING THE OBJECTIVES—SPECIFIC APPLICATIONS

In addition to understanding these general safety procedures, the instructor, as well as the students, should recognize their specific application to the entire physical education program. The instructor must be fully aware of the particular hazards associated with each activity, the methods by which avoidable hazards can be removed, and the steps that should be taken to compensate for necessary risks inherent in various sports.

Teachers, coaches, equipment manufacturers, and other sports and recreational leaders have been untiring in their efforts to promote safety in sports participation. Few unavoidable hazards remain in even the most potentially dangerous activities. Improved protective devices, more stringent safety rules, and better-trained instructors have overcome many of the risks once considered inevitable. In the early days of baseball and hockey players did not wear the helmets that have since become standard equipment. The body shock caused by tackling and blocking in football has been greatly reduced by adequate padding. Punishing holds have been generally eliminated in wrestling, and careful spotting in tumbling has removed many gymnastic accidents. Further improvements may be expected, as the attention given to safety continues to increase. The day may come when the helmets boxers now wear in training will be required during competitive bouts.

SAFEGUARDING THE HEALTH OF THE ATHLETE[12]

Participation in athletics is a privilege involving both responsibilities and rights. The athlete's responsibilities are to play fair, to keep in training, and to conduct himself with credit to his sport and his school. In turn he has the right to optimal protection against injury as this may be assured through good conditioning and technical instruction, proper regulation and conditions of play, and adequate health supervision.

Periodic evaluation of each of these factors will help to assure a safe and healthful experience for players. The check list below contains the kinds of questions to be answered in such an appraisal.

Proper Conditioning helps to prevent injuries by hardening the body and increasing resistance to fatigue.
1 Are prospective players given directions and activities for preseason conditioning?
2 Is there a minimum of three weeks of practice before the first game or contest?
3 Are precautions taken to prevent heat exhaustion and heat stroke?
4 Is each player required to warm up thoroughly prior to participation?
5 Are substitutions made without hesitation when players evidence disability?

Careful Coaching leads to skillful performance, which lowers the incidence of injuries.
1 Is emphasis given to safety in teaching techniques and elements of play?
2 Are injuries analyzed to determine causes and to suggest preventive programs?
3 Are tactics discouraged that may increase the hazards and thus the incidence of injuries?
4 Are practice periods carefully planned and of reasonable duration?

Good Officiating promotes enjoyment of the game and the protection of players.
1 Are players as well as coaches thoroughly schooled in the rules of the game?
2 Are rules and regulations strictly enforced in practice periods as well as in games?
3 Are officials qualified both emotionally and technically for their responsibilities?
4 Do players and coaches respect the decisions of officals?

Right Equipment and Facilities serve a unique purpose in protection of players.
1 Is the best protective equipment provided for contact sports?
2 Is careful attention given to proper fitting and adjustment of equipment?

[12]American Medical Association, *Tips on Athletic Training*, VIII, 1969, p. 23.

3 Is equipment properly maintained, and are worn and outmoded items discarded?
4 Are proper areas of play provided and carefully maintained?

Adequate Medical Care is a necessity in the prevention and control of injuries.
   1 Is there a thorough preseason health history and medical examination?
   2 Is a physician present at contests and readily available during practice sessions?
   3 Does the physician make the decision as to whether an athlete should return to play following injury during games?
   4 Is authority from a physician required before an athlete can return to practice after being out of play because of disabling injury?
   5 Is the care given athletes by coach or trainer limited to first aid and medically prescribed services?

BASKETBALL

Basketball is considered a noncontact game. It was so intended by its originator, Dr. James A. Naismith, when he introduced the game in 1871. As basketball developed, it became less of a noncontact sport. Players today are bigger, faster, stronger, and in better condition, and the action is much rougher. There is a great deal of body contact and very little equipment to protect against injuries. Today's game involves intense nervous strain and requires great endurance. For these reasons, a participant must be in good physical condition if he or she is to play effectively and safely.

Although it is strenuous, basketball has a relatively low incidence of serious accidents in comparison with football and other physically demanding sports. Every season, however, a number of injuries result from collisions between players, poor physical condition, unnecessary roughness, poor officiating, inadequate personal equipment, slippery floors (from perspiration, dirt, or debris), inadequate play areas, tripping over play equipment, and more recently the unsportsmanlike conduct of spectators.

Agility, quickness, coordination, and desire are important qualities of a good basketball player. But the player must also be adequately conditioned to carry on assignments without undue fatigue, which often contributes to accidents. It would be wise to employ a strength-development program in conjunction with preseason or prepractice drills. Many coaches have found that such programs result in improved jumping ability, endurance, stamina, and confidence.

As basketball for women has evolved into a modern game, it has become a sport characterized by almost continuous running. Before a woman is ready to perform adequately in the modern game she must attain a high state of physical fitness. She must be well conditioned. Another important consideration for women players is proper rest and nutrition. A well-balanced diet of normal foods will provide all the protein an athlete needs for peak performance. This applies particulary to women players, who may be more concerned about weight problems than are male participants.

Suggestions to help minimize injuries during participation may be found in other sections of this chapter. Specific information dealing with personal gear, the physical plant and field equipment, practice and game routine, and general administrative precautions are presented.

TACKLE FOOTBALL

It has been estimated that close to 2 million young men participate in tackle football. The range extends from sandlot or semi-organized football to the highly organized professional, college, and university levels. It has been estimated that as many as half of the participants receive at least slight injuries each season. The U.S. Consumer Product Safety Commission estimates that each year over 230,000 people receive hospital emergency-room treatment for injuries associated with football and football equipment, with most injuries occurring at the high school and college levels.[13]

With trained coaches now employed to ensure adequate training for all players, with competent officiating, safe equipment, and equal competition, and with studies constantly in progress to improve safety measures, the risks involved in football are being reduced each year.

Since it is now widely recognized that organic vigor, muscular strength, and general good health, including freedom from even minor ailments, are required for safe participation in football, a preseason medical and dental examination is usually provided for all players. The current emphasis on conditioning procedures geared to the specific needs of participants and on adequate practice periods before actual competition has also helped prevent injuries. Muscles and joints that have grown weak from relative disuse are now gradually strengthened through carefully planned conditioning programs. Performing leg-extension exercises against resistance, for example, helps to develop strong thigh muscles and thus lessens the possibility of knee injuries.

In training players in fundamental football skills, the coach gives special attention to the methods of tackling, blocking, dodging, and falling that are least likely to cause injury. "Spearing," or driving the head directly into the chest of an opponent when blocking or tackling, has been condemned and prohibited. Adequate time must be given to the thorough learning of these fundamental skills. The coach is careful to teach students a type of game that is consistent with their ability, realizing that simple plays, well executed, are less likely to cause injury and more likely to result in victory than complicated plays poorly performed.

Football helmets are constantly being improved to offer greater protection against brain injury. Adequate shoulder and pelvic protectors have reduced the body shock that was once a major football hazard. Protective devices for the teeth, similar to the boxer's rubber mouthpiece, are now available for football players.

[13]U.S. Consumer Product Safety Commission Fact Sheet No. 42, *Football and Football Equipment,* October, 1974.

Keeping the playing field smooth and placing flexible yard markers and players' benches well behind the sidelines are additional safety measures that are now generally observed. The care taken to ensure competent officiating and to impress players with the importance of adhering strictly to the rules of the game has reduced the number of injuries attributed to unnecessary roughness. It is now standard practice to have a physician in attendance at all games and a stretcher in readiness. Most coaches understand that any team member who is hurt during the game should not be allowed to return to the playing field until the doctor has given approval.

Despite the progress made in reducing the number of football casualties, some preventable injuries still occur because of improper leadership. Presumably, examples of administrative negligence will become increasingly less common as more coaches recognize the causes of football accidents and the measures that can be taken to eliminate them. Players sometimes suffer ankle and knee injuries when they are furnished with football cleats unsuitable to the condition of the turf. Other casualties result from the coach's failure to remove team members from the game when they show signs of strain, to restrict practice periods to a reasonable length, and to see that all players remain active and warm during the entire session. "Warm-up" activities should be performed before a player is permitted to enter a game or practice. Adequate intake of salt water is recommended for replacement of fluid loss.

Planning too rigorous a football schedule may also increase the risks in the game. Conscientious coaches will avoid exploiting their teams by refusing to schedule games with larger schools that have heavier, more skillful players. Unequal competition, such as a contest between freshmen and seniors, often results in a high incidence of accidents among younger children, who are likely to suffer serious leg injuries as the result of the joint abuse endured in heavy body contact. The number of games scheduled during a season should be kept to a reasonable limit. In most instances postseason games should be avoided, not only because of the additional strain but because of the unfavorable weather conditions likely to prevail late in the year. Most of the safety principles recommended for football are applicable to such games as touch football, soccer, and field hockey.

TOUCH FOOTBALL

More people are playing touch football than ever before. Men and women, young and old, are playing touch football on pick-up teams, after school, and as weekend recreational activity. The informal nature of the game, together with the wide range of ability, experience, and physical condition of participants, creates potential accident situations. The field of play may be an open area which has the potential for accidents (chuck holes, tin cans, broken bottles, etc.).

Organized touch football as played in intramural, physical education, and recreation programs does have specific rules and regulations. However, many games are played on an informal basis, and rules are sometimes ignored. Little regard is given to physical fitness, and the mixture of younger and older players is conducive to mishaps.

There is little accurate information available upon which to base an accident-prevention program. There is some evidence that players who are equipped with protective garb, teamed according to size and ability, and instructed in proper play and safety techniques, adherence to rules and good officiating will have a lower accident potential. NAIRS is compiling additional data to prove this point. Touch football provides many individuals with an inexpensive recreational activity. It is relatively safe when played according to rules and regulations. Lack of respect for rules and of regard for other participants can make it a dangerous sport.[14]

BASEBALL AND SOFTBALL

Baseball activity with its related equipment, ranks fourth as a cause of sports accidents according to the U.S. Consumer Product Safety Commission. An analysis of the activities involved in the game is necessary if we are to understand how participation may be made safer.

According to one study, the most common baseball hazards are: running body contact, risk from bat and ball, hard throwing and swinging motion, and the barriers enclosing the field of play. Another study found the following types of injuries most prevalent: sprains, strains, contusions, pulled muscles, and fractures. These injuries were most commonly caused by: sliding and running between bases, throwing and running between bases, being struck by a pitched ball, collision between players, throwing, and sliding and being struck by a pitched ball.

According to baseball experts, knowledge of fundamentals and the specific skills necessary for each position is a deterrent to baseball accidents. The player who executes a play properly, who knows how to throw and slide as well as the overall strategy of playing, has reduced the potential for accidents.

Lack of proper physical conditioning also creates possibilities for accidents. Because the sport does not demand strenuous effort from most players throughout the game, this phase is sometimes neglected. In many cases this neglect is a direct cause of injury. Instructors, coaches, and managers must keep emphasizing the importance of staying "in shape" during the off-season as well as the playing season.

Proper supervision of play and practice is also necessary to keep accidents and injuries at a minimum. Equipment scattered on the ground, spectators crowding the playing area, loosely organized practices, and participants who "horse around" all contribute to the potential for accidents.

Proper equipment and facilities are needed if the sport is to be played safely. In organized programs, the furnishing of equipment and safe facilities is

[14]Joseph Dzenowages, "Touch and Flag Football," in *Safety in Team Sports,* American School and Community Safety Association Monograph No. 3, chap. 5, p. 33, 1977.

the responsibility of those conducting the activity. When the sport is played on an informal basis, playground instructors, supervisors, recreation leaders, and parents should assume responsibility. This is particularly true for Little League baseball.

Where to locate a field in reference to the sun; the location of light poles, fences, and fence posts; grass versus artificial turf; tools for care of the playing field; clean and well-ventilated shower and locker rooms—all these matters must be considered to ensure safe participation.

For additional detailed information describing the skills necessary for each position see "Baseball and Softball".[15]

GYMNASTICS

Young people are great imitators. They are likely to endanger themselves by attempting the gymnastic feats they have seen in the movies or at the circus. Watching such a performance gives one the impression that the routine is easy, as indeed it is for a trained acrobat. Students must be taught, therefore, that safe, competent gymnastic work requires a high degree of skill, which can be gained only through experience and much strenuous practice.

The instructor can help prevent injuries in the gymnastics class by regularly inspecting all apparatus and seeing that ropes, metal connections, and cable fastenings are kept in good condition. Instructors should make sure that mats are placed in strategic positions, that students wear hand guards to prevent blisters, and that ample space is provided between gymnastic apparatus and tumbling areas. They must be thoroughly familiar with the ability of each participant. No one should be allowed to attempt a feat for which he or she lacks the requisite degree of physical fitness and skill. All participants must understand that they are not to perform any stunt without the instructors permission.

THE TRAMPOLINE

Each year more than 19,000 people are treated in hospital emergency rooms for injuries associated with trampolines.[16] These injuries indicate that the trampoline can be a dangerous piece of equipment.

If the school owns a trampoline, extreme care must be taken to ensure its proper use. Because the trained trampoline performer seems to bound and soar high in the air and land easily, individuals tend to overlook the high degree of balancing skill, muscular control, and coordination required to avoid landing on the metal frame or hitting the canvas in a way likely to cause an injury. If these dangers are explained, performers should be willing to abide by the necessary safety measures. The trampoline looks like a great deal of fun, and individuals will be eager to use it. The wise instructor will make it clear that they will be permitted to do so only if they observe the proper precautions.

---

[15]Warren J. Huffman, in *Safety In Team Sports,* op cit., pp. 1–14.
[16]U.S. Consumer Product Safety Commission, Fact Sheet No. 85, *Trampoline,* February, 1976.

In using the trampoline, participants must be taught to "kill" the spring by bending their knees slightly immediately upon landing on the canvas, so that they will be able to control their bounce. Safety pads should be attached to the metal frame. Performers should be required to wear safety belts when learning new stunts, which should be attempted only after the basic preliminary bounces have been thoroughly mastered.

The trampoline should not be considered a back-yard toy or activity, but rather a piece of gymnasium equipment to be furnished with a proper safety frame and spring padding. There should be adequate personnel for spotting. All spotters should be instructed on how they can be most effective in preventing injuries. There should be at least one spotter on each side of the trampoline.

When supervised use of the equipment is over, the equipment should be locked and secured to prevent unathorized and unattended use.

A recent development regarding the trampoline has been the position of the American Academy of Pediatrics. Because trampoline accidents, stemming primarily from improper use of a somersault, have resulted in a significant number of cases of quadriplegics, the academy warns against all use of the trampoline in schools and colleges.

As a result of the above action, the American Alliance for Health, Physical Education and Recreation formulated and adopted the following statements at its national convention on April 10, 1978.

The use of trampoline for the development of competitive skills in sport

The controlled use of the trampoline as a training device for athletes in related sports (e.g., diving, gymnastics, pole vaulting) warrants clarification in lieu of the current concerns of appropriate safety considerations. The 1978 American Alliance for Health, Physical Education and Recreation Statement of the trampoline in physical education and recreational programs precludes the use of the somersault except for advanced students who are controlled by a safety harness.

However, the practice of utilizing the trampoline by varsity athletes for skill development have definable performance standards which exceed that justified for physical education and recreational programs. Further, the apparent safety record accompanying such use is admirable.

Consequently, the American Alliance for Health, Physical Education and Recreation extends to the organizations who are responsible for the conduct of sport its support of the following guidelines for those coaches who choose to utilize the trampoline for these purposes.

Continuous conscious attention must be given to the control of the risks accepted by proficient athletes pursuing the benefits of the trampoline in skill development for related sports. As is recommended for its controlled use in physical education, the trampoline should constitute an elective activity by the athlete requiring competent coaching supervision, skilled spotters aware of the routine being practiced, competent use of the safety harness while learning skills involving the somersault, security against unsupervised use, proper erecting and maintenance of the apparatus, a plan for emergency care should an accident occur, and the documentation of participation and any accidents which occur.

It should be emphasized that without the safety harness the best of spotting cannot intervene effectively to prevent serious neck injury and quadriplegia if an athlete lands incorrectly from a poorly executed skill. Yet, it is acknowledged that the competitive athlete at times requires freedom from the safety harness to refine and ready his/her skills for competition in another sport.

The use of trampolines and minitramps in physical education

Over the years, trampoline accidents have resulted in a significant number of cases of quadriplegia. The annual frequency appears to be low yet persistent. Late in 1977, the American Academy of Pediatrics took a public position that the trampoline was posing an undue risk of serious injury and therefore warned that it should not be utilized as a competitive sport nor as an activity within physical education.

Subsequently, further examination of injury patterns and the benefits justifying selective inclusion of the trampoline within a physical education program, whether in educational institutions or recreational settings, has permitted the American Alliance for Health, Physical Education and Recreation to formulate the following statement.

Risk of injury, including serious injury, accompanies many physical activities enjoyed by young persons, even under the best of conditions. The vast majority of known cases of quadriplegia resulting from trampoline accidents have stemmed from improper execution of a somersault. While there is little encouragement for trampolining as an interscholastic or intercollegiate event, the use of the trampoline in physical education classes does not apparently constitute an unreasonable risk of serious injury providing that the following controls are ensured:

1 That the program be offered as an elective. No student should be required to engage in trampolining. It follows that all new participants should be helped to appreciate the risks of this activity and the measures being taken to control those risks.

2 That the program be supervised by an instructor with professional preparation in teaching trampolining. This implies that the selection of skills being taught are commensurate with the readiness of the student in a proper progressive manner, and that reminders of injury control measures are incorporated in the teaching process. By supervision is meant direct observation of the activity plus intervention capabilities when warranted.

3 That spotters be in position whenever the trampoline is being used and that all students (and teaching aides, if used) be trained by the instructor in the principles and techniques of spotting.

4 That the somersault not be permitted to be attempted in regular classes. If special opportunities exist in the physical education program for advanced students with demonstrated proficiency, the foot-to-foot somersault may be taught if the safety harness is used and if the objective clearly is not to wean the student away from the harness to execute skills involving the somersault. The safety harness must be controlled by persons trained by the instructor and capable for this task.

5 That the apparatus be locked, and otherwise secured as best the facilities provide, to prevent unauthorized and unsupervised use.

6 That the apparatus be erected, inspected, and maintained in accordance with the manufacturer's recommendations.

7 That policies for emergency care be preplanned and actively understood by all affected personnel. This includes first aid competence at hand, class supervision during the initial management of the injured student, communicative accessibility to appropriate medical assistance when needed, and transportation capability to appropriate medical facility when needed.

8 That participation and accident records be maintained for the trampoline and other gymnastic apparatuses and periodically be analyzed.

The Trampolette (Minitramp). The minitramp, while different in nature and purpose from the trampoline, shares its association with risk of spinal cord injury from poorly executed somersaults. The best of mats do not provide substantial protection from the minitramp accident that leads to quadriplegia. As recommended for trampoline safety, the minitramp should constitute an elective activity requiring competent instruction and supervision, spotters trained for that function, emphasis on the danger of somersaults and dive-rolls, security against unsupervised use, proper erection and maintenance of the apparatus, a plan for emergency care should an accident occur, and documentation of participation and of any accidents which occur.

In addition to that stipulated in the preceding paragraph, the following constitute the controlled conditions to be ensured.

1. No multiple somersault be attempted.
2. No single somersault be attempted unless:
    a. the intended result is a foot-landing
    b. the student has demonstrated reasonable ability for such on the trampoline with a safety harness, off the diving board of a swimming pool, or in tumbling.
    c. a competent spotter(s) is in position, knowing the skill which the student is attempting, and physically capable of handling an improper execution. If the safety harness is employed, the instructor must be satisfied that it is controlled competently.
    d. the minitramp is reasonably secured to help prevent slipping at the time of execution.
    e. a mat should be utilized, sufficiently wide and long to prevent a landing on the mat's edge and provide for proper footing of the spotter(s).

CAMPING AND HIKING

Camping and hiking are relatively safe activities when they are carefully planned and all participants recognize and compensate for the risks involved. Camping in the great out-of-doors formerly involved many hazards and few comforts. Today carefully run camps provide an organized recreational program with trained personnel to take care of most of the chores and to supervise all potentially dangerous activities. Even those who prefer a more rugged type of camping can be spared many of the hazards formerly associated with outdoor life—unduly rough terrain, unimproved swimming facilities, mosquitoes, poison ivy—for such dangers have been or are being eliminated in most camping areas.

The principal danger in camping today lies in attempting to enjoy the outdoor life without observing the safety measures recommended by camp authorities. Current literature on camping includes detailed explanations of the proper procedures for using equipment, building a fire, and guarding against various kinds of injuries. Unfortunately too many campers are still ignorant of these procedures or careless about observing them.[17]

Camp-age children are at "a daredevil time of life," a time of great enthusiasm, high adventure, and often reckless daring, without the background and experience for judgment making. To guard against the child's tendency to get into dangerous situations, most camps for young people have set up thoroughgoing safety programs which provide a careful health examination for prospective campers, prompt and reliable medical care, protection against mosquitoes, a campsite cleared of poison ivy and other poisonous plants, inspection of drinking water, a sanitary, protected swimming area, well-enforced swimming and boating regulations, intelligent leadership by trained counselors, well-supervised arts and crafts shops, carefully planned hikes and

---

[17]"How to Keep Camping Carefree," *Family Safety,* vol. 28, no. 1, pp. 7–9, Spring, 1966.

trips, and instruction and practice in self-care under the rugged conditions of outdoor living.

In planning a camping and hiking trip, the organizers should restrict the group to those who are in good physical condition and who are similar in age, physical capacity, and interests. Before undertaking the trip, they should instruct potential campers in the hazards of outdoor life and the necessary precautions, and then assist the campers in formulating their own code for safe camping, based on their understanding of the risks involved. With the proper guidance, campers can easily appreciate the necessity of observing the following regulations:

1 Select a safe hiking trail.

2 Keep with your group.

3 When walking on a highway, stay on the extreme left-hand side of the road, facing oncoming traffic.

4 Avoid walking on the highway after dark.

5 Do not drink untested water.

6 Carry pure water with you.

7 Do not eat any fruit or other vegetation that you cannot definitely identify.

8 Learn to recognize poison ivy, poison oak, and poison sumac.

9 Avoid undue exposure to the sun. Wear a hat if you must be in the sun for a prolonged period.

10 Do not swim in rivers or lakes that have not been approved for this purpose.

Each camper should have comfortable, sturdy shoes; soft, woolen socks, including an extra pair in his or her pack; and a raincoat or poncho, regardless of weather predictions. Flashlights, matches, an ax, a compass, and a first-aid kit are also standard equipment.

A good campsite near enough to be reached comfortably before dark should be carefully chosen in advance, after permission to use it has been secured. The park or conservation commission in most states will gladly furnish information on public facilities suitable for camping. A careful inspection should be made to ensure that there are no poisonous plants or dangerous holes in the area. Water taken from a natural source at the site should be boiled for at least 1 minute before it is used for drinking. A simpler method is the use of water-purification tablets purchased at many drug stores and camp suppliers. The campfire should be built on a bare spot, free of leaves and other flammable underbrush. It must be thoroughly extinguished with plenty of water when no longer needed. It should be started early enough to provide a small bed of coals with a minimum of flame for preparing the meal, since a roaring fire would seriously endanger the cook as well as the dinner. All campers must understand and observe the safety rules governing the use of the ax and other camping implements. They should be taught to keep dangerous knives sheathed when not in use and to carry heavy equipment properly in order to minimize strain.

All special activities undertaken as part of the camping trip should be carefully planned and well organized, and the usual safety measures governing such activity should be faithfully observed. If a nearby mountain or hill is to be climbed, a competent leader should be selected, as well as someone to bring up the rear of the party and see that no one strays off or lags behind. No one should go swimming unless facilities have been investigated in advance and a qualified instructor is on hand. Even then, due care should be exercised in venturing into strange water. Its depth must be determined before any diving is allowed. The roll-call or buddy system should be used to ensure that all members of the group are present and safe.

At least one member of every camping group should be qualified to administer first aid, and any cuts or bruises should receive immediate attention. Since the soil of many fields is highly contaminated by tetanus organisms, improper cleansing of even the slightest wound may cause serious complications. If campers have had an immunization dose of tetanus toxoid early in life and if all cuts receive prompt and adequate treatment (which should include giving a booster shot of tetanus toxoid as soon as possible after the injury), the danger of this disease is slight. Although every effort should be made to avoid selecting a campsite in an area known to be inhabited by poisonous snakes, a snake-bite kit should be included with the first-aid equipment as an added precaution.

For mountain climbers, poor weather conditions constitute an important safety factor when visibility is limited and natural hazards may be hidden. Knowing how to act in the following weather conditions is important to survival; wind, rain, blizzards, white-out, dense fog, darkness, sun (desert), and lightning. Before attempting an extensive mountain-climbing trip, check local weather conditions and consult local authorities; rangers, mountain rescue units, etc.

HUNTING

Each fall millions of people take to the outdoors in search of game. More people participate in hunting in this country than in any other sport, with the possible exception of fishing. It is perhaps remarkable that only about 500 accidental deaths each year are directly attributable to hunting, especially since in most states anyone of legal age can obtain a license to own a gun by paying a small fee. Weapon manufacturers have done much to keep accident figures low by publicizing safety measures, but more intensive instruction in the proper use of firearms will undoubtedly result in an even better safety record.

Through the persistent efforts of the National Rifle Association, the Hunter Safety Training Program has been adopted with the aid of legislation in several states and voluntarily in others. In addition to offering instruction in the use of firearms and in handling firearms in the hunting field, the movement aims toward legislation which will limit the granting of hunting licenses to persons under sixteen years old (New York has raised the age to twenty-one) to those who have taken and passed a course in safe gun handling.

Education in firearms and in their use in hunting is a relatively new technique for making hunting safe. The favorable reception accorded to the program by educators, conservation leaders, and fish-and-game law-enforcement personnel is indicative of a constructive public attitude toward firearms education.

Instruction in firearms is sometimes discouraged at the high school level on the assumption that it arouses curiosity about guns and thus fosters their use by irresponsible adolescents. It is true that the victims of most firearms accidents are between the ages of fifteen and twenty-four, but this fact indicates a need for more, not less, training. Records show that young people who have been taught how to handle weapons properly usually operate them safely, but those who merely assume that they know how to use a gun are most often responsible for accidents.

Firearms accidents are commonly attributed to such human faults as handling loaded guns in and around the home and moving into the line of fire without giving warning, and to such mechanical hazards as weapons "accidentally" discharging and bullets ricocheting from a hard surface.

An analysis of hunting accidents conducted by the National Rifle Association several years ago showed that faulty judgment (victim out of sight of shooter, shooter swinging at game, victim mistaken for game, victim moving into line of fire) was a major contributing factor in 37 percent of the cases. Lack of skill and aptitude (stumbling or falling with weapon, trigger catching on an object, unloading weapon, loading weapon) caused 21 percent of the accidents. Violating rules and laws (removing weapon from vehicle, weapon falling from insecure rest, riding with loaded weapon, improper crossing of obstacles, horseplay with loaded weapon, clubbing cover or game) accounted for 14 percent and defective weapons and other unknown causes brought about the remaining 28 percent. Today, the percentages have probably changed, but it still can be stated that the underlying cause of most hunting casualties is inadequate knowledge of firearms. Too few hunters realize, for example, that a bullet fired from a .22-caliber rifle can travel as far as 500 yards after glancing off a flat surface. It can also crash through a 9-inch board. The familiar excuse, "I didn't know the gun was loaded," is further evidence of general ignorance concerning the proper use of firearms. The first step in handling any gun is to assume that it is loaded, point it in a safe direction, examine it at the breach, and remove any shells or cartridges. A gun should always be kept unloaded until it is time to use it, and then it should be kept on safety until just before it is aimed at the target.

President John F. Kennedy's assassination by gunfire kindled intensive debate regarding guns and the increase in armed crimes. The debate became even more heated after the assassinations of the Reverend Martin Luther King Jr. and Senator Robert F. Kennedy. The National Rifle Association maintains that it is not a gun problem but a *crime* problem, for people can be strangled or killed with a knife. Control of the *misuse* of guns continues to be a problem. The National Firearms Act (1934) outlaws machineguns, sawed-off shotguns, and rifles except by special license. The U.S. Post Office regulations ban the shipment of pistols to the general public. But undesirables obtain guns regardless. Guns can be lethal weapons whether considered as a form of protection, used in hunting or target practice, or regarded as collectors' items. Our problem is to encourage the proper use of these weapons and at the same time keep them out of the hands of undesirables.

Youngsters should be taught to use good judgment in playing with toy guns that shoot rubber-tipped projectiles. As they grow older and graduate to a BB gun and finally a .22 rifle, they will know where and where not to point a gun. The adult should take every opportunity to help them understand the precautions that must be taken in using a weapon, to ensure their own safety and that of others in their group. A visit to an archery range may impress a child with the importance of good "range hygiene," especially if attention is called to the care for group safety that participants exercise in waiting to retrieve their arrows until all shooting has ceased and everyone has laid down his or her bow.

Through proper instruction and supervised practice, youth can learn to remove all the unnecessary hazards associated with hunting and compensate for the unavoidable dangers connected with the actual firing of the weapon. In developing their own rules for the proper use of firearms, they should be guided by the following "Ten Commandments of Gun Safety."[18]

1 Treat every gun with the respect due a loaded gun. This is the cardinal rule of gun safety.

2 Carry only empty guns taken down or with the action open, into your automobile, camp, or home.

3 Always be sure that the barrel and action are clear of obstructions.

4 Always carry your gun so that you can control the direction of the muzzle, even if you stumble. Keep the safety on until you are ready to shoot. [Figure 5-4]

5 Be sure of your target before you pull the trigger.

6 Never point a gun at anything you do not want to shoot.

7 Never leave your gun unattended unless you unload it first.

8 Never climb a tree or fence with a loaded gun.

9 Never shoot at a flat, hard surface or the surface of water.

10 Avoid alcoholic drinks before or during shooting.

Guns are not the only hazards that face hunters.

For example more deer hunters die from heart attacks than from gun-shot wounds. Overexertion, falls, drownings, and exposure all take their toll.

A swig of spirits may seem to have a warming effect on a cold day, but its value is short lasting. Alcohol actually lowers skin temperature and also impairs judgment and coordination.

Hunting can be a dangerous sport, but if one is equipped with hunting and firearm safety information and competency, it need not result in an accident.[19]

---

[18]National Safety Council, Safety Education Data Sheet No. 3, rev., *Firearms*, National Safety Council, Chicago.

[19]National Safety Council, *Farm Safety Review*, pp. 9–10, September–October, 1977.

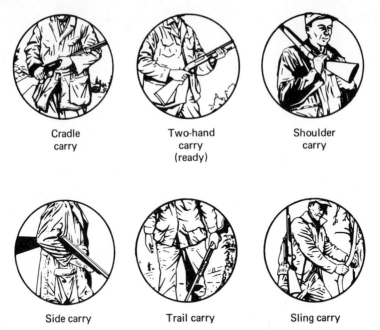

Cradle carry	Two-hand carry (ready)	Shoulder carry
Side carry	Trail carry	Sling carry

Figure 5-4 Safe gun carries. (Source: National Rifle Association Instructor's Manual, 1973, p. 85, Hunter Safety and Conservation Program, the National Rifle Association of America, Washington, D.C.)

PLAYGROUND ACTIVITIES

"The U.S. Consumer Product Safety Commission has estimated that more than 100,000 individuals are injured annually in accidents involving public and home playground equipment—injuries so serious that they require hospital emergency room treatment."[20] Most of these injuries are incurred by children between the ages of five and ten, followed by ages two to four and ten to fourteen.

The injured parts of the body were the areas above the neck, feet and hands, and the trunk. The most frequent types of injury were lacerations, fractures, contusions, and abrasions.

Swings, swing-set frames, gliders, horizontal bars, climbing apparatus, standing too close to moving equipment, exposed bolts and screws, and sharp edges—all these were factors in accidents. Horizontal bars and jungle gyms were the factor most commonly involved in the more serious injuries.[21]

Promoting safety in the playground, at school, and at home is largely a matter of providing well-planned and quality facilities and adequate supervision. Led by curiosity and propelled by abundant energy, young children are more than likely to fall victim to the various hazards in the play area, if not to create new hazards. The director or parent must exercise constant vigilance, immediately put a stop to any dangerous practices, and help offenders understand why their behavior is not acceptable. Young children will respect a firm

[20]U.S. Consumer Product Safety Commission, Fact Sheet No. 22, *Playground Equipment,* September, 1974.
[21] National Safety Council, *Accident Facts.* 1974 and 1975 eds., p. 84.

and sympathetic supervisor who understands their needs. A recreational program that appeals to a variety of interests requiring skills within the performers' range, and that offers children opportunities to satisfy their desire for fun and accomplishment through safe activities can do much to prevent them from experimenting on their own.

It is important that children learn to use good judgment in deciding where and how to play, lest they become dependent on the direction of the teacher or the patrol leader to keep them out of harm's way. Instruction in playground safety should be given early. The incidence of accidents in this area rises steadily as children grow older, reaching a peak when they are in the sixth and seventh grades. If youngsters are to refrain from dangerous acts voluntarily, they must be given every opportunity while in the lower grades to develop a sense of responsibility for their own safety and that of others.

Children should understand that safety regulations and the rules of good sportsmanship are intended to ensure fun for everyone. The supervisor who takes the time to explain the reason for rules in terms of the various playground hazards and the consequent need for proper behavior will find that children will be more cooperative. Although regulations should be posted as reminders, safety notices are not an adequate substitute for the supervisor's guidance.

In explaining how to play safely on swings, teeterboards, and other playground apparatus, the instructor should emphasize correct procedures rather than practices to be avoided. In using swings, for example, children must learn to take turns, remain seated, hold firmly to the ropes, and—when they leave the swing—to walk straight ahead, and not wander into the path of another swing.

Appointing an older student as a "safety person" (Figure 5-5) to assist youngsters in using playground apparatus will help prevent the many accidents that result from children's eagerness to play on certain types of apparatus

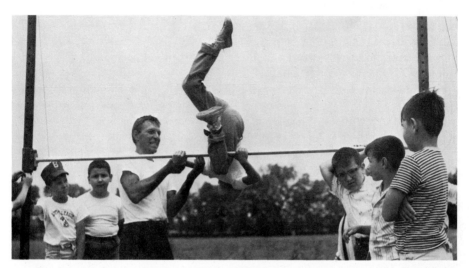

Figure 5-5   The safety man, either a teacher or an older student, makes certain that a child will not fall when he uses playground apparatus. (Source: Wide World Photo.)

before they have enough skill to do so safely. Every effort should be made to discourage small children from using equipment intended for an older group. If possible, youngsters in the lower grades should have a special play area at some distance from the large swings, high slides, and other equipment provided for older children.

Children are easily distracted. The supervisor should stress the need for alertness in all play activities and help youngsters develop the habit of always looking where they are going and giving full attention to whatever they are doing. Too often children are hurt when jumping off a swing or colliding with some piece of equipment in their haste to join a friend who has called to them excitedly.

The supervisor is responsible not only for regulating children's behavior but for keeping their environment as safe as possible. The playground surfacing should be designed to minimize the danger of falls. The play area should be checked daily to ensure that any pieces of broken glass or other sharp objects are removed, that ruts are filled in, and that slide landings are leveled with sand or sawdust. All apparatus should be inspected regularly, and children should be encouraged to report any defective equipment. Having each boy and girl take part in an opening cleanup keeps them safety-conscious and develops a feeling of pride in *their* playground.

Since some accidents are inevitable despite the most conscientious preventive measures, adequate first-aid equipment should be readily available at the playground, and the supervisor must be thoroughly trained in giving the proper emergency treatment for all types of injury. Children should be urged to report any cuts or bruises at once.

The basic principles of safety in public playgrounds are applicable to play areas around the home and to other areas where parents must assume responsibility for supervision.

Playground surfaces have been a problem for school administrators and recreation departments for many years. When school and recreation departments started to resurface playgrounds with asphalt and concrete to decrease maintenance and increase durability, numerous serious accidents began to occur involving individuals who fell from permanent-type equipment.

Grassy-type surfaces are satisfactory under normal conditions. They are difficult to maintain because of alternating periods of rain, snow, mud, dust, and dampness, which make the play area unfit for use during many days of the school year. In an effort to solve some of the problems of turf, permanent-type surfaces have been installed.

Permanent-type surfaces have solved some of the problems of housekeeping, cleanliness, and maintenance, but they have increased the incidence of broken bones, concussions, and in a few cases, fatalities. Because of these fatalities several different materials have been tried to provide a softer surface. Rubber-asphalt and cork, tanbark, wood shavings, sand, sawdust, cork, etc., have been used, but all have various shortcomings. It has been shown that when playground apparatus is removed youngsters run more, fall more often, and have more collisions.

Various studies of the problem have shown that a 1-inch-thick cushion, made from new rubber, provided the most protection. This type of safety cushion proved to be durable, clean, resilient, and easy to maintain. It is manufactured in interlocking blocks, is easily installed, and provides maximum deceleration for both light and heavy children.

In studies conducted in California, where the rubber cushion has been extensively used, no serious injuries were reported, minor abrasions practically disappeared, and there was an increase in the use of playground apparatus.[22]

SWIMMING AND OTHER AQUATIC SPORTS

Considering that swimming, boating, surfboard riding, water skiing, canoeing, skating, and scuba and skin diving are all very popular sports, it is amazing that the figure of slightly under 8,000 drownings annually isn't much greater. Considerable credit for the relatively low casualty rate in this area must be given to the American Red Cross, the Boy Scouts of America, and the YWCA and YMCA, which for many years have promoted, conducted, and supported intensive educational programs in aquatic safety. In no other sport has there been such insistence upon accident-prevention measures. The fatality figures would undoubtedly be higher if it were not for the excellent work done by the alert, well-trained lifeguards stationed at swimming pools and waterfront resorts.

Drowning, nevertheless, is the second-ranking cause of death for people from the ages of one to forty-four and the third leading cause of all accidental deaths (Table 5-6). Of the millions who frequent backyard, motel, and apartment pools as well as bathing beaches every summer, fewer than 10 percent are really skillful swimmers capable of caring for themselves in all the swimming situations they are likely to encounter. With over 700,000 permanent pools and 2½ million portables, the number of pool drownings may soon surpass the 1971 total of 644. (Table 5-7) There is unquestionably a need for more persistent safety education in aquatics. The protection afforded in supervised swimming and boating areas may not always be available when a water accident occurs.

Many private agencies offer excellent swimming instruction, but the public schools, which are obviously in the best position to reach adolescents, have not assumed enough responsibility in this area. More than half of all high school students are unable to swim 50 yards.[23] Even when swimming instruction is included in the physical education program, students often acquire only enough skill to expose themselves to danger. The ability to pass a beginner's swimming test is no assurance that one can care for oneself, and possibly others, in the event of a serious water accident.

Good swimming ability and good physical condition can do much to compensate for many aquatic hazards, for the skillful swimmer expends a minimum of effort and thus runs relatively little risk of overtaxing his or her endurance. The major objective of the school's aquatic program must be to

[22]Mitchill Royal Division Industries, San Fernando Road, Los Angeles, Calif. 90065.
[23]J. W. Clemensen et al., *Your Health and Safety,* 4th ed., Harcourt, Brace & World, Inc., New York, 1957, chap. 8.

TABLE 5-5
Accidental Deaths by Age, Sex, and Type, 1975

Age and Sex	All Types	Motor-Vehicle	Falls	Drowning†	Fires, Burns	Ingest. of Food, Object	Firearms	Poison (solid, liquid)	Poison by Gas	% Male All Types
All Ages	103,030	45,853	14,896	8,000	6,071	3,106	2,380	4,694	1,577	70%
Under 5	4,948	1,576	197	800	752	504	71	114	38	58%
5 to 14	6,818	3,286	137	1,300	580	77	424	49	81	70%
15 to 24	24,121	15,672	497	2,520	502	223	758	1,332	357	81%
25 to 34	13,823	7,680	428	1,080	500	218	359	1,215	263	81%
35 to 44	9,054	4,289	530	660	461	241	249	638	208	77%
45 to 54	9,993	4,089	1,057	630	757	369	215	545	216	74%
55 to 64	9,650	3,574	1,392	490	845	429	143	381	176	71%
65 to 74	9,220	3,047	2,148	310	795	451	115	233	139	63%
75 & over	15,403	2,640	8,510	210	879	594	46	187	99	47%
Male	72,376	33,597	7,696	6,782	3,733	1,829	2,042	3,147	1,165	
Female	30,654	12,256	7,200	1,218	2,338	1,277	338	1,547	412	
Percent male	70%	73%	52%	85%	61%	59%	86%	67%	74%	

Source: *Accident Facts*, National Safety Council, Chicago, 1977, p. 14.

TABLE 5-6
Swimming Pool Drownings—Type of Pool and Age of Victim, United States, 1971

Type of Pool	All Ages	Number of Deaths by Age										
		Under 1	1–4	5–9	10–14	15–19	20–24	25–34	35–44	45–54	55–64	65 and Over
Total	644	14	242	103	92	65	29	20	22	26	15	16
Home	259	12	164	24	9	10	6	5	9	11	3	6
In-ground	210	6	135	21	6	8	4	4	8	9	3	6
Above-ground	40	4	27	3	1	1	1	1	1	1	...	...
Unknown	9	2	2	...	2	1	1	...	...	1	...	...
Public	168	...	9	44	58	33	12	3	4	2	1	2
Apartment	103	...	40	14	4	6	5	7	6	9	8	4
Hotel or motel	61	2	14	9	11	7	5	4	3	3	2	1
Fish, decorative	17	...	12	...	...	2	...	...	...	1	...	2
Group, private club	14	...	3	3	4	2	1	...	...	...	1	...
Youth athletic organization	13	...	...	8	1	3	...	...	...	...	...	1
School	9	...	...	1	5	2	...	1	...	...	...	...

Source: Unpublished data from the Bureau of Community Environmental Management (since abolished), United States Department of Health, Education, and Welfare. From *Metropolitan Life Insurance Statistical Bulletin*, July–August, 1977, p. 5.

TABLE 5-7

Accidental Drownings—Activity and Proximate Cause, United States, 1971

Activity	All Causes	Proximate Cause							
		Exhaustion	Swept into Deep Water	Sinking of Support	Trapped or Entangled	Cramp or Other Attack	Struck Object	Caught in Flood	Other
Total	4,767	1,034	772	481	257	202	137	60	1,824
Recreational									
Swimming	1,137	807	107	3	14	132	51	...	23
Unorganized facility	934	669	98	2	9	107	28	...	21
Organized facility	187	123	9	1	5	25	23	...	1
Underwater	16	15	...	...	...	...	...	...	1
Bathing, wading	537	56	431	...	1	17	3	1	28
Unorganized facility	361	6	326	...	1	7	...	...	21
Organized facility	176	50	105	...	...	10	3	1	7
Playing adjacent to water	689	1	35	...	1	1	...	4	647
Standing, walking near water	547	2	13	1	...	11	...	3	517
Playing on raft, float	94	4	4	36	...	2	...	...	48
Playing on flotation tube or toy	67	4	6	17	...	1	2	...	37
Playing on ice	56	...	1	1	...	...	...	2	52
Fishing from boat	335	1	1	208	...	3	14	3	105
Boating									
Powerboat	147	1	...	64	2	1	22	...	57
Rowboat	107	5	1	58	1	2	1	2	37
Canoe	47	...	...	39	...	...	3	...	5
Sailboat	36	1	...	22	...	...	3	...	10
Surfing	13	...	2	3	...	2	1	1	4
Hunting	40	...	14	13	3	...	...	...	10
Scuba diving	47	30	1	...	14	1	...	...	1
Skin diving	27	22	1	...	3	...	1	...	...
Nonrecreational									
Motor vehicle occupant	359	7	108	...	200	...	25	1	18
Attempting rescue	143	88	28	2	7	3	...	5	10
Taking bath	86	...	1	...	...	20	...	...	65
All other	253	5	18	14	11	6	11	38	150

Source: Unpublished data from the Bureau of Community Environmental Management (since abolished), United States Department of Health, Education, and Welfare. From Metropolitan Life Insurance Statistical Bulletin, June, 1977, p. 10.

teach students to swim and dive skillfully enough to protect themselves under all conditions. They should also be thoroughly trained in the approved methods of water rescue and artificial respiration so that they will be able to safeguard others as well as themselves (Figure 5-6). All should be familiar with the procedures recommended by the American Red Cross for protection at the waterfront.

The number of reports involving nonswimmers who drowned when their canoe or boat capsized and swimmers who became exhausted when they were too far from shore to return safely indicates that many people do not fully appreciate aquatic hazards. More than 50 percent of drowning accidents occur during nonswimming activities (falling from boat, etc.) (Table 5-8). If knowledge of these hazards were more widespread, fewer might be willing to participate without first learning how to swim well. Undoubtedly the fun of water sports tends to make participants disregard such dangers as high breakers and steep sloping shores, which can make surf bathing extremely perilous, undertow and rip tides, which can easily carry a person far out beyond his depth and beyond his or her ability to swim back to safety. The majority of drownings can be attributed to a disregard of the recognized rules of safe aquatics.

Since an understanding of aquatic hazards, including the common, and often fatal, errors of swimmers and nonswimmers, should make participants amenable to safety rules, the instructor of any water sport should see that all students are thoroughly familiar with the principal causes of drowning, and where they occur. (Figure 5-7 and Table 5-7)

The causes of drowning may be classified as follows:

Psychological	Mechanical	Physiological
1. Overestimation of ability	1. Stepping off into deep water	1. Organic upset or failure
2. Attempts at swimming rescue, panic, etc.	2. Failure of supporting devices in deep water	2. Exhaustion, cramps, cold, allergy, etc.
3. Attempting long swims alone or from overturned boats or canoes	3. Hitting bottom, floating or submerged objects	
4. Lack of knowledge regarding bathing, swimming, diving, and boating conditions	4. Inability to use overturned boats or canoes for support	
5. Daring, showing off, taking chances	5. Diving from high boards and landing badly	
	6. Falling into deep water from docks, boats, or canoes	

If these causes are to be eliminated, safety instruction must be an integral part of a participant's training in any water sport. The instructor should try to convince the class that safety regulations do not curtail fun but rather enhance it by ensuring that enjoyment will not end in tragedy. When instructing students not to dive into water of unknown depth, the instructor should explain that this

Chest Pressure—Arm Lift Method

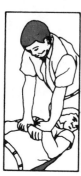

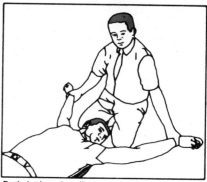

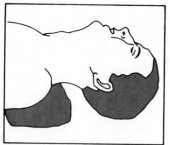

Lay victim on back with padding under shoulder and neck to help tilt head back.

Rock backward, pull arms up and out to move air into lungs. Repeat process.

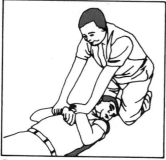

Turn to side and place forearms on chest.

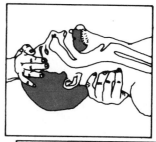

Lay the victim on the back and tilt head backward to open air passage.

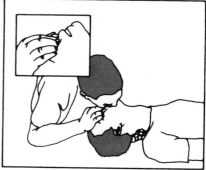

Rock forward and push down victim's forearms and chest.

Pinch the nose closed, form a tight seal with your mouth over the victim's mouth and blow your air in.

When using either of these artificial respiration methods, the victim should receive a breath *every five seconds*. Recovery may be quick, but sometimes may take hours. Do not give up quickly. Check often for obstructions. Stop only after the victim is finally breathing regularly.

Figure 5-6 Saving a life. [Source: National Rifle Association Student Manual, 1973 (revised 1976), p. 49, Hunter Safety and Conservation Program, the National Rifle Association of America, Washington, D.C.]

rule is intended to protect swimmers from the possibility of hitting their heads on the bottom or striking a submerged object—accidents which may cause serious cuts or bruises, unconsciousness, paralysis, or even a broken back or neck.

Warning participants of the dangers involved in disregarding a safety rule, however, may not always be enough to guarantee their obedience. Diving, after all, is a great deal of fun. If young people are not taught specific procedures for determining the depth of the water, such as wading to the waist and then swimming, they will be tempted merely to take a chance, assume that the water is deep enough, and dive. All too many spinal-cord lesions have resulted from diving accidents. Striking the head on an obstruction in the water can cripple the diver for life. Although the negative approach may be used effectively, positive instruction must receive primary stress. Swimmers should be taught not only to avoid venturing alone far out from shore but to swim relatively near and parallel to the shore if they want to take a long swim, so that they will be able to reach safety easily if they should become exhausted.

Using this combined positive and negative approach, the instructor should try to make participants understand and accept all safety rules pertinent to the sport of their choice. Students in the swimming course, for example, should be familiar with the following regulations:

1 Swim only in areas supervised by a lifeguard.
2 Do not go into the water too soon after eating.

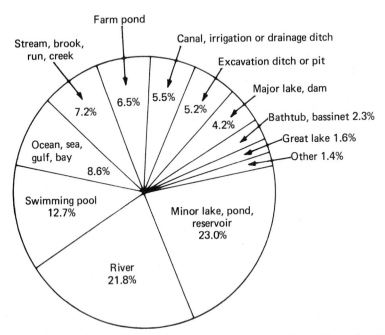

Figure 5-7 Accidental drownings—by site, United States, 1971. (Source: Metropolitan Life Insurance Statistical Bulletin, June 1977, p. 11.)

3 Never swim alone.

4 Cooperate with the lifeguard by staying inside the safety lines.

5 Stay out of deep water unless you are sure of your swimming ability.

6 Do not swim unless you are in good physical condition, free of even minor ailments.

If instruction in canoeing or boating is included in the program, participants should be taught how to prevent the vessel from capsizing. They should learn to sit, not stand, in the boat and to enter and leave the vessel without tipping it. The boating course is usually restricted to swimmers, but if nonswimmers are included they must understand the necessity of wearing a life jacket and of staying with the boat if it should overturn.

Participants in any aquatic sport must be instructed in the procedures to be followed in the event of an accident. Ice skating is not a hazardous activity under ideal conditions, but skaters should know what to do in case of ice failure. The importance of avoiding panic cannot be stressed too strongly. All students must understand that people in distress should float or tread water, not exhaust their energies by wildly waving their arms and trying to climb out of the water.

Lifesaving techniques should also be taught in connection with all water sports (See Figure 5-8). Familiarity with the American Red Cross slogan, "Throw, row, go, tow," should prevent students from making heroic but foolish attempts to rescue people in distress by swimming out to them. This procedure is least likely to be effective and should be resorted to only when no pole, rope, or buoy is available.

A water safety program should stress the following:

1 Seeing that all participants learn to swim—not just a little, but well enough to take care of themselves in an emergency

2 Learning, by practice, to stay afloat with clothes on

3 Swimming only where there are lifeguards

4 Swimming with others—never alone

5 Furnishing all boats with enough life preservers to supply one to each occupant

6 Learning to give mouth-to-mouth respiration

7 Educating and enlightening a public, so that it will be aware of the hazards of aquatics but willing to practice aquatic safety at all times

Safety education in general should be concerned with helping students develop a sense of responsibility for their own welfare and that of others. The swimming program offers the instructor numerous opportunities to impress students with the importance of this objective. Participants should be taught that making a voluntary effort to care for themselves and others at the waterfront is one way of putting their democratic ideals into action. Even if they are willing to risk their own safety, they should realize that they have no right to endanger others by behaving recklessly. Students should understand that their responsi-

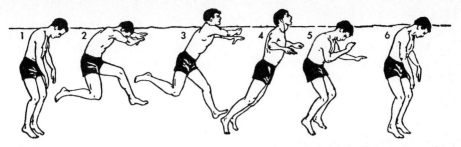

1. **Rest**—Take a deep breath and sink vertically beneath the surface, relax your arms and legs, keep chin down and allow fingertips to brush against knees. Keep neck relaxed and back of head above the surface.

2. **Get set**—Gently raise arms to a crossed position with back of wrists touching forehead. At the same time step forward with one leg and backward with the other.

3. **Lift head, exhale**—Without moving your arms and legs from the *get set* position raise your head quickly but smoothly to the vertical and *exhale through your nose.*

4. **Stroke and kick, inhale**—To support your head above the surface while you *inhale through your mouth*—gently sweep the arms outward and downward and step downward with both feet.

5. **Head down, press**—As you drop beneath the surface put your *head down* and press downward with your arms and hands to arrest your fall.

6. **Rest! rest! rest!**—Relax completely as in Step #1 for 6 to 10 seconds. *Always* breathe from choice—*never* from necessity.

Adapted with permission by E.J. Smyke, Emory University, Atlanta, Georgia

For sale by the Superintendent of Documents, U.S. Government Printing Office, Washington, D.C. 20402

SEEK DROWNPROOFING INSTRUCTION AT YOUR LOCAL POOL, SWIM CLUB, OR SWIMMING ORGANIZATION

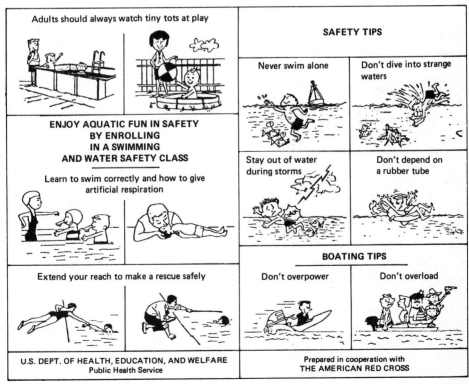

Figure 5-8 Learn Fred Lanoue's "Drownproofing" technique—it may save your life!

bility to others consists not only of avoiding improper conduct but of rendering positive assistance whenever the need arises. Swimmers are called upon to rescue someone in distress more often than most people realize, and the inability to do so may prove disastrous.

Because of its many physical, social, and emotional benefits, swimming has been rated as a valuable sports activity. Sound educational procedures and eternal vigilance are necessary to prevent the loss of these benefits. It is strongly recommended that swimming be included in the physical education program. Whenever such instruction is offered, the following health and safety measures must be instituted to ensure that students will not be exposed to needless risks:

1 No student with any infection, such as a cold, a skin disease, nasal drainage, or discharging ears, should be permitted to use the pool.

2 Sanitary conditions must be maintained in and around the pool and in the adjacent rooms.

3 Pool attendants and instructors must be fully qualified lifeguards, proficient in the accepted method of administering artificial respiration.

4 No bather should be allowed to enter the pool room unless an attendant is present.

5 When the pool has been drained, no one except the attendant should be allowed to enter the room.

6 Students should understand that they are to use the toilet and to bathe thoroughly, removing all their clothes and using warm water and soap, before entering the pool.

7 Spitting, spouting water, and blowing the nose should be strictly prohibited in the pool. Bathers should be instructed to use the scum gutter for expectoration.

8 Boisterous or rough play, except in supervised water sports, should be strictly prohibited in the pool, in dressing and shower rooms, and on the runways, diving board, float, and platform. Students should also be instructed not to run on the tile walk bordering the pool, which is likely to be wet and slippery.

9 The entire pool must be adequately illuminated whenever it is in use.

10 Nonswimmers should be required to wear brightly colored bathing caps as identification. The roll call or buddy system should be used to make sure that all students are present and accounted for at all times.

11 The diving area must be kept clear for diving. Swimming in this area must be prohibited except for divers swimming to the edge of the pool.

With officials estimating that swimming will be our number-one recreational activity by 1980, there can be no question of its importance as a life-saving activity. Swimming can and should be within the reach of everyone, and it opens the doors to many other water-related activities.

SWIMMING POOL DROWNINGS

The substantial increase in swimming pools, particularly of the home variety, has brought corresponding increase in home pool drownings. A significantly high proportion of the victims have been very young (Table 5-6). More than half (359) of all pool drownings occurred among children under ten years of age, and of these drownings about 40 percent were incurred by children from one to four. There is no question that constant, responsible supervision is necessary for this age group.

The very young often drown after unintentionally falling or slipping into the pool. Youngsters have drowned in rainwater that accumulated in the deep end of a pool after the pool had been drained. Youngsters attempting to retrieve objects such as toys and boats have also suffered fatalities.

In all pool drownings, the most frequently reported proximate cause (the factor considered to have the greatest involvement in the fatality) was exhaustion. Other proximate causes were stepping or falling into deep water, a cramp or other attack, striking an object, and collapse or loss of a flotation device. Outstanding primary causes, in order of importance, were inability to swim, overestimation of swimming ability, overt trespassing, preexisting physical impairments and failure to heed or obey warnings.[24]

Inadequate fencing is also a major factor in home pool drownings.

Constant, responsible adult supervision is necessary every minute that youngsters are playing in home or other swimming pools.

"Of special interest is the fact that more pool drownings occurred in regions consisting of the states of Arizona, California, Hawaii and Nevada than in any other area of the country. About 200, or nearly one-third of the 644 pool drownings occurred in these states."[25]

The following safety tips from the National Safety Council can provide home pool owners with a safe summer of swimming:[26]

1 Secure the pool with an adequate enclosure at least four feet high. Keep the gate locked.

2 Provide responsible supervision of all swimmers at all times.

3 Firmly enforce pool rules that prohibit roughhousing.

4 Make sure all pool users understand the proper use of diving boards and slides.

5 Mark water depths at various intervals on the deck or edge of the pool for safe diving and swimming.

6 Use the floating life line that comes with the pool to indicate where the pool's bottom drops off.

7 Never allow anyone to swim alone.

---

[24] *Metropolitan Life Insurance Statistical Bulletin,* vol. 58, pp. 4–5, July–August 1977.
[25] *Ibid.*
[26] "Pool Problems are Little Ones," *Family Safety,* vol. 34, no. 2, pp. 4–5, National Safety Council, Summer, 1975.

BOATING

There has been a tremendous increase in recreational boating in recent years. Table 5-8 illustrates the rapid rise in registered boats and gives a conservative estimate of the number of unregistered boats. With close to 10 million boats in use, it is estimated that at least 50 million people have turned to boating for relaxation and recreation.

Boating has become a hazardous activity. A good number of our 9 million pleasure craft are equipped with motors that produce well over 25 horsepower. The fatalities reported to and investigated by the Coast Guard show a rise from 36 in 1952 to 200 in 1967 and 1,264 in 1976 (Tables 5-8 and 5-9). No estimate can be made of unreported near accidents or of accidents which cause property damage of less than $100.

State and federal laws require that boating accidents involving personal injury, loss of life, or property damage over $100 be reported to the nearest Coast Guard office. It has been estimated that only 10 percent of nonfatal accidents involving injury or damage over $100 are presently being reported. Failure to report accidents is self-defeating. Data from accidents are needed for research into the causes of accidents, and for planning preventive safety programs, improving standards of boat design, and building safety equipment. Many of the present programs involving equipment, accessory modification, education, and instruction have developed from in-depth analysis of boating accidents.

Reports tell of fourteen- to sixteen-year-old novices who lose control of their boats and ram other craft with demolishing force, or plow into nearby swimmers. High-powered boats often buzz and sometimes swamp peaceful fishermen. Propeller blades can rip through a person's thigh or back with fatal results.

TABLE 5–8
Recreational Boating in the United States, 1970–1976

Year	Numbered Boats*	Actual Boats in Use†	Number of Fatalities	Fatality Rate per 100,00 Boats in Use
1970	5,128,345	7,400,000	1,418	19.2
1971	5,510,092	7,700,000	1,582	20.5
1972	5,910,794	8,000,000	1,437	18.0
1973	6,339,678	8,340,000	1,754	21.0
1974	6,830,456	8,550,000	1,446	16.9
1975	7,303,286	8,850,000	1,466	16.6
1976	7,671,213	9,150,000	1,264	13.8

*Numbered boats are undocumented vessels numbered by: (1) a state with an approved numbering system, or (2) by the Coast Guard under the Federal Boating Act of 1958 or the Federal Boat Safety Act of 1971.
†Coast Guard estimate of actual boats in use. Includes documented vessels, as well as numbered vessels, and unnumbered watercraft.
Source: Reports of United States Coast Guard. Reprinted in *Metropolitan Life Insurance Statistical Bulletin*, vol. 58, September, 1977, pp. 5–6.

TABLE 5–9
Fatalities in Recreational Boating in the United States, 1970–1976

Operation At Time of Accident	Number of Fatalities						
	1970	1971	1972	1973	1974	1975	1976
Cruising/Sailing	606	622	639	684	540	555	489
Fishing	331	318	231	277	255	344	264
Hunting	20	46	38	31	23	11	37
Swimming/Skin diving	1	6	0	1	1	2	2
Maneuvering	47	36	57	85	35	36	37
Waterskiing	31	38	36	44	30	39	34
Racing	17	9	7	14	14	5	8
Towing/Being towed	9	6	5	16	12	8	12
Drifting	137	130	135	206	186	218	148
Fueling	9	7	10	22	1	5	2
At anchor/Docked	49	77	74	76	69	41	50
Other	57	124	39	67	132	86	72
Unknown	104	163	166	231	148	116	109
Total	1,418	1,582	1,437	1,754	1,446	1,466	1,264

Source: Reports of United States Coast Guard. Reprinted in *Metropolitan Life Insurance Statistical Bulletin,* vol. 58, September, 1977, pp. 5–6.

Investigations of boating fatalities reveal that the most common causes are:

1. Lack of experience in boating
   a. Failure to understand the proper manipulation of the craft. (A yachting cap does not necessarily signify a skilled operator of a boat.)
   b. Failure to understand the ever-changing winds and waves, which result in dangerous "rough water."
   c. Failure to learn and/or obey the "rules of the road."
2. Lack of ability, knowledge, and experience in handling oneself (and others) in a water emergency; specifically, poor swimming ability and lack of knowledge of the best lifesaving methods. A recent survey by the American Red Cross shows that 40 to 50 percent of those engaged in boating activities cannot swim well enough to save themselves or others.
3. Unsafe boat; overloading; no life preservers
4. Unsafe behavior
   a. Standing in a boat.
   b. Attempting to tow a skier and manipulate the craft when alone in the boat.
   c. Allowing fuel vapors to accumulate in the lower part of the boat. An electric spark or lit cigarette could cause a disastrous explosion and fire. (A half-pint of gasoline in the bilge may create a potential explosive force of 5 pounds of dynamite.)
5. Unsportsmanlike conduct and/or disregard for others
6. High-speed turns

There have been increased restrictions recently in who may operate motor boats. However, almost anywhere in the United States a person can legally hop into a powerful boat and take off with no test of skill, no license, no check-out, no age limitation, no required liability insurance, and no preparation. Recently, the state of Illinois placed restrictions on motorboat operators between the ages of twelve and seventeen. Such persons can now operate a boat only under the supervision of a parent, guardian, or someone at least eighteen years old who has been selected by a parent. Without such supervision, they must hold a boating safety certificate issued by the state department of conservation.

Such certificates can be earned by taking an 8-hour boating safety course that is approved by the department and offered by organizations, school systems, and volunteers throughout the state. The new law also bars anyone nine years old or under from operating a motorboat.

If the millions of boat operators are to become safe operators of all types of craft, they must regulate themselves. All boaters should learn to swim well, and should take one or more courses in safe boat handling from organizations such as the United States Power Squadrons, American Red Cross, state departments of conservation, and the Coast Guard Auxiliary. Where programs are not available, new boat owners should seek advice from experienced operators and marine dealers before venturing into waters by themselves.

The craft most often involved in accidents are outboard-powered boats. We offer the following suggestions for safety:

SUGGESTIONS FOR SAFETY[27]

1 Gasoline vapors are explosive and, being heavier than air, will settle in the lower parts of a boat. All doors, hatches, and ports should be closed while fueling, galley fires and pilot lights extinguished, smoking strictly prohibited, and the filling nozzle kept in contact with the fill pipe to prevent static spark. Avoid spilling. Do not use gasoline stoves, heaters, or lights on board. Polyethylene or plastic containers should NOT be used for gasoline. The heat in the covered bow can easily cause an explosion.

2 After fueling thoroughly, ventilate all compartments and check the machinery and fueltank areas for fumes before attempting to start the motor. Remember that the electrical ignition and starting system could supply the ignition to any accumulation of explosive vapors. Take time to be safe. Keep fuel lines tight and bilges always clean.

3 Do not overload. Maintain adequate freeboard at all times; consider the sea conditions, the duration of the trip, and the predicted weather.

4 Keep an alert lookout. Serious accidents have resulted from failure in this respect. And it pays dividends—not only in avoiding collision with other boats, but also with objects that could damage your hull or propeller.

5 Be especially careful when operating in any area where swimmers might be. They are often difficult to see when there is glare on the water or if it is a bit choppy.

6 Watch your wake. It might capsize a small craft; it an damage boats or property along the shore. You are responsible. Pass through anchorages only at minimum speed because a violent rolling may spill dishes or coffee, awaken sleepers, or cause other resented nuisance.

7 Keep fire-fighting and lifesaving equipment in good condition and readily available at all times. The first few seconds are often the most important.

8 Obey the Rules of the Road. Neglect of this is the greatest single cause of collision.

---

[27]U.S. Coast Guard, Treasury Department, *Pleasure Craft,* C.G.-290.

Rules of the road

In boating, just as in driving a car, certain basic, safe operating practices must be followed. Learn them—they are your key to years of boating pleasure.

In the "rules" that follow, the terms "port" and "starboard" are used to refer to left and right. Notice that "port" and "left" have four letters. This is a good way to remember their relationship.

1. Powered boats yield the right of way to all boats without motors except when being overtaken. (See rule 3).

2. When meeting another boat head on, keep to starboard unless you are too far to port to make this practical.

3. When overtaking another boat, the right of way belongs to the boat being overtaken. If your boat is being passed, you must maintain course and speed.

4. When two boats approach at an angle and there is danger of collison, the boat to port must give way to the boat to starboard.

5. Always keep to starboard in a narrow channel or canal.

6. Boats underway must stay clear of vessels fishing with nets, lines or trawls. (Fishing boats are not allowed to fish in channels or to obstruct navigation, however.)

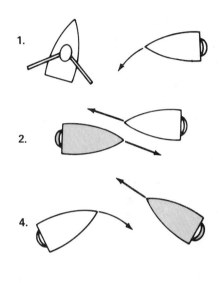

Figure 5-9 Rules of the road. (Source: Safety Ahoy, p. 4, Aetna Life and Casualty, Hartford, Conn.)

There is no excuse for ignorance, as copies of these Rules are available free; furthermore, instruction in all phases of small-boat seamanship, may be obtained through the Coast Guard Auxiliary. [See Figure 5-9]

9 For their safety—and your peace of mind—have children wear life preservers. Never hesitate to have "all hands" wear life preservers whenever the weather, a dangerous bar, or other circumstances cause the slightest doubt of safety. For a description of various types of Personal Floating Devices, PFD's, see the National Safety Councils booklet, *Splashdown With Safety*.

10 Know the fuel-tank capacity and the cruising radius of that supply. If it is necessary to carry additional gasoline, do so only in proper containers and take special precautions respecting stowage to prevent the release and accumulation of such vapor in confined spaces.

11 If you ever capsize, remember that if the boat continues to float it is usually best to remain with it. You are more easily located by a search plane or boat, and attempts to swim to a distant shore are so often unsuccessful.

12 Good housekeeping is even more important afloat than ashore. You have less room on a boat for storage, and may need something in a hurry. Have a place for everything—and everything in its place. This also makes for cleanliness, which diminishes the probability of fire.

13 Know the meanings of the buoys—what they mark, and what their peculiar markings indicate. Learn how they should be passed—on which side, whether close aboard or well clear; the significance of their lights, by color and characteristics. And never, never, moor to one. It is a Federal offense for which a penalty of $500 could be imposed. [See Figure 5-10]

14 Consider what action you would take under various emergency conditions—man overboard, fog, fire, a stove-in plank or other bad leak, motor breakdown, bad storm, collision. If you don't know, or are in doubt, look into it.

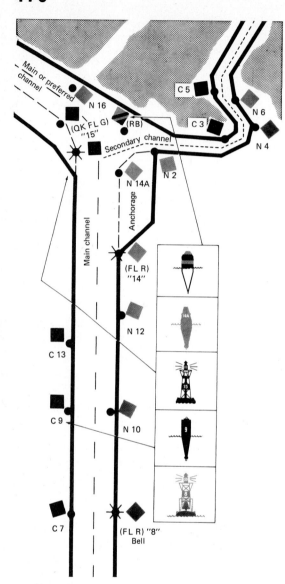

BUOYS ARE AIDS TO SAFE NAVIGATION

They warn of danger and indicate approaches, entrances, turns, and side limits of channels. Learn to identify them—they are just as necessary as highway route markers and warning signs.

The channel shown on this page illustrates some of the principal buoys you will encounter as you enter from seaward. A brief study of this channel will help you to review and remember the major characteristics of buoys.

Important Reminder: Color of paint is the only characteristic which has the same meaning on all buoys. Red buoys, for instance, always indicate the starboard side of the channel when entering from seaward (inward bound). That's why you can always trust that old sailing maxim, "Red Right Returning" which means: keep the red buoys on your right (starboard) when returning from the sea.

Typical Buoys

1. **NUN:** A typical nun buoy. Indicates the starboard side of the channel when entering from seaward (inward bound).
   SHAPE: conical
   COLOR: red
   NUMBER: even
   When a nun buoy is painted with red and black horizontal bands (top band red) and not numbered, it marks an obstruction with the recommended or principal channel to the left of the buoy when entering from seaward.

2. **LIGHTED BUOY (BLACK):** Buoy with quick flashing green light. Indicates the port side of the channel when entering from seaward (inward bound). Quick flashing light means special caution is required.

3. **CAN:** A typical can buoy. Indicates the port side of the channel when entering from seaward (inward bound).
   SHAPE: cylindrical
   COLOR: black
   NUMBER: odd
   When a can buoy is painted with red and black horizontal bands (top band black) and not numbered, it marks and obstruction with the recommended or principal channel to the right of the buoy when entering from seaward.

4. **LIGHTED BUOY (RED):** Buoy with flashing red light and a bell. Indicates starboard side of the channel when entering from seaward (inward bound). Note: Lighted buoys may have bells, gongs, whistles, horns or no sound.

Always Remember
"Red Right Returning"

Figure 5-10 Buoys are aids to safe navigation. (Source: Safety Ahoy, pp. 4–5, Aetna Life and Casualty, Hartford, Conn.)

15 Have an adequate anchor and sufficient cable to assure good holding in a blow, considering the maximum depth of water where you will be operating. And take care against stowage which would cause line to deteriorate.

16 Boat hooks are not required equipment but they are valuable when mooring or when needed to retrieve pets, preservers (and people) "over the side." It is good practice to have a body harness on pets especially if your deck is well above water.

17 Know the various distress signals. You may need help or have an opportunity to help others who are signaling for it.

18 Storm signals are for your information and safety. Learn them and be guided accordingly. A compass and a small transistor radio for receiving weather reports are essential.

19 Water skiing is great sport, but only when you are well clear of all other boats, bathers, and obstructions and there are two persons in the boat to maintain a proper lookout.

20 Falls are the greatest cause of injury both afloat and ashore. Eliminate every tripping hazard where possible, make conspicuous those which must remain, have adequate grab-rails, and pay particular attention to the slipping qualities of footwear used aboard.

21 Have a chart (or charts) of your area. You may know it well, but you'll be surprised how much more the chart will disclose.

22 Always instruct at least one other person on board of the rudiments of boat handling in case you are disabled—or fall overboard.

23 Keep electrical equipment and wiring in good condition. No knife switches or other arcing devices should be in fuel or engine compartments. Allow ample ventilation around batteries.

24 Check your fuel-supply system; see that the tanks are vented outboard, that the fill pipes are located outboard of coaming and extend to the bottom of the tank. Have an adequate filter on the fuel line.

25 Do not use kapok-filled preservers to sit upon. Such action compresses the filler and reduces its efficiency.

26 Never operate a boat while intoxicated.

Numerous accidents and fatalities also occur in canoes, rowboats, and sailboats. The most common unsafe practices in operating these craft are:

1 Improper loading and overloading
2. Standing up
3 Lack of boat- and canoe-handling skills
4 Disregard of weather and water conditions
5 Failure to use life-saving equipment when indicated

For more detailed information regarding small craft safety, readers may wish to refer to the appropriate section in The American Alliance for Health, Physical Education And Recreation book Sports Safety or to Monograph No. 5 of the American School and Community Safety Association of AAHPER, which is concerned with safety in aquatic sports.

The National Association of State Boating Law Administrators recently (January 1978) adopted national standards for boating safety education. Copies of the standards are available from state offices of the boating law administrator.

WATERSKIING

Waterskiing is a safe, clean, and enjoyable outdoor sport. Thousands of beginners take to the water each summer and, become skilled enough to enjoy the activity, after a few lessons, regardless of previous athletic accomplishments.

Waterskiing is basically safe. Few fatalities and serious accidents occur to an estimated 20 million annual skiers. But when high-horsepower boats take the skier skimming over the waves, waterskiing becomes potentially dangerous.

Too often a motorboat operator is trying to find out the skier's limit of skill—whether the skier can stay above water as the boat goes through questionable maneuvers. And these water cowboys are oblivious of the fact that small fishing craft, other boats hauling skiers, and even swimmers may be in the vicinity.

Unfortunately, legislation is slow to prohibit such abuses. It behooves skiers to set up their own safety regulations.

The majority of waterskiing accidents involve the beginner who has not had proper instruction, or the reckless boat operator. The five elements of safety in waterskiing are: (1) the skiier, (2) skiing gear, (3) the boat driver, (4) the boat and water, and (5) the water. The following regulations will help make water skiing safe and enjoyable.

For safe and courteous boat operators

1 All passengers must sit on a seat while the boat is under way.

2 Know and obey the rules of the road; when in doubt, let courtesy rule.

3 Practice the skills necessary for safe ski-boat operation before attempting ro pull a skier.

4 Be alert for traffic conditions and your skier's success in remaining on the skis.

5 As a boat operator, you must make sure of a safe right of way. You must keep eyes front, and a second person in the boat must take the responsibility for the skier's safety. An understanding of this combined responsibility is important.

6 While backing into position to throw the tow rope to the skier, do not back straight toward the skier; back the boat to one side of the skier.

7 Keep at least 100 yards behind another boat that is pulling a skier.

8 Do not turn a boat in close quarters in such a way that the skier might swing too close to a bridge, dock, or shore line.

9 When the skier falls, immediately turn around and get your boat close enough to the skier, on the downwind side, to protect him or her from other moving boats, and so a gust of wind won't blow the boat too close to the skier.

For safe and courteous skiers

1 Unless you are a well-qualified swimmer, do not attempt skiing.

2 Wear a life jacket or belt regardless of your swimming or skiing ability.

3 When making a start, be sure that the tow rope is not tangled around your body, your leg, or a ski. Raise the tow bar up and out of the water to make sure that it is clear.

4 Do not swing close to another boat, dock, or person standing on the shore.

5 When skiing under a bridge or through a congested area of boats, follow a straight course behind your boat.

6 After falling, hold clasped hands up in the air as a signal that you are all right—or hold up a ski.

SPEED OKAY

The okay signal, with thumb and forefinger making an "O." No motion of head if both hands are in use.

START

Shout "HIT IT" or nod head.

FASTER

Palm up - motion upwards, or nod head if both hands are in use.

SLOWER

Palm down - motion downward, or shake head if both hands are in use.

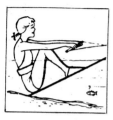
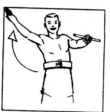
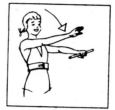
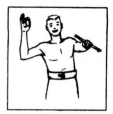

TURN

Palm vertical, describe curving motion with hand in direction desired.

WHIP OFF

Point at direction and then give quick circular motions with hand.

JUMP

Raise hand sharply imitating jumping arc.

STOP

Hand up, fingers outstretched — policeman style.

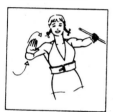
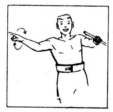
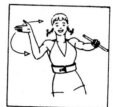
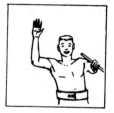

BACK TO DOCK

With bent elbow, point forefinger downward.   Still pointing, extend arm downward sharply.

CUT MOTOR

Draw finger across windpipe in cutting motion.

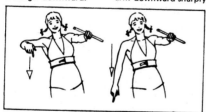
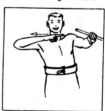

While on land the Ski Instructor should demonstrate all Skier's Signals as part of his "Dry Land Instruction". To pass the Intermediate rating of the National Water Ski Association, campers must be able to demonstrate on land all ten of the Skiers' Signals; therefore, signals should be used while riding whenever appropriate. These ten signals seem to be commonly accepted and universally used; however, Ski Instructors can develop additional signals as they see fit.

Figure 5-11 Skiers' signals. (Source: American Association for Health, Physical Education and Recreation, Sports Safety, Division of Safety of the Association, 1971, p. 204.)

7 Do not release the tow rope and coast into or toward any obstruction; coast free into an unobstructed and clear right-of-way area.

8 Assume your share of responsibility to make waterskiing a sport which can be enjoyable to the participant and without objection to other users of the waterway.

9 Know the waterskiing signals (see Figure 5-11).

SNOWMOBILES

Snowmobiling is one of the fastest growing winter sports and recreational activities in North America. Like many mushrooming activities, it has grown without a great deal of control at the local or state level. This rapid growth and the ease with which one can participate can lead to accidents and personal injury. The increased occurrence of accidents has proved the need for safer use of snowmobiles.

Snowmobiles are motorized vehicles capable of moving over ice and snow at great speed. There is no doubt that they provide pleasant, exciting winter recreational activity.

Today the snowmobile provides hunter, fishers, naturalists, and other outdoor enthusiasts with easy transportation to out-of-the-way places. It is also used for search and rescue work and for delivering supplies to snowbound areas.

Like any other piece of moving equipment, the snowmobile is only as safe as the person operating it. The key to safe operation is learning how to operate the vehicle skillfully, knowledge of the vehicle itself, courtesy, and good judgment.

THE SNOWMOBILER'S RESPONSIBILITY. The following safety suggestions have been developed by the International Snowmobile Industry Association and the Ontario Safety League.[28]

1 *Basic training is required for the safe operation of snowmobiles.* Despite the simplicity of controls and handling, everyone should obtain some training.

2 *Know your legal status regarding snowmobiles.* If in doubt, contact the nearest motor vehicle office of your state government, police or highway department or the department of conservation. In addition to traffic regulations, a knowledge of legal responsibility pertaining to public liability and property damage when trailering or operating a snowmobile is important.

3 *Treat a snowmobile with the respect and care due any power-driven vehicle.* Common sense, handling and proper maintenance will pay off in added safety and pleasure in the use of your machine.

4 *Show proper courtesy and respect for other people and their property.* Obtain consent of property owners before snowmobiling on their private lands. Do not damage landscaping such as shrubs and trees or fences and gates. Check with park officials before using public lands and conform to all rules and regulations. Respect the privacy of others. A snowmobile creates sufficient noise to disturb people who want peace and quietness.

---

[28]International Snowmobile Industry Association, Minneapolis, Minn. Ontario Safety League, 208 King Street W., Toronto 1, Canada.

Operation

1 It is important to study your Owner's Manual carefully. Learn as much as possible concerning the mechanical operation of your snowmobile. A knowledge of some minor repairs and adjustments is a practical necessity when on extended safaris and a convenience at any time.

2 A snowmobile is not a magic carpet, it is a mechanical means of transportation designed to travel over snow and ice-covered areas within the limits of its ability. Learn and respect these limitations.

3 Recognize your own limitations as a driver. Start cautiously and increase your snowmobiling activities as experience and knowledge are acquired.

Hazards

1 Certain conditions can make snowmobiling difficult and even hazardous.

2 Rough terrain and uneven snow surfaces can result in overturned machines and spills if travelled at too great a speed.

3 Mild weather with resultant wet snow and slush creates the worst conditions for snowmobile operations. Below freezing temperatures are necessary for the best snowmobiling.

4 Ice-travel is the most hazardous of all snowmobile operations. Most snowmobile fatalities have been drownings as a result of machines breaking through thin or rotten ice. Snowmobilers should never travel on frozen lakes or rivers without an intimate knowledge of ice conditions and water currents. The latter is of utmost importance as currents can cut away the underside of an ice surface, making it unsafe at that particular spot. A check made even a few feet away from this area could show ice of a safe thickness. The shoreline of a lake is often the most hazardous because of currents created by contributary streams and rivers.

5 It is advisable to use the 'buddy system,' two machines or more, when travelling any distance away from snow-ploughed roads or patrolled trails. Do not attempt distant safaris into remote areas without an experienced person in the group.

6 Avoid public thoroughfares and when necessary cross at right angles using extreme caution.

7 When travelling in wooded areas slow down and watch for snow-covered stumps and fallen trees which could be a hazard.

Clothing

1 Proper clothing is the most important factor in the enjoyment of any outdoor winter recreation and snowmobiling is no exception.

2 It should be warm and windproof, yet light and sufficiently flexible not to impede movement.

3 Insulated footwear is a great comfort and fleecelined or insulated leather or plastic mitts are the most practical.

4 A heavy wool toque with attached face mask and shatterproof, tinted goggles are necessary in cold weather operation.

5 If operating over rough country or in heavily wooded areas, a safety helmet worn over a wool liner is a good precaution against head injury.

6 Do not wear loose scarves or clothing which could become tangled in moving parts.

7 Take every precaution to keep clothing and footwear dry. Do not become over-heated. Loosen clothing at the throat to allow warm air to escape as necessary.

8 Watch for frostbites when out in freezing temperatures. They will appear as white spots most frequently on exposed parts such as ears, nose and cheeks. It is advisable for members of a party to watch each other for these danger signs.

9 Minor frostbites can be thawed out with the heat from a warm hand or a warm compress if available. Do not rub with snow or massage as this will damage the frozen skin tissue. Extensive frostbite should have expert medical treatment as soon as possible.

Equipment

An extra drive-belt should be carried like a spare tire, plus spark plugs with the necessary tools for installation. This is basic equipment for even casual snowmobiling within ready reach of outside assistance. But for distant safaris in remote areas, the list is much longer.

1 A pair of snowshoes or skis for each passenger. This is just as necessary as lifejackets in a boat if stranded miles from the nearest snow-ploughed road.

2 Emergency fuel supply.

3 A light-weight block and tackle with 50 feet of ¼-inch nylon rope. This could mean the difference between abandoning your machine or continuing your trek if badly stuck.

4 Topographical map of area to be travelled and compass.

5 Hand-axe, hunting knife, waterproof container of matches and a small pan or kettle.

6 Dehydrated emergency rations and some tea bags. Black tea is more energizing than coffee for most people. Always keep these in reserve for an emergency.

7 A compact first aid medical kit.

8 A small-sized, waterproof tarpaulin and space-type survival blanket.

Note: On distant safaris it is best to trailer supplies and equipment. A snowmobile will haul the extra weight more efficiently than carrying it.

Survival

If an emergency should arise such as a breakdown or becoming lost which requires existence under winter survival conditions the first important rule is—DON'T PANIC! This is vital to survival.

1 Conserve food and energy, and take careful stock of the situation.

2 Light a fire. This will keep you warm and attract the attention of rescuers on the ground or in the air.

3 If a shelter is needed, it can be made with snow, poles, evergreen boughs or anything that will break the wind. A person can be quite comfortable with a fire built to reflect into an emergency shelter even in sub-zero temperatures.

4 A hundred-foot circle tramped in the snow with paths radiating from the centre like spokes in a wheel can be readily seen from a search plane during daylight hours. Evergreen boughs placed upright in the snow beside the paths are helpful. They will cast shadows on a sunny day.

INJURIES AND FATALITIES.
The National Safety Council reported that 154 snowmobile-related deaths in a recent year were caused by collisions with fixed objects, collisions with moving motor vehicles, and drownings. In nonfatal-injury accidents, the most frequent causes were collisions with fixed objects, collisions with moving snowmobiles and other motor vehicles, and overturns.

DRIVER EDUCATION FOR SNOWMOBILES?
Snowmobiles increase in popularity each year, particularly in areas with long winters. The need for a driver education program, particularly for young operators, is being discussed in different parts of the country.

At a recent conference it was shown that such a program can bring positive results. A Wisconsin study reported a 12 percent decrease in serious snowmobile-related injuries in a single year. Several states now require a snowmobile safety course for young drivers.

Safety educators may wish to provide driver-education programs on a voluntary basis on nonschool time.

There are various state agencies and major manufacturers of snowmobiles that can provide assistance in formulating driver education and safety programs. Those seeking more information should contact one of the following agencies: the department of natural resources, department of motor vehicles, department of public safety, division of wildlife, department of parks and recreation, and the department of conservation.

SKATEBOARDS

The U.S. Consumer Product Safety Commission has estimated that more than 375,000 individuals per year will be injured in skateboard accidents. This is a substantial rise from 3,200 in 1974. More injuries will occur in this activity than in scholastic, collegiate, and backyard football. The commission stated that no other product under its jurisdiction has demonstrated such dramatic growth in the number of associated injuries.

The tremendous increase in injuries caused by the use of skateboards has become a major concern of state, local, and national officials. Recently skateboard injuries increased 159 percent from one year to the next.

One manufacturer of skateboards recently reported that it had boosted production of skateboard wheels from 80,000 a month to 20,000 a day, and that the demand still could not be met.

This dramatic increase in the use of skateboards, along with twenty-eight skateboard fatalities since 1975, has caused the industry and the federal government to look into possible accident-prevention programs. An analysis of skateboard accidents reveals the following:

1 In almost all cases investigated, accident victims did not wear protective equipment such as helmets, padding, and special gloves.

2 The 28 fatalities occurred in one of two ways: victims fell and struck their heads, or they were hit by motor vehicles.

3 The majority of accidents occurred to males. Approximately 54 percent of the injuries were to the ten to fourteen age group, and 21 percent were to the fifteen to nineteen age group.

4 Fractures were the most common injury, accounting for about one-third of all injuries. More than half the fractures were to the lower arm or lower leg. Most of the other injuries were lacerations, contusions, and abrasions.

5 One out of three accidents occurred when skateboards struck irregularities in the riding surface. One out of four accidents involved victims who lost their balance.

6 In slightly more than 1 percent of the injuries, the skateboard was directly responsible, for example, when the wheels fell off.

7 One-third of those injured had been skateboarding less than 1 week.

A summary of the principal causes reveals that 32 percent of the accidents were caused by irregularity in riding surface; 26 percent by loss of balance; 16 percent by slipping off the board; 13 percent by other causes, such as being pushed; and 9 percent by the board slipping out from under the victim.

A skateboard can sustain a speed of up to 35 miles per hour on asphalt pavement, without brakes and with no protective equipment. The risks are clear, particularly for the beginner.

The following steps are recommended for reducing accidents and fatalities.

1 Use protective gear such as helmets, padding, and special gloves.
2 Avoid using public streets and highways. Skate only in a controlled environment.
3 Learn how to fall correctly in order to minimize injury. (Consult physical education teacher or gymnastics instructor.)
4 Learn to perform the basic maneuvers well before attempting more complicated or "trick" moves.
5 Choose a sturdy skateboard with only enough play in the wheels to turn corners. Too much wheel wobble causes instability.

Some communities, for example, Malibu West, California, have banned skateboards. Others have considered a ban because skateboards interfere with traffic and contribute to accidents.

Some authorities believe that "skateboard riders under 13 years of age may not have adequate muscular coordination to maintain balance and sufficient maturity to exercise judgement about types of maneuvers to attempt on skateboards."[29]

EVALUATION

The physical education, athletics, and recreational programs should be evaluated at regular intervals to determine what progress has been made toward achieving their safety objectives. A reduction in the number of injuries in the gymnasium and on the playing field may seem encouraging, but it may merely indicate that fewer students are participating in potentially dangerous sports. The incidence of accidents is a valid means of judging safety efforts only if statistics are carefully analyzed and interpreted.

The evaluation process should include appraisals of instructors, facilities, and equipment, but primary emphasis should be given to estimating students' progress in developing the attitudes and skills conducive to safe participation in the activities. The instructor should try to determine the extent to which they recognize specific hazards and manifest a sense of personal responsibility for their own safety and the safety of others.

Because of the rapidly increasing popularity of many recreational sports, it

[29]Consumer Product Safety Commission, Fact Sheet No. 84, *Roller Skates, Ice Skates and Skateboards*, 1976, p.1.

becomes more and more important for participants themselves to take steps to make their sports safer. Courses in some activities have been suggested for the schools. Courses are offered by people who have an interest in the sport. How is the public responding? How well are the directors of press, radio, and television covering the subject? How well are prominent sports participants responding to information about known hazards, to the possibility of removing them or of counteracting the hazards which cannot be removed? Is there evidence of a growing safety consciousness as more and more people turn to these recreational activities? Can they make wise and safe use of their leisure time?

LEARNING EXPERIENCES

The following assignments are designed to supplement the study of this chapter by helping potential teachers, coaches, and recreational leaders increase their understanding of the hazards of various activities.

1 Study the chief causes of accidents in one or more of the sports not covered in this chapter, such as golf, tennis, horseback riding, wrestling, soccer, or fishing. Develop a safety code or a set of safety principles for the sport or sports you select.

2 Invite a well-known local hunter to address your class on safety in hunting and to demonstrate the correct procedures for handling firearms.

3 Request brochures from several reputable camps, and note all potentially hazardous activities included in their programs and all references to safety measures.

4 Prepare a list of safety principles to govern each of five common camp activities.

5 Analyze the accident record of a nearby school, noting the type and frequency of accidents in the physical education program. Discuss the accident trend revealed by this study.

6 With the help of the student council or safety committee, inspect the various physical education and athletic areas of a nearby school or recreation area. Suggest procedures for eliminating or compensating for any hazardous conditions you observe.

7 Write a 500-word paper showing how good sportsmanship, which is generally considered essential to safe participation in sports, can reduce accidents in other activities.

8 Determine the primary cause and any contributory causes of a sports accident reported in the newspaper. Explain how this accident might have been prevented.

9 List the opportunities that might be given students participating in a given sport to assume responsibility for their own safety and the safety of others.

10 Request information from your state high school athletic association on your state athletic benefit or accident insurance plan. Describe its benefits and compare them with those offered in the plans discussed by other members of the class.

11 Invite the coaches of various sports in a nearby school to talk to your class on the place of safety in their sports.

12 Be prepared to discuss the advantages and disadvantages of black-top, concrete, grass, gravel, and rubberized playground surfacing.

13 Request a swimming coach or your local Red Cross representative to discuss the newer methods of artificial respiration.

14 Survey a community that has backyard swimming pools. Analyze the safe and unsafe features of the pool and surrounding area.

SELECTED REFERENCES

Abend, Albert. "The Need For Driver Education for Snowmobilers," *Concept for Traffic Safety,* vol. 7, no. 2, pp. 10–12, Aetna Life & Casualty, Hartford, Conn., Fall-Winter, 1974.

Accident Facts, National Safety Council, Chicago. Yearly

American Red Cross, Washington:
Advanced First Aid and Emergency Care, 1973.
Basic Canoeing, 1965
Basic Outboard Boating
Basic Rescue and Water Safety, 1975
Basic Rowing, 1964
Basic Sailing, 1966
Canoeing, 1977
Cardiopulmonary Resuscitation (CPR), 1974
First Aid for Foreign Body Obstruction of Airway, 1976
Lifesaving Rescue and Water Safety, 1975
Standard First Aid and Personal Safety, 1976
Swimming and Water Safety, 1976

American School and Community Safety Association, an Association of the American Alliance for Health, Physical Education and Recreation, Sports Safety Series Monographs.
No. 1, *Administration and Supervision for Safety in Sports,* 1977
No. 2, *Accident Surveillance System for Sports,* 1977
No. 3, *Safety in Team Sports,* 1977
No. 4, *Safety in Individual and Dual Sports,* 1978
No. 5, *Safety in Aquatics,* 1978
No. 6, *Safety in Outdoor and Recreational Sports,* 1978

Blyth, Carl S., and David C. Arnold: *The Forty-Fifth Annual Survey of Football Fatalities 1931–1975,* National Collegiate Athletic Association, Mission, Kansas, 1976.

Blyth, Carl S., and Frederick Muller: "When and Where Players Get Hurt," *The Physician and Sports Medicine,* pp. 45–52, September, 1974.

Clarke, Kennith, and Allan S. Braslow: "Football Fatalities in Actuarial Perspective," *Medicine and Science.* 1978.

Combes, Harry, and A. E. "Joe" Florio: "Basketball Safety." in *Sports Safety,* American Association for Health, Physical, Education, and Recreation, Washington, 1970, pp. 86–89.

Consumer Product Safety Commission, Washington, Fact Sheets:
No. 8, *Swimming Pools*
No. 22, *Playground Equipment*
No. 42, *Football and Football Equipment*
No. 84, *Rollerskates, Ice Skates, and Skateboards*
No. 85, *Trampolines*

Florio, A. E. "Joe": *Basketball, Safety in Team Sports,* Sports Safety Series, Monograph No. 3, American School and Community Safety Association, an Association of the American Alliance for Health, Physical Education and Recreation, 1977, pp. 15–19.

Garrick, James G., and Leonard T. Kurkland: "The Epidemiologic Significance of Unreported Ski Injuries," *Journal of Safety Research,* pp 182–187, December, 1971.

Grieve, Andrew: "Safety of Facilities," *Journal of Health, Physical Education and Recreation,* pp. 24–25, October, 1974.

Hartman. Betty G.: "The Female Athlete: Safeguards and Injury Controls," *Current Sports Medicine Issues,* Proceedings of the National Sports Congress, February, 1973.

"The Hazards of Hunting," Farm Safety Review, vol. 35, no. 5, September–October, 1977.

Kretzler, Harry H.: "Artificial Turf and Football Injuries," *Annual Safety Education Review,* pp. 61–70, American Alliance for Health, Physical Education and Recreation, Washington, 1972.

National Safety Council, Chicago, Data Sheets:
    No. 3, *Firearms*
    No. 18, *Camping*
    No. 22, *Gymnasium, Safety in the*
    No. 27. *Swimming*
    No. 28, *Small Craft*
    No. 29, *Play Areas*
    No. 43, *Hiking and Climbing*
    No. 44, *Fishing Hook and Line*
    No. 69, *Playground Apparatus*
    No. 71, *Baseball Safety*
    No. 72, *Football Safety*
    No. 74, *Playground Surfaces*
    No. 75, *General Safety*
    No. 77, *Basketball Safety*
    No. 89, *Track and Field Events*
    No. 100, *Snow Mobiles*
    Happy Hunting
    Operation Water Proof

National Safety Council, Chicago, *Family Safety Magazine:*
    "An Eye for Sports" (eye injuries), pp. 24–25, Fall, 1976
    "Are Organized Sports Child's Play?" pp. 18–20, Winter, 1973–74
    "Heads You Lose" (football) pp. 4–7, Spring, 1972
    "How to Dive and Survive," pp. 4–6, Spring, 1974
    "How to Avoid That Sinking Feeling" (life preservers) pp. 12–13, Summer, 1972
    "Keep Up on Water Skiing," pp. 24–25, Summer, 1976
    "Pool Problems Are Little Ones," pp. 4–5, Summer, 1975
    "Skateboards Are Alive and. . . . Well?" p. 29, Fall, 1975
    "Summer Is a Sometime Trap," pp. 28–30, Summer, 1970
    "Sure You Can Get Hurt," pp. 11–13, Summer, 1976
    "The Alluring but Alarming Snowmobile," pp. 4–6, Winter, 1969
    "Things You Can't See In the Sea," pp. 6–8, Summer, 1974
    "Wanted, High School Football Trainers," pp. 22–24, Fall, 1973
    "Your Daughter the Fullback," pp. 4–6, Fall, 1974
    NEISS Data Highlights, U. S. Consumer Product Safety Commission, Washington. Monthly and annual.

Robey, Carl S., Carl S. Blyth, and Frederick Mueller: "Athletic Injuries, Application of Epidemologic Methods," *The Journal of the American Medical Association,* vol. 217, no. 2, pp. 184–189, July 12, 1971.

Yost, Charles Peter: "Total Fitness and Prevention of Accidents," *The Journal of Health, Physical Education and Recreation,* pp. 32–37, March, 1967.

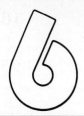

Traffic Safety Education

OVERALL OBJECTIVE:

The student of safety should be able to comprehend the problem of highway traffic safety, and state how traffic safety education programs can alleviate this problem.

INSTRUCTIONAL OBJECTIVES:

After completing this chapter the student will be able to:

1 List the significant factors that contribute to the highway safety problem.
2 List the specific kinds of improper driving habits that cause accidents.
3 Correlate improper driving to different age groups.
4 Explain why traffic safety education should start early in life.
5 Explain the Highway Safety Act of 1966, and the responsibilities of the Department of Transportation, National Highway Traffic Safety Administration.
6 List the federal highway program standards.
7 Outline the basic elements in a high school driver and traffic safety education program.
8 List the responsibilities of the state office of education in implementing a traffic safety education program.
9 Define the following terms: driver education, classroom phase, laboratory phase, multimedia mode, electronic simulator mode, off-street multiple-car driving range mode, and performance objective.
10 Discuss the implications of physical growth, mental growth, and emotional maturity to driver and traffic safety.
11 Describe the standards and administrative procedures needed for an approved driver education course.

TRAFFIC SAFETY EDUCATION

Today, traffic safety is a major public health problem involving a variety of interacting elements. "Motor vehicle accidents claim more lives annually than all crimes of violence, more than natural catastrophes, more than any of the diseases except heart, cancer, stroke, and pneumonia. Motor vehicle accidents account for more than 90 percent of the dead from all forms of transportation combined."[1]

Medical science has made extensive progress in curing disease and keeping our citizens healthy, but no vaccine has been discovered to prevent an annual toll of over 47,000 deaths and close to 2 million disabling injuries. More than 2 million Americans have died in traffic accidents since the advent of the automobile, and each year thousands are added to this figure. When war deaths are compared with motor-vehicle fatalities, it can be said that one's chances of survival are greater on the battlefield[2] (Table 1-3, Chapter 1).

With a population of over 200 million people, including more than 134 million licensed drivers, and with over 140 million motor vehicles, 100 million bicyclists, and 3½ million young people reaching driving age each year, the nation must regard traffic accidents as a major social problem. At the present rate, one out of every two Americans will suffer death or injury from traffic accidents.

Today, 62 percent of the American population depend upon the motor vehicle for their livelihood, particularly workers such as sales and delivery people and intercity bus and truck drivers. The figure also includes people who commute to work by private vehicle and people who rely on motor vehicles to get to school, run errands, and take vacations. There is no question that the motor vehicle plays an important part in the economy of this nation. We are a nation on wheels.

In recent years a greater effort has been made to encourage drivers to save fuel by sharing rides, joining car and van pools, and exploring other modes of transportation. The vast majority of people still prefer the flexibility of their private cars. Energy conservation and the increased cost of fuel may change the figures slightly, but there is no indication that a massive shift from private to public transportation will occur (Figure 6-1).

What can be done about this problem? Is it possible to make our streets and highways safe? Only continued effort on the part of our citizens will make traffic safety a reality. Much has been accomplished in the past and a great deal of emphasis is being placed on the problem today, but much still remains to be done. We must increase qualitative research efforts aimed specifically toward solution of the accident problem.

How may our safety keep pace with our amazingly accelerated mobility?

---

[1] U.S. Department of Transportation, National Highway Traffic Safety Administration: *Federal Highway Administration Traffic Safety,* 1974, part 1, p. 3, "A Report on Activities under the Highway Safety Act of 1966," 1974.
[2] *Accident Facts,* National Safety Council, Chicago, 1977, p. 49.

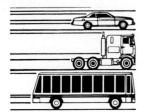

Most Commuters Get to Work by Private Vehicle

Privately owned motor vehicles are by far the top choice of Americans in getting to and from work. A new U.S. Census Bureau survey finds 86 percent of job commuters in 21 metropolitan areas using private cars or trucks.

More American job commuters in these areas car-pooled by private vehicle than rode in all forms of public transportation combined. About 18 percent shared the ride by car or truck and only 12 percent rode buses, street cars, commuter trains, subways or elevated rail cars to and from work. Some 68 percent of the commuting workers drove alone.

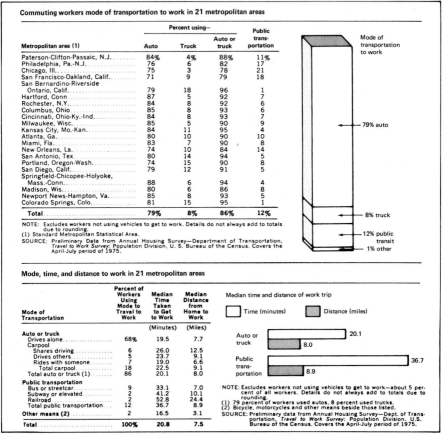

Commuting workers mode of transportation to work in 21 metropolitan areas

Metropolitan area (1)	Percent using—			Public trans- portation
	Auto	Truck	Auto or truck	
Paterson-Clifton-Passaic, N.J.	84%	4%	88%	11%
Philadelphia, Pa.-N.J.	76	6	82	17
Chicago, Ill.	75	3	78	21
San Francisco-Oakland, Calif.	71	9	79	18
San Bernardino-Riverside Ontario, Calif.	79	18	96	1
Hartford, Conn.	87	5	92	7
Rochester, N.Y.	84	8	92	6
Columbus, Ohio	85	8	93	6
Cincinnati, Ohio-Ky.-Ind.	84	8	93	7
Milwaukee, Wisc.	85	5	90	9
Kansas City, Mo.-Kan.	84	11	95	4
Atlanta, Ga.	80	10	90	10
Miami, Fla.	83	7	90	8
New Orleans, La.	74	10	84	14
San Antonio, Tex.	80	14	94	5
Portland, Oregon-Wash.	74	15	90	8
San Diego, Calif.	79	12	91	5
Springfield-Chicopee-Holyoke, Mass.-Conn.	88	6	94	4
Madison, Wis.	80	6	86	8
Newport News-Hampton, Va.	85	8	93	5
Colorado Springs, Colo.	81	15	95	1
Total	**79%**	**8%**	**86%**	**12%**

NOTE: Excludes workers not using vehicles to get to work. Details do not always add to totals due to rounding.
(1) Standard Metropolitan Statistical Area.
SOURCE: Preliminary Data from Annual Housing Survey—Department of Transportation, *Travel to Work Survey*; Population Division, U. S. Bureau of the Census. Covers the April-July period of 1975.

Mode of transportation to work

- 79% auto
- 8% truck
- 12% public transit
- 1% other

Mode, time, and distance to work in 21 metropolitan areas

Mode of Transportation	Percent of Workers Using Mode to Travel to Work	Median Time Taken to Get to Work (Minutes)	Median Distance from Home to Work (Miles)
Auto or truck			
Drives alone	68%	19.5	7.7
Carpool			
Shares driving	6	26.0	12.5
Drives others	5	23.7	9.1
Rides with someone	7	19.0	6.6
Total carpool	18	22.5	9.1
Total auto or truck (1)	86	20.1	8.0
Public transportation			
Bus or streetcar	9	33.1	7.0
Subway or elevated	2	41.2	10.1
Railroad	2	52.8	24.4
Total public transportation	12	36.7	8.9
Other means (2)	2	16.5	3.1
Total	**100%**	**20.8**	**7.5**

Median time and distance of work trip

☐ Time (minutes)   ▨ Distance (miles)

- Auto or truck: 20.1 / 8.0
- Public transportation: 36.7 / 8.9

NOTE: Excludes workers not using vehicles to get to work—about 5 percent of all workers. Details do not always add to totals due to rounding.
(1) 79 percent of workers used autos, 8 percent used trucks.
(2) Bicycle, motorcycles and other means beside those listed.
SOURCE: Preliminary data from Annual Housing Survey—Dept. of Transportation, *Travel to Work Survey*; Population Division, U.S. Bureau of the Census. Covers the April-July period of 1975.

Figure 6-1 Modes, time, and distance of commuting workers. (Source: Motor Vehicle Facts and Figures, 1977, p. 50, Motor Vehicle Manufacturers Association, Detroit, Mich.)

There is no simple answer, no panacea. Human nature is of such complexity that improvement of behavior is a gradual and continuing process. Traffic safety entails a long, steady education of drivers, pedestrians, cyclists, traffic and highway engineers, law enforcers, and automobile designers and manufacturers. Nevertheless, if the toll of traffic accidents is to be significantly reduced, there must be a broad and effective approach to educating the individual.

Ralph Nadar, in *Unsafe at Any Speed,* made the public aware of how unsafe motor vehicles are and how automobile manufacturers have failed to

TABLE 6–1
Improper Driving Reported in Accidents, 1976

Kind of Improper Driving	Fatal Accidents			Injury Accidents			All Accidents*		
	Total	Urban	Rural	Total	Urban	Rural	Total	Urban	Rural
Total	100.0%	100.0%	100.0%	100.0%	100.0%	100.0%	100.0%	100.0%	100.0%
Improper driving	76.8	78.4	76.4	83.4	83.3	83.7	86.9	86.6	87.0
Speed too fast†	32.1	26.4	34.0	19.2	14.2	26.7	17.1	12.2	27.1
Right of way	16.5	24.3	14.0	27.1	32.1	19.7	25.8	27.4	22.1
Failed to yield	11.4	15.7	10.0	19.3	21.3	16.2	19.0	18.8	19.1
Passed stop sign	2.8	2.3	3.0	2.5	2.7	2.2	2.3	2.5	1.9
Disregarded signal	2.3	6.3	1.0	5.3	8.1	1.3	4.5	6.1	1.1
Drove left of center	12.9	5.4	15.4	4.3	2.8	6.5	4.1	2.8	6.6
Improper overtaking	1.7	0.9	2.0	1.7	1.3	2.3	3.1	3.0	3.3
Made improper turn	0.9	0.9	0.8	2.6	3.0	2.0	4.4	4.9	3.4
Followed too closely	0.7	1.3	0.6	8.2	10.2	5.2	10.2	12.1	6.3
Other improper driving	12.0	19.2	9.6	20.3	19.7	21.3	22.2	24.2	18.2
No improper driving stated	23.2	21.6	23.6	16.6	16.7	16.3	13.1	13.4	13.0

*Principally property damage accidents, but also includes fatal and injury accidents.
†Includes "speed too fast for conditions".
Source: Reports of state and city traffic authorities, as follows: Urban—40 cities; Rural—10 states; Total—NSC estimates based on Urban and Rural reports. Reported in *Accident Facts*, National Safety Council, Chicago, 1977.

make cars safe. His thesis that it is easier to redesign automobiles to make them safe than to change the nature of the people who drive them is not the opinion of the authors. The tendency to put most of the blame for our traffic safety problem on the automobile instead of on the driver does not get at the core of the problem. Improvements in enforcement, education, legislation, and engineering are necessary factors in reducing the accident rate.

The National Traffic and Motor Vehicle Safety Act of 1966 is an excellent piece of legislation. It established automobile safety standards that were long overdue. There is no doubt that these standards reduce the possibility of injury when a collision occurs, but they do not prevent the initial collision, which is usually caused by the human element.

As we have indicated in Chapter 1, road conditions and mechanical defects combined do not account for a majority of all motor-vehicle accidents. Most traffic accidents are caused by improper driving and traffic violations, the most common of which are exceeding speed limits, driving on the wrong side of the road, following too closely, illegally seizing the right of way, driving under the influence of alcohol, passing improperly, and disregarding traffic-control devices[3] (Tables 6-1 and 6-2).

IMPROPER DRIVING

In most accidents, factors are present relating to the driver, the vehicle, and the road. It is the interaction of these factors which often sets up the series of events which culminates in a mishap.

[3] *Accident Facts*, National Safety Council, Chicago, 1977.

TABLE 6-2

Improper Driving by Age of Driver in Fatal Accidents, 1975

Kind of Improper Driving	All Ages	Age of Driver							
		15–19	20–24	25–34	35–44	45–54	55–64	65–74	75 and Over
Total	100.0%	100.0%	100.0%	100.0%	100.0%	100.0%	100.0%	100.0%	100.0%
Speed too fast†	36.7	43.8	41.9	39.7	34.8	29.4	23.8	13.3	8.5
Right of way	17.3	13.5	12.3	13.8	17.0	21.5	27.2	40.2	50.1
Failed to yield	10.9	7.8	7.0	8.4	10.4	14.5	18.7	27.8	35.9
Disregarded traffic controls	6.4	5.7	5.3	5.4	6.6	7.0	8.5	12.4	14.2
Improper lane or ran off road	24.1	24.0	23.8	24.3	25.2	26.0	25.1	21.8	16.6
Improper or erratic lane changes	0.8	0.7	0.8	0.8	0.9	1.1	0.9	0.9	0.7
Improper overtaking	2.4	2.7	2.6	2.4	2.0	1.9	1.8	2.2	2.1
Improper turn	1.5	1.1	1.0	1.1	1.5	1.9	2.5	3.5	4.3
Followed improperly	1.1	0.9	1.1	1.1	1.4	1.3	1.3	1.3	0.7
Other violation	16.1	13.3	16.5	16.8	17.2	16.9	17.4	16.8	17.0

†Includes "speed too fast for conditions."

Source: Based on National Highway Traffic Safety Administration 1975 Fatal Accident Reporting System. Reported in *Accident Facts*, National Safety Council, Chicago, 1977.

Table 6-1 relates just to the driver and shows the principal kinds of improper driving which were factors in accidents. Correcting these improper practices could have an important effect on accident occurrences. This does not mean that road and vehicle conditions can be disregarded.

The percentages of speeding violations in fatal accidents decrease steadily from 44 percent for drivers aged fifteen to nineteen to about 9 percent for drivers seventy-five and over, according to data from the National Highway Traffic Safety Administration 1975 Fatal Accident Reporting System. Right-of-way violations increased from 12 percent for twenty- to twenty-four-year-old drivers to 50 percent for those seventy-five and over. These and other violations involved in fatal accidents nationally are shown in Table 6-2.

TRAFFIC SAFETY STARTS EARLY

General safety education must begin at an early age, when children can be taught desirable attitudes toward risk taking and highway aggressiveness. Attitudes toward highway safety are more deeply instilled when they are developed during a continuous traffic safety education program. Traffic safety involves more than personal use of automobiles and consideration of their relationship to other objects on the road. Traffic safety starts with the preschool child, or when the youngster becomes a pedestrian, roller skater, bicyclist, tricyclist, or Moped operator.

Parents should assume preschool traffic safety responsibility, with formal instruction to begin the day a youngster starts school. "Many educators have long recognized that traffic safety education is an important responsibility of the school, presumably because of the importance of the underlying objective: to preserve and enhance the capability of the individual to achieve their potential as human beings in all respects."[4]

An early traffic safety education program can prepare our children and youth for the sudden emergencies that may arise when they are on their own and when they are responsible for getting to and from school, home, the grocery store, playground, business district, and the entire community.

First experiences are more likely to leave lasting impressions than are later experiences, and early traffic safety education should be an essential part of the school curriculum. It should be stressed at every grade level from elementary school through high school.

Today, many states are adopting the total traffic safety education concept and are developing and implementing kindergarten-through-twelfth-grade safety programs.[5] At these levels traffic safety may be integrated with everyday learning projects. These projects include a definite set of behavioral objectives

---

[4]*Traffic Safety Education for Schools,* American Automobile Association Foundation for Traffic Safety, Washington, 1965, p. 1.
[5]See the next section of this chapter for an example of what one state did in initiating a kindergarten to ninth grade traffic safety education program.

that will describe to students, teachers, and parents the expected outcome of the learning process, and determine whether the learning has been achieved.[6]

Formal education may be supplemented by school activities such as student safety councils, traffic safety patrols, bicycle safety clubs, and student traffic courts.

The chapters on bicycle safety, pedestrian safety, a safe school environment, teaching safety, and planning a school safety program describe the materials and procedures that may be used in teaching traffic safety at all grade levels. The following general objectives have been suggested by the Insurance Institute for Highway Safety. Although the objectives are not stated in terms of measurable human behavior, they give an overview of what an early traffic safety program should accomplish. Among the objectives are to:

1 Reduce the toll of traffic accidents

2 Develop a recognition of situations involving traffic hazards

3 Develop a sense of responsibility for the safety of oneself and others, whether they be pedestrians, bicyclists, Moped drivers, or passengers in motor vehicles

4 Develop an appreciation of the work of police officers, school patrols, adult crossing guards, traffic and highway engineers, and others who are constantly striving to make communities safer places to live

5 Develop an appreciation for the need for obeying school patrols, adult crossing guards, traffic officers, traffic signs, signals, and road markings

6 Use the safest routes to and from school, play area, business district, church, and other areas frequented by school-age youth

7 Study the causes of traffic accidents and what is being done to reduce them

Effective learning experiences in early traffic safety education programs will aid immeasurably in developing attitudes of social responsibility in future drivers. See Appendix A (P. 460) for North Carolina's safety program.

THE HIGHWAY SAFETY ACT OF 1966

To reduce motor-vehicle accidents, injuries, and fatalities, the federal government established a national highway safety program under the Highway Safety Act of 1966. This program required the establishment of uniform highway safety program standards upon which states and communities could organize their programs.

This act provided federal grants to aid states in conducting a comprehensive highway safety program. There have been modifications to the original act, and additional changes will probably be made in the future. In fact, there is

[6](See Ralph W. Tyler, *Basic Principles of Curriculum Construction,* The University of Chicago Press, 1969; Thorwald Eshensen, "Writing Instructional Objectives," *Phi Delta Kappan Journal,* 1967; and Robert F. Mager, *Preparing Instructional Objectives,* Fearon Publishers, Belmont, Cal., 1962.)

some question as to whether or not current standards will remain in force, at least in their present form.

NATIONAL HIGHWAY SAFETY PROGRAM STANDARDS[7]

Section 402 of The Highway Safety Act is as follows:

(a) Each State shall have a highway safety program approved by the Secretary, designed to reduce traffic accidents and deaths, injuries, and property damage resulting therefrom. Such programs shall be in accordance with uniform standards promulgated by the Secretary. Such uniform standards shall be expressed in terms of performance criteria. Such uniform standards shall be promulgated by the Secretary so as to improve driver performance (including, but not limited to, driver education, driver testing to determine proficiency to operate motor vehicles, driver examinations (both physical and mental) and driver licensing) and to improve pedestrian performance. In addition such uniform standards shall include, but not be limited to, provisions for an effective record system of accidents (including injuries and deaths resulting therefrom), accident investigations to determine the probable causes of accidents, injuries, and deaths, vehicle registration, operation, and inspection, highway design and maintenance (including lighting, markings, and surface treatment), traffic control, vehicle codes and laws, surveillance of traffic for detection and correction of high or potentially high accident locations, and emergency services. Such standards as are applicable to State highway safety programs shall, to the extent determined appropriate by the Secretary, be applicable to federally administered areas where a Federal department or agency controls the highway or supervises traffic operations. The Secretary shall be authorized to amend or waive standards on a temporary basis for the purpose of evaluating new or different highway safety programs instituted on an experimental, pilot, or demonstration basis by one or more States, where the Secretary finds that the public interest would be served by such amendment or waiver.

(b) (1) The Secretary shall not approve any State highway safety program under this section which does not—

(A) provide that the Governor of the State shall be responsible for the administration of the program.

(B) authorize political subdivisions of such State to carry out local highway safety programs within their jurisdictions as a part of the State highway safety program if such local highway safety programs are approved by the Governor and are in accordance with the uniform standards of the Secretary promulgated under this section.

(C) provide that at least 40 per centum of all Federal funds apportioned under this section to such State for any fiscal year will be expended by the political subdivisions of such State in carrying out local highway safety programs authorized in accordance with subparagraph (B) of this paragraph.

(D) provide that the aggregate expenditure of funds of the State and political subdivisions thereof, exclusive of Federal funds, for highway safety programs will be maintained at a level which does not fall below the average level of such expenditures for its last two full fiscal years preceding the date of enactment of this section.

(E) provide for comprehensive driver training programs, including (1) the initiation of a State program for driver education in the school systems or for a significant expansion and improvement of such a program already in existence, to be administered by appropriate school officials under the supervision of the Governor as set forth in subparagraph (A) of this paragraph; (2) the training of qualified school instructors and their certification; (3) appropriate regulation of other driver training schools, including licensing of the schools and certification of their instructors, (4) adult driver training programs, and programs for the retraining of

---

[7]United States Code 1964, *Title 23,* § 401 et seq., Sept. 9, 1966, Pub. L. 89-564,80 Stat. 731.

selected drivers; and (5) adequate research, development and procurement of practice driving facilities, simulators, and other similar teaching aids for both school and other driver training use.

After the establishment of the National Highway Safety Bureau—now National Highway Traffic Safety Administration—the staff began to develop a series of program standards based upon the interpretation of Section 402. Ultimately 18 standards were developed. They are:

  1 Periodic Motor Vehicle Inspection.
  2 Motor Vehicle Registration.
  3 Motorcycle Safety.
  4 Driver Education.
  5 Driver Licensing.
  6 Codes and Laws.
  7 Traffic Courts.
  8 Alcohol in Relation to Highway Safety.
  9 Identification and Surveillance of Accident Locations.
  10 Traffic Records.
  11 Emergency Medical Services.
  12 Highway Design, Construction, and Maintenance.
  13 Traffic Control Devices.
  14 Pedestrian Safety.
  15 Police Traffic Services.
  16 Debris Hazard Control and Cleanup.
  17 Pupil Transportation.
  18 Accident Investigation and Reporting.

The purpose and a brief description of the standards follow.[8]

1. Periodic motor vehicle inspection:

Purpose: The purpose of Highway Safety Program Standard Number 1, Periodic Motor Vehicle Inspection, is to increase, through periodic vehicle inspection, the likelihood that every vehicle operating on the public highways is properly equipped and is being maintained in a reasonably safe working condition.

The Standard calls for (1) at least an annual inspection of all motor vehicles, or the conduct of an experimental, pilot or demonstration program, (2) inspection by trained and certified inspectors, (3) coverage of systems, subsystems, and components having substantial relation to safe vehicle performance, (4) inspection in accordance with NHTSA-issued inspection criteria and procedures, and (5) annual compilation of data by vehicle make and model.

2. Motor vehicle registration:

Purpose: The purpose of Highway Safety Program Standard Number 2, Motor Vehicle Registration (MVR) is as follows: "To provide a means of identifying the owner and type,

---

[8]*An Evaluation of The Highway Safety Program,* A Report to the Congress from the Secretary of Transportation, U.S. Department of Transportation, National Highway Traffic Safety Administration. Washington, 1977, pp. III-3 to III-64.

weight, size and carrying capacity of every vehicle licensed to operate in the State, and to make such data available for traffic safety studies and research, accident investigation, enforcement, and other operational users; and to provide a means for aggregating ownership and vehicle information for: (a) accident research; (b) planning and development of streets, highways and related facilities; and (c) other operational uses."

The Standard requires that "each State shall have a motor vehicle registration program, which shall provide for rapid identification of each vehicle and its owner; and shall make available pertinent data for accident research and safety program development."

3. Motorcycle safety:

Purpose: The purpose of Highway Safety Standard Number 3, Motorcycle Safety, is to assure that motorcycles, motorcycle operators, and their passengers meet standards which contribute to safe operation and to the reduction of deaths and injuries.

The elements of the Standard address basic safety problems: Preventing or reducing the severity of head injuries, determining whether novice motorcyclists have the basic skills, and assuring that the vehicles have minimum safety equipment and maintenance. Different elements require the wearing of helmets by operators and passengers, eye protection for operators, special tests and license for operators, and special inspection criteria for motorcycles.

4. Driver education:

Purpose: The Highway Safety Program Standard Number 4, Driver Education, aims to insure the availability and quality of curricula in public and commercial driver schools, for adults as well as young beginning drivers, with the overall purpose of reducing the accident involvement of drivers who lack proper knowledge and skills.

Elements of the Standard describe the basic curriculum objective and subject matter for youths, require certification of instructors according to State criteria including instructors at commercial schools, insure the provision of adult training and retraining, and encourage an overall State research and procurement program to support driver education.

5. Driver licensing:

Purpose: The purpose of the Highway Safety Program Standard Number 5, Driver Licensing, is to reduce accidents involving drivers who lack the knowledge, skills, and physical or mental ability to operate a motor vehicle, principally by ensuring uniform licensing procedures aimed at detecting driving incompetence.

The major elements of this Standard deal with the initial driving examination, driver records, license renewal, and driver improvement programs. Other elements describe requirements for driver competence, procedures for determining driver incompetence, and necessary characteristics of a data system dealing with driver licensing, including creation of a single State agency to administer the program.

6. Codes and laws:

Purpose: The purpose of the Highway Safety Program Standard Number 6, Codes and Laws, is to encourage uniformity in traffic codes, laws, and ordinances within a State, and to foster further adoption by all States of the Rules of the Road Chapter of the *Uniform Vehicle Code* (UVC).

The elements of this brief Standard simply restate its purpose, requiring each State to have a program aimed at achieving uniformity within its boundaries and consistency with other States with respect to the traffic rules of the road.

7. Traffic courts:

Purpose: The purpose of the Highway Safety Program Standard Number 7, Traffic Courts, is to promote prompt, impartial adjudication of proceedings involving motor vehicle law, and to recommend a minimal uniformity among the practices of the traffic courts within a State.

The Standard has only one requirement: That all convictions for any moving violation be reported to the State traffic records system. It also makes six recommendations, one designed to ensure a court appearance for all persons charged with hazardous moving violations, the others aimed at improving the independence, quality, and uniformity of traffic courts.

8. Alcohol in relation to highway safety:

Purpose: The stated purpose of Highway Safety Program Standard Number 8, Alcohol in Relation to Highway Safety, is to broaden the scope and number of activities directed at reducing the frequency of alcohol-related accidents.

The Standard's elements contain the basic structure which now underlies the drinking–driving laws of all 50 States, providing for (1) the use of chemical tests, (2) establishment of a BAC value (.10%) which is presumptive evidence of intoxication, and (3) "implied consent" of a motorist to submit to a chemical test. Other elements relate to the collection of data on fatalities, the control of the chemical test program, and evaluation of the Standard.

9. Identification and surveillance of accident locations:

Purpose: The purpose of Highway Safety Program Standard Number 9, Identification and Surveillance of Accident Locations, is to identify specific locations or sections of streets and highways which have high or potentially high accident experience, as a basis for establishing priorities for improvement, selective enforcement, or other operational practices that will eliminate or reduce the hazards at the location so identified.

The Standard calls for (1) an accident analysis program based on uniformly reported data, (2) during the identification phase, accident locations are pinpointed and recorded, (3) surveillance should include both record reviews and prevention-oriented examination of the highway network, and (4) accident location surveillance, follow-up surveillance, and assignment of priorities for corrective measures.

10. Traffic records:

Purpose: The purpose of the Highway Safety Program Standard Number 10, Traffic Records, is to provide guidance for the State creation of comprehensive, efficient, and uniform traffic record systems containing appropriate information on drivers, vehicles, highways, and accidents. The data from these systems must be available to provide the information base for identifying safety problems, developing corrective measures, and evaluating actions taken.

The overall thrust of the elements is to emphasize the application of record systems in identifying problems. Most elements describe the basic requirements for identifying problems through relevant data, including collection and input of information, analysis of data, and retrieval and output capabilities. Various elements specify information needs about drivers, vehicles, and accidents.

11. Emergency medical services:

Purpose: The purpose of the Highway Safety Program Standard Number 11, Emergency Medical Services, is to create an emergency care system capable of responding quickly to accidents, providing appropriate care at the scene of the accident and in transit, and providing the necessary transportation and communications to bring medical care so quickly as to reduce the likelihood of death and further injury.

The elements of the Standard aim at setting requirements for qualified and trained personnel, for the right types and numbers of vehicles, and for communication and coordination with the rest of the medical care system. All these are to be encompassed in a comprehensive statewide plan for emergency medical services.

12. Highway design, construction and maintenance:

Purpose: The purpose of Highway Safety Program Standard Number 12, Highway Design, Construction and Maintenance, is to assure that existing streets and highways are maintained in a condition that promotes safety; that capital improvements, either to modernize existing roads or to provide new facilities, meet approved safety standards; and that appropriate precautions are taken to protect passing motorists, as well as highway workers, from accident involvement at highway construction sites.

13. Traffic engineering services:

Purpose: The purpose of Highway Safety Program Standard Number 13, Traffic Engineering Services, is to assure the full and proper application of modern traffic engineering principles and uniform standards for traffic control, to reduce the likelihood and severity of traffic accidents.

The main thrust of this standard is that each State, in cooperation with its political subdivisions, and each Federal department or agency which controls highways open to public travel or supervises traffic operations, shall have a program for applying traffic-engineering measures and techniques, including the use of traffic-control devices, to reduce the number and severity of traffic accidents.

14. Pedestrian safety:

Purpose: The purpose of this Highway Safety Program Standard Number 14, Pedestrian Safety, is to recognize pedestrian safety as a significant feature in the overall highway safety program, and to reduce accidents involving pedestrians by encouraging regular State attention to the problem.

The elements of the Standard emphasize, first, identifying the pedestrian problem, then taking countermeasures involving attention to (a) environments, (b) driver response, and (c) the pedestrian population, especially school children.

15. Police traffic services:

Purpose: The purpose of Highway Safety Program Standard Number 15, Police Traffic Services, is to reduce accidents by strengthening and improving all police traffic services from accident prevention all the way to the arrest process. The Standard emphasizes use of police patrols to enforce traffic laws, improve traffic flow, prevent accidents, aid the injured, document individual accidents, supervise cleanup, and restore traffic flow.

The Standard's elements aim at providing basic needs in a State program: uniform training procedures, records, and reporting systems; inservice training; selective assignment; coordination with other agencies regarding traffic problems; and achievement of uniformity between neighboring jurisdictions.

16. Debris hazard control and cleanup:

Purpose: The purpose of Highway Safety Program Standard Number 16, Debris Hazard Control and Cleanup, is to reduce accidents due to debris on the highway. It seeks to establish proper responsibilities and procedures for removing debris and for restoring the location to a safe condition.

The elements of the Standard require that a State have a program with established procedures for training rescue and salvage personnel, speeding their arrival at an accident site, improving their ability to rescue trapped persons and removing debris, and setting up an appropriate communications system.

17. Pupil transportation safety:

Purpose: Highway Safety Program Standard Number 17, Pupil Transportation Safety, has as its purpose the reduction of death and injury to school children while they are being transported to and from school.

To achieve this purpose, various elements of the Standard cover the operation and maintenance of vehicles, the qualifications, training and conduct of the drivers, and passenger behavior. The objectives of these components are to ensure driver competency, promote safe passenger behavior and ensure adequate vehicle quality and transportation procedures.

18. Accident investigation and reporting:

Purpose: The objective of the Highway Safety Program Standard Number 18, Accident Investigation and Reporting, is to promote comprehensive, efficient, and uniform accident investigation procedures and systems. The Standard emphasizes both the gathering of accident information, and its entry and storage for use in planning highway safety programs.

The main thrust of the Standard is thus the promotion of comprehensive and uniform reporting systems, emphasizing completeness and accuracy of data, and efficiency in retrieval and use of that data. The Standard emphasizes cooperation between agencies within a jurisdiction, the need for compatibility between the data from different jurisdictions, the training and qualifications of accident investigators, and the use of data to determine accident causation and improve highway safety programs. The Standard is closely interrelated to two other Standards: Police Traffic Services (No. 15) and Traffic Records (No. 10).

The Highway Safety Act places emphasis on secondary school driver education as an integral part of effective programming for traffic safety. The bill provides millions of dollars to help finance these programs. On a matching basis, state and local governmental officials may use these funds to (1) initiate, expand, and improve high school driver education programs; (2) prepare driver education teachers; (3) procure equipment, practice-driving facilities, and other teaching aids; and (4) conduct research designed to improve the effectiveness of instruction.

Of special interest to educators, one section of the act states:

The secretary shall not approve any state highway safety program which does not provide for comprehensive driver education programs, including the initiation of a state program for driver education in the school system or for a significant expansion and improvement of such a program already in existence, to be administered by appropriate school officials under the supervision of the Governor.

Driver education, now recognized through federal legislation, makes millions of dollars available to help state and local governments expand and improve this important area of the traffic safety program.

Crashes are usually caused by the interaction of three factors: people, vehicles, and roadways. Driver education seeks to teach future drivers the knowledge, skills, and attitudes most important to safe driving.

Formal driver education began in the late 1930s. It has been improved over the past 30 years through the knowledge and experience obtained since the first National Conference on Driver Education Standards in 1949. Today the elements of the standards describe the basic curriculum, objectives, and subject matter for youth; require certification of instructors, including those at commercial schools, according to each state's requirements; ensure the provisions of adult training and retraining; and encourage an overall state research and procurement program to support driver education.

DRIVER AND TRAFFIC SAFETY EDUCATION

Leadership in traffic safety should come from the state department of education. The department should be directly responsible for the leadership, coordination, supervision, and promotion of traffic safety education programs for schools under their jurisdiction. The following policies indicate the responsibilities of state departments of education for implementing traffic safety education programs:[9]

- Encourage development of traffic safety education as part of the total educational program.
- Provide advisory and consultative services to help school systems improve and expand their programs.
- Aid school systems in developing effective methods for administering and supervising comprehensive traffic safety education programs.
- Establish and promulgate standards for traffic safety education including high school driver education.
- Develop teacher-certification requirements with adequate standards for qualification.
- Encourage teacher-preparation institutions to develop and implement high-quality, competency-based teacher-preparation programs.
- Develop and distribute resource materials, i.e., curriculum guides, administrative handbooks, and other pertinent information.
- Develop appropriate procedures to assist school systems in purchasing or otherwise obtaining automobiles and other equipment for laboratory instruction, including plans for the preventive maintenance of such equipment and its periodic replacement.
- Advise school systems on matters of insurance and legal responsibilities related to administration and operation of school safety programs.
- Stimulate school systems to undertake in-service activities for teachers and encourage teachers to acquire additional professional preparation.
- Serve as liaison between representatives of teacher-education institutions and professional associations of driver education teachers.
- Develop effective means of utilizing the advisory services of qualified individuals and groups.
- Aid and encourage those conducting appropriate research studies.
- Stimulate and conduct effective community relations activities at state and local levels.
- Study and recommend needed legislation, cooperating closely with groups actively concerned with its adoption.
- Counsel on specifications and design of facilities and equipment.
- Compile and make available lists of colleges and universities which offer courses in traffic safety education.
- Evaluate state and local program effectiveness.

[9] *Policies and Guidelines for Driver and Traffic Safety Education,* American Driver and Traffic Safety Education Association, National Education Association, Washington, 1974, pp. 5–6.

ORGANIZATION AT THE STATE, DISTRICT, AND SCHOOL LEVELS

Within each state department of education there should be a sufficient number of qualified specialists and available consultants to administer and supervise the total traffic safety program. One person should be designated as the head of the unit, responsible for the statewide program.

At the local school level, the district superintendent of education is the key person in the implementation of a successful traffic safety education program. In many school systems this responsibility is delegated to a supervisor. Financial resources, facilities, selection of staff, establishment of standards of performance, and sufficient time, effort, and enthusiasm are important elements of a quality driver and traffic safety program.

At the school level, individual principals have direct responsibility for implementing the program, with a member of the faculty designated as the safety chairperson or coordinator. The faculty member can also be responsible for coordinating and supervising the kindergarten-through-twelfth-grade safety-education program for the school system. The quality of the program will depend largely on the competence, interest, enthusiasm, dedication, and capability of the school safety coordinator and the faculty members selected to conduct the program.

In senior high schools, driver education should be a separate subject in the curriculum. Traffic safety may still be integrated with other subjects in the curriculum. It can be taught on a unit basis in the social, behavioral, physical, and biological sciences, or in health education. These units would supplement the instruction given in driver education courses.

The course should be offered to students as they are approaching or have reached legal driving age. The recommended driver education course is presented in two phases, preferably concurrently. The first phase consists of learning activities in the classroom. The second is the laboratory phase, usually called the practice-driving phase. It provides for actual behind-the-wheel driving instruction in a dual-control automobile on public streets or highways or on an established driving range. Additional laboratory work can be provided by means of classroom driving simulators. Both parts of the program should be taught by a well-prepared, qualified, and certified high school driver education teacher meeting the minium standards recommended by the National Conference on Policies and Guidelines for Driver and Traffic Safety Education.[10]

The task of driver education is to provide young people with the knowledge, skills, and, most importantly, the proper attitudes and a sound understanding of our social responsibility for the safe use of streets and highways. No agency is better qualified to prepare these students than our nation's schools,

[10]Ibid., pp. 22–23.

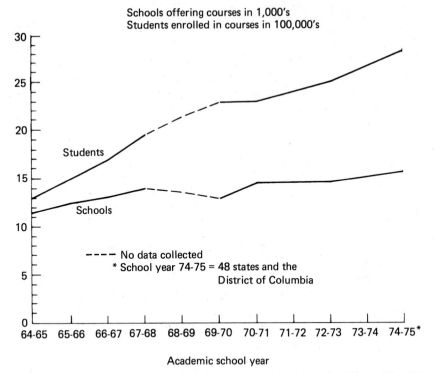

Schools offering courses in 1,000's
Students enrolled in courses in 100,000's

Figure 6-2 Relationship between schools offering courses and students enrolled. (Source: Driver Education Status Report, 1976, p. 1, National Safety Council, Chicago, Ill.)

for every year over 3 million students are potential candidates for driver's licenses.

According to a recent survey (1974-1975) of driver education programs conducted by the National Safety Council, 15,984 out of 19,127 public, private, and parochial high schools (84 percent) were providing driver education programs meeting minimum national standards. Of the 3,728,192 students eligible for driver education annually, 2,814,604 were receiving minimum instruction.

Figure 6-2 illustrates the growth of driver education since 1964. Despite the rapid progress, there is still room for expansion. Education in traffic safety should be available at all grade levels in elementary and secondary schools, in institutions of higher learning, and in adult education programs. "Because the core problem is one of human behavior, the proper education of as many persons as can possibly be reached *before they are licensed to drive* is our greatest hope for helping man adapt himself more successfully to his use of the motor vehicle."[11]

[11]*Policies and Practices for Driver Education,* National Commission on Safety Education, National Education Association, Washington, 1960, p. 9.

OBJECTIVES OF DRIVER AND TRAFFIC SAFETY EDUCATION

A central statement of purpose that considers the needs of both education and the highway transportation system must be part of an effective high school driver education program. The ultimate purpose of the program is to provide educational experiences that will give beginning drivers the competency to become socially responsible drivers. Each educational system will want to formulate its own specific objectives. The following objectives were developed at the most recent national conference on driver and traffic safety education.

GENERAL OBJECTIVES[12]

Upon completion of a high school driver education course, students will be able to:

- Describe or, under simulated conditions, demonstrate techniques for coping with critical driving situations
- Formulate a set of guidelines for avoiding harmful highway consequences resulting from misuse of alcohol or other drugs
- List the primary components of a comprehensive highway safety program and identify the general purpose of each component.

After identifying explicit objectives for the entire course, each objective should be assigned to a mode of instruction such as classroom, multimedia, simulator, range, or on-street, where learning best can take place. Examples of mode objectives are given below. Lesson plans or modules built around logical clusters of objectives should then be developed. These should be followed by a variety of learning activities associated with the concerned objectives. Evaluation techniques for determining whether students have acquired essential performance traits should also be developed.

Regular classroom mode objectives

To enable students to:
- Develop a set of strategies for preventing various psychological, physiological, social or other factors from having an adverse effect on one's ability to perform the driving task
- Define the legal and moral responsibilities of highway users.

Electronic simulator mode objectives

To enable students to:
- Perceive common and unusual traffic hazards
- Respond correctly to selected driving emergencies.

Off-street multiple-car driving range mode objectives

The multiple-car range unit addresses itself to two broad categories of objectives; those that are involved with basic control (manipulation) and those that are involved with decision-making for conflict avoidance.

---

[12]*Policies and Guidelines for Driver and Traffic Safety Education,* American Driver and Traffic Safety Education Association, National Educational Association, Washington, 1974, p. 14.

On-street mode objectives

To enable students to:

• Demonstrate a level of proficiency in the human functions (identification, prediction, decision, and execution) sufficient to perform legally and safely as they interact with other highway users in routine and difficult system environments

• In the driver education car, demonstrate the ability to deal with oncoming vehicles by choice of traffic lane, position within the lane, and speed adjustment to avoid collisions.

GUIDELINES FOR BEGINNING COURSES

The following are some of the recommended guidelines for implementing the course within a school district.[13]

Driver education courses provided within school districts for youthful beginners should:

• Be based on current curriculum guides approved by the state department of education

• Be offered at the grade or age level where most students are closely approaching or have just reached the minimum legal driver licensing age

• Be scheduled so that a sufficient number of courses are provided during the regular school day and, as necessary, at other times so that every youth within the school jurisdiction has an opportunity to enroll

• Consist of 90 hours of structured learning experiences, scheduled over a full term or more, including laboratory instruction with in-car driving experience for each student

• Be conducted in facilities designed to provide learning experiences appropriate to and/or required by course objectives

• Provide students with no more than two hours of classroom instruction and one hour of behind-the-wheel instruction during any 24-hour period. Where simulation and/or off-street multiple-car driving ranges are utilized, not more than one additional hour per student per day should be allowed

• Provide laboratory instruction only to students who are currently participating in the classroom instruction

• Use only those practice vehicles that are equipped according to standards established by the appropriate state agency and are covered by property, liability, and medical-payment insurance sufficient to recover damages to the school, teachers, students, general public, the vehicles, and their owners

• Use as managers of student learning in driver education, only regularly employed and certificated teachers who are on the district salary schedule, and who are supervised by school officials responsible for the program.

Driver education teachers should instruct a maximum of six hours per day.

CONSIDERING STUDENTS' NEEDS

Driver education instructors, must understand the interests, needs, and capabilities of their students if they are to plan a program that will be meaningful to them and that will stimulate effective learning. The young people in high school driver education courses are at a critical stage of their development. The

[13]Ibid., p. 15

"growing pains" occasioned by the physical, mental, and emotional changes taking place during this period may give rise to serious psychological difficulties and undesirable behavior patterns. No longer children but not yet adults, adolescents are likely to find the problems of personal adjustment particularly complicated. Many teen-agers will need sympathetic guidance in working out satisfactory solutions.

The driver education instructor should review the personality traits associated with adolescence and study their significance for driver education. Many of these traits have both positive and negative implications. Some characteristics that are potentially conducive to reckless behavior may become assets rather than liabilities if students are properly motivated. A brief summary of several important aspects of adolescent development is offered here. The teacher should understand how the changes in this process are likely to affect driving ability and how driver education can help students solve the psychological problems created by these changes.

IMPLICATIONS OF PHYSICAL GROWTH. Adolescents of seventeen or eighteen are physically adults, but they retain much of the abundant vitality of a healthy child. They are thus ready and eager for challenging adventure. This desire for thrills and excitement, which is strengthened by some of the emotional and mental characteristics of adolescence, often manifests itself in hot-rod races and other dangerous pursuits. The driver education instructor who understands the cause of such behavior can try to prevent recklessness by pointing out to students that mastery of basic skills is a prerequisite to real adventure, and that learning to drive well will increase their opportunities for stimulating experiences. The "excess" vitality of most young people makes them well able to take a driver education course in addition to their regular curriculum load. The extra course may, in fact, serve as a desirable outlet for their exuberance.

Adolescents, for all practical purposes, have attained physical maturity. They tend to think of themselves as adults and to demand the recognition and the privileges that they associate with adult status. The girl who is old enough to marry and the boy who is nearly eligible for military service quite naturally feel that they should be free of the restrictions imposed on children. They may belligerently proclaim their independence by rebelling against rules and regulations.

But adolescents claim adult privileges without recognizing and accepting adult responsibilities, for mental and emotional maturity does not automatically accompany physical maturation. Young people need to be given responsible, challenging tasks if they are to become mature in other than the physical sense, but adults are reluctant to entrust important jobs to teen-agers who continue to behave like children. This situation illustrates the proverbial vicious circle: restrictions induce rebellious behavior, and rebelliousness is countered with further restrictions.

The driver education instructor, however, is in an excellent position to help students develop good judgment and the sense of responsibility that are the earmarks of true maturity. In learning to drive, young people are participating in an adult activity and acquiring skills that will help establish their independence. They are therefore motivated to learn and to be receptive to instruction. The teacher can make them understand that the privilege of operating a car carries with it the obligation to drive in a way that will not endanger themselves or others, that traffic regulations are designed for their own protection, and that the ability to drive efficiently and safely indicates their competence and reliability and thus entitles them to the respect and approval of society. When this approach is adopted, students usually make a determined effort to acquire good driving skills and demonstrate their trustworthiness.

IMPLICATIONS OF MENTAL GROWTH. Although young people rarely attain full intellectual development during adolescence, their curiosity about themselves and their environment is intensified, their interests become broader, and their ability to reason increases. As they approach adulthood and look forward to the time when they will face the world on their own, their choice of a vocation, their relationship with the opposite sex, and various religious, ethical, and political issues become serious problems for them.

Adolescents have left the world of childhood, where the prevailing order was firmly established and their status was fixed and accepted, but they have not yet entered the world of adults. The interim period is often one of chaos, yet the doubts and questions that arise stimulate mental growth. The thinking of young people is often motivated, at least subconsciously, by the desire to discover a new order to govern their lives.

The adolescent's awakened curiosity, of course, is a stimulus to learning. The driver education teacher, like all other high school teachers, should take advantage of it. Since students are likely to exhibit a growing interest in civic affairs, the teacher should give them opportunity to discuss local traffic conditions and the means of coping with them, and should guide them in recognizing the value of law-enforcement agencies and the logical basis for traffic rules and regulations.

Classroom discussion of traffic laws in relation to democratic principles should (1) strengthen reasoning ability and help develop good judgment, (2) prevent students from using their growing intellectual powers to find loopholes in existing regulations and from allowing their curiosity to stimulate such dangerous experiments as trying to see how fast a car can go, and (3) help students understand their responsibilities as drivers and thus recognize their relationship to society and their place in the adult world. By teaching students to operate an automobile efficiently, a driver education course may increase the vocational possibilities open to them and their opportunities to participate in social activities.

IMPLICATIONS OF EMOTIONAL DEVELOPMENT. For the reasons already mentioned, adolescence is likely to be a period of frustration. High school students are physically ready for adult experiences, but they are encompassed by prohibitions. They want the respect and approval of society, but they are not entrusted with responsibility. Half adult and half child, the adolescent is between two camps, in a no-man's-land of doubts and insecurities. It is not surprising that many young people develop a sense of inferiority and fail to acquire emotional stability.

The driver education instructor should recognize that it is the lack of self-confidence and of emotional control that makes many adolescents poor risks as drivers. The highly emotional person is easily distracted from the task at hand, and a driver must be constantly alert to hazards. Drivers with little self-confidence tend to become disconcerted by traffic conditions and thus incapable of the sure, quick, and accurate decisions that a motorist must often make. On the other hand, drivers who feel inferior sometimes exploit the temporary sense of power they acquire when they are behind the wheel by performing dangerous, aggressive acts in an attempt to compensate for their personal inadequacy.

A well-conducted driver education course can help students develop safe driving habits so that they will follow the proper procedures automatically, even when under emotional stress. Competent instruction should also instill such a strong sense of responsibility for safety that insecure young people will seek less dangerous substitutes for emotional satisfaction than fast and reckless driving.

Ideally, of course, the instructor should try not only to prevent students' maladjustments from interfering with their driving but to guide them in overcoming these maladjustments. A driver education course is an excellent means of helping adolescents gain emotional maturity and social responsibility. The ability to drive well, in addition to developing self-respect and gaining the respect of others, may provide opportunities for worthwhile experiences that will satisfy the need for adventure and aid in personality development. Provisions must be made for the handicapped. Many mentally retarded, culturally and educationally deprived, emotionally disturbed, physically handicapped, and hearing- and visually-impaired persons can profit from instruction in traffic safety education.

ORGANIZATION OF COURSE CONTENT

At the first national conference on driver education, held at Jackson's Mill, West Virginia, October, 1949, representatives of forty-three states and the District of Columbia decided on the following standard terms to be used in discussing driver education programs:[14]

- *Driver education* refers to all those learning experiences provided by the school for the purpose of helping students to learn to use motor vehicles safely and efficiently.
- *Classroom instruction* in driver education programs refers to those learning experiences which are provided elsewhere than in an automobile.
- *Practice driving* refers to those learning experiences in driver education provided for the student as an observer and a student driver in an automobile.

[14]*High School Driver Education: Policies and Recommendations,* National Commission on Safety Education, National Education Association, Washington, 1950.

At the second and third conferences, these terms were reaffirmed and expanded. At the fourth conference in 1963 the terms were described as follows:[15]

• *Driver and Traffic Safety Education* are learning experiences provided by the school for the purpose of helping students to become good traffic citizens and to use motor vehicles safely and efficiently.

Standard Course is one which includes both classroom and laboratory instruction and meets all minimum standards as set forth in the conference.

• *Classroom Instruction* is group instruction which covers such content areas as traffic citizenship, laws and regulations, characteristics of drivers, role of government, automobile use, and traffic problems.

• *Psychophysical Equipment* is testing devices used to demonstrate varying abilities related to field of vision, visual acuity, distance judgment, reaction time, color discrimination, etc.

• *Laboratory Instruction* is an extension of classroom instruction which provides students with opportunities for traffic experiences under real or simulated conditions.

• *Dual-Control Car* is a car equipped with an extra brake and, where necessary, an extra clutch pedal.

• *In-Car Practice* is supervised student experience at the controls of a practice driving car either on-street or on a multiple-car driving range.

• *Observation Time* includes students' time spent in the vehicle other than at the controls and involves group discussion and assessment of the driving task.

• *Driving Simulation* is a teaching method employing both films and electromechanical devices designed to represent the driver's compartment of the automobile through which students develop proper judgment and behavior responses as well as manipulative skills.

• *Multiple-Car Driving Range* is an off-street area on which a number of cars are used simultaneously to provide laboratory instruction under the supervision of one or more teachers. The area includes:

a. space for the development of fundamental skills
b. road surfaces wide enough for two-way and multiple-lane traffic
c. intersections, curves, and grades
d. lane markings, signs, and signals
e. a method of communication between teacher and students by radio, loud speaker, or other effective means

• *Driver Improvement Course* is a special course conducted for traffic law violators, traffic accident repeaters, and volunteers for the purpose of re-education in traffic responsibilities.

At the most recent conference held in 1973 the following terms were adopted.[16]

• *Driver education.* Classroom and laboratory student learning experiences designed to enable motor vehicle operators to become safer and more efficient highway users and to acquire knowledge about the highway transportation system so that they may contribute to its improvement.

---

[15] *Policies and Practices for Driver and Traffic Safety Education,* National Commission on Safety Education, National Education Association, Washington, 1964.
[16] *Policies and Guidelines for Driver and Traffic Safety Education,* American Driver and Traffic Safety Education Association, National Education Association, Washington, 1974, pp. vii and viii.

- *Classroom phase.* That portion of driver education course, based in a classroom environment, which is characterized by student learning under the management of a teacher or teachers.
- *Regular classroom mode.* Group or individualized student learning experiences which take place in a teacher-managed classroom environment without utilization of an electronic or mechanical student response system.
- *Multimedia classroom mode.* Group student learning experiences which take place in a teacher-managed classroom environment utilizing audio-visuals and featuring student response to multiple-choice test items depicted on a screen.
- *Laboratory phase.* That portion of a driver education course, covering motor vehicle operation under real or simulated conditions, characterized by student learning experiences arising from use of electronic driving simulation equipment, an off-street multiple car driving range, and/or on-street driving practice in a dual-controlled car under the direction of a teacher.
- *Electronic simulator mode.* Group student learning experiences which permit individuals to operate vehicular controls in response to audio-visual depictations of traffic environments and driving emergencies. The electromechanical equipment provides for evaluation (by a teacher) of perceptual, judgmental, and decision-making performance of individuals and groups.
- *Off-street multiple-car driving-range mode.* Student learning experiences which take place on an off-street area on which a number of cars are used simultaneously under the direct supervision of one or more teachers for the purpose of improving perceptual judgment, decision-making, and psychomotor skills.
- *On-street mode.* Student learning experiences which are supervised by a teacher and take place in a dual-controlled motor vehicle while operating on streets and highways.
- *Learning activity package.* A lesson plan for use by students and/or teachers which contains one or more performance objectives stated in terms of measurable human behavior, related student learning activities, and procedures for determining whether learners have achieved the objective or objectives.
- *Performance objective.* A statement of learning intent which attempts to describe specific levels of expected outcomes and identifies the conditions under which the performance will be demonstrated.

INSTRUCTIONAL OBJECTIVES AND COURSE CONTENT

Much has happened in recent years to cause changes in the course content of driver and traffic safety education. Several studies have analyzed the three E's (education, enforcement, and engineering) of traffic safety to determine exactly what is involved in driving a motor vehicle. This analysis of the driving task, along with the formulation of instructional objectives to meet the needs of a task-analysis approach, has stimulated many changes in the program.

The Automotive Safety Foundation's Resource Curriculum of 1970, followed by the studies of the Human Resources Research Organization (HumRRO) and others, was instrumental in making significant changes in the driver education curriculum. Today the instructional program is based on a task-analysis approach rather than the accident-causation approach. The approach of new high school driver education text books is based on this concept. Many new state guides have also been developed from the task-analysis approach. (See Appendix B (p. 465) for an example of how one state developed a guide for its driver education curriculum.) The plan describes in detail the:

1 Highway transportation system

2 Official plan for controlling the highway transportation system safety problem

3 Approach for development of the driver education program

4 A driving task model

5 Implications for driver education

6 General objectives for driver education

The four major categories and the twelve units of instruction deal with:

The nature of the driving task

Unit   1

The basic knowledge

Unit 2.   Traffic laws and rules for driving performance

Unit 3.   Vehicle performance and control capabilities

Unit 4.   Habits and skills for vehicle operation and maneuvers

Driving strategies and tactics

Unit 5.   Perception of system events

Unit 6.   Judgment of system events

Unit 7.   Decision making for a plan of action

Highway users' responsibilities

Unit 8.   Driver condition and behavior

Unit 9.   Alcohol and other drugs

Unit 10. Obedience to and enforcement of traffic laws

Unit 11. Post-crash procedures and responsibilities

Unit 12. Selection, inspection, and maintenance of Safe Vehicles

In a recently published teacher's edition of a high school driver education textbook, the following topics were covered:

1   New approaches to driver education

2 Organization of the text

3 Materials Accompanying the Text

4 Using the Teacher's Edition

Chapters of the textbook covered these additional topics:

1 You and the highway system

2 Preparing to drive

3 Basic maneuvers

4 Decision making and driving

5 Driving laws

6 Highway conditions

7 Vehicle performance

8 Other highway users

9 System failures

10 Driver performances

11 Motorcycles
12 Career opportunities

After extensive research that analyzed the many tasks involved in driving a motor vehicle, HumRRO developed a list of instructional objectives. A detailed description of each subject, the learning activities to be performed, the knowledge and degree of skill required, and an evaluation instrument are found in Table 6-3.

TEACHING METHODS

A variety of teaching methods and teaching techniques have been presented in Chapter 4, and space will not permit a full description of the methods and techniques used in teaching driver education. There are several teacher-education textbooks that go into detail about the various techniques used in the classroom and laboratory phases of driver and traffic safety education.

You may wish to refer to *Driving Task Instruction,* Aaron and Strasser, The Macmillan Company, New York; *Driver and Traffic Safety Education,* 2d ed., by the same authors; or *In-Car Instruction Methods and Contents,* 2d ed., William Anderson, Addison-Wesley, Reading, Mass., for a detailed presentation of teaching methods and techniques.

Time factors may require the teacher to select the most effective methods of supplying experiences that can foster the skills, knowledge, and attitudinal traits needed by youthful drivers. It is important that professional preparation provide a thorough foundation in the various disciplines dealing with human behavior and development.

The following guidelines may assist the teacher in selecting methods for presenting facts, concepts, principles, and generalizations.[17]

- One cannot effectively "tell" another how he shall think, feel, or act during a lifetime of independent operation in the traffic environment
- Authoritative approaches or implied force seldom produce permanent changes in driver behavior
- The value of lecture is often limited to providing students with factual information
- When development of desirable traffic behavior patterns is the primary purpose of a specific lesson, student-centered activities encourage participants to examine a variety of insights, reveal attitudes and beliefs, discuss probable results and arrive at a choice based on reasoning
- Individual differences among students should encourage teachers to use a variety of presentation techniques and methods
- Extensive or repeated presentations of gruesome collision scenes do more harm than good

---

[17] *Policies and Guidelines fo Driver and Traffic Safety Education,* American Driver and Traffic Safety Education Association, National Education Association, 1974, pp. 23–24.

TABLE 6–3
Driver Education Instructional Objectives

Subject	Purpose
Preparation	To enable the student to prepare the car and its occupants for a safe and comfortable trip.
Starting	To enable the student to start the car.
Accelerating	To enable the student to accelerate smoothly and safely from a standing position.
Starting on grades	To enable the student to start a car on an upgrade and on a downgrade from a standing position.
Steering—lane keeping	To enable the student to maintain proper position in required lane.
Steering—turning	To enable the student to make a safe, comfortable turn.
Speed control	To enable the student to adjust speed to existing traffic conditions to account for variations in traffic flow and legal speed limits.
Downshifting	To enable the student to downshift to maintain speed or reduce speed, before starting down a hill, in heavy, slow-moving traffic, or in emergency situations.
Stopping	To enable the student to come to a normal safe stop on level roadways and on hills and to make required rapid stops.
Backing	To enable the student to back up safely and smoothly.
Skid control	To enable the student to prevent and stop a skid.
Surveillance	To enable the student to maintain a complete and accurate understanding of the driving environment and to identify any critical changes that might affect his driving.
Urban driving	To enable the student to drive safely in an urban area and react appropriately to pedestrians and to other traffic.
Highway driving	To enable the student to drive in a safe, efficient manner in open country and mountainous terrain.
Freeway driving	To enable the student to safely enter, drive on, and exit from a freeway.
Car following	To enable the student to maintain an adequate separation between the car and the vehicle ahead.
Passing	To enable the student to make sound passing decisions and to complete passes safely without interference to other road users.
Entering traffic	To enable the student to enter traffic without interfering with other vehicles.
Leaving traffic	To enable the student to leave the line of traffic with minimal interference to the vehicles behind and to the side of the car.
Lane changing	To enable the student to change lanes safely and without obstructing the flow of traffic.
Parking	To enable the student to park the car safely and legally, and to exit from the car, with minimal interference with other vehicular or pedestrian traffic.
Leaving a parking space	To enable the student to leave a parking space safely without obstructing other vehicular or pedestrian traffic.
Pedestrians, cyclists, and animals	To enable the student to respond with safe and cautious actions when encountering pedestrians, cyclists, and animals.

207

TABLE 6–3 (*continued*)
Driver Education Instructional Objectives

Subject	Purpose
Emergency areas	To enable the student to drive safely through or by an attended emergency area, or to provide necessary assistance when he is the first to reach a severe accident.
Parked cars	To enable the student to drive safely alongside parked and parking vehicles.
Being passed	To enable the student to accommodate a passing vehicle by adjusting the car's speed and/or position as necessary for the other vehicle to complete the pass quickly.
Being followed	To enable the student to drive ahead of other vehicles with a minimum risk of rear-end collision.
Oncoming cars	To enable the student to adjust his course as necessary when meeting oncoming vehicles, and to take evasive action when necessary to avoid a head-on collision.
Overtaking	To enable the student to safely overtake a vehicle ahead and to avoid having to initiate emergency maneuvers.
Special vehicles	To enable the student to act safely when in the vicinity of special vehicles, viz., school buses, police, fire, and other emergency vehicles.
Intersections— approaching	To enable the student to approach an intersection and to react appropriately to other traffic and traffic controls.
Intersections— through	To enable the student to proceed through an intersection prepared to react to changing traffic conditions.
Intersections—right turn	To enable the student to safely make a right turn at an intersection.
Intersections—left turn	To enable the student to safely make a left turn at an intersection.
Traffic circles	To enable the student to negotiate traffic circles safely.
On-ramps	To enable the student to safely enter a roadway from an entrance ramp with or without an acceleration lane.
Off-ramps	To enable the student to exit safely from the main roadway.
Hills	To enable the student to negotiate hills safely and effectively.
Curves	To enable the student to negotiate highway curves safely and comfortably.
Lane usage	To enable the student to select the appropriate lane for driving.
Road surfaces	To enable the student to drive safely on different types of road surfaces; to enable the student to adjust his driving according to road surface conditions.
Wet roads	To enable the student to drive safely on a wet surface.
Road shoulders	To enable the student to deal effectively and safely with road shoulders.
Obstructions	To enable the student to deal safely with roadway obstructions and barricades.
Snow	To enable the student to drive, stop, and park safely on ice- and snow-covered roadways.
Sand	To enable the student to drive safely on sand-covered roadways.
U-turns	To enable the student to perform a U-turn where legally permissible.

208

TABLE 6–3 (*continued*)
Driver Education Instructional Objectives

Subject	Purpose
Two- and three-point turns	To enable the student to turn around by means of a three-point turn, or a two-point turn using a driveway.
Entering off-street areas	To enable the student to approach and enter off-street areas in a safe and efficient manner.
Off-street driving	To enable the student to drive safely in and around off-street areas without impeding traffic flow.
Railroad crossings	To enable the student to safely cross railroad crossings and to respond to possible dangers at such crossings.
Bridges and tunnels	To enable the student to enter, drive through or across, and leave a tunnel or bridge safely and expeditiously.
Toll plazas	To enable the student to negotiate toll plazas in a safe and expeditious manner.
Limited visibility	To enable the student to drive during weather conditions that limit visibility.
Climate	To enable the student to drive safely and comfortably during extremely hot or extremely cold weather.
Wind	To enable the student to maintain directional control during a high crosswind.
Night driving	To enable the student to drive safely during darkness.
Towing	To enable the student to adjust his driving behavior to compensate for the effects of towing a trailer.
Hauling loads	To enable the student to adjust his driving behavior to compensate for the effects of hauling heavy loads within or on top of the car.
Car emergencies	To enable the student to react safely when a car's malfunction endangers its occupants and other road users.
Mechanical problems	To enable the student to respond appropriately to malfunction indications although the apparent malfunction may be unlikely to affect the safety of the driver or other road users.
Disabled cars	To enable the student to deal safely with breakdowns that disable the car while on the road.
Dealing with breakdowns	To educate the student to remedy various on-road emergency malfunctions.
Pushing cars	To educate the student in the methods, procedures, and hazards involved when being pushed or pushing another vehicle.
Trip planning	To educate the student in the planning and preparation which precede driving and in navigational activities.
Loading	To enable the student to load objects securely in the passenger area, trunk, and on the roof.
Trailers	To enable the student to attach a trailer to the car and load the trailer properly.
Alcohol and drugs	To educate the student on the effects that drugs and alcohol have on driving safety and performance.
Physical and emotional conditions	To enable the student to become aware of physical and emotional conditions that may affect driving ability and how to compensate for such conditions.
Maintenance	To educate the student to maintain the car in sound operating condition through routine care and servicing.

209

TABLE 6–3 (continued)
Driver Education Instructional Objectives

Subject	Purpose
Inspection and servicing	To educate the student to have the car inspected and serviced in accordance with the recommendations of the manufacturer.
Repair	To educate the student to have the car repaired in response to breakdowns, symptoms of malfunctions, and deficiencies noted during inspection and servicing.
Certification	To inform the student about driver and car certification.
Accidents	To educate the student on the post-accident responsibilities of the driver.

Source: A. James McKnight and Alan G. Hunt, *Driver Education Task Analysis: Instructional Objectives,* HumRRO Safety Series, Human Resources Research Organization, Alexandria, Va., March, 1971.

• Safety concepts should be presented to students with a positive accent rather than a negative one
• Instructional techniques for in-car teaching should be flexible, with full recognition of individual differences in previous driving experience, eagerness to learn, physical coordination, composure, confidence, attitude, etc.

COURSE STANDARDS AND ADMINISTRATIVE PROCEDURES

Qualifications for Teachers

In the past, teachers of driver education have had backgrounds representing almost every subject in the high school curriculum. Many of these teachers did a remarkable job in light of the material that was available. Driver education goes beyond the mere teaching of driving skill, rules and regulations, and safe practices. The teacher has the unique opportunity to help students develop desirable traits such as courtesy, cooperation, and acceptance of responsibility, traits which will make them better citizens as well as competent drivers.

The fund of knowledge concerning traffic safety has increased significantly in the last decade. Today a teacher must be able to define objectives precisely, select the proper methods and content for guiding students toward the accomplishment of these objectives, and formulate and use criterion tests to measure student accomplishment of these objectives. To achieve the objectives of driver and traffic safety education, teachers in this area must have the same basic qualifications as teachers in any other field. A teacher of driver education should have preservice experiences consisting of an undergraduate teaching major in driver or safety education, with no less than a minor in the field. Basic professional education, including psychology and sociology, is desirable and is already included among many state certification standards.

The ultimate success of any traffic safety education program depends upon the teachers. Professional preparation, character, personality, and complete dedication to the subject are primary requisites for a good driver and traffic safety teachers.

All teachers of driver and traffic safety education should be qualified according to the standards developed by the American Driver and Traffic Safety Education Association, which is a department of the National Education Association. The association's qualifications are as follows:[18]

Efficiency in the driving task requires that motor vehicle operators develop a set of complex perceptual skills which are adaptable to a wide range of situations. These perceptual-motor skills should be accompanied by instantly recallable knowledge and behavior that is semi-automatic.

For these and other reasons, school districts should employ and assign driver education teachers who have met high-level teacher preparation and certification standards and who have:

- Desirable physical and mental capabilities for teaching driver education as determined
- by screening examinations and other evaluative tools.
- A bachelor's degree or its equivalent from an accredited institution of higher education.
- A valid state driver license with a satisfactory driving record as defined by the state department of education (In determining what is satisfactory, the driving record should be checked at least annually).
- At least a teaching minor (or equivalent) of 18–22 semester units in driver or safety education.
- Competencies essential to successful performance as a driver education teacher.
- Preservice preparation and direct experience or supervised student teaching with experiences in both classroom and laboratory phases of instruction.
- Specific knowledge of the dual controlled car plan, electronic simulation systems, off-street multiple car driving ranges, multimedia response systems, and related literature.

Formal preparation should also provide teachers with competencies to perform the following functions:[19]

The desirable type of teacher of driver and/or safety education:

- Adapts safety curricula provided by state or local boards of education to his or her school's program in accordance with local needs and resources.
- Demonstrates ability to identify key elements in complex situations, predict risk involvement, and execute safe decisions.
- Provides students with learning experiences in the cognitive, psychomotor, and affective domains which will help them to perform safely within the highway transportation system and other technological environments.
- Selects and conducts learning activities, from simple to complex, which corresponds with the learners' mental, physical, and emotional performance capabilities.
- Selects routes for on-street and on-site lessons to facilitate learning experiences in a systematic manner.

---

[18]Ibid., pp. 22–23.
[19]*Policies and Guidelines for Preparation and Certification of School Safety Personnel,* American Driver and Traffic Safety Education Association, Washington, 1974, pp. 8–9.

• Enlists and utilizes community safety resources which enhance the instructional program (i.e., police, courts, auto dealers and clubs, safety councils, driver licensing, and insurance agencies).

• Selects or develops evaluation devices which measure the behavior sought in specified objectives.

• Interprets the school safety program to the public.

• Participates in activities leading to professional growth, such as graduate study, workshops, and activities of professional associations.

Preparation of a teacher of driver education or safety education should include preservice experiences consisting of an undergraduate teaching major in driver or safety education with no less than a minor in the area.

Driver and safety education teachers should meet the established certification requirements and should have successfully completed a program that includes:

• General professional education
• Core experiences including general principles of accident causation and prevention

A broad driver and safety education teacher preparation program should include those experiences which provide the prospective teacher with appropriate capability in the following areas:

• Ability to structure and implement driver education learning experiences and to identify and develop support materials related to the following modes:
Regular classroom
Multi-media
Driving simulation
Off-street multiple car driving range
On-street

• Ability to assist students in examining and clarifying their beliefs, attitudes, and values as they relate to safety

• An understanding of the basic principles of motor vehicle systems, dynamics, and maintenance

• An understanding of the interaction of all highway transportation system elements
• Procedures and conditions for activating an emergency medical services system
• Demonstrated competence in motor vehicle operation and on-street instruction
• An understanding of the physiological and psychological influences of alcohol and drug abuse as they relate to the highway transportation system
• An understanding of due processes in the application of laws
• Ability to communicate effectively with appropriate agencies concerned with safety
• Understanding the frequency, severity, nature, and directions for prevention of accidents which occur to age groups while participating in various life activities.

SCHEDULING

Factors affecting scheduling vary so much from school to school that no single scheduling pattern can be recommended. Each school must schedule driver and traffic safety to meet its own needs. In fitting the course in the curriculum, the following considerations should be taken into account:

1 The number of students to be accommodated

2 The type of course to be offered

a. Single phase—classroom only

b. Two-phase—classroom, and on-street practice driving

c. Three-Phase—classroom, simulation or range, and on-street practice driving

d. Four-Phase—classroom, simulation, range, and on-street practice driving

3 The number of weeks required to complete the course or, in some instances, the number of weeks allocated to the course: six, twelve, or full semester

4 The number of vehicles available for practice driving

5 The number of simulators available: 10, 12, 16, or 20

6 The type and size of the multiple-car driving range

7 School course requirements (some schools require driver education for graduation)

8 (many states prescribe a minimum period of instruction, and some have made driver education a prerequisite to a driver's license)

9 The funds available

10 The number of qualified and certified teachers available

To achieve the ultimate objectives of driver and traffic safety education, educators should formulate a schedule that includes a full-semester course covering all phases of the program—classroom, laboratory, simulation, and range—concurrently. The school administrator and the teaching staff should formulate a schedule that permits effective teaching and learning in the time allocated to the program. A scheduling committee could be established to assist in this process.

PROCUREMENT AND USE OF DRIVER EDUCATION VEHICLES

The cars used in high school driver education programs can be obtained in the following ways:

1 *Purchase.* When possible the school should purchase its own car with its own funds, just as it purchases other educational equipment.

2 *Loan.* Through the cooperation of the automobile industry and local automobile dealers, vehicles can be obtained on loan. When vehicles are obtained on this basis, there must be a clear understanding of responsibilities: the length of time the car is to be loaned, maintenance and storage arrangements, amount of insurance coverage needed, and responsibility for returning the vehicle in conditions acceptable to the dealer. Loan agreement forms and assistance for this program may be obtained through the American Automobile Association and through its affiliated automobile clubs. Local dealers are reimbursed from $250 to $500 for cooperating in the local high school programs. The majority of vehicles used in driver education today are obtained on a loan basis from local dealers.

3 *Rental or lease.* In some cases it may be desirable for the local school district to obtain a vehicle by monthly rental. The dealer takes care of all the expenses involved, and the school pays the dealer a designated monthly fee.

4 *Gift.* On rare occasions service clubs, local insurance agencies, area automobile dealers, and other community groups donate a car for driver education purposes.

The school district should formulate strict policies governing the use of the car. In most agreements signed by the local dealer and school it specifies that the vehicle should be used only for driver education and the agreement can be terminated if the agreement is violated. Other policies as to what personnel is authorized to use the car and when and where it is to be operated should also be stated.

LIABILITY AND INSURANCE

Liability of school personnel for student accidents is discussed in detail in Chapter 4. General recommendations are offered here for avoiding legal entanglements in connection with driver education. There have been few court decisions involving the liability of teachers and/or school districts in cases of student accidents. There is little risk to all concerned when the following criteria are observed:

1 A competent, well-trained, certified teacher conducts the program.

2 Practice-driving vehicles are used solely for their intended purpose and are kept in good mechanical condition.

3 The school has formulated sound policies governing the use of the car and what to do in case of injuries and accidents.

4 There is continuous supervision in the classroom, simulation laboratory, and driving range.

5 Lessons are taught on a logical, sequential basis.

6 Instructors use common sense in deciding whether or not to hold practice driving during bad weather. Students are taught how to handle a car under all conditions, but only when they have the competency to do so without the risk of incurring an accident.

The possibility of casualties in a driver education course cannot be entirely eliminated. The board of education should carry insurance giving complete financial coverage for accidents. The school's insurance adviser and legal counsel can suggest the proper coverage for all personnel involved. The individual driver education teacher may wish to seek additional information about insurance coverage and any additional protection that may be desired.

OTHER CONSIDERATIONS

Other aspects of the driver education program that should be considered are:

1. *Cost and financing of the program.* There are approximately 35 states that provide financial support for driver education. Federal funds are also available to help support the program.
2. *Records and reports.* The purpose of keeping records and reports is to reflect standards, improve instruction, record and control costs, show progress of the student, provide a source of data for research, and verify students' accomplishments upon course completion. It is also important to have accident report forms available in each of the practice-driving vehicles and an accurate and complete file of all accident reports.
3. *Selecting students.* The school should provide driver education for every eligible student at the time requested. If it is necessary to select students on a priority basis, the following criteria may be used:
   a. Students who are the only person eligible to drive in their immediate families
   b. Students with a vocational need to drive
   c. Students who are approaching or have passed the legal driving age
   d. Students who have been referred to the class by the traffic courts
4. *Liaison with state agencies.* Local school districts should establish direct contact with the various state agencies that have a relationship to traffic safety education:
   a. The safety unit or division of the office of education, in order to be apprised of policy changes and new requirements.
   b. The driver's licensing division of the motor vehicle department. Many schools in cooperation with this division assist in procuring instruction permits for driver education students.
   c. The governor's department of transportation and, specifically, the governor's representative to the Federal Highway Safety Program. These agencies make federal funds available for local driver and traffic safety programs.
   d. State police traffic safety units. These groups may assist local driver education programs in reference to various aspects of law enforcement, such as demonstrations of breathalyzer tests and radar equipment.
5. *Liaison with the private sectors.* Insurance company accident-prevention divisions, local and national safety councils, and automobile clubs often provide services to local driver education programs.

EVALUATION

Driver education is subject to the same evaluative criteria as other school subjects.

> Evaluation is the process by which the objectives of the program are assessed. It aims to determine in which way and to what extent the long and short range objectives of the program are being achieved. It involves the examination of the administrative policies and instructional procedures, progress and achievement of the student, and the continuing follow-up of the effectiveness of the program.
>
> The importance of this aspect of driver education cannot be overemphasized. There is a place for informal type research conducted by teachers and/or their administrators, or a more detailed sophisticated type done by the research staff of a school system or state departments of education.[20]

It is difficult to measure objectively the long-range effect of driver education because of the many variables involved. Nevertheless, local, state, federal, and other agencies must make concerted efforts to develop reliable instruments to measure the effectiveness of the program. Only through effective evaluation can the quality of traffic education programs be assured.

LEARNING EXPERIENCES

The following learning activities should enhance the student's knowledge of traffic safety education:

1 Develop a paper to justify why traffic safety education should begin early in the life of a school child.

2 Outline a talk, to be delivered before an interested group, on "What is driver education?"

3 Develop a paper describing the differences between traditional driver education programs and the newer task-analysis-based program.

4 Analyze several high school driver education programs in terms of state and national course standards.

5 Develop an original visual aid that can be used in either the classroom or laboratory phase of instruction.

6 Select several high school driver education text books from the university library and analyze their content. Evaluate them as tools for achieving the objectives of a high school driver education program.

7 Write to several state departments of education to find the type of traffic safety education programs they recommend for their various school districts. Give your own evaluation of the programs.

8 Develop a paper describing the Traffic Safety Act of 1966 and how it will affect traffic safety programs.

[20] *Driver Education for Illinois Youth,* Office of Superintendent of Public Instruction (now Office of Education), State of Illinois, Springfield, Ill., 1972, p. 41.

9 Evaluate the eighteen federal traffic safety standards and list them in order of importance in reducing traffic accidents.

10 Observe the habits of motorists, pedestrians, and bicyclists at a busy intersection near a high school for a 30-minute period. Report your findings to the class.

11 Visit a local traffic court for observation of court procedures.

SELECTED REFERENCES

Aaron, James E., and Marland K. Strasser: *Driver and Traffic Safety Education,* The Macmillan Company, New York, 1977, p. 502.

————: *Driving Task Instruction, Dual Control, Simulation and Multiple Car,* The Macmillan Company, New York, 1974, p. 429.

American Automobile Association, Falls Church, Va.:
   Behind the Wheel Driving Guides
   Behind the Wheel Guide for Sportsmanlike Driving
   Digest of Motor Laws, Annual
   Free Materials and Services for Driver Education Courses
   How to Drive, adult education text, p. 218
   Project Workbook for Sportsmanlike Driving
   Sportsmanlike Driving, teacher's edition
   Tests for Sportsmanlike Driving
   Traffic Education Resources Catalog 7th ed.

American Driver and Traffic Safety Education Association, Washington:
   Policies and Guidelines for a School Safety Program, 1974
   Policies and Guidelines for Driver and Traffic Safety Education, 1974
   Policies and Guidelines for Preparation and Certification of School Safety Personnel, 1974

Anderson, William G.: *In-Car Instruction Methods and Contents,* 2d ed., Addison-Wesley Co., Reading, Mass., 1977, p. 353.

Automobile Facts and Figures, Automobile Manufacturers Association, Detroit, Mich., Yearly.

Automotive Safety Foundation, Washington:
   The Multiple-Car Method: Exploring Its Use in Driver and Traffic Safety Education, 1972 (also available from the American Driver and Traffic Safety Association)

A Resources Curriculum in Driver and Traffic Safety Education, 1970.

Bishop, Richard W., et. al.: *Driving: A Task Analysis Approach,* Rand McNally & Company, New York, 1975.

Halsey, Maxwell, et al.: *Let's Drive Right,* teacher's annotated edition, 5th ed., Scott, Foresman & Company, Glenview, Ill., 1972.

Marshall, Robert L., et. al. *Safe Performance Driving,* Ginn & Company, Lexington, Mass., 1976.

McNight, A. James, and Bert B. Adams: *Education Task Analysis,* vol. 1: *Task Descriptions,* Department of Transportation, Washington, HS800—367, 1970.

————and Alan G. Hunt: *Driver Education Task Analysis: Instructional Objectives,* HumRRO Safety Series, Human Resources Research Organization, Alexandria, Va., 1971.

National Committee on Uniform Traffic Laws and Ordinances: *Uniform Vehicle Code,* 1968, *Model Ordinance,* 1968, and *Supplement II,* 1976, Washington.

National Highway Traffic Safety Administration, Washington: *Guide for Teacher Preparation in Driver Education,* secondary school ed., 1974.

Highway Safety Program Manual, vol. 4, *Driver Education,* 1969.

The Driver Education Evaluation Program (DEEP), 1975.

National Safety Council, Chicago:

Accident Facts, 1977 edition

Driver Education Status Report, 1976

Guide to Traffic Safety Literature, current edition

School and College Transactions, 1974, vol. 23

Traffic Safety Magazine

State of Illinois: *Driver Education for Illinois* Youth Safety Education Section, Office of Superintendent of Public Instruction (now Office of Education), Springfield, Ill., 1972, p. 195.

U.S. Department of Transportation, National Highway Traffic Safety Administration: *An Evaluation of the Highway Safety Program,* A Report to the Congress from the Secretary of Transportation, July, 1977, p. 131.

7

Legal Liability

OVERALL OBJECTIVE:

The student should understand the legal implications of individual behavior.

INSTRUCTIONAL OBJECTIVES:

After completing this chapter the student will be able to:

1 Explain the legal considerations that determine whether a tort has been committed.
2 Discuss the implications of Good Samaritan laws.
3 Determine the standard of care owed to another person, based upon one's relationship to that person.
4 Understand the legal terminology associated with the law of torts.
5 Explain the legal defenses against tort.
6 Understand that most legal decisions reflect the "commonsense" standard held by most people.
7 Discuss the relationship of insurance and personal liability.

LIABILITY FOR ACCIDENTS

The prevention of accidents is an ethical obligation that can become a legal responsibility. Individuals such as teachers, recreation leaders, coaches, and physicians are legally at risk because of their occupation. But all private citizens are legally accountable for actions or inactions which harmfully affect others. A realistic concept of liability can promote personal safety. It can alleviate the unreasonable fear which occasionally prevents an individual from becoming involved with other people. Understanding the basic concepts, principles, and terminology associated with legal liability can help people anticipate risks and defend themselves against the possibility of legal claims and judgments.

The broad area of law which includes liability is known as tort. The word *tort* is derived from the Latin "tortus" meaning "twisted." In translation, it means

219

"a wrongful act." A tort is a civil wrong, other than a breach of contract, for which the court will provide compensation to the injured party (plaintiff). The court's purpose is to adjust the loss and compensate for injuries. Theoretically, the plaintiff, after adjudication, is placed in the same position he or she would have been in if the tort had not occurred.

Although criminal behavior is an offense against the entire public, tort law provides protection against injury to private individuals, their property, or their reputations. Criminal adjudication requires proof beyond a reasonable doubt, but in tort law judgments are awarded on the basis of the evidence presented on behalf of each party. The burden of proof rests necessarily with the plaintiff. For the courts to provide redress, the plaintiff must demonstrate that the commission or omission of an act caused damage. In and of itself, a wrongful act does not constitute a tortious situation. The action (or lack of action) must be both wrongful and harmful.

The legal test for tort consists of four questions. They must be answered in the affirmative for a tort to have occurred.

1 Did the defendant have a duty or responsibility to the plaintiff? Was there an obligation to protect the plaintiff against unreasonable risk of harm?

2 Was there a failure to conform to the required standard of care owed the plaintiff? This question establishes the existence of negligence, which is the dominant principle of tort law.

3 Was there a causal connection between failure to provide adequate care and resulting injury (proximate cause)?

4 Did an actual loss or damage result from the commission or omission of an action by the defendant?[1]

DUTY

The first question centers on an issue known as standard of care. In some situations there is absolutely no legal duty, although there may be a moral duty to protect another human being from unreasonable harm. If you see a stranger engaged in a dangerous situation which you suspect might lead to injury, and injury eventually occurs, no action can be brought against you. In such situations no legal standard of care exists. In an emergency situation, unless you have some relationship to the injured party, you are not legally obligated to render first aid. If you decide to become involved and begin to administer first aid, a relationship is established, and you become legally responsible for exercising reasonable judgment and providing an adequate standard of care.

GOOD SAMARITAN LAWS

There seems to be a great deal of confusion surrounding the Good Samaritan laws which exist in some states. New Mexico's law is reprinted at the end of this section. The purpose of the law is to encourage the administration of first aid by

[1] William L. Prosser, *Handbook of the Law of Torts,* 4th ed., West Publishing Company, St. Paul, Minn., 1971, p. 143.

offering protection to good citizens against groundless civil litigation. The law protects those who render first aid in a reasonably prudent fashion. Reasonable prudence might be defined as good judgment applied to action, carefulness, and precaution. The law does not, and was never intended to, provide immunity against negligent individual behavior.

If a person (doctor, nurse, certified first-aider, etc.) possesses knowledge, skill, or intelligence beyond the capacity of the ordinary person, the law will demand a higher standard of care. Such individuals are expected to exercise reasonable care consistent with their level of knowledge and ability. A person who is certified in first aid by the American Red Cross is expected to provide accurate and beneficial assistance. Although this may seem an inducement to avoid certification as a first-aider, nothing could be further from the truth. Even though their standard of care is higher, first-aiders are trained to exercise reasonable judgment and appropriate care. If their behavior should fall below the standard expected of others with similar training, the consequences suffered by the injured party will probably be minor rather than major. If first aid is rendered according to the procedures taught by the American Red Cross, the first-aider will have a valuable ally in proving that his or her behavior was prudent.

TWENTY-SIXTH LEGISLATURE, STATE OF NEW MEXICO, HOUSE JUDICIARY COMMITTEE SUBSTITUTE FOR SENATE BILL NO. 6

To Relieve From Civil Liability Those Persons Who Render Emergency Care; Providing Exceptions, and Defining Terms. Be It Enacted By The Legislature Of The State Of New Mexico:

Section 1. No person who shall administer emergency care in good faith at or near the scene of an emergency, as defined herein, shall be liable for any civil damages as a result of any action or omission by such person in administering said care, except for gross negligence; provided that nothing herein shall apply to the administering of such care where the same is rendered for remuneration or is rendered by any person or agent of a principal who was at the scene of the accident or emergency because he or his principal was soliciting business or performing or seeking to perform some service for remuneration.

Section 2. As used in this act "emergency" means an unexpected occurrence involving injury or illness to persons, including motor vehicle accidents and collisions, disasters, and other accidents and events of similar nature occuring in public or private places.

LICENSEE AND INVITEE

Sometimes the standard of care is determined by whether one's relationship to another person is that of a *licensee* or an *invitee*. If a person enters your property in pursuit of his or her own convenience, pleasure, or business, without your express or implied invitation, your only legal duty is to refrain from intentionally harming the visitor.[2] A *licensee* must accept your premises as they are found. The obvious exception to this principle occurs when visitors,

[2]Henry Campbell Black, *Black's Law Dictionary,* 4th ed., West Publishing Company, St. Paul, Minn., 1951, p. 1070.

because of age or other limiting conditions, require a greater standard of care involving positive efforts on your part to protect their well-being.

An *invitee* enters your premises as a result of direct or implied invitation. However, a three-year-old child who wanders onto your property, allured by a swimming pool, is considered an invitee by virtue of the *attractive nuisance.* An attractive nuisance is an object so enticing that it could reasonably be expected to attract the curiosity of one who lacks the intelligence, maturity, or experience to appreciate the danger it poses. The standard of care demanded for an invitee is one of positive and reasonable propriety for protection against harm. Others who may be classified as invitees are students attending public schools, postal delivery workers, meter readers, and social acquaintances. The difference in the standard of care required for a licensee or an invitee depends upon the general concept of invitation.

The guiding principle in determining standard of care is that the greater the relationship, the greater the obligation to provide positive protection. Teachers, for example, are held to a high standard of care. The student is considered an invitee because of compulsory attendance laws. Because of the age, maturity, and experience limitations of most students, and because teachers stand *in loco parentis* (in the place of a parent), schools are expected to provide a safe environment and establish reasonable behavior for the protection of students. Teachers are experts on the nature of children; they are licensed by the state to offer their services as properly trained professionals. Therefore, the expectation for protection is well above the expectation for the ordinary citizen. We encourage every teacher to enroll in at least one course in safety education and a course in first aid.

FORESEEABILITY

One consideration in determining negligence is the concept of *foreseeability.* If the defendant could not reasonably foresee any harm as the result of his or her conduct, or if the behavior was reasonable in light of what could have been anticipated, there is no negligence and no liability.[3] The test of foreseeability is the ability of a prudent person in the exercise of ordinary care to foresee that injury or harm will naturally or probably result.[4]

LAST CLEAR CHANCE

Another way to determine negligence is the doctrine of *last clear chance,* also known as the humanitarian doctrine and the doctrine of discovered peril. The party who has the last clear chance to avoid danger or injury is liable for the consequences of a situation. Depending on the standard of care owed to the plaintiff, the defendant has a duty to intervene in order to prevent injury. Even if

[3]Prosser, op. cit., p. 250.
[4]74 AM. JUR. 2d *Torts* §10 (1974), footnote 91, *Drum v. Miller,* 135 N.C. 204, 47 S.E. 421.

the plaintiff's negligence continues until the injurious occurrence, the defendant may be considered negligent if, after learning of the impending peril, he or she took no action to avert the injury. Foreseeability and the opportunity of last clear chance entail a legal obligation to accept responsibility for the well-being of persons to whom a standard of care is owed.[5]

EMERGENCY SITUATIONS

An individual confronted by an emergency is ordinarily held to the same standard of care applied to other people in similar situations. An emergency is defined as a sudden or unanticipated event which necessitates immediate action. A person in an emergency situation cannot be held to the same standard of care as one who has had time to reflect. Even if it later appears that the defendant made a decision which no reasonable person could possibly have made after careful deliberation, there is no negligence. The choice may have been inappropriate, but it was prudent under the circumstances created by the emergency.[6]

Many emergencies are avoidable through appropriate preventive behavior. When a potentially dangerous situation exists, which the defendant has knowledge of and opportunity to correct, the defendant becomes liable for those consequences which arise from his or her failure to provide adequate protection. Negligence would govern this issue, and a defense utilizing the emergency doctrine would be inappropriate. The emergency situation was created as a result of negligence, or failure to act for the reasonable protection of others. Educational systems as well as teachers have an obligation to prevent emergencies through adequate planning, implementation, and evaluation of safety programs (see Chapters 3 and 4).

PROXIMATE CAUSE

There is no commonly accepted definition of proximate cause. In essence, the defendant's negligence must be a substantial factor in producing the damage. The harm must be a natural or probable consequence of the defendant's act. Furthermore, a negligent person is legally responsible for only the harm which is caused by his or her negligence. The plaintiff must be able to demonstrate an unbroken chain of events between the act and the damage. Thus, a person can be negligent but will not be held liable when his or her negligence is not the proximate cause of the harm. In an automobile accident where a person suffers internal injuries and a broken arm, and a first-aider incorrectly applies a splint to the fracture, the first-aider is liable only for the consequences of his or her negligent behavior. If the victim dies as a result of the internal injuries, the plaintiff, in order to collect damages, would have to demonstrate a relationship of proximate cause between the improper splint and the subsequent death.

---

[5]Black, op. cit., p. 1025.
[6]Prosser, op. cit., p. 169.

DAMAGE RELATED TO NEGLIGENCE

The determination of whether or not a tort has occurred is based on statutory and judicial law. The awarding of damages commensurate with the consequences of the tort constitutes subjective settlement by the judge or jury. Damages are dependent upon the magnitude of harm suffered by the plaintiff, the extent of negligence by the defendant, and the strength of the relationship between the defendant's negligent behavior and the injury. If the negligence is direct and the consequences severe, the damages will be high. If the actual harm caused by the negligent behavior is minor, the damages will be lower, reflecting the relationship between the negligence and its consequences. It is worth repeating that the purpose of tort law is to adjust losses. The intent is to return the injured party to the same position he or she would have occupied if the tort had not occurred.

LEGAL DEFENSES AGAINST TORT

ASSUMPTION OF RISK

In this defense, the plaintiff must consent in advance to relieve the defendant of an obligation or duty toward the plaintiff.[7] The injured party must voluntarily accept the risks inherent in the activity. It is essential that the consenter perceive and understand the risks, and that the choice to accept these risks be voluntarily accepted. When these conditions are met, the defendant is absolved of all legal duty and cannot be charged with negligence. Factors such as age, maturity, and intelligence are important considerations.

Contrary to popular belief, a signed parent permission slip does not constitute a waiver of liability. Such documents indicate that parents or guardians are aware of an activity and agree to permit a child to participate. If the child is subsequently injured through the normal and predictable hazards of the activity, and there is no negligent behavior, the permission slip becomes a defense against a parental claim that the child should not have engaged in that activity.

Negligence is not among the risks accepted by parents on behalf of their children. As an illustration, suppose that a parent allows a child to participate in a swimming party. If, in walking to the locker room, the child trips and falls against the deck of the pool and suffers a concussion, there would be no valid grounds for suit. This sequence of events would legally be termed a *pure accident.* If the children, while unsupervised, engage in a game of tag on the pool's deck, and someone falls, negligence might well be proved. In this instance, the signed permission slip is no defense against liability. Assumption of risk means the acceptance of the foreseeable dangers associated with an activity.

[7]Ibid., p. 440.

CONTRIBUTORY NEGLIGENCE

The burden of proving contributory negligence is on the defendant. It is necessary to demonstrate that the conduct of the plaintiff contributed as a legal cause to the injury suffered. The defendant must show a causal relationship between the plaintiff's negligence and the harm. The principle of this defense is that plaintiffs have a standard of care and a duty to protect themselves from injury. When contributory negligence can be proved, there will usually be no recovery of damages. Contributory negligence does not constitute an effective legal defense when the plaintiff, because of age or other limiting factors, has essentially no standard of care.[8]

COMPARATIVE NEGLIGENCE

Statutes have been enacted in some states to award damages on the basis of comparative negligence. The extent of recovery depends on the proportion of blame. When the defendant is largely at fault, the recovery will be extensive. As comparative negligence shifts toward the plaintiff, recovery will be correspondingly lower.

LIABILITY AND TEACHERS

It is incorrect to assume that someone is liable for every injury sustained in school. The fact that a student gets hurt does not, in itself, mean that the teacher in charge is liable.[9] A Louisiana court ruled that although the school board is expected to take reasonable precaution and care to avoid injury to students, the board is not an ensurer of the lives and safety of children.[10] Legally defined, pure accidents cannot be foreseen or avoided by reasonable precaution.

Some areas of the school program are obviously more dangerous than others. Gymnasiums, pools, shops, laboratories, field trips, student transportation, school patrols, and play areas are phases of the school program that require thorough instruction and close supervision. When the potential for harm is conspicuous, the teacher must be especially careful and take advantage of every opportunity to provide adequate protection to the students. The courts expect conduct consistent with the behavior of similarly trained professionals of good standing. For a teacher, the best legal defense against liability is the prevention of injury through competent instruction and adequate supervision.

Some teachers have expressed the mistaken belief that they are not permitted to render first aid to injured students. However, teachers owe students an exceptionally high standard of care. Because teachers stand *in loco parentis,* first aid, provided correctly, is not only permissible but expected. It is

---

[8]LeRoy J. Peterson, Richard A. Rossmiller, and Marlin M. Volz, *The Law and Public School Operation,* Harper & Row, Publishers, Incorporated, New York, 1969, p. 293.
[9]Ibid., p. 316.
[10]*Whitfield v. East Baton Rouge Parish School Board,* 43 SO 2d 47 (La. 1949).

reasonable to anticipate that injuries will occur to young people while in shcool, and the district should adopt definite policies about emergencies. Teachers are not expected to possess expert knowledge of first aid, but they should have basic training and should follow the emergency plan established by the school district. "The courts can give no redress for hardship to an individual resulting from action reasonably calculated to achieve a lawful end by lawful means."[11] An action may not be maintained "for damages resulting to individuals from acts done by persons in the execution of a public trust or for the public benefit, acting with due skill and caution and within the scope of their authority."[12]

INADEQUATE INSTRUCTION

A fourteen-year-old freshman was injured while jumping over a gymnastic horse in a compulsory physical education class. The teacher was an accredited physical education instructor who had explained the correct way to vault the horse, demonstrated the jump, described the dangers of the activity, and told the class that the maneuver should not be attempted by individuals who were not confident of their ability to successfully and safely perform the vault. Mats were placed around the area for protection, and all jumps were supervised. The court ruled in favor of the teacher.[13]

Junior high school girls were playing a game of line soccer as a compulsory activity in physical education. Eight inexperienced and inadequately prepared girls of varying sizes were competing for possession of the ball at the time of the injury. The district curriculum guide noted that lead-up activities should precede this game and that only a limited number of students should contend for the ball at one time. An expert witness testified that skills such as kicking, dribbling, and passing were needed to play the game adequately. The court ruled that, under the circumstances, although the injury was not inevitable, it was foreseeable. The teacher was held liable for the injury.[14]

QUALITY OF SUPERVISION

A plaintiff brought charges against a school district for injuries sustained when a kindergarten pupil had his finger cut off by a playground gate. Although the teacher was not immediately present at the time of the injury, she had previously warned students not to swing on the gate. The design and condition of the gate were not defective, and the student's finger was cut off while he was swinging on the gate. The court stated that "The standard of care required of any officer or employee of a school is that which a person of ordinary prudence, charged with

---

[11] 2 AM. JUR. 2d *Actions* §71 (1962), footnote 13, *O'Keefe v. Local 463, United Assoc. P. & G.,* 277 N.Y. 300, 14 N.E. 2d 77, 117 ALR 817.

[12] 2 AM. JUR. 2d *Actions* §71 (1962), footnote 17, *Tinsman v. Belvidere Delaware R. Co.,* 26 NJL 148, *Cleveland & P.R. Co. v. Speer,* 56 Pa. 325.

[13] *Sayers v. Ranger,* 83 A 2d 775 (W.J. 1951).

[14] *Keesee v. the Board of Education of the City of New York,* 235 N.Y.S. 2d 300 (1962).

his duties, would exercise under the same circumstances. The fact that the teacher was not immediately present did not constitute negligence and was not the proximate cause of the student's injuries."[15]

A young girl was walking to school after having had lunch at home. While entering the school premises she was struck in the face by a snowball. The court noted that "The school is not liable for every thoughtless or careless act by which one pupil may injure another. . . . It is unreasonable to demand or expect perfection of supervision from ordinary teachers or ordinary school management, and a fair test of reasonable care does not demand it."[16]

In another case, the teacher was apparently out of the classroom for more than 25 minutes. During about 5 to 10 minutes of that time one student was wielding a knife. Eventually another student was stabbed. The court ruled that the third-party act was not an event which was equally likely to occur in the presence or absence of the teacher. Had the incident been the result of an impulsive act, the issues of foreseeability and last clear chance might have worked in favor of the teacher, notwithstanding her extended period of absence from the classroom. The court ruled that the teacher's absence was negligent behavior which constituted the proximate cause of injury to the student.[17]

FORESEEABILITY

The following case is a classic, since it involves an accident that occurred during the teaching of safety. A shop teacher was holding class outdoors and going over a test on safety which had been given several days before. The teacher read the questions and then looked up as responses came from the class, which was sitting in a semicircle in front of him. Testimony revealed that one boy was flipping a knife into the ground for about 20 minutes. On one occasion, the knife glanced off a clipboard and struck another pupil in the eye. The central issue was whether the teacher knew, or should have known, about the dangerous activity. The teacher testified that he was unaware of the knife flipping. The court ruled that if the teacher had used ordinary care in observing the class, the injury would not have occurred. The plaintiff won the case.[18]

During a football scrimmage the quarterback was tackled and a massive pile-up followed. After the play, the student complained of a neck injury and did not get up from the ground. At that time he could, however, move his fingers. The coach ordered eight players to remove the injured player from the field without using a stretcher. Subsequently, the young man became a quadriplegic. Testimony revealed that if the paralysis had been a result of the original injury, the boy would not have been able to move his fingers. In awarding the plaintiff $325,000, the court said that "The amount of caution used by the ordinary prudent person varies in direct proportion to the danger known to be

[15]*Luna v. Needles Elementary School District,* 316 P 2d 773 (C.H. 1957).
[16]*Lawes v. Board of Education of the City of New York,* 213 NE 2d 667 (N.Y. 1965).
[17]*Christofides v. Hellenic Eastern Orthodox Christian Church of New York,* 227 N.Y.S. 2d 946 (1962).
[18]*Lileanthal v. San Leandro Unified School District,* P 2d 889 (Cal. 1956).

involved. . . ."[19] In this case, the amount of caution exercised by the teacher was inadequate to the accident situation.

INSURANCE

The insurance industry in this country has developed as a result of the high economic risk associated with certain activities. Its principal purpose is to reduce the extent of personal loss by transferring the uncertainty to a company which insures many people against the same risks. Actuarial techniques accurately predict the extent of a loss and redistribute its cost, in the form of premiums, throughout a large population of policy holders. The insured person is substituting a small known fee for a potentially large and unpredictable amount of money. The basic purposes of insurance are to reduce the uncertainty, transfer the risk, and reimburse (indemnify) the economic loss sustained by paid policy holders.

LIABILITY INSURANCE

An individual or a business can be held economically accountable for injury to another person or to that person's property. This is the reason for liability insurance. The concept of insurance is thousands of years old, but liability insurance originated in the late 1800s. Automobile liability insurance was first issued in 1888 as an extension of the coverage offered to owners of horse-drawn carriages.[20] Liability insurance for business firms developed shortly thereafter. Product liability and worker's compensation liability were established shortly after the turn of the century. Other types of liability coverage now available to the public include professional, officers and directors, marine, and fire-hazard insurance.

Liability insurance companies agree to pay, to the limit of the policy, those sums for which the policy holder is held legally liable. The company does not make payments directly to the insured, but to the injured party; therefore, policies of this type are sometimes referred to as third-party insurance. Ordinarily, judgment must be rendered in a court of law before payment is made, but the insurer, at its option, may choose to settle with the injured party out of court. This might occur when the amount claimed is so small that defense costs would surpass the claim, or when the facts clearly indicate liability so that the defense would represent an additional cost.[21]

The insurer agrees to defend or settle all claims covered by the contract which allege negligence on the part of the insured. Whether the claims are substantiated or not, the insurer will provide the legal defense against lawsuits. The insurance company pays for all court costs including the costs of wit-

---

[19]*Welch v. Dunsmuir Joint Union High School District*, 326 P 2d 633 (Cal. 1958).
[20]Irving Pfeffer and David R. Klock, *Perspectives on Insurance*, Prentice-Hall, Inc., Englewood Cliffs, N.J., 1974, p. 38.
[21]S. Huebner, Kenneth Black, Jr., and Robert S. Cline, *Property and Insurance Liability*, Appleton-Century-Crofts, New York, 1968, p. 374.

nesses, evidence, and related expenditures. In the settlement or judgment, the amount payable by the insurer cannot exceed the limits of the policy, although court costs and the costs of defense may be added.

Property and liability insurance have grown at an astounding rate. In 1946 the industry collected premiums in excess of $3 billion. By 1970 the amount had jumped to $27 billion.[22] Several factors account for the increased demand for this type of protection. Inflation has raised the level of financial risk significantly. Juries, unsophisticated in legal technicalities, have often awarded unreasonable sums, rationalizing that because the insurance company is paying no one really loses. Injured parties are becoming more aware of their legal right to compensation. In this age of consumerism, many people are aware of the economic loss associated with liability and have chosen to minimize the level of uncertainty through insurance.

Comprehensive personal liability insurance protects an individual or family against lawsuits involving personal actions or property owned or used by the insured. Typically, the policy protects the insured against personal liability, personal medical payments, and physical damage to property. Coverage ordinarily extends to the person named on the policy. If that person is head of a household, the policy includes his or her spouse, relatives, and others under the age of twenty-one in the insured's care. Intentional acts which lead to physical harm or property damage are excluded from the coverage.

The broad-form homeowner's policy is divided into two parts. The first section is property insurance, which covers the dwelling, additional structures not part of the dwelling, personal contents, and added living expenses. The second section is liability insurance, which covers personal liability for damages to other persons or property, and medical payments to others who are on the insured's property with permission, or who are injured elsewhere, if the accident was caused by the insured or an animal owned by the insured.

Personal liability is regularly covered by the homeowner's insurance policy. The purposes and general coverage benefits are quite similar. If an individual has homeowner's insurance, it is unnecessary to also carry a comprehensive personal liability policy. The homeowner's policy offers multiperil protection that covers most risks associated with home ownership. The dwelling and contents are covered against fire and other perils as well as theft. People who rent a place to live may obtain similar coverage to protect their personal property and to protect themselves against personal liability.

LEARNING EXPERIENCES

The following activities are designed to supplement the study of this chapter.

1 Prepare several fictitious lawsuits claiming legal liability. Identify the major factors influencing the outcome of each case. Using additional cases, conduct a "mock" courtroom trial with students assuming the roles of plaintiff,

---

[22]Pfeffer and Klock, op. cit., p. 147.

defendant, witnesses, defense attorney, attorney for the plaintiff, judge, and jury.

2 Invite a local lawyer to address the class on tort. The lawyer might discuss actual cases, using false names, and identify the factors which helped determine the outcome of the suit. Good Samaritan laws and their implications for administering first aid could also be discussed.

3 Invite an insurance agent to speak to the class on liability insurance. Identify the major factors one should consider when selecting a liability policy. Discuss the factors which enable one to calculate the amount of coverage considered "adequate."

4 Visit a local court for the purpose of observing judicial procedures. Follow the visit with classroom discussion.

5 Brainstorm the issue of liability insurance for professionals such as teachers and recreation leaders. Describe the protection that needs to be offered in such a policy. Discuss what steps can be taken to reduce the number of unwarranted claims against professionals.

6 Because so many childhood accidents occur in public schools, analyze the type of insurance made available to students, such as athletic or accident coverage. Study some of the dangerous areas in schools and identify potential sources of lawsuits directed at teachers.

7 Go to a university or law library and ask for help in locating information on tort law. Research five liability cases and abstract the essentials of each. Read the information to the class and ask for opinions about the outcome and the factors which were considered in determining the outcome.

SELECTED REFERENCES

American Jurisprudence 2d, West Publishing Company, St. Paul, Minn.

Black, Henry Campbell: *Black's Law Dictionary,* 4th ed., West Publishing Company, St. Paul, Minn., 1951.

Henderson, James A., Jr., and Richard N. Pearson: *The Torts Process,* Little, Brown & Company, Boston, 1975.

Huebner, S. S., Kenneth Black, Jr., and Robert S. Cline: *Property and Liability Insurance,* Appleton-Century-Crofts, New York, 1968.

Peterson, Le Roy J., Richard A. Rossmiller, and Marlin M. Volz: *The Law and Public School Operation,* Harper & Row, Publishers, Incorporated, New York, 1969

Pfeffer, Irving, and David R. Klock: *Perspectives on Insurance,* Prentice-Hall, Inc., Englewood Cliffs, N.J., 1974.

Prosser, William Lloyd: *Handbook of the Law of Torts,* 4th ed., West Publishing Company, St. Paul, Minn., 1971.

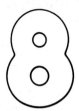

Pedestrian Safety

OVERALL OBJECTIVE:

Students of safety should understand the magnitude of the accident problem and the trends in pedestrian accidents. They should be able to identify accident causes in order to develop units for teachers of pedestrian conduct and accident avoidance.

INSTRUCTIONAL OBJECTIVES:

After completing this chapter the student will be able to:

1 List the significant death and injury figures from current and past years. Using these data, infer and discuss trends in pedestrian safety problems.
2 List the major causes of pedestrian accidents as they relate specifically to preschool, student, middle-aged, and older pedestrians.
3 Explain the laws and ordinances (local, state, and federal) that relate to the rights and duties of the pedestrian.
4 Discuss and recommend behavioral changes that would lead to safe pedestrian practices.
5 Organize material that could be used in teaching a unit on pedestrian safety at a specific grade level.
6 List two specific learning activities for each grade, 1 through 8, that would encourage pedestrian safety.
7 Formulate a pedestrian safety program for senior citizens.
8 List the eighteen federal highway pedestrian safety standards.

PEDESTRIAN SAFETY

Probably the most ignored element in traffic safety programs is the pedestrian, the highway user who is on foot. The pedestrian problem might be completely forgotten if not for the adult crossing guards and the school traffic patrols that we see helping youngsters get to and from school safely every day. When analyzing accident figures, one realizes that the pedestrian-accident problem has not been solved. "Since 1928 when national statistics first became available, approximately 480,000 pedestrians have died in traffic accidents. Unless strong action such as widespread education, increased enforcement, and improved engineering is taken, that figure will reach 580,000 by 1980. Plus an astronomical number of serious injuries."[1]

As more and more motor vehicles choke our streets and highways, and as their speed constantly increases, pedestrian accidents continue to be a serious problem. Almost everyone in this country is a pedestrian. Since about two out of every four pedestrians are drivers, it is evident that problems between drivers and pedestrians are everybody's business. Although for a number of years pedestrian fatalities decreased, for the past several years they have shown an increase, averaging close to 10,000 annually. Pedestrian deaths account for approximately one-fifth of all traffic fatalities. The number of injuries continues to be around 120,000 annually.[2] With a population of over 200 million in the United States, one can see that constant attention must be given to pedestrian safety.

Pedestrians are currently subject to much greater risk than they were 30 years ago, not only because of the millions of additional vehicles on the road but because of the great population shift from rural sections to urban centers. With most of the nation's motor vehicles and pedestrians concentrated in relatively small areas, traffic conditions are naturally far more congested and dangerous than they would be if the increased automobile production had been absorbed evenly throughout the country. In a recent study conducted by the American Automobile Association, it was found that nearly 85 percent of pedestrian accidents and 67 percent of pedestrian fatalities occur in urban areas. In cities with over 200,000 people, 33 to 50 percent of all traffic fatalities occur to pedestrians. Although there are fewer pedestrian accidents in rural areas, the accidents are usually more serious because of higher speeds of vehicles, poor lighting, and lack of sidewalks and emergency-care facilities. These facts illustrate the need for greatly expanded and more effective work in both urban and rural areas.

The increased speed of the modern car has also helped raise the pedestrian-accident toll. An automobile traveling at the once usual rate of 24 miles per hour is moving eight times faster than a pedestrian normally walks (Figure 8-1). At 60 miles per hour, a car is traveling twenty times faster. The pedestrian today has very little time to get out of the path of a rapidly approaching car. In a collision the pedestrian is obviously the one to suffer—160 pounds and $\frac{1}{5}$ horsepower clearly have no chance against a 3,000-pound automobile with a 200-horsepower engine. Although only one of every four nonpedestrian traffic accidents results in a casualty, someone is hurt in nearly every pedestrian accident, and one of every thirteen pedestrians injured in a traffic accident dies.

[1]*How to Make Pedestrians Safer,* Highway Users Federation for Safety and Mobility, Washington.
[2]*Accident Facts,* National Safety Council, Chicago, 1977. Unless otherwise noted, all statistics in this chapter are drawn from this source.

For each 1 yard a
pedestrian walks,

A car goes 8 yards
at 24 m.p.h.

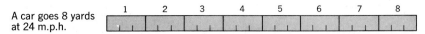

Figure 8-1 Car speed versus walking speed. Adult pedestrians walk at about 3 miles per hour. To figure out the ratio of car speed to pedestrian speed divide the speed of the car in miles per hour by 3. (Source: Sportsmanlike Driving 2d ed., 1948, p. 115, American Automobile Association, Falls Church, Va. See also 5th ed., 1965, Chapter 12.)

PLANNING A PEDESTRIAN SAFETY PROGRAM

When drivers take an examination for a driver's license, they must show that they have mastered certain skills in handling an automobile and that they know the rules of the road. We cannot license pedestrians before we permit them to walk on our streets and highways. But we can protect individuals by teaching them the fundamentals of pedestrian safety in an education program that will make them good pedestrians.

Various studies of the accident problem have shown that education can be effective in promoting highway safety. The overall reduction in the pedestrian toll must be attributed at least in part to the safety efforts of the school, particularly to the work of student traffic patrols. Despite the encouraging results thus far achieved, the pedestrian education program must be strengthened and expanded. A well-organized campaign to prevent traffic accidents requires the cooperation not only of all pupils, teachers, and parents, but also of all other members of the community, particularly law-enforcement personnel.

IDENTIFYING ACCIDENT CAUSES

An analysis of pedestrian traffic accidents in an average year reveals the following significant facts[3] which may serve as a basis for determining the causes of such accidents and planning preventive measures (Figure 8-2):

• Approximately 45 percent of the pedestrians killed in accidents are more than forty-five years old, yet only one-sixth of the nation's population is in this age group.
• Of the pedestrians killed, approximately 25 percent are under fifteen years of age.
• Among the adult population, 20 to 25 percent of all pedestrians killed have been drinking.
• Of the pedestrians killed, 95 percent are nondrivers.
• Six out of ten pedestrian deaths and injuries happen while pedestrians

[3]*Manual on Pedestrian Safety*, American Automobile Association, Washington, 1964, p. 8.

cross or enter streets. Two-fifths of all accidents occur between intersections, but the proportion varies among age groups.

• The majority of pedestrian accidents and fatalities occur in urban areas, especially in cities with populations of over 200,000.

• Although most pedestrian accidents occur in urban areas, rural pedestrian accidents are often more serious. Vehicle speeds in rural areas are generally higher. Driver visibility is limited, and pedestrians do not walk facing traffic or wear light-colored clothing. The probability of a fatality in an urban pedestrian accident is one in twenty. In rural accidents the probability is one in five.

Rain is another contributor to pedestrian accidents. It reduces the driver's visibility, and also cuts the pedestrian's visibility by means of umbrellas, rain hats, and other gear.

Like drivers, pedestrians must be able to judge gaps in traffic and know their own abilities and limitations. Depending on their age and physical condition, pedestrians may need as much as 10 seconds to cross a two-lane street (Figure 8-1).

Some of the characteristics and conditions that help cause pedestrian accidents are shown in Table 1-6 and Table 1-7. The high proportion of aged victims suggests that poor reflexes, impaired vision and hearing, degeneration of the nervous system, and other physical disabilities cause many accidents. The correlation between safety violations and accidents indicates that ignorance of pedestrian regulations or failure to recognize their importance can be another common cause. Ignorance of how an automobile functions increases a pedestrian's vulnerability to accidents, for most victims are nondrivers who presumably know very little about the operation of a car.

	Death total	Change from 1975	Death rate	
Pedestrian accidents	**8,300**	**−1%**	**3.9**	Includes all deaths of persons struck by
Urban	5,800	−5%		motor vehicles, either on or off a street or
Rural	2,500	+9%		highway, regardless of the circumstances of the accident.

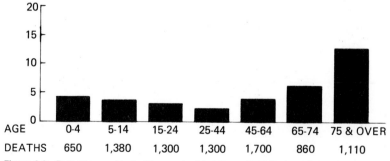

DEATH RATE (per 100,000 population in each age group)

AGE	0-4	5-14	15-24	25-44	45-64	65-74	75 & OVER
DEATHS	650	1,380	1,300	1,300	1,700	860	1,110

Figure 8-2 Pedestrian accidents. (Source: Accident Facts, 1977, National Safety Council, Chicago.)

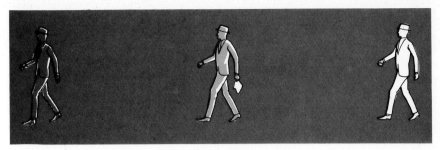

Tested distances at which pedestrian was seen by driver

Black clothes	With white handkerchief	Large white area
Visible 95-195 ft.	Visible 164-291 ft.	Visible 206-377 ft.

Figure 8-3 Night visibility of pedestrians varies with amount of white showing. (Source: Pedestrian Protection, p. 7, American Automobile Association, Falls Church, Va.)

The pedestrian's unfamiliarity with the problems of the motorist is a particularly significant point. Because pedestrians can "stop on a dime," they may not realize that an automobile requires well over 100 feet to come to a full stop, even at only 40 miles per hour. Because they can easily dodge an object in their path by quickly changing direction, they may underestimate the difficulty of manipulating a motor vehicle. Failing to understand the swift approach of a car, pedestrians may not recognize the danger to which their unsafe acts expose them; they rely too much on the driver's ability to avoid hitting them. Pedestrians may feel that avoiding accidents is exclusively the driver's responsibility. This attitude, coupled with ignorance of the driver's limitations, is undoubtedly responsible for many pedestrian accidents, particularly during hours of diminished light.

People walking after dark are often unaware that they can usually see an oncoming car long before the driver can see them (see Figure 8-3). The bright headlights on most modern automobiles do not guarantee that the driver can spot a pedestrian at a great distance. Unless the person on foot is carrying some object that reflects light or is wearing very light-colored clothing, he or she is almost invisible to the driver until the car is dangerously close.

Some additional facts concerning the pedestrian problem at night also deserve consideration:[4]

- Darkness increases the general pedestrian hazard by 63 percent.
- Darkness almost doubles the hazard of pedestrians in the 15 to 39 year age group.
- Darkness almost triples the hazard of pedestrians in the 40 to 64 year age group.
- Adequate street lighting is helpful in increasing the driver's ability to see pedestrians.
- Poor lighting of the highway is worse than none at all.
- Efficient headlights greatly increase the distance at which drivers see clothing or reflector buttons.

[4]*Sportsmanlike Driving*, 2d ed., American Automobile Association, Washington, chap. 8. See also 3d ed., chap. 19, 4th ed., chap. 12, and 7th ed., chap. 8.

REFLECTORIZATION.   Today, various vehicles have reflectors that glow at night. Automobiles and motorcycles have reflectorized license plates. Most bicycles have reflectorized lights, pedals, tires, and plastic discs on spokes to protect them from being hit at night by motorists. But what protects the pedestrian? In most cases nothing.

In many European countries pedestrians wear reflective material on their clothing, but in this country it is not very common. Half of all pedestrian fatalities occur at night. Because such accidents are the largest single cause of death for children between the ages of five and fourteen, greater emphasis must be placed on the use of reflectorized materials. Pedestrians must be aware of the fact that many drivers have limited vision at night.

When nighttime pedestrian accidents and fatalities occur, the reason usually given is "I didn't see him!" In one survey, 87 percent of the drivers who struck pedestrians at night stated that they did not see the victim in time. Some didn't see the victim until after the impact.

Reflective tape and fabric would help reduce nighttime accidents. A pedestrian wearing reflective material can be seen at 500 feet or more in a vehicle's headlights. A driver going 50 miles per hour needs 185 feet to stop. A pedestrian wearing white is visible at 180 feet. In dark clothing, the pedestrian is not visible until he or she is only 55 feet away, provided the driver's lights and windshield are free of dirt and mud.

Reflectorized materials are now available in many varieties. There is no reason for pedestrians not to use this method of protecting themselves at night.

SETTING OBJECTIVES

The overall objective of a school's pedestrian safety program is to prevent pedestrian accidents by removing their causes. When the causes have been identified through study of available accident records, the students themselves, with the assistance of the teacher, should formulate specific objectives in the light of their particular needs, abilities, and interests. The following list of suggested objectives is offered as a guide:

1 To acquire knowledge, understanding, and appreciation of the traffic rules and regulations designed to ensure safe use of streets and highways by pedestrians and motorists

2 To recognize pedestrian privileges, responsibilities, and duties in the use of streets and highways

3 To practice sound pedestrian behavior at all times

4 To understand the special pedestrian problems of foreigners, the aged, and the handicapped

Since the student's list of objectives must be developed to suit his or her particular needs, it will probably be much more detailed than the example given here. A list prepared by an elementary school group, for example, might include such items as "to learn the meaning of traffic signs and signals," "to develop the habit of playing only in safe areas," and "to follow the proper procedures in going to and from school."

ACHIEVING THE OBJECTIVES

People are most likely to comply with a safety rule if they understand its purpose and realize that it is intended for their protection. The teacher should make certain that students are not only familiar with all pedestrian regulations but also recognize and appreciate the logic and value of these regulations.

Students should be taught that traffic regulations are intended to give the person on foot a "break." If a pedestrian is already in a street intersection uncontrolled by a traffic light when a car approaches, he or she has the right to continue across the street. The pedestrian is not expected to stand in the middle of the intersection until the car passes, rather, the driver must stop and wait until the pedestrian reaches the curb safely.[5] Students should be taught that in return for this concession pedestrians crossing a street at any place other than an intersection must yield the right of way to motorists. The area between intersections is drivers' territory; it is not intended for pedestrians. Through group discussion of such traffic rules, students can learn to appreciate the need for mutual understanding between pedestrians and drivers and to recognize the fact that the person in the street, as well as the driver of a car, is responsible for highway safety.

EXPLAINING PEDESTRIAN REGULATIONS

For students to have a common starting point in studying pedestrian safety regulations, teachers should acquaint them with the pedestrian rights and duties listed in the *Model Traffic Ordinance,* a suggested guide to rules of the road that has been developed over a period of years by committees from various organizations interested in promoting highway safety. The ordinance, which represents an attempt to establish uniformity in traffic laws, is generally recognized as a valuable contribution to the nation's accident-prevention efforts. The original rules have been revised where necessary to take into account new developments and accumulated experiences. The following standards may be considered up to date:

Article II. Traffic-control devices

Sec. 11-202. *Traffic-control signal legend*

Whenever traffic is controlled by traffic-control signals exhibiting different colored lights, or colored light arrows, successively one at a time or in combination, only the colors green, red

---

[5]See *Model Traffic Ordinance,* National Committee on Uniform Traffic Laws and Ordinances, Washington, rev., 1962, rev., 1968, and Supplement II, 1976.

and yellow shall be used, except for special pedestrian signals carrying a word legend, and said lights shall indicate and apply to drivers of vehicles and pedestrians as follows:

a Green indication:

1 Vehicular traffic facing a circular green signal may proceed straight through or turn right or left unless a sign at such place prohibits either such turn. But vehicular traffic, including vehicles turning right or left, shall yield the right of way to other vehicles and to pedestrians lawfully within the intersection or an adjacent crosswalk at the time such signal is exhibited.

2 Vehicular traffic facing a green arrow signal, shown alone or in combination with another indication, may cautiously enter the intersection only to make the movement indicated by such arrow, or such other movement as is permitted by other indications shown at the same time. Such vehicular traffic shall yield the right of way to pedestrians lawfully within an adjacent crosswalk and to other traffic lawfully using the intersection.

3 Unless otherwise directed by a pedestrian-control signal as provided in Sec. 11-203, pedestrians facing any green signal, except when the sole green signal is a turn arrow, may proceed across the roadway within any marked or unmarked crosswalk.

b Steady yellow indication:

1 Vehicular traffic facing a steady circular yellow or yellow arrow signal is thereby warned that the related green movement is being terminated or that a red indication will be exhibited immediately thereafter. (Revised, 1975.)

2 Pedestrians facing a steady circular yellow or yellow arrow signal, unless otherwise directed by a pedestrian-control signal as provided in Sec. 11-203, are thereby advised that there is insufficient time to cross the roadway before a red indication is shown and no pedestrian shall then start to cross the roadway. (Revised, 1975.)

c Steady red indication

1 Vehicular traffic facing a steady circular red signal alone shall stop at a clearly marked stop line, but if none, before entering the crosswalk on the near side of the intersection, or if none, then before entering the intersection and shall remain standing until an indication to proceed is shown except as provided in subsection (c)3. (Revised, 1975.)

2 Vehicular traffic facing a steady red arrow signal shall not enter the intersection to make the movement indicated by the arrow and, unless entering the intersection to make a movement permitted by another signal, shall stop at a clearly marked stop line, but if none, before entering the crosswalk on the near side of the intersection, or if none, then before entering the intersection and shall remain standing until an indication permitting the movement indicated by such red arrow is shown except as provided in subsection (c)3. (New, 1975.)

3 Except when a sign is in place prohibiting a turn, vehicular traffic facing any steady red signal may cautiously enter the intersection to turn right, or to turn left from a one-way street into a one-way street, after stopping as required by subsection (c)1 or subsection (c)2. Such vehicular traffic shall yield the right of way to pedestrians lawfully within an adjacent crosswalk and to other traffic lawfully using the intersection. (Revised and renumbered, 1975.)

4 Unless otherwise directed by a pedestrian-control signal as provided in Sec. 11-203, pedestrians facing a steady circular red or red arrow signal alone shall not enter the roadway. (Revised and renumbered, 1975.)

Sec. 11-203. *Pedestrian-control signals*

Whenever special pedestrian-control signals exhibiting the words "Walk" or "Don't Walk" are in place such signals shall indicate as follows:

a *Flashing or Steady Walk.*—Any pedestrian facing the signal may proceed across the roadway in the direction of the signal and every driver of a vehicle shall yield the right of way to him.

b *Flashing or Steady Don't Walk.*—No pedestrian shall start to cross the roadway in the direction of the signal, but any pedestrian who has partially completed his crossing on the walk signal shall proceed to a sidewalk or safety island while the don't walk signal is showing. (Section revised, 1975.)

Article V. Pedestrians' rights and duties

Sec. 11-501. *Pedestrian obedience to traffic-control devices and traffic regulations*

a A pedestrian shall obey the instructions of any official traffic-control device specifically applicable to him, unless otherwise directed by a police officer. (New, 1969.)

b Pedestrians shall be subject to traffic and pedestrian-control signals as provided in §§ 11-202 and 11-203. (Revised, 1968.)

c At all other places, pedestrians shall be accorded the privileges and shall be subject to the restrictions stated in this chapter.

Sec. 11-502. *Pedestrians' right of way in crosswalks*

a When traffic-control signals are not in place or not in operation the driver of a vehicle shall yield the right of way, slowing down or stopping if need be to so yield, to a pedestrian crossing the roadway within a crosswalk when the pedestrian is upon the half of the roadway upon which the vehicle is traveling, or when the pedestrian is approaching so closely from the opposite half of the roadway as to be in danger. [See Figure 8-4.]

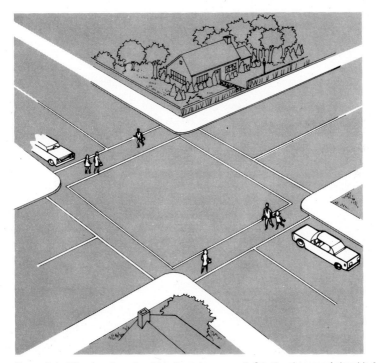

Figure 8-4 Who does have the right of way in crosswalks? In the absence of signal indications, drivers shall yield to any pedestrian within a crosswalk when the pedestrian is upon the half of the roadway upon which the vehicle is traveling or when the pedestrian is approaching so closely from the other half of the roadway as to be in danger. Though you may legally have the right of way it may not be safe to insist upon taking it. (Source: Planned Pedestrian Program, Foundation for Traffic Safety, American Automobile Association, Falls Church, Va.)

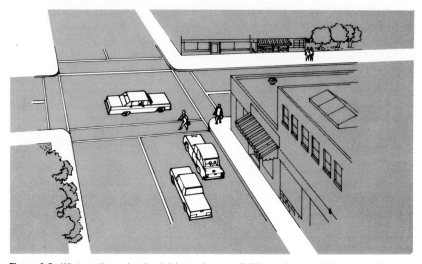

Figure 8-5 What are the pedestrians' rights and responsibilities as they reach the crosswalk, as covered by provisions in the *Uniform Vehicle Code* and the *Model Traffic Ordinance?* No pedestrian shall leave a curb or other place of safety and walk or run into the path of a vehicle which is so close as to make it impossible for the driver to yield. Whenever a vehicle is stopped at an intersection crosswalk to permit a pedestrian crossing, no other driver is allowed to overtake and pass the stopped vehicle; however, it doesn't mean that he won't. (Source: Planned Pedestrian Program, Foundation for Traffic Safety, American Automobile Association, Falls Church, Va.)

b No pedestrian shall suddenly leave a curb or other place of safety and walk or run into the path of a vehicle which is so close as to constitute an immediate hazard. (Revised, 1971.) [See Figure 8-5.]

c Paragraph (a) shall not apply under the conditions stated in 11-503(b).

d Whenever any vehicle is stopped at a marked crosswalk or at any unmarked crosswalk at an intersection to permit a pedestrian to cross the roadway, the driver of any other vehicle approaching from the rear shall not overtake and pass such stopped vehicle.

Sec. 11-503. *Crossing at other than crosswalks*

a Every pedestrian crossing a roadway at any point other than within a marked crosswalk or within an unmarked crosswalk at an intersection shall yield the right of way to all vehicles upon the roadway. [See Figure 8-6.]

b Any pedestrian crossing a roadway at a point where a pedestrian tunnel or overhead pedestrian crossing has been provided shall yield the right of way to all vehicles upon the roadway.

c Between adjacent intersections at which traffic-control signals are in operation pedestrians shall not cross at any place except in a marked crosswalk. [See Figure 8-7.]

d No pedestrian shall cross a roadway intersection diagonally unless authorized by official traffic-control devices; and when authorized to cross diagonally, pedestrians shall cross only in accordance with the official traffic-control devices pertaining to such crossing movements.

Sec. 11-504. *Drivers to exercise due care*

Notwithstanding other provisions of this chapter or the provisions of any local ordinance, every driver of a vehicle shall exercise due care to avoid colliding with any pedestrian or any person propelling a human powered vehicle and shall give an audible signal when necessary and shall exercise proper precaution upon observing any child or any obviously confused, incapacitated or intoxicated person. (Revised, 1971 & 1975.) [See Figure 8-8.]

Sec. 11-505. *Pedestrians to use right half of crosswalks*

Pedestrians shall move, whenever practicable, upon the right half of crosswalks. [See Figure 8-9.]

Sec. 11-506. *Pedestrians on highways*

a Where a sidewalk is provided and its use is practicable, it shall be unlawful for any pedestrian to walk along and upon an adjacent roadway.

b Where a sidewalk is not available, any pedestrian walking along and upon a highway shall walk only on a shoulder, as far as practicable from the edge of the roadway.

c Where neither a sidewalk nor a shoulder is available, any pedestrian walking along and upon a highway shall walk as near as practicable to an outside edge of the roadway, and, if on a two-way roadway, shall walk only on the left side of the roadway.

d Except as otherwise provided in this chapter, any pedestrian upon a roadway shall yield

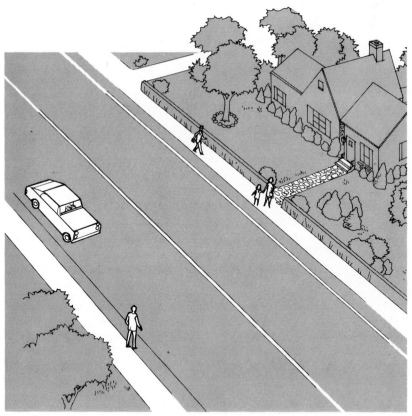

Figure 8-6   Jaywalking is dangerous; you are much safer crossing at the crosswalk. Pedestrians crossing at places other than a crosswalk, marked or unmarked, shall yield the right of way to vehicles. Remember, a driver is not expecting you to cross in the middle of the block. (Source: Planned Pedestrian Program, Foundation for Traffic Safety, American Automobile Association, Falls Church, Va.)

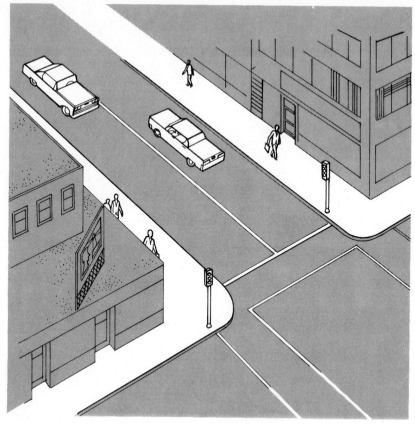

Figure 8-7 The signals are for your protection. Pedestrians shall not be permitted to cross between adjacent intersections where signals are in operation. Obeying the traffic signal is a sign of mature judgment. (Source: Planned Pedestrian Program, Foundation for Traffic Safety, American Automobile Association, Falls Church, Va.)

the right of way to all vehicles upon the roadway. (Section revised; Subsection (d) New, 1971.) [See Figure 8-10.]

Sec. 11-507. *Pedestrians soliciting rides or business*

a No person shall stand in a roadway for the purpose of soliciting a ride.
b No person shall stand on a highway for the purpose of soliciting employment, business, or contributions from the occupant of any vehicle.
c No person shall stand on or in proximity to a street or highway for the purpose of soliciting the watching or guarding of any vehicle while parked or about to be parked on a street or highway. [See Figure 8-11.]

Sec. 11-508. *Driving through safety zone prohibited*

No vehicle shall at any time be driven through or within a safety zone.

Sec. 11-509. *Pedestrians' right of way on sidewalks*

The driver of a vehicle crossing a sidewalk shall yield the right of way to any pedestrian and all other traffic on the sidewalk. (Revised, 1971 & 1975.)

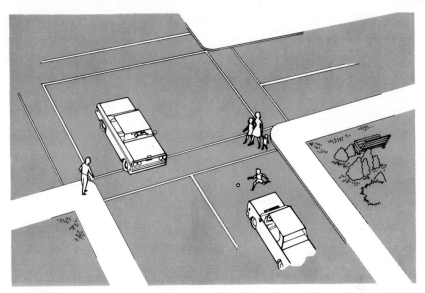

Figure 8-8 Drivers are to exercise due care to avoid colliding with pedestrians under any circumstances and shall use their horn when necessary, giving special consideration to children and any confused or incapacitated person upon the roadway. Drivers should watch out in particular for the young, old, and the blind. The pedestrian is no match for a moving vehicle. (Source: Planned Pedestrian Program, Foundation for Traffic Safety, American Automobile Association, Falls Church, Va.)

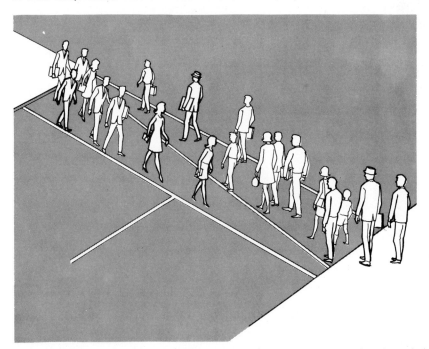

Figure 8-9 There are also rules of the road for pedestrians. Pedestrians shall use, insofar as is practicable, the right half of the crosswalk and shall cross the street at right angles except as otherwise directed by crosswalk markings. Staying on your side is an act of courtesy and avoids conflicts. (Source: Planned Pedestrian Program, Foundation for Traffic Safety, American Automobile Association, Falls Church, Va.)

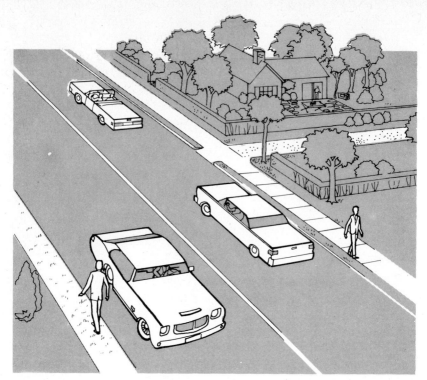

Figure 8-10 Walk only where the motorist expects you to walk. Where sidewalks are provided, pedestrians shall not walk along and upon an adjacent roadway. Where there are no sidewalks, pedestrians shall, when practicable, walk only on the left side of the roadway or shoulder, facing approaching traffic. Walk facing the traffic when on a roadway or where there are no sidewalks. (Source: Planned Pedestrian Program, Foundation for Traffic Safety, American Automobile Association, Falls Church, Va.)

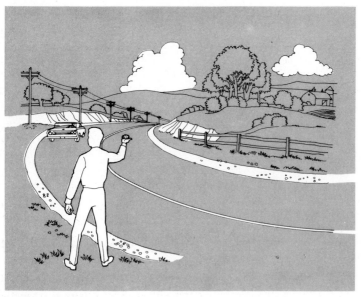

Figure 8-11 Pedestrians shall not stand in the roadway for the purpose of soliciting a ride. Hitchhiking is illegal and could be dangerous for the driver. It is good policy to avoid hitchhikers. (Source: Planned Pedestrian Program, Foundation for Traffic Safety, American Automobile Association, Falls Church, Va.)

244

Sec. 11-510. *Pedestrians yield to authorized emergency vehicles*

a Upon the immediate approach of an authorized emergency vehicle making use of an audible signal meeting the requirements of Sec. 12-401 (d) and visual signals meeting the requirements of Sec. 12-218 of this act, or of a police vehicle properly and lawfully making use of an audible signal only, every pedestrian shall yield the right of way to the authorized emergency vehicle.

b This section shall not relieve the driver of an authorized emergency vehicle from the duty to drive with due regard for the safety of all persons using the highway nor from the duty to exercise due care to avoid colliding with any pedestrian. (NEW SECTION, 1971.)

Sec. 11-511. *Blind pedestrian right of way*

The driver of a vehicle shall yield the right of way to any blind pedestrian carrying a clearly visible white cane or accompanied by a guide dog. (New, 1971.)

Sec. 11-512. *Pedestrians under influence of alcohol or drugs*

A pedestrian who is under the influence of alcohol or any drug to a degree which renders himself a hazard shall not walk or be upon a highway except on a sidewalk. (New, 1971.)

Sec. 11-513. *Bridge and railroad signals*

a No pedestrian shall enter or remain upon any bridge or approach thereto beyond the bridge signal, gate, or barrier after a bridge operation signal indication has been given.

b No pedestrian shall pass through, around, over, or under any crossing gate or barrier at a railroad grade crossing or bridge while such gate or barrier is closed or is being opened or closed. (New section, 1971.)

PRESCHOOL PEDESTRIAN SAFETY

Before conducting a pedestrian safety program in a school situation, we must realize that safety education should begin at home. The responsibility for early training rests with parents and guardians. Such training can begin as soon as the child learns to walk. Youngsters should be taken out into traffic situations and taught safe pedestrian practices. Parents can conduct and supervise learning activities that will instill practical knowledge and habits of safe pedestrian behavior. The American Automobile Association has developed an excellent "Pre-School Children in Traffic Program" for parents of youngsters from 2½ to 6 years of age.

SAFETY TOWN

Another program that helps preschool children acquire confidence and self-responsibility is called Safety Town.[6] This program is usually sponsored by a local agency in the community. It is offered to youngsters who will be attending school for the first time. It is usually conducted during the summer months, and provides experiences of traffic situations in a simulated village (see Figure 8-12).

[6]*Safety Town,* Traffic Engineering and Safety Department, American Automobile Association, Falls Church, Va., 1968.

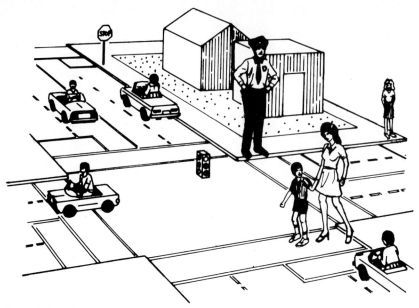

Figure 8-12 Safety town.

TEACHING SAFE PEDESTRIAN PRACTICES

When students have become familiar with the rights and duties of the pedestrian, the teacher should help them recognize the type of conduct that is in keeping with these regulations and assist them in formulating a code of behavior for the pedestrian. The following list of safe practices exemplifies such a code. It is suitable for all age groups but should be used to guide students in developing their own standards. Students should not be required to memorize it, for they are far more likely to learn and obey rules that they themselves have devised than rules imposed on them by others. Therefore, the teacher should always explain the reasons for safe behavior.

The careful pedestrian:

1 Selects safe play areas away from streets.

2 Understands and follows the directions of safety-patrol members and/or traffic officers.

3 When there are alternative routes to school, chooses to cross streets where traffic is relatively light.

4 Crosses the street only at crosswalks.

5 Looks for traffic in all directions, watching especially for turning cars, before crossing an intersection.

6 Considers the width of the street and the speed of approaching cars before stepping into the street. Waits on the curb or in the safety zone if there is any doubt that he or she has ample time to reach the opposite curb safely.

7 Never dawdles in crossing a street but walks directly to the opposite curb, keeping to the right half of the crosswalk.

8 Sets an example by obeying traffic laws, street signs, traffic signals, and road markings.

9 Never enters a street from behind or between parked cars.

10 Watches for backing and turning cars before stepping into the street.

11 Stands in safety zones until the path to the curb is clear and then proceeds to the curb directly opposite.

12 Gets out of an automobile, bus, or streetcar on the curb side and watches for oncoming traffic before crossing the street.

13 Never crosses in front of a vehicle from which he or she has just alighted.

14 Walks on the left side of a street, highway, or rural road if there is no sidewalk. Steps off the road, if possible, when a motor vehicle approaches.

15 Uses the overpass or underpass, whenever one is provided, to reach the opposite side of the street.

16 Redoubles caution when the weather is bad, when streets are crowded, or when other conditions increase hazards.

17 Carries an umbrella in a way that does not obstruct the view of traffic.

18 Takes special care when in a hurry, when carrying bundles, when not feeling well, or when distracted or worried.

19 Does not try to hitch onto moving vehicles.

20 Does not always insist on his or her rights as a pedestrian.

21 Uses common sense and remains alert at all times.

22 Wears white after dark.

PROVIDING LEARNING EXPERIENCES

Students can learn sound pedestrian practices most effectively when they are given opportunities to put into practice the knowledge and skills they have been taught in the classroom. The following assignments will enable them to participate actively in the pedestrian safety program and thus to learn by doing:

1 Study the rights and duties of the pedestrian listed in the *Model Traffic Ordinance* and discuss them in class.

2 Under the guidance of the teacher, demonstrate the proper way to cross streets en route to and from school.

3 Secure a list of local pedestrian laws and ordinances from the police department and discuss them in class.

4 Invite a local traffic officer to talk to your class on the proper pedestrian procedures at busy intersections controlled by the school patrol.

5 Have members of the school patrol explain their functions to the younger children.

6 Construct safety signs, such as STOP, GO, CAUTION, LEFT TURN, RIGHT TURN, WAIT, WALK, and DON'T WALK. Explain the proper interpretation of each sign.

7 Assemble information on pedestrian safety by writing to safety organizations, insurance companies, motor clubs, etc., to request copies of their pertinent publications.

8 Examine and discuss pictures, posters, and reading materials pertaining to pedestrian safety.

9 Discuss the good and bad habits demonstrated in the pedestrian safety films that you have been shown.

10 List the discourteous, unsafe pedestrian habits that you have observed in the halls and on the stairs in your school. Discuss proper pedestrian habits in these areas.

11 Secure an accident spot map from the local police or highway department, and study pedestrian accidents that have occurred in your community over a given period of time. List the places where the accidents most frequently occurred, the hours at which they happened, their causes, and the ages of the victims. Note how many of these accidents were due to pedestrian violations of traffic rules.

12 Analyze *your* conduct as a pedestrian during the past week, and list your pedestrian violations. Compare the advantages you gained by your unsafe behavior with the degree of danger you incurred.

13 Participate in student discussions dealing with such topics as: "The Pedestrian and the Automobile" "The Pedestrian at Night" "How to Formulate a Pedestrian Code" "How to Cross Crowded Intersections Safely" "Understanding Traffic Signs and Signals" "Comparing the Pedestrian Violations Occurring in Different Age Groups" "Jaywalking."

14 Observe a busy intersection in your community. List and compare the pedestrian violations committed by adults and by students.

15 Observing the same intersection, record the number of times you witness each of the common pedestrian violations, such as crossing between intersections, disregarding traffic signals, and stepping out into the street behind or between parked automobiles.

16 Observe an intersection in the vicinity of your school and note *(a)* how many students look to the left before leaving the curb, *(b)* how many look to the right, *(c)* how many look to the left, to the right, and to the left again, and *(d)* how many look in neither direction.

17 List the physical defects, such as impaired hearing or vision, that may cause improper pedestrian acts.

18 List some traffic-engineering accomplishments that help protect pedestrians.

19 List five specific pedestrian practices that you consider essential to safety and that, if followed faithfully, could greatly reduce the number of pedestrian accidents.

20 Write a radio or dramatic sketch or a television presentation on proper pedestrian procedures, and plan to present it before the entire school.

21 Prepare a series of articles on sound pedestrianism for publication in the school or community newspaper.

22 List pedestrian acts that irritate motorists and discuss ways of eliminating these practices.

23 List drivers' acts that irritate pedestrians and discuss ways of eliminating these practices.

24 Have students construct original pedestrian safety posters.

OLDER ADULT PEDESTRIAN SAFETY

Older adults, whose lives span the years from horse-and-buggy days to the space age, have difficulty in today's ever-changing, complex traffic situation. Persons sixty-five years of age or older are involved in more than 40 percent of all pedestrian deaths in this country.

Older adults, who grew up and formed their habits and attitudes in the early years of the motor age, are too frequently involved in fatal accidents because they do not know how to be safe pedestrians in today's fast-moving, congested traffic. The problem may get worse as we consider the fact that this age group is growing at a faster rate than any other age group. "By 1980 over ten percent of our population, or some 25 million citizens, will be 65 years of age or older."[7] Therefore, it is the responsibility of the community, school, home, church, safety council, and civic and other organizations to do everything possible to help our older citizens live safely and securely in our motorized age. Through these various organizations, including driver-refresher programs, efforts must be made to orient older pedestrians and motorists to their physical capabilities and teach them to compensate for any short-comings.

Probably the main reasons for the increased older pedestrian problem are the physical changes that occur with aging:

1 Older people are likely to have hearing and vision impairments. They have less accurate depth perception and lateral field of vision, which make it more difficult to judge distances of objects to the side when looking straight ahead.

2 The perceptions and responses of older persons are slower. It takes longer for the older person to perceive a dangerous situation and react to it in time to avoid an accident.

3 Older people have more difficulty in learning, particularly when it is necessary to counteract an old, established habit or attitude.

Although the above factors contribute to the accident problem, it must be pointed out that older pedestrians are probably more cautious and are increasingly safety-minded as they attempt to compensate for the physical and mental changes which come with age.

Special studies show that pedestrian accidents to the elderly are different from overall pedestrian accidents. Most pedestrian accidents result when the

[7]*Older Adult Pedestrian Safety,* American Automobile Association, Falls Church, Va., 1965, p. 3.

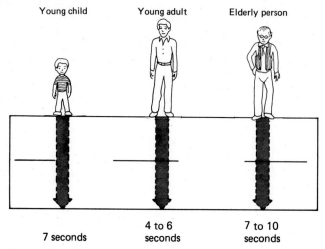

Young child   Young adult   Elderly person

7 seconds   4 to 6 seconds   7 to 10 seconds

Figure 8-13 Elderly pedestrians take longer. Although young people may take a shorter period of time to cross streets and highways, the potential risk involves those youngsters who dart unexpectedly into the street and highway.

pedestrian commits a violation or an unsafe walking practice. It was also found that alcohol is a significant factor in many adult accidents. The following describe the nature and causes of older pedestrian accidents.[8]

1 Seven out of ten older adult pedestrian accidents occurred at intersections while the pedestrian was crossing in a crosswalk, and almost half of these occurred as the pedestrian crossed with a signal. One-third of all older adult accidents were considered to be in violation or doing something unsafe. More than half of all intersection accidents involved turning vehicles. There would seem to be some relationship here to an older person's slower pace, slower reaction time, less accurate distance judgement and possibly a narrower field of vision. Depending on their age and physical condition, the older pedestrian may need as much as 10 seconds to cross a two-lane road. [see Figure 8-13]

2 Nightime and dusk are particularly hazardous times for older pedestrians even though many older people avoid walking at night. When they do they should always wear something white so they can be seen more readily. It may also take the eyes of the older person a longer period of time to adjust to night conditions.

3 Older males fare badly as pedestrians, even though they are outnumbered by women in this age bracket.

4 Accident records show that one of every four pedestrians in the 25–55 age bracket had been drinking. However, in very few older adult pedestrian accidents was alcohol to be found a contributing factor.

Pedestrian safety programs for older adults can do a great deal to reduce the number of deaths and injuries. The three E's of traffic safety—education, enforcement, and engineering—along with legislation can be the basic starting points. Start out by getting the facts. Study accident records and find out where, why, and how older adults are involved in pedestrian accidents. Pinpoint the

[8]Ibid., pp. 7–8.

specific needs for education, enforcement, and engineering. Perhaps a different timing for signals, lower curbs with ramps, and refuge islands may aid in solving the problem. Last but not least, use the experience and wisdom of older adults.

Older adults are usually safety-conscious. They are willing to learn if someone is willing to take the time to aid them. A defensive pedestrian safety program utilizing local clubs, churches, safety councils, police departments, senior citizen clubs, etc., can be very effective in combating the problem. The program could emphasize safe walking practices such as those illustrated in Figure 8-14.

Older pedestrians are involved in the largest proportion of pedestrian deaths, but studies show that this group is making the greatest improvement. "In 1937 the death rate per 100,000 population for pedestrians 65 years of age and older was 47.0. In recent years it was down to 14.0, a 70 percent reduction."[9] A continued improvement can and should be made by older citizens.

EVALUATION

Educators must be concerned with measuring the effectiveness of the school's pedestrian safety program. Accurate evaluation is essential to continued improvement. Whatever method of evaluation is selected should meet the following standards:

1 It should show how much the students have gained in knowledge and how much they have improved in performance.

2 It should indicate the extent to which the stated objectives of the program have been achieved.

3 It should be a continuous process with enough flexibility to meet changing conditions.

4 It should raise and attempt to answer the following specific questions:

a. Has the student learned how to cross streets and roads properly? Does the student understand and habitually obey traffic signs, signals, and road markings?

b. Has the student learned how to be a safe pedestrian under all conditions, in bad weather as well as in good, at night as well as during the day?

c. Has the student developed a wholesome attitude toward motorists and an understanding of their problems?

d. Does the student appreciate the pedestrian problems of the older adult and the handicapped?

No one method of evaluation can answer all these questions. If several means are used—testing, observation, and interview—the teacher should be

[9]Ibid, p. 14.

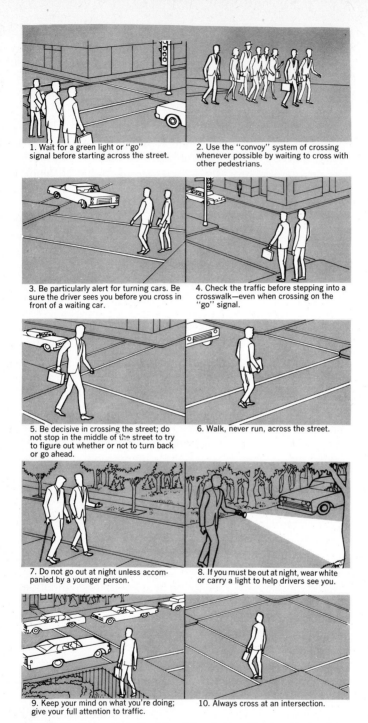

1. Wait for a green light or "go" signal before starting across the street.

2. Use the "convoy" system of crossing whenever possible by waiting to cross with other pedestrians.

3. Be particularly alert for turning cars. Be sure the driver sees you before you cross in front of a waiting car.

4. Check the traffic before stepping into a crosswalk—even when crossing on the "go" signal.

5. Be decisive in crossing the street; do not stop in the middle of the street to try to figure out whether or not to turn back or go ahead.

6. Walk, never run, across the street.

7. Do not go out at night unless accompanied by a younger person.

8. If you must be out at night, wear white or carry a light to help drivers see you.

9. Keep your mind on what you're doing; give your full attention to traffic.

10. Always cross at an intersection.

Figure 8-14 Safety rules for the older adult pedestrian. Attention with alert observation is the key for older adults in safe crossing of streets and highways. (Source: Older Adult Pedestrian Safety, 1970, p. 30, Automobile Association, Falls Church, Va.)

able to measure the degree of improvement in students' knowledge, skills, and attitudes. The classroom test, probably the most commonly used measuring device, is clearly the simplest means of determining students' knowledge and attitudes. Tests are most valuable as evaluation tools if they are given before and after students have been trained in pedestrian safety, so that the teacher can estimate the extent to which the instruction provided has resulted in greater knowledge and better attitudes. Tests cannot show whether or not students are *utilizing* the knowledge they have acquired. They have only limited value as an indication of the school's effectiveness in promoting pedestrian safety. In the final analysis, teachers must turn to accident statistics to discover how well pedestrian education is accomplishing its major objective.

Educators, particularly those assigned specific responsibility for safety, such as safety supervisors, coordinators, and director, should frequently analyze school and community records of pedestrian accidents, and interview some of the victims to determine how, where, when, and to whom these accidents occur. Such data may reveal that a particular age group has an unusually high pedestrian-accident rate, that a particular intersection is the scene of many accidents, or that most pedestrians are injured in violating a particular safety regulation. On the basis of this information, teachers can define the areas in which pedestrian education should be strengthened. Subsequent studies of accident records should indicate whether or not the school's efforts to improve its program have been effective.

FEDERAL HIGHWAY PEDESTRIAN SAFETY STANDARDS

A recent development that relates to standards and evaluation is the U.S. Department of Transportation's Highway Safety Program Standard 14, which deals with pedestrian safety. Compliance with this standard is an effective method of evaluating a statewide pedestrian safety program. The purpose and seven components of Standard 14 are as follows:

Purpose

To emphasize the need to recognize pedestrian safety as an integral, constant and important element in community planning and all aspects of highway transportation and to insure a continuing program to improve such safety by each State and its political subdivisions.

Standard

Every State in cooperation with its political subdivisions shall develop and implement a program to insure the safety of pedestrians of all ages. The program shall provide, as a minimum, that:

I. There is a continuing Statewide inventory of pedestrian-motor vehicle accidents, identifying specifically:
   A. The locations and times of all such accidents.
   B. The age of all of the pedestrians injured or killed.
   C. Where feasible, to determine whether the exterior features of the vehicle produced or aggravated an injury.

    D. The color and shade of clothing worn by pedestrians when injured or killed, and the visibility conditions which prevailed at the time.

    E. The extent to which alcohol is present in the blood of fatally injured pedestrians 16 years of age and older.

    F. Where possible, to determine the extent to which pedestrians involved in accidents have physical or mental disabilities.

II. There are established Statewide operational procedures for improving the protection of pedestrians through reduction of potential conflicts with vehicles:

    A. By application of traffic engineering practices including pedestrian signals, signs, Markings, parking regulations and other pedestrian and vehicle traffic-control devices.

    B. By land-use planning in new and redevelopment areas for safe pedestrian movement.

    C. By provision of pedestrian bridges, barriers, sidewalks and other means of physically separating pedestrian and vehicle pathways.

    D. By provision of environmental illumination at high pedestrian volume and/or potentially hazardous pedestrian crossings.

III. There is established a Statewide program for familiarizing drivers with the pedestrian problem and with ways to avoid pedestrian collisions.

    A. The program content shall include emphasis on

        (1) Behavior characteristics of the three types of pedestrians most commonly involved in accidents with vehicles: (i) children; (ii) persons under the influence of alcohol; (iii) the elderly

        (2) Accident avoidance techniques that take into account the hazardous conditions, and behavior characteristics displayed by each of the three high risk pedestrian groups listed in subparagraph (1)

    B. Emphasis on this program content shall be included in:

        (1) all driver education and training courses

        (2) driver improvement courses

        (3) driver license examinations

IV. There are Statewide programs for training and educating all members of the public as to safe pedestrian behavior on or near streets and highways.

    A. For children, youths and adults enrolled in schools, beginning at the earliest possible age.

    B. For the general population via the public media.

V. There is a Statewide program for the protection of children walking to and from school, entering and leaving school buses, and in neighborhood play.

VI. There is a Statewide program for establishment and enforcement of traffic regulations designed to achieve orderly pedestrian and vehicle movement and to reduce vehicle-pedestrian conflicts.

VII. This program shall be periodically evaluated by the States, and the National Highway Traffic Safety Administration and the Federal Highway Administration shall be provided with an evaluation summary.

LEARNING EXPERIENCES

The following activities represent only a few of the many learning experiences that can be of value to the teacher of pedestrian safety.

    1 Develop a pretest, suitable for all grade levels, to determine students' knowledge, attitudes, and behavior patterns in regard to safe pedestrianism.

    2 Develop a lesson plan on jaywalking.

    3 Outline a talk, to be delivered before a parent-teacher group, a local board of education, or a civic organization, explaining a proposed pedestrian safety program.

4 With the aid of the National Safety Council, the local safety council, the local newspaper, and the local radio or television station, plan a pedestrian safety campaign for an elementary school, a high school, a community, and for older adults.

5 Prepare an article on pedestrian safety for the local newspaper or a magazine such as *School Safety* or *Traffic Safety*.

6 Analyze pedestrian accidents shown on the spot map in the local traffic bureau.

7 Plan improvements in legislation that would increase the protection afforded to pedestrians.

8 Write a paper on how uncooperative attitudes on the part of pedestrians and motorists can contribute to accidents.

9 Plan a field trip for your students that will give you, as a teacher, an opportunity to evaluate what the class has learned about pedestrian safety.

10 Plan a pedestrian-safety-slogan contest for an elementary school, a high school, a community, and a senior-citizens' club.

SELECTED REFERENCES

American Automobile Association, Falls Church, Va.:
> *Adult Crossing Guards,* 1964, p. 26
> *First Steps for Pedestrian Protection*
> *How Cities Protect Pedestrians*
> *Manual on Pedestrian Safety,* 1964, p. 162
> *Older Adult Pedestrian Safety,* 1970, p. 15
> *Parents, Safeguard Your Child*
> *Pedestrian Control Through Legislation and Enforcement,* 1965
> *Pedestrian Protection*
> *Pedestrian with Mileage,* 1964
> *Pedestrian Safety Check*
> *Play Yards Are Life Savers*
> *Safety Town*
> *Sportsmanlike Driving,* 7th ed., 1975, chap. 8.
> *Survey on Alcohol Testing and Pedestrian Accidents,* 1970.
> *The Young Pedestrian,* 1972, p. 16

Baker, Susan P., Leon S. Robertson, and Brian O'Neill: "Fatal Pedestrian Collisions," *American Journal of Public Health,* p. 318, April, 1974

Fleig, Peter H., and Daniel J. Duffy: "A Study of Pedestrian Safety Behavior Using Activity Samplings," *Traffic Safety Research Review,* December, 1967.

Highway Users Federation for Safety and Mobility, Washington: *How to Make Pedestrians Safer.*

Jones, Trevor O. and Brian S. Repa: "A General Overview of Pedestrian Accidents and Protective Countermeasures," *Proceedings of the Third International Congress on Automotive Safety,* vol. 1, 1974, pp. 1-6

Lawton, Alfred H., and Gordon Azar: "Some Observations of Behavior of Older Pedestrians," *Medical Times,* January, 1964.

Manual on Uniform Traffic Control Devices, U.S. Bureau of Public Roads, Washington, 1971.

Metropolitan Life Insurance Company, New York:
 Accident Hazards of School-age Children
 Be Safe for Life's Adventure
 Help Them to Safety
 Help Your Child to Safety
 How Parents Can Help in Safety Education
 Play It Safe
Model Traffic Ordinance, National Committee on Uniform Traffic Laws and Ordinances, Washington, rev., 1968, p. 20, supplement II, 1976.
National Safety Council, Chicago:
 Accident Facts, yearly
 Dead Right
 Much to Do about Safety
 Pedestrian Safety, rev.
 Railroad Trespassing, rev.
 Safe on Foot
 Safeguarding the Pedestrian (Report of the Committee on Pedestrian Control and Protection)
 A Safety Program for High Schools
 A Safety Program for the Elementary and Junior High Schools
 To and From School
 Traffic-control Devices
 Walk Safely Too
 Winter Walking
School Pedestrian Safety Program, Automotive Safety Foundation, Washington, 1965, p. 32.
The Skandia Report, A Report on Children in Traffic, Report I, September 1971, Report II, June 1974. Skandia Insurance Company, Stockholm 3, Sweden
Transportation and Traffic Engineering Handbook, Prentice-Hall, Inc., Englewood Cliffs, N.J., 1976, pp. 58–65
Uniform Vehicle Code and Model Traffic Ordinance, National Committee on Uniform Traffic Laws and Ordinances, Washington, rev., 1968, supplement II, 1976.
U.S. Department of Transportation, Washington:
 A New Look at Pedestrian Safety
 Pedestrian Safety Standards, July, 1973

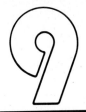

Bicycle Safety

OVERALL OBJECTIVE:

The student should understand the problems associated with bicycling in mixed traffic, and understand the conditions that cause bicycle accidents. The student should be able to suggest preventive methods and programs.

INSTRUCTIONAL OBJECTIVES:

After completing this chapter the student will be able to:

1 Discuss the magnitude of the bicycle-accident problem, giving specific figures.
2 List twelve of the seventeen bicycling practices that most often cause accidents.
3 Formulate specific objectives that can best achieve a reduction in cycle accidents.
4 List at least thirty items appropriate for inclusion in a bicycle code.
5 List the five correct positions that determine if a bicycle is the proper size for its rider.
6 Identify from a bicycle or bicycle photograph the items of preventive maintenance that should be inspected on a regular basis.
7 Conduct a bicycle-skills-test rodeo.
8 Explain the laws and ordinances (local, state, and federal) as they relate to the rights and duties of the bicyclist.
9 Use a bicycle as a mode of transportation, with due consideration for safety.

BICYCLE SAFETY

There has been a spectacular increase in the use of the bicycle since World War II. In 1945 there were approximately 9 million bicycles in the United States. Today there are close to 100 million bicycle riders, from preschool youngsters to their grandparents. This cult of the bicycle will continue to grow, and the reasons for this are not difficult to explain. Bicycling is an inexpensive mode of transportation. It provides recreation and promotes physical fitness. With the current emphasis on environmental pollution, gasoline conservation, and congestion caused by motor vehicles, one can easily understand the popularity of bicycling. Increased use of the bicycle as a mode of transportation is reflected in the growing proportion of adult drivers in recent years.

The surge in bicycle driving has been accompanied by an increase in accidents. As shown in Table 1-5, the number of bicycle–motor-vehicle deaths, which account for 90 percent of all bicycle fatalities, has more than doubled since 1935. It has been estimated that 1 million bicyclists have been injured annually, with approximately 400,000 requiring hospital emergency-room treatment. Since 1960 there has been a significant increase in the number of fatalities occurring to young adults and adults. Persons fifteen years of age and older incurred more than half of the fatalities in 1975, as compared with about one-fifth in 1960. Nevertheless, 50 percent of bicycle fatalities occur to pre-school children and to the five-to-fourteen age group (see Figure 9-1). The problem of bicycle safety should command the attention of students, parents, and teachers throughout the country. Although various agencies should participate in bicycle safety programs, there is no question that the largest number of bicycle drivers can be reached through school educational programs, including adult continuing education. The effectiveness of education in preventing accidents has been repeatedly demonstrated since safety was introduced into the school curriculum in the early 1920s. Through an education program, the cyclist can gain competencies in safe cycling and can learn and understand the laws and ordinances that govern cycling. The youngster can also be taught to perceive and recognize dangerous situations.

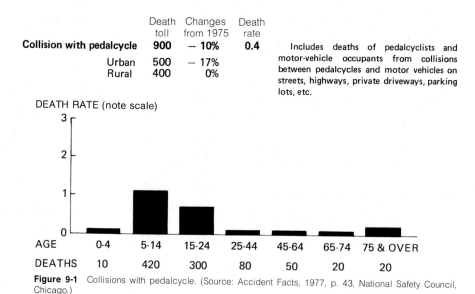

	Death toll	Changes from 1975	Death rate	
Collision with pedalcycle	**900**	**− 10%**	**0.4**	Includes deaths of pedalcyclists and motor-vehicle occupants from collisions between pedalcycles and motor vehicles on streets, highways, private driveways, parking lots, etc.
Urban	500	− 17%		
Rural	400	0%		

DEATH RATE (note scale)

AGE	0-4	5-14	15-24	25-44	45-64	65-74	75 & OVER
DEATHS	10	420	300	80	50	20	20

Figure 9-1 Collisions with pedalcycle. (Source: Accident Facts, 1977, p. 43, National Safety Council, Chicago.)

A bicycle safety program can help provide accident-prevention training for the many future operators of motorcycles, motorized bicycles (Mopeds), and automobiles. To a large extent, the many competencies needed for becoming a responsible traffic safety citizen can be initiated in a bicycle safety program. In collisions between bicycles and motor vehicles, the bicyclists violated traffic laws in half the cases studied. We are doing a disservice to young bicyclists if we do not prepare them to cope with the everyday traffic to which they will be exposed.

BICYCLING PRACTICES THAT CAUSE ACCIDENTS

Some recent research has started to pinpoint specific critical behaviors that lead to collisions between bicycles and automobiles. Some of the most common bicycling practices which most often cause accidents are:

1 Making improper turns
2 Disregarding traffic signs or signals
3 Failing to yield right of way
4 Driving too fast for conditions
5 Driving in the middle of the street
6 Carrying passengers
7 Cutting in and out of traffic
8 Running into opened automobile doors
9 Running into parked cars
10 Driving abreast of other cyclists
11 Driving against traffic
12 Entering streets without first stopping or slowing down to look
13 Driving between motor vehicles and the curb
14 Showing off on the bicycle
15 Driving on the sidewalk

This analysis shows that bicycle accidents are primarily caused by ignorance or misunderstanding of the basic and commonsense rules of the road, ignorance or defiance of laws and ordinances, and lack of skill and experience in traffic conditions.

Other facts that shed light on the bicycle safety problem are:

1 Approximately 50 percent of bicycle–motor-vehicle accidents occur at intersections.
2 Seventy percent occur during daylight hours.
3 Eighty percent of the bicyclists killed or injured in traffic accidents are violating traffic laws at the time of the accident.
4 Fifty percent of the motor-vehicle–bicycle accidents involve a violation on the part of the motor-vehicle operator.

5 Twenty percent of the bicycles involved in accidents have some mechanical defect.

6 Parking lots, playgrounds, bicycle paths, and bicycle size are also factors in bicycle safety.

Responsibility for bicycle safety education rests with several groups. Educational systems, including state departments of education, colleges and universities, and local school districts; federal governmental agencies; civic groups; and bicycle manufacturers are all responsible for promoting and implementing a bicycle safety education program. The program should provide learning experiences that give bicyclists the general competencies shown in Figures 9-9 through 9-15.

BICYCLE SAFETY PROGRAM

The ability to drive a bicycle safely can be gained only through an educational and training program that provides learning experiences that give bicyclists many general competencies. Among the components of the program are:

1. The bicyclist must know and obey rules of the road, particularly the rules of the community in which he or she drives.
2. The bicyclist must know the state and local laws and ordinances that pertain specifically to bicycles. Bicyclists must understand that bicycles, unless otherwise designated, are legally considered vehicles, and that the driver must obey all state and local laws and ordinances that apply to vehicles.
3. The bicyclist must have competence in skills and techniques for all driving situations:
    a. The bicyclist must conform to traffic, weather, road, pedestrian, and environmental conditions.
    b. The bicyclist must develop skill in balancing, pedaling, steering, and avoiding dangerous situations such as objects on the road, pedestrians, animals, and fixed objects.
    c. The bicyclist must know and use proper hand signals (see Figure 9-2). The bicyclist must give signals well in advance so that motorists behind and ahead know the cyclist's intentions. This is especially important when the cycle has hand brakes. A bell or horn should be used as a warning device (sirens are illegal).
    d. The bicyclist must ride *with* the flow of traffic, *not* against it. This is a legal requirement, and it provides the driver greater opportunity for evasive action.
    e. The bicyclist must know, understand, and obey all traffic signs, signals, and road markings (see Figures 9-3, 9-4, and 9-5).
    f. When driving on a public street or highway, cyclists should always

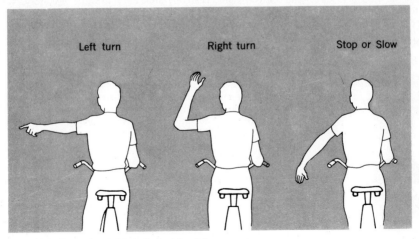

Left turn   Right turn   Stop or Slow

Figure 9-2   Proper hand signals for the bicyclist.

    drive in single file. In places such as designated bicycle paths, driving two abreast may be permitted.

g. The bicyclist should perform all stunt and trick driving in restricted areas to avoid collisions with other cyclists, pedestrians, and fixed objects.

h. The bicyclist should realize riding with more persons than the bicycle is intended for is dangerous. It decreases vision and maneuverability. It is also illegal. Exceptions are made for adults who wish to carry young children securely fastened to their persons or in a special carrier. This too may be a dangerous practice.

i. The bicyclist should avoid, if possible, heavy and high-speed vehicular traffic. At heavily traveled and busy intersections, the cyclist should dismount and proceed as a pedestrian by walking the cycle across the intersection.

j. Bicyclists must anticipate the actions of motorists in parked vehicles by allowing adequate space for doors which may open in their path.

k. The bicyclist should always slow down and look in all directions when leaving a driveway, school yard, alley, parking lot, etc.

l. When driving at night, cyclists should wear light-colored clothing. They should make sure that the headlight and rear reflector are functioning properly. The use of reflectorized tape and clothing will increase the bicyclist's ability to be seen by other drivers.

m. The bicyclist must watch out for drain grates, soft shoulders, potholes, and loose sand and gravel, particularly at corners.

4. The bicyclist should know the procedures to follow after an accident. This information is important in case of legal action and for insurance purposes.

TRAFFIC SIGNS

Bicyclists must obey street and highway signs. There are three kinds of signs: regulatory, warning, and guide. There are seven basic shapes and eight basic colors. Once you learn the colors and shapes, you can identify them at a glance.

Regulatory Signs

Stop. An eight-sided, or octagon, sign always means stop. Slowing down is not enough—the stop must be complete, at the marked stop line. Or, if there is no stop line, before the marked crosswalk. If the crosswalk is not marked, stop before entering the intersection, at a point from which you can observe oncoming traffic. Give way to the oncoming traffic *and* to pedestrians before moving on.

Do not enter. This sign is found on one-way and "dead end" streets. It means exactly what it says. Do not ride a bicycle into a street where you see such a sign.

Yield. This triangular shape always means that you must slow down to make sure there is no oncoming traffic, or pedestrians crossing. You must stop, if necessary, since the right-of-way belongs to other traffic or pedestrians.

Wrong Way. This sign may be used in addition to the "Do Not Enter" sign. It means you are going the wrong direction. You should pull to the side and stop. When traffic is clear, turn around and return to the road on which you were traveling.

One Way. You may ride *only* in the direction the arrow points.

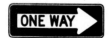

No Bicycles. A red circle with a red bar through the center means NO. This specific sign means bicycles are not allowed. Do not ride where you see the sign.

No Right Turn. Here again, the red circle with a red slash through the middle means NO—in this case no right turn.

No U Turn. Another circle and slash—this time meaning no U turn.

Figure 9-3 Traffic signs the bicyclist should understand. (Source: Illinois Bicycle Rules of the Road, Office of the Secretary of State, Springfield, Ill.)

End One Way, and **Two Way Traffic Ahead.** This sign warns that a one-way street is changing to two-way. Move into the proper lane and be alert for traffic coming toward you.

 Obey Your Signal Only. Busy intersections often have traffic light signals to control movement of cars and bicycles more effectively. When you see this sign, watch and obey only the signal facing you.

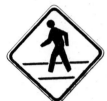 **Keep Right.** Signs such as this tell you where to ride as you are approaching traffic islands, median strips, or obstructions. You must ride to the side indicated by the arrow.

Also, in most states, expressways and tollways are posted, and signs forbid use of these highways by all slower-moving vehicles such as bicycles, motor-bicycles, farm equipment, and so on.

 Warning Signs

Warning signs will help you ride safely by telling you what to watch out for ahead.

Ped Xing on the right warns you that there is a crosswalk ahead.

All of the signs are easy to understand. Watch for them. . .let them alert you to what is up ahead.

Guide Signs

Guide signs include route markers, information signs and distance and location signs.

Of chief interest to you as a cyclist will be *Bike Route* signs, and *Parking* directions, if you ride in a larger city where parking may be a problem.

Figure 9-3 *(Continued)*

263

PAVEMENT MARKINGS

In many cases, traffic signs are painted right on the pavement. Bicyclists must observe these signs. They include:

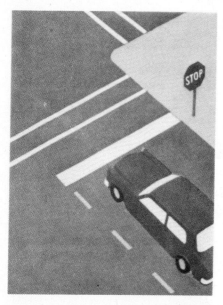

White Stop Line. This shows you where you must stop for a traffic light or stop sign.

Pedestrian Crosswalks. Most intersections have white lines which show pedestrian crosswalks. Watch for people walking between these lines. They have the right of way.

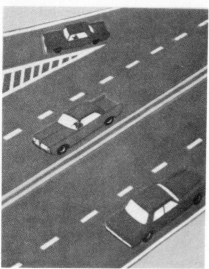

Center Lines. A double yellow center stripe means do not cross the stripe (except to turn into a driveway or alley). The double line indicates there is more than one lane of traffic moving in both directions. White dashes mark the lane separations on either side of the double yellow stripe. You should ride on the right side of the right lane, except to pass or to make a left turn.

Where there is only one lane for traffic in each direction, and passing is permitted, the center of the street is marked with a broken yellow stripe.

Figure 9-4 Pavement markings.

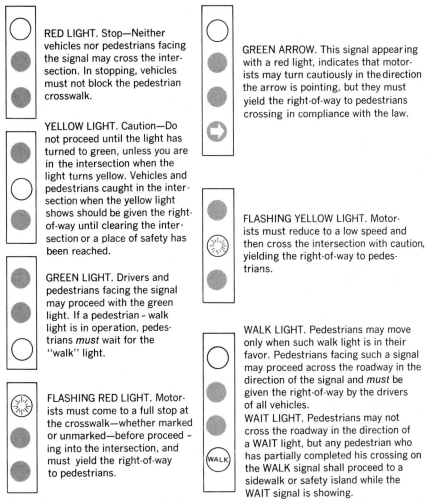

RED LIGHT. Stop—Neither vehicles nor pedestrians facing the signal may cross the intersection. In stopping, vehicles must not block the pedestrian crosswalk.

YELLOW LIGHT. Caution—Do not proceed until the light has turned to green, unless you are in the intersection when the light turns yellow. Vehicles and pedestrians caught in the intersection when the yellow light shows should be given the right-of-way until clearing the intersection or a place of safety has been reached.

GREEN LIGHT. Drivers and pedestrians facing the signal may proceed with the green light. If a pedestrian–walk light is in operation, pedestrians *must* wait for the "walk" light.

FLASHING RED LIGHT. Motorists must come to a full stop at the crosswalk—whether marked or unmarked—before proceeding into the intersection, and must yield the right-of-way to pedestrians.

GREEN ARROW. This signal appearing with a red light, indicates that motorists may turn cautiously in the direction the arrow is pointing, but they must yield the right-of-way to pedestrians crossing in compliance with the law.

FLASHING YELLOW LIGHT. Motorists must reduce to a low speed and then cross the intersection with caution, yielding the right-of-way to pedestrians.

WALK LIGHT. Pedestrians may move only when such walk light is in their favor. Pedestrians facing such a signal may proceed across the roadway in the direction of the signal and *must* be given the right-of-way by the drivers of all vehicles.
WAIT LIGHT. Pedestrians may not cross the roadway in the direction of a WAIT light, but any pedestrian who has partially completed his crossing on the WALK signal shall proceed to a sidewalk or safety island while the WAIT signal is showing.

Figure 9-5 Bicyclists should obey traffic-light signals. The "signalized intersection" has traffic lights to control the traffic. The lights are three different colors: red, yellow, and green. Each color has a definite message for the bicycle driver.

5. The bicyclist should carry some means of identification on his or her person or cycle, in case the cyclist loses consciousness.
6. Bicyclists should leave bicycles in an upright position, locked and properly parked when not in use, so that they do not create a hazard and are not exposed to damage.
7. The bicyclist should always give pedestrians the right of way and should know the regulations for driving on sidewalks.
8. Bicyclists must develop an attitude of sportsmanlike conduct if they wish to become competent drivers on streets and highways and in designated bicycle paths and trailways.

These competencies will help bicyclists become responsible traffic safety citizens as they take their place in today's traffic scene.

It is evident that the major cause of accidents is unsafe behavior by bicyclists and motor-vehicle drivers, and that there is a need for a comprehensive bicycle safety program.

MODEL BICYCLE ORDINANCE

The tremendous increase in the bicycle population in recent years has stimulated a great deal of interest in providing proper laws and ordinances to aid and guide the cyclist. A *Uniform Vehicle Code and Model Traffic Ordinance,* which should be implemented by states and municipalities, has been developed by the National Committee on Uniform Traffic Laws and Ordinances. The following section reproduces in its entirety a booklet distributed by the AAA, which includes the code and ordinance.

Preface

This booklet suggesting traffic regulations duplicates sections in the *Uniform Vehicle Code* and *Model Traffic Ordinance* that contain special provisions applicable to bicycles and other vehicles moved by human power. Copies of the basic documents may be purchased from the National Committee on Uniform Traffic Laws and Ordinances, 1776 Massachusetts Avenue, N.W., Washington, D.C. 20036. The main volume (1968) costs $5.00 and the 1976 supplement, which contains significant changes relating to bicycles, costs another $3.00.

Bicyclists must generally comply with the same rules of the road as the drivers of other kinds of vehicles. For instance, cyclists must comply with red lights, stop signs, and yield signs. Cyclists must obey speed limits and ride on the right half of the roadway with traffic. Motorists facing stop or yield signs must yield to cyclists on intersecting roadways. All rules of the road for motorists and cyclists are not, however, duplicated in this booklet because it is devoted more to rules which supplement the general rules of the road. If you are interested in all rules of the road, you should consider securing material describing them from your state department of motor vehicles or you may want to read your state vehicle code. The Rules of the Road Chapter of the *Uniform Vehicle Code* has served as the pattern for most of our state traffic laws and still serves as a guide for quality and uniformity.

In addition to sections in this document, municipalities should consider their state traffic laws and any model traffic ordinance which, may have been developed for use in their state. References in this booklet to a chapter, article, section, subsection, lettered or numbered paragraph or footnote originate in the whole *Uniform Vehicle Code* or *Model Traffic Ordinance* (main volume, 1968 and supplement, 1976).

Uniform vehicle code

*Model statutes for state
motor vehicle and traffic laws*

Chapter 1. *Words and phrases defined*
   1-105 **Bicycle***   Every vehicle propelled solely by human power upon which any person may ride, having two tandem wheels, except scooters and similar devices.

*Bicycles were included in the definition of "vehicle" at the National Committee on Uniform Traffic Laws and Ordinances meeting, July 23–25, 1975.

1-114 **Driver**   Every person who drives or is in actual physical control of a vehicle.

1-184 **Vehicle**   Every device in, upon or by which any person or property is or may be transported or drawn upon a highway, excepting devices used exclusively upon stationary rails or tracks. (A bicycle is a vehicle.)*

Chapter 3. *Certificates of title and registration of vehicles*

3-102 **Exclusions**   No certificate of title need be obtained for: 5. A vehicle moved solely by human or animal power.

Chapter 4. *Anti-theft laws*

4-101 **Exceptions from provisions of this chapter**   This chapter does not apply to the following unless a title or registration has been issued on such vehicles under this act: 1. A vehicle moved solely by human or animal power.

Chapter 7. *Financial responsibility*

7-103 **Exempt vehicles**   The following vehicles and their drivers are exempt from this article:

7. A vehicle moved solely by human or animal power.

Chapter 9. *Civil liability*

9-401 **Negligence of children**   A violation of any provision of this act by a child under the age of 14 shall not constitute negligence per se although a violation may be considered as evidence of negligence.

Chapter 11. *Rules of the Road*

11-313 **Restrictions on use of controlled-access roadway**   (a) The (State highway commission) by resolution or order entered in its minutes, and local authorities by ordinance, may regulate or prohibit the use of any controlled-access roadway (or highway) within their respective jurisdictions by any class or kind of traffic which is found to be incompatible with the normal and safe movement of traffic.

(b) The (State highway commission) or the local authority adopting any such prohibition shall erect and maintain official traffic-control devices on the controlled-access highway on which such prohibitions are applicable and when in place no person shall disobey the restrictions stated on such devices.

11-504 **Drivers to exercise due care**   Notwithstanding other provisions of this chapter or the provisions of any local ordinance, every driver of a vehicle shall exercise due care to avoid colliding with any pedestrian or any person propelling a human-powered vehicle and shall give an audible signal when necessary and shall exercise proper precaution upon observing any child or any obviously confused, incapacitated or intoxicated person.

11-509 **Pedestrians' right of way on sidewalks**   The driver of a vehicle crossing a sidewalk shall yield the right of way to any pedestrian and all other traffic on the sidewalk.

11-1103 **Driving upon sidewalk**   No person shall drive any vehicle other than by human power upon a sidewalk or sidewalk area except upon a permanent or duly authorized temporary driveway.

11-1105 **Opening and closing vehicle doors**   No person shall open any door on a motor vehicle unless and until it is reasonably safe to do so and can be done without interfering with the movement of other traffic, nor shall any person leave a door open on a side of a vehicle available to moving traffic for a period of time longer than necessary to load or unload passengers.

Article XII—operation of bicycles and other human-powered vehicles

11-1201 Effect of regulations (a) It is a misdemeanor for any person to do any act forbidden or fail to perform any act required in this article.

(b) The parent of any child and the guardian of any ward shall not authorize or knowingly permit any such child or ward to violate any of the provisions of this act.

11-1202 Traffic laws apply to persons on bicycles and other human-powered vehicles Every person propelling a vehicle by human power or riding a bicycle shall have all of the rights and all of the duties applicable to the driver of any other vehicle under chapters 10 and 11, except as to special regulations in this article and except as to those provisions which by their nature can have no application.

11-1203 Riding on bicycles No bicycle shall be used to carry more persons at one time than the number for which it is designed or equipped, except that an adult rider may carry a child securely attached to his person in a back pack or sling.

11-1204 Clinging to vehicles (a) No person riding upon any bicycle, coaster, roller skates, sled or toy vehicle shall attach the same or himself to any (streetcar or) vehicle upon a roadway.

(b) This section shall not prohibit attaching a bicycle trailer or bicycle semitrailer to a bicycle if that trailer or semitrailer has been designed for such attachment.

11-1205 Riding on roadways and bicycle paths (a) Every person operating a bicycle upon a roadway shall ride as near to the right side of the roadway as practicable, exercising due care when passing a standing vehicle or one proceeding in the same direction.

(b) Persons riding bicycles upon a roadway shall not ride more than two abreast except on paths or parts of roadways set aside for the exclusive use of bicycles. Persons riding two abreast shall not impede the normal and reasonable movement of traffic and, on a laned roadway, shall ride within a single lane.

(c) Wherever a usable path for bicycles has been provided adjacent to a roadway, bicycle riders shall use such path and shall not use the roadway.

11-1206 Carrying articles No person operating a bicycle shall carry any package, bundle or article which prevents the use of both hands in the control and operation of the bicycle. A person operating a bicycle shall keep at least one hand on the handlebars at all times.

11-1207 Left turns (a) A person riding a bicycle intending to turn left shall follow a course described in § 11-601 or in subsection (b).

(b) A person riding a bicycle intending to turn left shall approach the turn as close as practicable to the right curb or edge of the roadway. After proceeding across the intersecting roadway, the turn shall be made as close as practicable to the curb or edge of the roadway on the far side of the intersection. After turning, the bicyclist shall comply with any official traffic control device or police officer regulating traffic on the highway along which he intends to proceed.

(c) Notwithstanding the foregoing provisions, the state highway commission and local authorities in their respective jurisdictions may cause official traffic-control devices to be placed and thereby require and direct that a specific course be traveled by turning bicycles, and when such devices are so placed, no person shall turn a bicycle other than as directed and required by such devices.

11-1208 Turn and stop signals (a) Except as provided in this section, a person riding a bicycle shall comply with § 11-604.

(b) A signal of intention to turn right or left when required shall be given continuously during not less than the last 100 feet traveled by the bicycle before turning, and shall be given while the bicycle is stopped waiting to turn. A signal by hand and arm need not be given continuously if the hand is needed in the control or operation of the bicycle.

11-1209 Bicycles and human-powered vehicles on sidewalks (a) A person propelling a bicycle upon and along a sidewalk, or across a roadway upon and along a crosswalk, shall yield the right of way to any pedestrian and shall give audible signal before overtaking and passing such pedestrian.

(b) A person shall not ride a bicycle upon and along a sidewalk, or across a roadway upon and along a crosswalk, where such use of bicycles is prohibited by official traffic-control devices.

(c) A person propelling a vehicle by human power upon and along a sidewalk, or across a roadway upon and along a crosswalk, shall have all the rights and duties applicable to a pedestrian under the same circumstances.

11-1210 **Bicycle parking** (a) A person may park a bicycle on a sidewalk unless prohibited or restricted by an official traffic control device.

(b) A bicycle parked on a sidewalk shall not impede the normal and reasonable movement of pedestrian or other traffic.

(c) A bicycle may be parked on the roadway at any angle to the curb or edge of the roadway at any location where parking is allowed.

(d) A bicycle may be parked on the roadway abreast of another bicycle or bicycles near the side of the roadway at any location where parking is allowed.

(e) A person shall not park a bicycle on a roadway in such a manner as to obstruct the movement of a legally parked motor vehicle.

(f) In all other respects, bicycles parked anywhere on a highway shall conform with the provisions of article 10 regulating the parking of vehicles.

11-1211 **Bicycle racing** (a) Bicycle racing on the highways is prohibited by § 11-808 except as authorized in this section. (b) Bicycle racing on a highway shall not be unlawful when a racing event has been approved by state or local authorities on any highway under their respective jurisdictions. Approval of bicycle highway racing events shall be granted only under conditions which assure reasonable safety for all race participants, spectators and other highway users, and which prevent unreasonable interference with traffic flow which would seriously inconvenience other highway users.

(c) By agreement with the approving authority, participants in an approved bicycle highway racing event may be exempted from compliance with any traffic laws otherwise applicable thereto, provided that traffic control is adequate to assure the safety of all highway users.

Chapter 12. *Equipment of vehicles*

12-101 **Scope and Effect of regulations** (e) The provisions of this chapter and regulations of the department shall not apply to vehicles moved solely by human power, except as specifically made applicable.

12-201 **When lighted lamps are required** Every vehicle upon a highway within this State at any time from a half hour after sunset to a half hour before sunrise and at any other time when, due to insufficient light or unfavorable atmospheric conditions, persons and vehicles on the highway are not clearly discernible at a distance of 1,000 feet ahead shall display lighted head and other lamps and illuminating devices as respectively required for different classes of vehicles, subject to exceptions with respect to parked vehicles, and further that stop lights, turn signals and other signaling devices shall be lighted as prescribed for the use of such devices.

Article VII—Bicycles

12-701 **Application of chapter to bicycles** No provision in this chapter shall apply to bicycles nor to equipment for use on bicycles except as to provisions in this article or unless a provision has been made specifically applicable to bicycles or their equipment.

12-702 **Head lamp required at night** Every bicycle in use at the times described in Sec. 12-201 shall be equipped with a lamp on the front emitting a white light visible from a distance of at least 500 feet to the front.

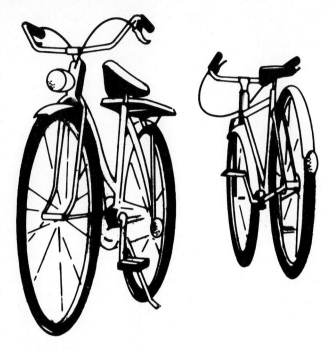

12-703 **Rear reflector required at all times**   Every bicycle shall be equipped with a red reflector of a type approved by the department which shall be visible for 600 feet to the rear when directly in front of lawful lower beams of head lamps on a motor vehicle.

12-704 **Side reflector or light required at night**   Every bicycle when in use at the times described in § 12-201 shall be equipped with reflective material of sufficient size and reflectivity to be visible from both sides for 600 feet when directly in front of lawful lower beams of head lamps on a motor vehicle, or, in lieu of such reflective material, with a lighted lamp visible from both sides from a distance of at least 500 feet.

12-705 **Additional lights or reflectors authorized**   A bicycle or its rider may be equipped with lights or reflectors in addition to those required by the foregoing sections.

12-706 **Brake required**   Every bicycle shall be equipped with a brake or brakes which will enable its driver to stop the bicycle within 25 feet from a speed of 10 miles per hour on dry, level, clean pavement.

12-707 **Sirens and whistles prohibited**   A bicycle shall not be equipped with, nor shall any person use upon a bicycle, any siren or whistle.

12-708 **Bicycle identifying number**   A person engaged in the business of selling bicycles at retail shall not sell any bicycle unless the bicycle has an identifying number permanently stamped or cast on its frame.

12-709 **Inspecting bicycles**   A uniformed police officer may at any time upon reasonable cause to believe that a bicycle is unsafe or not equipped as required by law, or that its equipment is not in proper adjustment or repair, require the person riding the bicycle to stop and submit the bicycle to an inspection and such test with reference thereto as may be appropriate.

Chapter 15. *Respective powers of state and local authorities*

15-101 **Provisions uniform throughout state**   The provisions of this act shall be applicable and uniform throughout this State and in all political subdivisions and municipalities therein and no local authority shall enact or enforce any ordinance on a matter covered by the provisions of such chapters unless expressly authorized.

15-102 **Powers of local authorities** (a) The provisions of this act shall not be deemed to prevent local authorities with respect to streets and highways under their jurisdiction and within the reasonable exercise of the police power from:

(b). Regulating the operation of bicycles and requiring the registration and inspection of same, including the requirement of registration fee.

Model traffic ordinance

For municipalities to implement or supplement provisions in the State Uniform Vehicle Code

Article XII-regulations for bicycles*

12-1 **Effect of regulations** (a) It is a misdemeanor for any person to do any act forbidden or fail to perform any act required in this article.

(b) The parent of any child and the guardian of any ward shall not authorize or knowingly permit any such child or ward to violate any of the provisions of this ordinance.

(c) These regulations applicable to bicycles shall apply whenever a bicycle is operated upon any highway or upon any path set aside for the exclusive use of bicycles subject to those exceptions stated herein.

12-2 **License required** No person who resides within this city shall ride or propel a bicycle on any street or upon any public path set aside for the exclusive use of bicycles unless such bicycle has been licensed and a license plate is attached thereto as provided herein.

12-3 **License application** Application for a bicycle license and license plate shall be made upon a form provided by the city and shall be made to the (chief of police). An annual license fee of_____shall be paid to the city before each license or renewal thereof is granted.

12-4 **Issuance of license** (a) The (chief of police) upon receiving proper application therefor is authorized to issue a bicycle license which shall be effective until (the next succeeding first day of July).

(b) The (chief of police) shall not issue a license for any bicycle when he knows or has reasonable ground to believe that the applicant is not the owner of or entitled to the possession of such bicycle.

(c) The (chief of police) shall keep a record of the number of each license, the date issued, the name and address of the person to whom issued, and the number on the frame of the bicycle for which issued, and a record of all bicycle license fees collected by him.

12-5 **Attachment of license plate** (a) The (chief of police) upon issuing a bicycle license shall also issue a license plate bearing the license number assigned to the bicycle, the name of the city, and (the calendar year for which issued) (the expiration date thereof).

(b) The (chief of police) shall cause such license plate to be firmly attached to the rear mudguard or frame of the bicycle for which issued in such position as to be plainly visible from the rear.

(c) No person shall remove a license plate from a bicycle during the period for which issued except upon a transfer of ownership or in the event the bicycle is dismantled and no longer operated upon any street in this city.

12-6 **Inspection of bicycles** The chief of police, or an officer assigned such responsibility, shall inspect each bicycle before licensing the same and shall refuse a license for any bicycle which he determines is in unsafe mechanical condition.

12-7 **Renewal of license** Upon the expiration of any bicycle license the same may be renewed upon application and payment of the same fee as upon an original application.

*The provisions in this article are authorized by UVC § 15-102(a)8.

12-8 **Transfer of ownership** Upon the sale or other transfer of a licensed bicycle the licensee shall remove the license plate and shall either surrender the same to the (chief of police) or may upon proper application but without payment of additional fee have said plate assigned to another bicycle owned by the applicant.

12-9 **Rental agencies** A rental agency shall not rent or offer any bicycle for rent unless the bicycle is licensed and a license plate is attached thereto as provided herein and such bicycle is equipped with the lamps and other equipment required by the State vehicle code.

12-11 **Traffic ordinances apply to persons riding bicycles** Every person riding a bicycle upon a roadway shall be granted all of the rights and shall be subject to all of the duties applicable to the driver of a vehicle by this ordinance, except as to special regulations in this article and except as to those provisions of this ordinance which by their nature can have no application.

12-14 **Attaching bicycle to poles** Any person may park near, and secure a bicycle to, any publicly owned pole or post for a period of not more than twelve consecutive hours, unless an official traffic-control device or any applicable law or ordinance prohibits parking or securing bicycles at that location. *No bicycle shall be secured to any tree, fire hydrant, or police or fire call box.* No bicycle shall be secured in any manner so as to impede the normal and reasonable movement of pedestrian or other traffic.

12-15 **Penalities** Every person convicted of a violation of any provision of this article shall be punished by a fine of not more than _____ dollars or by removal and detention of the license plate from such person's bicycle for a period not to exceed _____ days or by impounding of such person's bicycle for a period not to exceed _____ days or by any combination thereof.

An effective method of implementing the various sections of the ordinance would be a cooperative program including municipal governments, law enforcement agencies, courts, and school systems, with assistance from motor clubs, service organizations, local bicycle clubs, girl and boy scouts, 4-H groups, PTAs, and other interested groups.

FURTHER LEARNING EXPERIENCES

In addition to gaining the knowledge and skills previously described, young cyclists should participate in learning experiences designed to develop their sense of responsibility for bicycle safety, their driving skills, and their ability to keep a bicycle in good operating condition. The following list of suggested activities represents a few of the many possibilities:

1 Participate in student discussions dealing with such topics as "Should a School Court Be Established to Try Violators of the Bicycle Code?" and "The Goals of a Bicycle Club."

2 Practice specific skills that will enable you to control your bicycle under varying conditions.

3 Invite a reliable dealer to bring a bicycle to the school and demonstrate before your class how to adjust the seat and handlebars properly and how to keep the various parts of the bicycle in good running condition.

4 Invite a local police officer to explain to your class the purpose and method of properly registering and licensing bicycles.

5 Read selected pamphlets, books, and magazine articles pertaining to safe bicycling, and report on this material to your class.

6 Discuss the personal characteristics, other than age, that affect one's ability to ride a bicycle safely in the street.

THE BICYCLE

The bicycle safety instructor should make sure that students know how to select bicycles that are suited to their individual physical requirements. The instructor should discourage them from using bicycles that are the wrong size and hence difficult and dangerous to operate. If a bicycle is too large for the rider, it will be more difficult to control. The rider will be uncomfortable using it and may become injured by constantly straining to reach the pedals. Occasionally economy-minded parents who fail to realize this danger choose too large a bicycle in the hope that the child will not quickly outgrow it. Using an under-sized bicycle is preferable to using an oversized one. If the frame is too small for the rider, a satisfactory adjustment can sometimes be made by raising the seat and handlebars to give maximum comfort without sacrificing stability or safety.

There are five correct positions which determine whether a bicycle is properly adjusted to the rider's size and physical characteristics.[1]

    1 The leg, thigh and heel of the foot which is on the low pedal should form a straight line.
    2 The saddle should be parallel to the ground.
    3 The upper part of the body should be inclined slightly forward.
    4 The handle-bar grips should be at right angles to the handle-bar stem.
    5 The handle-bar grips should be approximately the same height as the saddle. [See Figure 9-6]

The above recommendations are primarily for conventional type bicycles. Some bicycles such as "hirisers" with smaller wheels and frames tend to make the driver sit erect with the hands well above the seat level and sport lightweight cycles will have dropped handle bars that bring the driver's hands below seat level. This crouched position is most comfortable for long distance driving and high speeds.[2]

TYPES OF BICYCLES

There are a great variety of bicycles available from a multitude of manufacturers. People must determine their individual needs before making a purchase. Price is often a determining factor. Bicycle costs range from $40 for the young cyclist to as much as $230 for the serious cycling enthusiast, who uses the cycle as a sports vehicle rather than for everyday transportation. A prospective

---

[1] *Bicycle Safety Tests,* Bicycle Institute of America, New York, now Bicycle Manufacturers Association, Washington, p. 15.
[2] *Bicycle Safety Education,* Data Sheet No. 1, rev., National Safety Council, Chicago, p. 4.

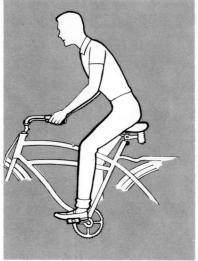

The upper part of the body should be inclined slightly forward

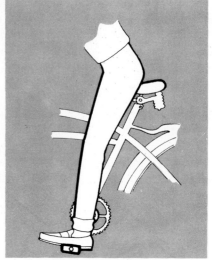

Leg, thigh, and heel of the foot which is on the low pedal should form a straight line (while seated)

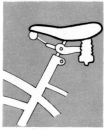

Saddle should be parallel to the ground

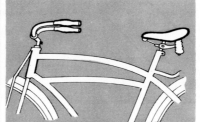

Handlebar grips should be approximately the same height as the saddle

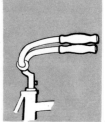

Handlebar grips should be at right angles to the handlebar stem

Figure 9-6 Correct bicycle-adjustment positions for conventional-type bicycles. (Source: Bicycle Safety Education Data Sheet No. 1, revised, p. 4, National Safety Council, Chicago.)

purchaser who is not familiar with the various qualities and features of a cycle should go to a reputable bicycle specialty shop. Some things to inquire about are:

1. Cost
2. Warranties and guarantees
3. Type of metal and construction
4. Needed accessories
5. Type of brakes (hand or coaster)
6. Hubs, rims, tires, frame, crank sets, pedals, handlebars, seats, and locks.

7. Number of speeds
   a. Three-speed
   b. Five-speed
   c. Ten-speed
   d. Single-speed

Space does not allow a more detailed description, but a reputable dealer should be able to explain the characteristics of the various items listed. A brief description of different types of cycles follows.

THREE-SPEED BICYCLES

Three-speed bicycles are desirable for short distances: trips to the store, driving to school, and leisurely driving. They are reliable, sturdy, and easy to operate, requiring minimal maintenance checks. They are somewhat heavier to ride and carry than other cycles.

FIVE-SPEED BICYCLES

Five-speed bicycles are "half-way bikes." Like three-speed bicycles, they are heavy. They require more maintenance. The advantages of a five-speed cycle include better climbing ability and easier long-distance riding.

TEN-SPEED BICYCLES

Ten-speed bicycles are appropriate for long-distance riding, high-speed driving, touring, and commutations of 10 miles or more. The ten-speed cycle requires driving techniques that use muscles of the torso and legs for increased power and efficiency. Only thigh muscles are involved in the upright position of three-speed and single-speed bicycles. Once you have decided on the type of cycle that fits your needs, it is a good policy to compare features and components of the various bicycles within your price range.

CORRECT RIDING TECHNIQUES

Correct riding techniques avoid muscular fatigue, which can lead riders to take their hands off the handlebars or shift their weight in the seat. These techniques enable riders to concentrate on road conditions and traffic and assure them of proper control of their bicycles in all emergencies.

Here are the five essentials of correct bicycle riding:[3]

   1 Always use the ball of the foot at contact point with the pedal.
   2 Pedal evenly. Rhythm is essential for good control and untiring bicycle riding.

---

[3] *Bike Safety Programs*, Bicycle Institute of America, New York, now Bicycle Manufacturers Association, Washington, p. 18.

3 Pedal straight. Knees should be kept parallel with the bicycle frame for effortless operation.

4 Elbows should be held in for better steering control.

5 Shoulders should be kept steady. Movement of the shoulders while pedaling is lost motion.

The following healthful hints will also contribute to safe cycling:

1 Avoid taking long rides on very hot days.

2 Never ride when you are ill or under medication.

3 Avoid riding immediately after eating; wait at least a half-hour.

Since one-fifth of all bicycle accidents are caused by mechanical defects, it is important that riders learn how to keep their bicycles in safe operating condition. Figure 9-7 indicates the essential parts of the bicycle that should be checked regularly to ensure safe riding. The following list summarizes the duties involved in the proper care and maintenance of bicycle (see Figure 9-8):

1 The bicycle should be cleaned and oiled according to the manufacturer's instructions, which are usually distributed with new bicycles.

2 Broken spokes should be replaced, loose spokes tightened, and bent spokes straightened.

3 The chain should occasionally be removed, cleaned thoroughly with kerosene, bathed in a good lubricating oil, and wiped dry. When it is replaced, the rear wheel should be carefully adjusted so that the chain is not too tight or too loose. The chain will operate smoothly if the inside, or sprocket side, is kept clean and well lubricated and the outside kept clean and dry. A few drops of oil on the chain will usually furnish sufficient lubrication.

4 The pedals and pedal bearings should be frequently taken apart (by removing the dust cap and nut on the outside end of the pedal), cleaned, oiled, and adjusted.

5 The paint and chromium work on the bicycle should be cleaned as often as necessary. A damp cloth will remove any dirt or mud caked on the frame. Any automobile wax can be used to protect the painted areas. Fender supports and other parts that may rust should be wiped occasionally with an oiled rag.

6 The wheel bearings should be repacked about once a year with ordinary cup grease.

7 The handlebars, grips, saddle, and pedals should be kept tight.

8 The chain and sprocket should have a protective covering so that they will not catch the rider's clothing.

9 The brake should be checked frequently to make sure that it takes hold quickly.

10 The bicycle should be equipped with a horn or bell that can be heard at a distance of at least 100 feet, a headlight visible at a distance of 500 feet, and a rear reflector visible at a distance of 300 feet.

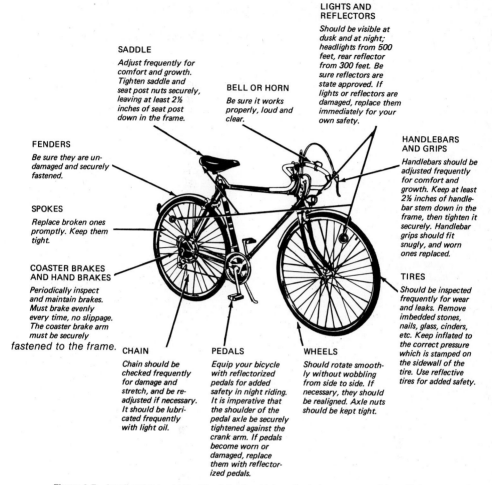

LIGHTS AND REFLECTORS

Should be visible at dusk and at night; headlights from 500 feet, rear reflector from 300 feet. Be sure reflectors are state approved. If lights or reflectors are damaged, replace them immediately for your own safety.

SADDLE

Adjust frequently for comfort and growth. Tighten saddle and seat post nuts securely, leaving at least 2½ inches of seat post down in the frame.

BELL OR HORN

Be sure it works properly, loud and clear.

FENDERS

Be sure they are undamaged and securely fastened.

SPOKES

Replace broken ones promptly. Keep them tight.

COASTER BRAKES AND HAND BRAKES

Periodically inspect and maintain brakes. Must brake evenly every time, no slippage. The coaster brake arm must be securely fastened to the frame.

HANDLEBARS AND GRIPS

Handlebars should be adjusted frequently for comfort and growth. Keep at least 2½ inches of handlebar stem down in the frame, then tighten it securely. Handlebar grips should fit snugly, and worn ones replaced.

TIRES

Should be inspected frequently for wear and leaks. Remove imbedded stones, nails, glass, cinders, etc. Keep inflated to the correct pressure which is stamped on the sidewall of the tire. Use reflective tires for added safety.

CHAIN

Chain should be checked frequently for damage and stretch, and be readjusted if necessary. It should be lubricated frequently with light oil.

PEDALS

Equip your bicycle with reflectorized pedals for added safety in night riding. It is imperative that the shoulder of the pedal axle be securely tightened against the crank arm. If pedals become worn or damaged, replace them with reflectorized pedals.

WHEELS

Should rotate smoothly without wobbling from side to side. If necessary, they should be realigned. Axle nuts should be kept tight.

Figure 9-7 A well-maintained bike, like defensive driving, also helps prevent accidents. To keep your bike in safe mechanical condition, follow the maintenance suggestions illustrated. (Courtesy of Bicycle Institute of America, Inc., now Bicycle Manufacturers Association, Washington.)

11 The tires should be checked every time the bicycle is used, tested with an air-pressure gauge at least once a week, and kept at the pressure indicated on the sidewalls. The sidewalls should be examined to make sure that they do not rub against the fork. The bicycle should never be jumped over curbs or other sharp elevations, for doing so may damage the wheels or tires.

12 Any damaged or worn part of the bicycle should be immediately replaced. This is the most important part of the rider's responsibility for the maintenance of his or her bicycle.

13 A reliable dealer or service person should be consulted about major repairs or adjustments.

Owner's name _____ Boy _____ Girl _____
Address _____ Age _____
Bicycle trade name _____
Color _____ Style: Boy's _____ Girl's _____
Size _____ Serial no. _____ License no. _____

Part	Condition	
	Satisfactory	Unsatisfactory
Brake		
Stops quickly	_____	_____
Stops evenly	_____	_____
Light and reflector		
Front light visible at 500 feet	_____	_____
Rear reflector visible at 300 feet	_____	_____
Warning device		
Horn or bell	_____	_____
Wheels and rims		
Run freely	_____	_____
Run true	_____	_____
Spokes straight and tight	_____	_____
Tires		
Treads	_____	_____
Inflation—correct pressure	_____	_____
Valves tight and capped	_____	_____
Handle bars		
Adjusted to body	_____	_____
Bars and grips tight	_____	_____
Saddle		
Adjusted to body	_____	_____
Tight	_____	_____
Crank assembly		
Hanger adjusted	_____	_____
Chain snug	_____	_____
Sprocket teeth present	_____	_____
Pedals with good tread	_____	_____
Chain guards tight	_____	_____
Frame and fenders		
Frame strength	_____	_____
Fenders tight	_____	_____
Spoke guards	_____	_____
Other factors		
Cleanliness	_____	_____
Lubrication	_____	_____

Approved _____ Inspector _____
Disapproved _____ School _____
Date _____ District _____

Figure 9-8 Suggested bicycle inspection report.

HIGH-RISE AND LIGHTWEIGHT BICYCLES

In addition to standard heavy-duty, middleweight, lightweight, touring, and sports cycles, a new type known as the "high rise" has recently appeared. This new design features small wheels, banana seats, and tall handlebars. This vehicle lends itself to antics and stunts not possible on a standard bike. As a result, clowning and stunting may lead to habits and skills that are basically unsafe. If care is taken and an appropriate place is selected (off the street) to perform these antics, the hazard factors can be minimized. If this type of cycle is purchased, parents must assume greater responsibility. They should direct their children to nearby parks, playgrounds, or empty parking lots for stunt and trick riding.

Lightweight bicycles have special characteristics aside from their weight. They are designed for smooth handling, speed, and durability. They are excellent for sports, touring, and recreational riding. They have high-pressure tires, a gear-shift mechanism that provides for different speeds, and front and rear caliper brakes which produce friction by forcing brake pads against the wheel rims. They are not as rugged as the heavier regular bike. All these characteristics have implications for the driver of the bicycle. The lightweights are capable of high speed, which can be hazardous for an inexperienced driver. Other moving vehicles and road surfaces must be constantly observed, since the time element for decision making grows shorter with increasing speed. Braking and turning must be avoided on slippery surfaces. Cyclists should maintain a firm grip on the handlebars when coasting through wet, slippery areas in order to maintain control. When braking, they should always apply the rear brakes first. In many cases it will not be necessary to use the front brakes at all. When both are applied, cyclists should release the front brakes first. Owing to the reduced stability of the lightweight cycle, drivers should always keep their fingers around the handle grips and not just resting on them.

EVALUATION

Although parents, school and local officials, and bicyclists appreciate and value a well-planned bicycle safety program, its effectiveness cannot be proved without evidence that riders are following safe practices at all times. Unfortunately, the conduct of cyclists while they are away from home and school cannot be directly measured without strong local law-enforcement and education programs. To some extent, their safe behavior at such times must be taken on faith. When the condition of bicycles and the riding practices observed at school appear satisfactory, such faith seems justified. Any evidence of a reduction in the bicycle-accident rate is a good indication that the program is achieving its objectives.

In addition to direct observation, effective law enforcement, and analysis of accident records, objective tests may be used to measure the extent to which students have acquired the knowledge, skill, and attitudes necessary for safe

Purpose: To show how to start and stop without wavering.

Test: Driver straddles bike, one foot on the ground, the other placed on opposite pedal, pedal placed 45 degrees above the horizontal, hands on handle grips. He should simultaneously push off, press down on the pedal and raise his body up and back onto the saddle. Driver then pedals a few turns and applies brake. When almost stopped, he should pull his body forward off the saddle, one foot on low pedal, opposite foot forward and down to engage the ground as his bicycle stops.

Scoring: Ten points if driver mounts, steers bicycle without losing balance or swerving from side to side erratically and gives his attention to a 180 degree area ahead, and then dismounts correctly. Deduct two points for each incorrect maneuver.

Significance: With proper saddle height, the inexperienced driver tends to start or stop while seated. Since his feet will not reach the ground, he tends to wobble into the traffic stream, or to fall to one side when stopping. If the pedal is not placed in the proper position for starting, insufficient speed may result in lack of control. This method gives full control at start and stop.

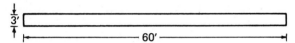

Figure 9-9 Mount and dismount.

bicycling. Good test results, even though they cannot prove that students are utilizing what they have learned, will at least show that students have the ability to ride safely. Poor results will clearly indicate the areas of the program that need to be strengthened. At present there are no comprehensive tests of this type. Each instructor must develop his or her own methods for measuring students' knowledge and attitudes in regard to traffic rules and maintenance

Purpose: To test balance and related sense of momentum, and the changes in balance required by intended changes in direction.

Test: Start 5' from the circle. Driver must enter circle at the opening and ride half-way around the first circle to his right, then change direction to ride to his left around the second circle. He reenters the first circle to his right, completing a figure 8. He repeats the procedure one more time, and returns to the meeting point of the circles for exit as marked.

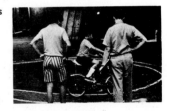

Scoring: Ten points is the best possible score. Deduct two points for each time the driver rides off the marked lane.

Significance: In traffic, there are many instances calling for a swerve in direction to avoid a pedestrian, a series of obstacles or a pothole in the road, or an oncoming vehicle. The rider must be able to change his direction in a precise manner, sometimes with little warning, so that the bicycle will go where he intends. The test develops precision of riding and confidence in the ability to control the bicycle, avoiding a spill or a collision.

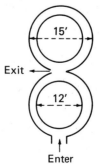

Figure 9-10 Circling and change in direction.

Purpose: To test poise and control in driving and to establish the ability to ride in a straight unwavering line as required on the road.

Test: Driver should start 20′ from the 60′ lane and the first pair of obstacles (blocks, weighted #1 cans or fist-size stones may be used as markers). The driver may go at any speed but must go between each of the pairs of markers without touching them. Markers may be placed at 5′ or 10′ intervals on opposite sides of the lane, 6 to 8 inches wide. The driver should turn to the outside of the marked lane and repeat the test. This time he should be directed by the judge to check traffic from the rear and to remove his left hand to make the proper arm signals for a left-hand turn, a right-hand turn, and slow or stop signal.

Scoring: Ten points if the driver steers his bicycle without veering between all markers, without touching them with the tires or stopping the bicycle, and signals correctly. Deduct two points for each faulty move.

Significance: For efficient cycling, the prime requisite is the ability to maintain perfect balance without a wavering path. The ability to drive a straight line permits the cyclist to maintain a position close to the road edge, out of the stream of traffic. It is necessary to watch for traffic approaching from the rear before making any maneuvers, without steering off the road or into the traffic. Signaling or gear-shifting requires removal of one hand without disturbing equilibrium.

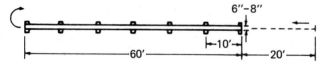

Figure 9-11 Straight line control.

techniques. Figures 9-9 through 9-15 illustrate skills tests that may be advantageously used by anyone conducting a bicycle safety program.*

MATERIALS AND FACILITIES NEEDED FOR ADMINISTERING SKILLS TESTS

1 A flat area large enough to accommodate the seven tests. Ideal sites include a school yard, shopping center, parking lot, playground, or blocked-off street. Hard-top surfaces are best.

2 Volunteers to run the skills-test stations, judges, registrars, etc.

3 A 50-foot tape measure

4 White plastic adhesive tape or chalk

5 Hammer, nails, and string to use as a swing arc to lay out circles

6 Traffic cones or quart cans filled with sand, or wooden blocks or boxes painted bright orange

7 Stop watches, clip boards, and scoring sheets

8 A public address system or power bullhorn

INSTRUCTIONAL PROGRAMS

Today there are many agencies that provide aid to people who wish to implement a bicycle safety education program. In most state offices of education or

*Permission granted by the Travelers Insurance Company. Hartford, Conn.

Purpose: To test the ability to change direction quickly, which requires balance and judgment.

Test: Driver should start 20' from the first obstacle, riding at normal speed and proceeding by going right of that obstacle, left of the second one, etc. Obstacles (blocks, weighted cans, or cones) should be 6' apart.

Scoring: Ten points if the driver does not hit any obstacles and if he goes alternately to the right and left of each one in the line. Deduct one point for each time he makes a wrong turn or touches an obstacle.

Significance: Hitting or missing an object in the road, whether it is a stone, a hole, or a pedestrian is a problem of instinct. A rider hits an obstacle because he is watching it, and naturally steers where he is looking. This test teaches the rider to focus on the clear path rather than on the obstacles.

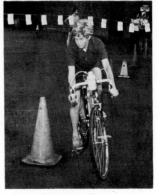

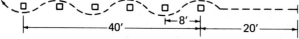

Figure 9-12 Weaving—maneuvering to avoid obstacles.

public instruction, formal bicycle units have been produced by safety divisions or curriculum departments. These units usually are developed for specific grade levels. They include such areas as:

    I. The accident problem as it relates to bicycle safety
       A. Statistical evidence
       B. Hazard factors
       C. Common traffic violations of the cyclist

Purpose: To test visual reactions in relation to momentum and to establish the driver's ability to stop in an emergency.

Test: Driver should go directly toward a cardboard box at a moderate speed and stop with the front part of the wheel 10" to 14" from the box. Brakes should be applied by the driver as he crosses the mark or line painted on the path as indicated. Judge should measure stopping distance.

Scoring: Ten points is the best possible score. Deduct two points if the driver touches the ground with either foot before bringing the bicycle to a stop or if his tires skid. Deduct one point for each 6" in excess of 14". Deduct 10 points if the rider touches or knocks over the box.

Significance: In the same way that the distance required to stop a car increases with speed, the distance required to stop a bicycle also increases. Frequently cyclists must stop in an emergency manner due to an on-coming car, a turning car, or a pedestrian who steps off the curb in their path. Sudden stops cause the weight to shift forward, allowing the bicycle to skid and lose control or to pitch the driver over the handlebars. It is necessary to learn to shift weight to the rear to avoid loss of control in a skid. This test is designed to teach riders to judge distance, according to speed, so they may stop their bikes before colliding with an obstruction.

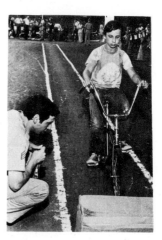

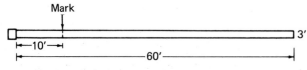

Figure 9-13 Stopping ability.

Purpose: To test the ability of the rider to turn his bicycle around easily and smoothly within a limited area.

Test: The rider travels within the marked lane following the S curves.

Scoring: Ten points is the best possible score. Deduct one point each time the driver touches the ground with either foot or rides over the border lines.

Significance: A rider is often called upon to turn around in a narrow street or constricted area. The successful completion of this test involves making smooth and easy turns without using the brake excessively, touching the ground with his feet or the border lines with either wheel of the bicycle.

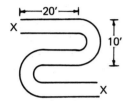

Figure 9-14 Short radius turning.

II. Use of the cycle
    A. Pleasure
    B. Errands
    C. Transportation
III. Selection of bicycles
    A. Size and type
    B. Construction
    C. Required accessories
IV. Care and maintenance
    A. Knowledge of the cycle
    B. Inspection and repairs
V. Development of skills in driving a cycle (see skills test)

Purpose: To test balancing at slow speed.

Test: Start with bicycle 15′ from a 60′ lane and drive slowly toward the lines. Driver should go between the lines of the lane as slowly as possible without touching either line. The judge begins timing the rider as he enters the lane. He should take at least thirty seconds or longer to reach the other end of the lane.

Scoring: Ten points if rider meets minimum time requirement of thirty seconds. Deduct two points each time he touches a line.

Significance: This test trains for straight driving, by developing a sense of balance as well as a sense of momentum of turning. The test emphasizes how a slight swing of the front wheel serves to reinstate the driver's balance when he starts to topple while pedaling at a slow speed.

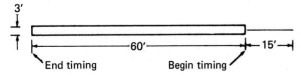

Figure 9-15 Slow speed.

VI. Traffic regulations governing bicycles (see model traffic ordinances)
    A. State laws
    B. Local laws
    C. Federal standards
VII. School activities promoting bicycle safety
    A. Assembly programs
    B. Parking regulations
    C. Parking facilities
    D. Bicycle courts
    E. Student bicycle patrols
    F. Safety surveys
    G. Field days, tours, and parades
    H. Bicycle rodeo
        1. Knowledge tests
        2. Skills tests

Agencies such as the National Safety Council, American Automobile Association, Bicycle Manufacturers Association of America, insurance companies, bicycle companies, the U.S. Consumer Product Safety Commission, provide educationally sound materials that can be used in any bicycle safety instructional program.

THE BICYCLE ON COLLEGE AND UNIVERSITY CAMPUSES

The bicycle is now one of the most popular methods of transportation on many college and university campuses. It is economical, noiseless, and easily stored. The construction of special lanes and parking facilities throughout the campus makes this mode of transportation increasingly popular.

Although control of bicycles on a university campus may seem simple, it is best to formulate some kind of bicycle code to protect the pedestrian as well as the cyclist. Usually the motor-vehicle division is vested with the powers, duties, and jurisdiction to administer such a code.

Space will not permit a detailed description of the items that should be included in a bicycle code, but the main classifications are presented here for guidance:

1 Definitions of terms in the code
2 Registration and licensing of bicycles
3 Equipment required
4 Operation of bicycle
5 Operation of bicycle paths
6 Bicycle-path control devices
7 Rules of the road
8 Parking
9 Penalties

10 Proper use of bicycle lanes
11 Proper use of bikeways

BICYCLE SAFETY RESEARCH

Recent studies have been conducted to analyze the bicycle-accident problem in depth. Vilardo and Anderson[4] of the National Safety Council of Chicago conducted a study that involved schools in six geographic areas, including urban and rural populations. A total of 60,700 questionnaires were distributed. A second sample was developed from an article on bicycle safety in an Ann Landers newspaper column. Parents reading the column requested a copy of the council's publication *Fun on a Bike.* A questionnaire was included with the pamphlet, with the returned data later included in the study.

The study was based on six program criteria:

1 Proper behavior at intersections
2 Matching bicycle and rider size
3 Bicycle usage
4 Stopping distance
5 Position in traffic (riding on right or left side)
6 Lighting of bicycle

The study attempted to evaluate the importance of these areas in terms of frequency of accidents. It also attempted to relate accident information to exposure in order to more clearly define the bicycle-accident problem. The study revealed that:

1 Boys are involved in more motor-vehicle accidents than girls.
2 There are fewer accidents at night, but nighttime accidents are usually more serious.
3 The type of accident depends on whether the bicycle is used as a toy or as a means of transportation. More motor-vehicle accidents occur when the bicycle is used as a means of transportation.
4 The relative safety of a bicycle is not determined by its style.
5 The size of the bicycle in relation to the size of the child may be an important factor in bicycle safety.
6 The side of the street on which a bicyclist rides does not seem to determine the frequency and type of accidents.

The Insurance Institute for Highway Safety completed a major report on bicycle accidents in order "to study characteristics of the operators involved relative to the probable responsibility for the collision of the bicyclist or motorist and/or their vehicle, based on pre-crash movements of the vehicle, and to determine the frequency of various types of collision configurations. An addi-

[4]Frank J. Vilardo, and Jane Anderson, *Bicycle Accidents to School Age Children,* Report No. 1/69, National Safety Council, Chicago, September, 1969, p. 80.

tional objective was to examine bicycle–motor-vehicle collisions in relation to bicyclist age."[5]

Some of the findings of the study were:

1. Ninety-nine percent of the involved bicyclists were injured. Of these, one percent fatally.

2. One percent of the motorists were injured to any degree.

3. Bicylists ages (886) in study:

280 (32 percent) were 4–9 years old
379 (43 percent) were 10–14 years old
151 (17 percent) were 15–19 years old
76 (9 percent) were 20 years of age or older

4. There was a strong relationship between bicyclist age and responsibility.

5. Young bicyclists may be less likely than adults to obey abstract traffic regulations, even if they understood them.

6. Young cyclists are also likely to have more difficulty than adults in controlling the bicycle because of lesser strength and coordination. Young cyclists are also less able than adults to localize sound, perceive movements in the periphery, read and interpret road signs and understand traffic terms.

7. Sixty-five percent of the collisions took place from 3:00 to 9:00 p.m. with 86 percent occurring during daylight, 7 percent during twilight and 7 percent in darkness.

8. Percentagewise, the following reasons for bicycle-motor vehicle collisions are:

a. Emerging from driveways, alleys, parking lots, etc., 23 percent
b. Ran through stop or yield sign, 20 percent
c. Intersected other vehicle traveling in same direction, 14 percent
d. Wrong way on a one-way street or in lane designated for traffic in opposite direction, 13 percent
e. Motorists responsible for 28 percent of accidents when they made a left turn and collided with an oncoming bicycle, and 28 percent when striking a bicycle from behind.

A study conducted by the Maryland State Department of Education analyzed 2,000 bicycle accidents. The study screened each individual accident report, and classified each critical maneuver by age-level involvement. A total of eighteen accident types were identified, but only those that accounted for at least 1 percent of the total were considered. Table 9-1 is a summary of these accident types and their percentages of occurrence for specific age groups.

A study called *Identifying Critical Behavior Leading to Collisions Between Bicycles and Motor Vehicles* was conducted in Santa Barbara, California, under the direction of the Santa Barbara Department of Public Works. The *principal* objective was to develop a cost-effective bicycle safety education program for school-age children, a program that would serve to reduce the incidence of accidents between bicycles and motor vehicles.

The study was based on three major premises. First, the education program must be based upon sound empirical data on the causes of bicycle–motor-vehicle accidents. Second, if bicycle safety education programs are to be implemented, they must be developed with full recognition of constraints on

[5]Insurance Institute for Highway Safety, *Status Report,* vol. 9, no. 22, December, 1974.

TABLE 9–1

Types and Percentage Occurrence of Bicycle Accidents for Specific Age Groups

Accident Type	Percentage Occurrence	Age Grouping
1. Cyclist exited driveway into motorist's path	15.0	5–14
2. Cyclist failed to stop/yield at controlled intersection	14.0	9–Adult
3. Motorist made improper left turn	10.6	9–Adult
4. Cyclist made improper left turn	10.0	9–14
5. Cyclist rode on wrong side of street	10.0	5–14 (Some adults)
6. Motorist collided with rear of cyclist	10.0	9–Adult
7. Motorist failed to stop/yield at controlled intersection	7.0 (In 16% of these, the bicycle had no lights)	9–Adult
8. Cyclist entered street from side of road other than intersection or driveway	5.4	5–Adult
9. Parking lot	3.2 (In 50%, the cyclist was responsible)	9–14
10. Motorist made improper right turn	3.1	9–Adult
11. Motorist exited driveway into cyclist's path	3.0	5–Adult
12. Other	2.7	5–Adult
13. Car sideswiped bicycle	2.7	5–Adult
14. Cyclist sideswiped car	2.1	9–Adult
15. Cyclist made improper right turn	1.4	9–14
16. Motorist opened car door into cyclist's path	1.2	9–Adult
17. Motorist failed to stop/yield at uncontrolled intersection	1.0	5–14
18. Cyclist failed to stop/yield at uncontrolled intersection	1.0 103.4%	5–14

Source: *School Safety World Newsletter*, National Safety Council, vol. 5, no. 2, Summer, 1977.

time and resources. Third, a feasible program can be developed only by taking full advantage of the knowledge and skills of other people who have been involved in bicycle safety training.

A secondary objective was to develop data that would be useful in the creation of a law-enforcement program that is cost-effective and compatible with the safety education program.

Some highlights of the study are:

1 The development of a concept of causation for the study was based on the premise that all accidents occur because operators behave in an inappropriate manner while in a traffic situation. Therefore, specific behavioral acts were the cause of the reported accidents.

2 Accidents can be curtailed through behavior modification of knowledge, skills, and attitudes, or by modification of the environment, or by a combination of the two.

3 Accident types were identified, and 91 percent of the accidents were sorted into ten major accident types.

4 The titles for the ten accident types and the pie-shaped figure (Figure 9-16) illustrate the relative proportion of the total accident sample that was categorized into each type. The illustration also indicates, for each accident type, whether the critical maneuver was executed by the cyclist or the motorist.

5 Another finding showed quite a difference in age range between male and female bicyclists. Female involvement began at six years of age up to twenty-five (90 percent of female participants were twenty-five years of age or younger). Male involvement began at about age four, two years younger than for females, and went to about thirty-four years of age, nearly nine years older than for females. The study also determined that the critical age at which males have the highest percentage of accidents is about thirteen, whereas for females it is about twenty.

The study also discussed when to start the educational program, fitting the program into a school schedule, grade levels, etc. Table 9-2 treats "pre-training accidents" as a function of the grade at which training is administered. It

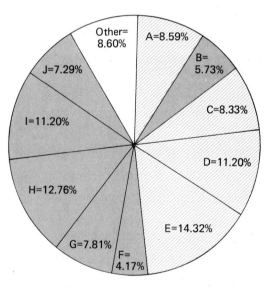

A. Cyclist exited driveway into motorist's path

B. Motorist exited driveway into cyclist's path

C. Cyclist failed to stop/yield at controlled intersection

D. Cyclist made improper left turn

E. Cyclist rode on wrong side of street

F. Motorist collided with rear of cyclist

G. Motorist failed to stop/yield at controlled intersection

H. Motorist made improper left turn

I. Motorist made improper right turn

J. Motorist opened car door into cyclist's path

KEY: Critical maneuver executed by cyclist

Critical maneuver executed by motorist

Figure 9-16 Breakdown of total accident sample by accident type.

TABLE 9-2

Estimated Pre-Training Accidents as a Function of Grade at Which Training is Administered

Type	Grade Level												
	K	1	2	3	4	5	6	7	8	9	10	11	12
Cyclist exited driveway into motorist's path	16%	22%	29%	36%	43%	52%	60%	67%	74%	82%	85%	88%	93%
Motorist exited driveway into cyclist's path	11%	16%	18%	27%	33%	38%	43%	47%	52%	55%	58%	65%	72%
Cyclist failed to stop/yield at controlled intersection	1%	6%	10%	15%	20%	28%	34%	38%	50%	65%	72%	76%	80%
Cyclist made improper left turn	1%	3%	8%	10%	15%	19%	27%	38%	46%	57%	63%	67%	72%
Cyclist rode on wrong side of street	1%	3%	6%	9%	13%	16%	18%	27%	39%	52%	58%	65%	71%
Motorist collided with rear of cyclist	0%	0%	0%	0%	0%	0%	3%	10%	16%	22%	26%	30%	45%
Motorist failed to stop/yield at controlled intersection	0%	0%	0%	1%	4%	5%	7%	8%	9%	15%	22%	26%	30%
Motorist made improper left turn	0%	0%	0%	0%	0%	1%	3%	4%	6%	10%	17%	23%	25%
Motorist made improper right turn	0%	0%	1%	3%	4%	4%	7%	10%	13%	17%	19%	23%	28%
Motorist opened car door into cyclist's path	0%	0%	0%	0%	0%	0%	0%	1%	6%	8%	13%	17%	21%

Source: Kenneth D. Cross, Anacapa Sciences, Inc., Santa Barbara, Calif.

illustrates that some types of countermeasure programs can be administered at higher grade levels without incurring an unreasonable number of accidents. (Note: the information describing this study was obtained from an abstract by Kenneth D. Cross of Anacapa Sciences, Inc., Santa Barbara, California). More research will be forthcoming from various public, private, and governmental agencies as solutions to the bicycle safety problem are sought.

These recent studies from Maryland and California indicate that specific accident-causation factors should be taught to specific age groups. The studies also support the idea that there is a need to develop a new, more advanced approach to bicycle safety education as a countermeasure. Basic fundamentals must be taught to the beginning cyclist. But the cyclist must also develop visual skills, including search and detection, and decision-making skills.

More emphasis should be placed on the motorist. This can be accomplished: in high school driver education programs; by including bicycle-safety content in a state's rules of the road; by including questions regarding the bicyclist and motorist in driver's licensing examinations; and by defensive-driving and driver-refresher courses, and driver-improvement programs.

Because of the high concentration of bicycles on college and university campuses and the increased use of bicycles by older adults, special emphasis should be placed on bicycle safety for these groups.

BIKEWAY SYSTEMS

The spectacular increase in the use of bicycles for recreation and transportation has created a demand for a safer and more accessible driving environment for cyclists in dense traffic situations. More than 100,000 bicycle–motor-vehicle accidents each year cause injuries and fatalities primarily to cyclists. A growing number of communities and states are seeking to curb cycle injuries and fatalities by improving the environment in which the cyclist operates. This can be accomplished by establishing bikeway systems. Such systems protect the bicyclist by physically separating bikes from motor vehicles or by making motorists more conscious of the presence of cyclists in the traffic mix.

Whether a cycle is used for recreation, errands, or general transportation, a properly designed bikeway can provide an effective shield against potential danger. If a community is concerned about bicycle accidents, the following general guidelines may assist in planning a feasible bikeway system.

There must be an organization for bikeway planning that includes transportation planners, political leaders, engineers (traffic and highway), urban planners, government executives, businessmen, and civic leaders. The committee would be concerned with:

    I. Developing a master plan
   II. Studying travel characteristics
       A. Generation of cycle trips
       B. Trip type and purpose
       C. Neighborhood driving

    D. Commuter driving
    E. Recreational driving
    F. Sports driving
III. Trip length and travel time
IV. Time of trips (time of day)
V. Joint-use development
    A. Bicyclists
    B. Hikers
    C. Equestrians
    D. Light, off-road motorcycles
    E. Mopeds
VI. Mixed-mode bicycle travel
    A. Commuters with other modes of travel
VII. Bicycle support systems (Long-distance, sports, and recreational cycling have greater need for a support system than neighborhood or commuter driving)
    A. Vehicle repair and storage
    B. Rest rooms, drinking fountains, telephones, campgrounds, information, etc.
VIII. Terminal facilities
    A. Secure and adequate storage facilities
IX. Bikeway types
    A. Exclusive bikeway
    B. Restricted bikeway
    C. Shared bikeway
X. Design criteria
    A. Outside-lane dimensions
    B. Parking
    C. Bikeway widths
    D. Vehicle speed
    E. Vehicle volume
XI. Warrants for bikeway types
XII. Bikeway capacities
XIII. Physical design criteria
    A. Design speed
    B. Radius of curve
    C. Grade capabilities
    D. Surface requirements
    E. Intersections and crossings
XIV. Bikeway signing
    A. Use of the *National Manual on Uniform Traffic Control Devices*
XV. Cross-section dimensions and clearance
    A. For exclusive bikeways
    B. For restricted bikeways
XVI. Costs
XVII. Financing bicycle facilities

Finding a type of bikeway that is economically and politically feasible for an individual community requires detailed planning. Support can be sought from both the state and the federal governments. Under current laws, states may obtain federal funds for bike-facility construction on a matching-fund basis. Many local communities are also receiving state and federal funds for bicycle safety programs.

The content outlined above has been obtained from the American Automobile Association booklet, *Planning Criteria for Bikeways*. Additional details are available in the *Transportation and Traffic Engineering Handbook*. Other information concerning the establishment of bicycle facilities is available from the Bicycle Manufacturers Association of America, state departments of transportation, the Federal Highway Administration, the National Safety Council, the League of American Wheelmen, and other organizations.

LEARNING EXPERIENCES

The following learning experiences should give prospective teachers of bicycle safety a better understanding of the problems involved in their field.

1 Develop a pretest for pupils in the elementary and secondary grades to determine their knowledge, attitudes, and practices in regard to bicycle safety.

2 Prepare a lesson plan on the proper care and maintenance of the bicycle.

3 Using records and additional pertinent data secured from the local police department and other sources, develop a graphic illustration of the bicycle accidents met with by elementary and high school students and adults in your community.

4 With the aid of the local newspaper and television and radio stations, the local safety council, and such national organizations as the Bicycle Manufacturers Association and the National Safety Council, plan a bicycle safety campaign for an elemenary school, a high school, and a community.

5 Outline a talk, to be given before a parent-teacher group, the local board of education, or a civic organization, explaining a proposed program of bicycle safety.

6 Prepare an article on bicycle safety for the local newspaper or the state educational magazine.

7 Plan a bicycle-skill contest as part of the school's annual play-day activities.

8 Plan a recreational bicycle trip for twenty-five students.

9 Analyze records of bicycle accidents during the past year, and discuss the accidents that might have been prevented.

10 Make a survey of hazardous bicycle situations in your community. Discuss possible means of eliminating them or at least of coping with them safely.

11 Prove mathematically that a bicyclist is safer riding in the same direction as an automobile by figuring out the coefficient of impact for car and bicycle when each is going at various speeds in the same and in opposite directions.

12 Check with various community agencies, and find out whether or not your community has a bicycle ordinance. If so, communicate the provisions of the ordinance to students and the community through newspapers, television, and radio.

13 Make a map of community, school, and college-campus bicycle paths.

14 Make a map illustrating where new bicycle paths should be constructed in your community.

15 Analyze bicycle accidents on a university campus and prescribe solutions to the problems.

SELECTED REFERENCES

Alth, Max.: *All about Bikes and Bicycling,* Hawthorne Books, Inc., New York, 1977
American Automobile Association, Falls Church, Va:
    Bicycle Hazards
    Bicycle Information Tests
    Bicycle Safety Kit
    Bicycle Skill Tests
    Bicycling is Great Fun
    Bike Basics
    Model Bicycle Ordinance
    Parents: Buying Your Child a Bicycle
    Special Survey on Bicycle Safety, 1972
    Sportsmanlike Driving, 7th ed., McGraw-Hill Book Company, New York, 1975
    Teacher's Guide to Bicycle Safety Activities and Projects
American Mutual Insurance Alliance Chicago: *Here's How to Develop a Bikeway System in Your Town.*
American Red Cross, Washington:
    American Red Cross Pamphlet 1075-1
    You and Your Bicycle
Bicycle Manufacturers Association of America, Inc., Washington:
    Bicycle Club Booklet
    Bicycle Safety Set
    Bicycle Safety Test Booklet
    Bicycling—Number One Sport
    Bike Ordinance in the Community
    Bike Quiz Guide
    Bike Safety Posters
    Pedal Primer
    So you Want a Bikeway
DeLong, Fred: *DeLong's Guide to Bicycles and Bicycling, The Art and Science,* Chilton Book Company, Radnor, Pa., 1974, p. 278
Hammond, Beverly J.: "Safety On Two Wheels," *Journal of Traffic Safety Education,* January, 1973
Illinois Office of Secretary of State: *Bicycle Rules of the Road,* 1978, Springfield, Ill.
League of American Wheelmen, Inc. A source of bicycle safety information. 19 South Bothwell Palatine, Ill. 60067

Licht, Kenneth F.: "A Bit of Heresy About Bike Safety Education," *Journal of Traffic Safety Education,* January, 1974

McIntyre, Bibs: *The Bike Book,* Harper & Row Publishers, Incorporated, New York, 1972.

Metropolitan Life Insurance Statistical Bulletin, "Cycling Accident Fatalities in the United States," June, 1976

Morse, Herbert W.: "Bicycle Safety-Education, Enforcement and Laws," *Journal of Traffic Safety Education,* April, 1977

National Committee on Uniform Traffic Laws and Ordinances, Washington:
  Uniform Vehicle Code, rev., 1968, pp. 168–170
  Model Traffic Ordinance, rev., 1968, 12, pp. 21–24
  Supplement II, 1976

National Safety Council, Chicago:
  Accident Facts, 1977
  All About Bikes
  Analyzing Bicycle Accident Reports, Memo 59
  Bicycle Accidents to School Age Children, Report No. 1/69
  Bicycle Safety in Action
  Bicycle Safety Tests
  Bicycles, Data Sheet No. 1
  Bicycles. Public Safety Memo 92
  Family Safety Magazine
    "Bike Boom and Boomerang," Summer, 1974
    "Babes on Bikes," Summer, 1975
    "A Motorist's Guide to Bicycle Safety," Spring, 1976
  Traffic Safety Magazine
    "This Cyclist Practices What He Preaches," December 1975

National Transportation Safety Board, Washington:
  Bicycle Use as a Highway Safety Problem, Special Study; Report No. NTSB-HSS-72-1: April, 1972
  Youth and Traffic Safety Education, Special Study; Report No. NTSB-STS-71-3, July 1, 1971

Popish, L. N. and R. B. Lyte: *A Study of Bicycle Motor Vehicle Accidents,* Department of Public Works Traffic Division, Santa Barbara, California, June 1973

Travelers Insurance Company: *Cycle Safety for P.P.P.—Skill Test Layout and Rodeo Guide,* Hartford, Conn., p. 8

Vilardo, F. J. and J. H. Anderson: *Bicycle Accidents to School-Age Children,* Report No. 1/69, National Safety Council, Chicago, September, 1969

U.S. Consumer Product Safety Commission, Washington:
  Fact Sheet No. 10: *Bicycles,* May, 1974
  Technical Fact Sheet No. 5: *The Bicycle Regulations,* April, 1976
  "This Cyclist Practices What He Preaches," Reprint from *Traffic Safety,* December, 1975, National Safety Council, Chicago

U.S. Department of Transportation: *Pedestrian and Bicycle Safety Study, Highway Safety Act of 1973 (Section 214),* Washington, March, 1975

Williams, Allen F.: "Factors in the Initiation of Bicycle Motor Vehicle Collisions," Insurance Institute for Highway Safety, *Status Report,* vol. 9, no. 22, December 10, 1974, Washington

Additional materials are available from insurance companies and bicycle manufacturers.

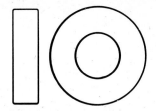

Motorcycle Safety

OVERALL OBJECTIVE:

The student should comprehend the magnitude of the motorcycle-accident problem and should know the changing trends in death and injury rates since motorcycles became an important part of the highway transportation system.

INSTRUCTIONAL OBJECTIVES:

After completing this chapter the student will be able to:

1 State the annual number of deaths and injuries that occur to motorcyclists.
2 Compare the death and injury rates of motorcyclists with those of other motor-vehicle operators.
3 List the most frequent causes of motorcycle accidents.
4 Describe a motorcycle education course for safety instructors
5 Implement a motorcycle driver education safety program.
6 Prepare motorcycle teaching units for classroom and practice-driving instruction.
7 Discuss the relationship between motorcycles and other vehicular traffic.
8 Discuss methods of integrating motorcycle education into a driver education curriculum.
9 Discuss the pros and cons of motorcycle helmet use laws
10 Discuss the question of licensing Moped operators.
11 Formulate a college and university motorcycle safety code.

MOTORCYCLE SAFETY

The rapid growth of motorcycle use in the past decade is a direct result of acceptance of motorcycles by the motorists of this country. The use of motorcycles as a means of transportation for commuting to work, touring, and recreation has reached a new peak of popularity in recent years. The National Safety

295

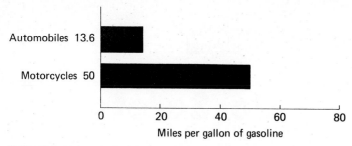

Figure 10-1 Motorcycles furnish economical transportation. (Source: *Guide to Safe Motorcycling*, 1973, p. 9, American Automobile Association, Washington, D.C.)

Council reports that the number of registered motorcycles has risen from 575,497 in 1960 to over 5 million in 1976 (Table 10-1). After analyzing the increases in the past decade, we can predict a 15 to 20 percent increase in the next decade, particularly if fuel increases in cost and becomes difficult to obtain.

Several factors have contributed to the popularity of motorcycles: the population explosion immediately after World War II, the relative prosperity of our era, the move to suburbia, crowded traffic conditions, lack of suitable parking for motor vehicles in congested areas, greater leisure time, the expansion of college and university campuses, the need for low-cost transportation (see Figure 10-2), and the development of a low-cost lightweight cycle.

The rapid rise in the use of motorcycles has been accompanied by an increase in the number of accidents, injuries, and fatalities suffered by motorcyclists (see Figure 10-1). In recent years the accident rate has risen at a slower pace, but deaths among drivers and passengers of motorcycles have more than doubled in the past decade and more than quadrupled since the early 1960s (Table 10-1). When the fatality rate is calculated on the basis of number of miles driven, the motorcycle emerges as the most hazardous motor vehicle on the highway.

Although the motorcycle is used by individuals of all age groups, the great majority of motorcycle fatalities are incurred by victims between the ages of sixteen and twenty-four, the prime educational years of our youth. "The majority of cycle operators in this age group have had less than 6 months of motorcycle driving experience. Over 90 percent of the drivers are male and approximately 80 percent of those killed or injured are male. Many of the females injured and killed are passengers."[1]

Among the many causes of motorcycle accidents, inexperience is the key factor. Some of the specific circumstances cited most frequently in special studies are failure to adhere to traffic laws or traffic signs, reckless driving, speeding, and failure to yield the right of way. Studies have also shown that many motorcycle accidents are the fault of automobile drivers rather than motorcyclists. Injuries resulting from motorcycle accidents are usually more

[1]National Safety Council, *Motorcycles*, Safety Education Data Sheet No. 98, rev., Chicago.

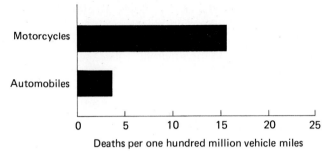

Figure 10-2 Motorcycle death rates four times that of passenger cars. (Source: *Guide to Safe Motorcycling*, 1973, p. 7, American Automobile Association, Washington, D.C.)

TABLE 10–1
Motorcycle and Total Motor-Vehicle Data, 1960–1976*

	Vehicles				Deaths			
	Motorcycles†		Total Motor Vehicles		Motorcycle Riders		All Motor Vehicle Occupants	
Year	No.	Yearly % Change	No.	Yearly % Change	No.	Yearly % Change	No.	Yearly % Change
1960	575,497		74,500,000		731			
1961	595,669	+ 3.5	76,400,000	+2.6	697	− 4.7	29,750	
1962	660,400	+10.9	79,700,000	+4.3	759	+ 8.9	29,860	+ 0.3
1963	786,318	+19.1	83,500,000	+4.8	882	+16.2	32,300	+ 8.2
1964	984,763	+25.2	87,300,000	+4.6	1,118	+26.8	34,700	+ 7.4
1965	1,381,956	+40.3	91,800,000	+5.2	1,515	+35.5	37,900	+ 9.2
1966	1,752,801	+26.8	95,900,000	+4.5	2,043	+34.9	39,450	+ 4.1
1967	1,953,022	+11.4	98,900,000	+3.1	1,971	− 3.5	42,800	+ 8.5
1968	2,100,547	+ 7.6	103,100,000	+4.2	1,900	− 3.6	42,700	− 0.2
1969	2,315,916	+10.3	107,700,000	+4.5	1,960	+ 3.2	44,100	+ 3.3
1960	2,814,730	+21.5	111,200,000	+3.2	2,330	+18.9	45,200	+ 2.5
1971	3,345,179	+18.8	116,300,000	+4.6	2,410	+ 3.4	43,500	− 3.8
1972	3,801,932	+13.7	122,300,000	+5.2	2,700	+12.0	43,200	− 0.7
1973	4,353,502	+14.5	129,800,000	+6.1	3,130	+15.9	44,700	+ 3.5
1974	4,966,132	+14.1	134,900,000	+3.9	3,160	+ 1.0	44,050	− 1.5
1975	4,966,844	+ ‡	138,000,000	+2.3	2,800	−11.4	36,400	−17.4
1976	5,110,000	+ 2.9	142,400,000	+3.2	3,000	+ 7.1	36,300	− 0.3

*The mileage death rate for motorcycle riders during 1975 is estimated to be about 11 deaths per 100 million miles of motorcycle travel. Based on data collected by the Federal Highway Administration, the 1975 rate represents a decrease from the 1974 rate of 14. The motorcycle mileage death rate of 11 compares with the overall motor-vehicle death rate of 3.5.

†Includes motor scooter, motorized bicycle, and motorized tricycle.

‡Less than 0.05 percent.

Source: Vehicles—Federal Highway Administration; motorcycle rider deaths, 1960–1967—National Center for Health Statistics; motorcycle rider deaths, 1968–1975, and motor-vehicle occupant deaths—National Safety Council. Reported in *Accident Facts*, National Safety Council, Chicago, 1977.

severe than those sustained in automobile accidents. A 300- to 400-pound cycle is no match for a 3,000- to 4,000-pound automobile.

The major circumstances that contribute to motorcycle accidents result from faulty human behavior rather than the environment or the condition of the vehicle. A motorcycle operator must assume the same degree of responsibility as the operator of any other mechanized vehicle. The safe operation of a motorcycle requires as many skills, although different, as are needed to drive an automobile. Yet most beginners usually teach themselves after a few hasty lessons from a dealer or friend.

DRIVER EDUCATION

Regardless of how a motorcycle is used, drivers need adequate initial instruction in vehicle operation and development of good driving attitudes, habits, and skills. Good habits must be learned and implemented from the beginning. In recent years there have been efforts to develop a formal motorcycle driver education course.

Because the motorcycle appeals to younger people, who incur the greatest number of deaths and injuries, the need for a systematic instructional program for beginning motorcyclists is obvious. Many motorcycle accidents seem to stem from the same causes as motor-vehicle accidents, and all states now provide high school driver education programs for beginning drivers. A similar program could easily be developed for the motorcyclist. The program could be developed as a separate course or in correlation with the driver education program.

RESPONSIBILITY FOR MOTORCYCLE EDUCATION

Educational systems, including state departments of education, colleges and universities, and local school districts; federal governmental agencies; civic groups; and motorcycle manufacturers all have a responsibility for promoting and implementing motorcycle education programs. The following guidelines for the agencies mentioned above have been developed by the American Driver and Traffic Safety Education Association.[2]

Responsibility for motorcycle education

The responsibility for motorcycle education rests with the education system, a number of civic groups, business and manufacturing concerns, and governmental agencies. State departments of education, colleges and universities, and local school districts all have a responsibility for providing quality motorcycle safety education programs.

State departments of education

Departments of education should establish procedures and criteria for (1) approval of courses in teacher preparation, (2) teacher certification standards, and (3) approval of courses

---

[2]American Driver and Traffic Safety Education Association, *Policies and Guidelines for Motorcycle Safety Education*, Washington, 1974, p. 39.

in motorcycle education offered by the local school districts. They should also provide consultant services to local school districts planning motorcycle education courses.

Colleges and universities

Institutions should prepare administrative and intructional personnel to conduct motorcycle education courses. Greater numbers of well-qualified teachers of motorcycle education will be needed during the next several years. Institutions of higher education with traffic safety education programs should expand their program offerings to include motorcycle education. In addition, the colleges and universities should conduct research and special studies in order to better meet the personnel requirements in motorcycle safety education.

Local school districts

School districts have the major responsibility for motorcycle education. Districts should implement motorcycle safety education programs which satisfy community needs and standards set by departments of education and other regulatory agencies.

The ultimate responsibility for motorcycle education falls upon the secondary schools. They are uniquely qualified to prepare youth, not only as competent motorcycle operators, but also as responsible participants in programs which affect safety in the highway transportation system. Furthermore, secondary schools are a logical place for motorcycle safety education programs. At this level of formal education, young people reach legal riding age in an environment that includes resources for learning under professionally prepared teachers. Additionally, students completing automobile driver education become an important audience, not only for learning safe practices of motorcycle riding, but also for gaining understanding of the coexistence and interaction necessary between motorcycle operators and other vehicles on the highways.

Motorcycle education is a natural extension of the school's traffic safety education program. Safety educators believe that properly designed and implemented secondary school programs in motorcycle education can be the *prime* factor in assuring that young people who choose to operate motorcycles do so safely.

MOTORCYCLE SAFETY FOUNDATION

The Motorcycle Safety Foundation began operation in 1973 to encourage and develop motorcycle safety education programs on a nationwide basis.

With tremendous growth annually in the number of registered motorcycles—from under one million in 1964 to over five million in 1976—and some 15 million motorcyclists now riding, the industry felt that a need existed for a nationally coordinated motorcycle safety effort.

As part of its initial program, the Foundation has developed *The Beginning Rider Course* which is available to schools and other interested organizations. Designed to train the beginning rider in the proper techniques of handling and riding a motorcycle, especially in traffic, the three-part instructional package consists of student textbook, student workbook, and instructor's guide. *The Beginning Rider Course* can serve as a basis for incorporating motorcycle safety education into a school's curriculum.

Some of the other projects sponsored by the Foundation include:

- Instructor Workshops held at colleges, universities, and military installations: effort to improve the quality and increase the quantity of motorcycle safety instructors.
- Research into skills required for safe motorcycle operation and traffic interaction: one

current study provides detailed knowledge of the rider's task as a basis for improving instruction.

• Liaison with state licensing authorities to upgrade the motorcycle operator licensing process: applicants should be able to demonstrate skills necessary for safe motorcycle operation.

• Public affairs programming in television, radio, and the press: to increase public awareness of the need for motorcycle safety education and necessity for motorists and motorcyclists to share the roadway safely.

• Technical assistance: to the limit of available resources, staff assists educators, the military, community groups, and others in organizing, implementing, and improving motorcycle safety and education efforts.

The Motorcycle Safety Foundation is a private, nonprofit organization sponsored by the leading motorcycle manufacturers: Honda, Yamaha, Suzuki, Kawasaki, and Harley Davidson. Its purpose is to enhance motorcycle safety through education and research. The primary mission of the Foundation is the development, evaluation, and promotion of quality motorcycle safety programs in the public interest.

In addition to specific programs in research, education, instructor preparation, and licensing improvement, the Foundation is establishing a clearinghouse on motorcycle safety education materials. For further information on Motorcycle Safety Foundation programs, publications, or services, please contact the Foundation at 6755 Elkridge Landing Road, Linthicum, Maryland.

An effective traffic safety education program requires a well-qualified, enthusiastic, and dedicated teacher. Although teachers with a safety background are desirable as motorcycle driver educators, any certified teacher, particularly one with motorcycle-driving experience, can become qualified as a motorcycle-driver educator. The Motorcycle Safety Foundation has been instrumental in initiating such programs, supporting them through financial grants, and providing instructional materials and instructors to many colleges and universities to implement their teacher-education programs. The materials developed by the Foundation staff for use in these programs are educationally sound. The following is a brief outline of the instructor preparation course:

Course objectives
1. Be familiar with course content and the instructional sequence of a novice motorcycle safety course.
   a. The motorcycle
   b. Basic cycle control
   c. Safe riding practices
   d. Complex situations
   e. Maintenance and insurance
   f. Operator fitness
   g. Off-road riding
2. Be able to demonstrate the knowledge and skills needed for motorcycle riding at a level of proficiency equal to that of novice rider course graduates.
   a. In-course tests
      1 Unit knowledge tests
      2 Range skill tests
      3 On-street performance tests

     b. Course evaluation tests
        1 Motorcycle safety education test, pretest
        2 Motorcycle safety education test, posttest
        3 Range skill test
        4 On-street performance test

3. Be able to organize lessons for classroom and laboratory instruction. Demonstrate teaching techniques and methods for novice motorcycle riders.
     a. Classroom instruction
     b. Range instruction
     c. On-street instruction

4. Be able to administer a test battery in a standardized manner. Use test results to aid students in mastering course content and to assess students' achievements of unit and course objectives.
     a. Knowledge evaluation
        1 Role and use
        2 Unit tests
        3 Pre- and post-course tests
        4 Student performance tests
     b. Skill evaluation
        1 Range test
        2 Daily laboratory progress
     c. Performance evaluation
        1 On-street test
        2 Daily laboratory progress

5. Be able to organize a course and successfully administer a program in motorcycle safety education.
     a. Administrative approval and rationale for motorcycle safety education
     b. Course schedule
     c. Instructional support
     d. Student schedule
     e. Program support
     f. Cycle procurement
     g. Community support and promotion

6. Be able to plan and administer instruction in secondary schools and at the community level to experienced motorcycle riders.[3]
     a. Protective equipment (See section on helmet-use law)
     b. Maintenance
     c. Perception and detectability
     d. Prediction and space utilization
     e. Complex situations
     f. Collision avoidance

---

[3] Motorcycle Safety Foundation, *Guidelines for Instructor Preparation*, Linthicum, Maryland 1975, p. 48.

Each unit contains an extensive list of student and teacher activities and unit resources.

The Motorcycle Safety Foundation's curriculum package for the motorcycle rider course is probably the finest that has ever been developed for a comprehensive student-teacher motorcycle safety program. It represents the culmination of extensive research efforts and is based on motorcycle task analysis and instructional objectives for motorcycle safety education.

In Illinois, a special motorcycle curriculum committee of the Safety Division of the Office of Public Instruction (now Office of Education) developed the motorcycle safety curriculum reprinted in Appendix C. The curriculum may be taught in conjunction with the high school classroom phase of the driver education course. The curriculum guide also describes a laboratory phase for schools that wish to implement a complete motorcycle safety education course.

MOTORCYCLE HELMET-USE LAWS

There are many questions concerning federal requirements for the use of motorcycle helmets. The effectiveness of wearing helmets can be determined by comparing the seriousness of motorcycle accidents in states with and without helmet laws.

The National Highway Safety Administration conducted a study of motorcycle accidents in Michigan, which had a helmet-use law, and in Illinois, which did not. The study compared the types and frequency of head injuries. It was found that the percentage of accidents that caused fatal and serious head injuries was *three* times greater in Ilinois than in Michigan. The percentage of accidents that caused any type of head injury was twice as great in Illinois as in Michigan. Helmets were found to be equally effective in all speed ranges.

The same study found that the law was effective in getting motorcyclists to wear helmets. In Michigan, 93 percent of motorcyclists involved in accidents were wearing helmets; in Illinois, only 24 percent of accident-involved riders were wearing helmets voluntarily.

An earlier study, conducted by the Illinois Department of Transportation, of motorcycle accidents in Illinois confirms the effectiveness of helmets. In 1968, the only full year in which the Illinois helmet-use law was in effect, motorcycle rider fatalities decreased about 27 percent. In the following year, after the law was declared unconstitutional by the Illinois Supreme Court, motorcycle fatalities increased 44 percent (Table 10-2).

The Highway Safety Act of 1966 *required* each state to have a highway safety program conforming to the standards developed by the Secretary of Transportation. One of the original thirteen standards dealt with motorcycle safety. One requirement of that standard was that each motorcyclist "wear an approved safety helmet." See Table 10-3 for helmet requirements by states.

In response to the standard, the number of states with helmet laws increased from 3 in 1966 to 48 and the District of Columbia and Puerto Rico in

TABLE 10–2
Effect of Motorcycle Helmet-Use Law in Illinois

	Number of Motorcycle Fatalities and Injuries and Percent of Changes 1966–1970				
	1966	1967	1968*	1969	1970
Killed	101	106	77	111	113
Percent change	....	+5.0	27.4	+44.2	+1.8
Injured	3,229	2,967	1,995	2,603	2,906
Percent change	....	7.5	33.2	+30.5	+11.6

*Only full year the state had a helmet law.
Source: Highway Users Federation, *Reporter,* Washington, June–July, 1977.

1975. Illinois and Nebraska adopted helmet-use laws, but their laws were declared unconstitutional by state supreme courts.

The rapid and favorable response by state legislators to the helmet-use standard has been followed by criticism of the regulation. At present the helmet-use law remains an issue, with safety professionals for the most part in favor and some organized groups of motorcyclists in opposition. The main question is whether or not the law infringes upon an individual's right to take risks. Many people contend that helmets do not reduce injuries but actually contribute to accidents and increase neck injuries.

The Secretary of Transportation attempted to impose sanctions by withholding federal safety funds from states that failed to implement a highway safety program. In 1976 Congress voted to prevent the imposition of sanctions by the Secretary, and prohibited any requirements for helmet use by riders over eighteen. Since then several states have repealed their helmet-use laws, and others have weakened their laws substantially (Figure 10-3).

Although many states have weakened their laws, repeal attempts have been defeated in several others. Many safety leaders and other people believe that the "individual rights" issue is a hollow one. They state that safety laws are intended to benefit all citizens and that such laws may restrict some individual rights by means of speed limits, building codes, etc.

A Massachusetts court told a motorcyclist objecting to the state's helmet-use laws (and the U.S. Supreme Court later affirmed):[4]

> While we agreed with plaintiff that the Act's only realistic purpose is the prevention of head injuries incurred in motorcycle mishaps, we cannot agree that the consequences of such injuries are limited to the individual who sustains the injury. The public has an interest in minimizing the resources directly involved. From the moment of the injury, society picks the person up off the highway; delivers him to a municipal hospital and municipal doctors; provides him with unemployment compensation if, after recovery, he cannot replace his lost job, and if the injury causes permanent disability, may assume the responsibility for his and

[4]"Motorcycle and Public Apathy," *American Journal of Public Health,* vol. 66, no. 5, May, 1976. See also, "Motorcycle Helmet Use Laws," *Facts on Vital Issues,* June–July, 1977, Highway Users Federation, Washington.

TABLE 10-3
Motorcycle Requirements by States

State	Special Driver License	Safety Helmet	Eye Protect.	Passenger Seat	Passenger Foot Rests	Mirror Required	Safety Inspection At Time of Reg.	Safety Inspection Periodically	Lights on all Times	Handlebar 15" Ht. Limit	Riding Prohibited Two Abreast	Riding Prohibited Between Lanes	Riding Prohibited Side Saddle
Alabama	X-A*	X		X									X
Alaska	X-B	X	X	X	X	X				X		X	X
Arizona	X	X	X	X	X	X				X	X	X	X
Arkansas		X	X	X	X		X						
California	X			X	X	X		X	X	X-E		X	X
Colorado	X	X	X			X		X-C	X-D		X	X	X
Connecticut	X-F	X	X	X	X	X		X					X
Delaware		X	X	X	X	X	X	X-C		X		X	X
Florida		X	X	X	X	X	X	X		X		X	X
Georgia	X	X	X	X	X	X	X	X	X	X		X	X
Hawaii	X	X	X	X	X		X	X				X	X
Idaho				X	X		X	X		X			X
Illinois	X			X	X	X			X	X	X	X	X
Indiana		X	X	X	X	X		X	X	X		X	X
Iowa		X		X	X	X	X-G			X		X	X
Kansas		X		X	X	X	X					X	X
Kentucky	X	X	X	X	X	X	X	X					X
Louisiana	X	X	X	X	X	X	X	X		X		X	X
Maine	X	X		X	X	X		X		X			X
Maryland	X	X	X	X	X	X	X			X	X	X	X
Massachusetts	X	X	X	X	X	X		X		X	X	X	X
Michigan	X	X	X-H	X		X						X	X
Minnesota	X	X	X	X	X	X		X		X-E			
Mississippi				X				X					
Missouri	X			X	X	X	X	X	X	X		X	
Montana		X		X	X	X		X					X

State	1	2	3	4	5	6	7	8	9	10	11	12	13	14
Nebraska	X	X	X	X	X			X			X			X
Nevada	X	X	X	X	X			X			X	X	X	X X X
New Hampshire	X	X	X	X	X			X			X	X	X	X X
New Jersey	X-I	X	X	X	X		X	X			X	X		
New Mexico	X	X	X	X	X		X	X		X	X	X	X	X X X
New York	X	X	X	X	X	X	X	X			X	X	X	X X
North Carolina			X	X	X		X	X				X		
North Dakota	X	X	X	X	X		X	X	X			X	X	X X X
Ohio	X	X	X	X	X			X	X		X	X	X	X X
Oklahoma	X-J	X	X	X	X		X-C	X	X-L			X		
Oregon	X	X	X	X				X			X-C	X		
Pennsylvania	X	X	X	X	X			X			X	X		
Rhode Island	X	X	X	X	X			X			X	X		
South Carolina	X	X	X	X	X		X	X			X	X	X	X X
South Dakota	X	X	X	X	X	X	X	X			X	X	X	X X X
Tennessee	X	X	X	X	X			X				X		X X X
Texas	X	X	X	X	X		X	X			X	X	X-E	X X
Utah	X-M	X-M	X	X	X		X	X	X-E		X	X		
Vermont	X	X	X	X	X	X	X	X			X	X	X	X X
Virginia	X	X	X	X	X		X	X			X	X		
Washington	X	X	X	X	X	X-N	X	X			X	X	X	X X
West Virginia		X	X	X	X	X	X	X			X	X	X	X X
Wisconsin	X	X	X	X	X			X	X		X	X	X	X
Wyoming			X	X	X			X			X	X		
Dist. of Col.	X	X	X	X	X		X	X			X	X	X	X

*A. Required if under 16 years
B. Required after July 1, 1973
C. Random Vehicle Inspection
D. Required after Jan. 1, 1975
E. Hand grips must be below shoulder height
F. Endorsement on license
G. First registration after sale
H. Required for speeds over 35 MPH
I. Operators & passengers under 18
J. 14–16 years old restricted as to hours, speed and horsepower
K. Operators & passengers under 21
L. Height limit 12 inches
M. On roads with speed limits over 35 MPH
N. At time of special endorsement on license

Source: *Guide to Safe Motorcycling*, American Automobile Association, Falls Church, Va., 1973, pp. 13, 14.

305

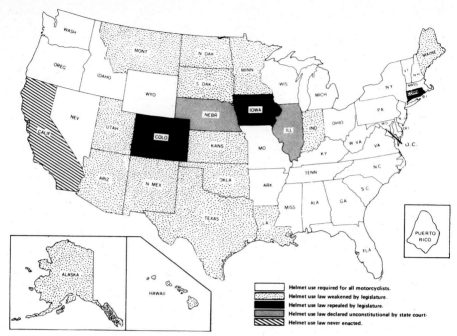

Figure 10-3 Motorcycle helmet-use laws. (Sources: *Accident Facts*, 1976, National Safety Council, Chicago,; *A Motorcycle Safety Helmet Study*, 1974, National Highway Traffic Safety Administration; *The Motorcycle in Traffic Accidents in Illinois*, March 1972, Illinois Department of Transportation; Highway Safety Acts of 1966 and 1976; Motorcycle Industry Council, Newport Beach, Calif.; Motorcycle Safety Foundation, Linthicum, Md.; Highway Users Federation, Reporter, Washington, June-July 1977.)

his family's subsistence. We do not understand a state of mind that permits plaintiffs to think that only he himself is concerned.

Head injuries account for the majority of motorcycle fatalities, and head protection is of critical importance. There is no doubt that helmet use reduces both the likelihood and severity of head injuries.

UNIFORM VEHICLE CODE AND MODEL TRAFFIC ORDINANCE, REVISED 1968[5]

ARTICLE XIII—Special rules for motorcycles (new, 1968.)

Sec. 11-1301—*Traffic laws apply to persons operating motorcycles*

Every person operating a motorcycle shall be granted all of the rights and shall be subject to all of the duties applicable to the driver of any other vehicle under this act, except as to special regulations in this article and except as to those provisions of this act which by their nature can have no application.

[5]National Committee on Uniform Traffic Laws and Ordinances, Washington, 1968.

Sec. 11-1302—*Riding on motorcycles*

a A person operating a motorcycle shall ride only upon the permanent and regular seat attached thereto, and such operator shall not carry any other person nor shall any other person ride on a motorcycle unless such motorcycle is designed to carry more than one person, in which event a passenger may ride upon the permanent and regular seat if designed for two persons, or upon another seat firmly attached to the motorcycle at the rear or side of the operator. (FORMERLY § 11-1103; REVISED, 1968.)

b A person shall ride upon a motorcycle only while sitting astride the seat, facing forward, with one leg on each side of the motorcycle.

c No person shall operate a motorcycle while carrying any package, bundle, or other article which prevents him from keeping both hands on the handlebars.

d No operator shall carry any person, nor shall any person ride, in a position that will interfere with the operation or control of the motorcycle or the view of the operator.

Sec. 11-1303—*Operating motorcycles on roadways laned for traffic*

a All motorcycles are entitled to full use of a lane and no motor vehicle shall be driven in such a manner as to deprive any motorcycle of the full use of a lane. This subsection shall not apply to motorcycles operated two abreast in a single lane.

b The operator of a motorcycle shall not overtake and pass in the same lane occupied by the vehicle being overtaken.

c No person shall operate a motorcycle between lanes of traffic or between adjacent lines or rows of vehicles.

d Motorcycles shall not be operated more than two abreast in a single lane.

e Subsections (b) and (c) shall not apply to police officers in the performance of their official duties.

Sec. 11-1304—*Clinging to other vehicles*

No person riding upon a motorcycle shall attach himself or the motorcycle to any other vehicle (or streetcar) on a roadway.

Sec. 11-1305—*Footrests and handlebars*

a Any motorcycle carrying a passenger, other than in a sidecar or enclosed cab, shall be equipped with footrests for such passenger.

b No person shall operate any motorcycle with handlebars more than 15 inches in height above that portion of the seat occupied by the operator.

Sec. 11-1306—*Equipment for motorcycle riders*

a No person shall operate or ride upon a motorcycle unless he is wearing protective headgear which complies with standards established by the commissioner.

b No person shall operate a motorcycle unless he is wearing an eye-protective device of a type approved by the commissioner, except when the motorcycle is equipped with a windscreen.

c This section shall not apply to persons riding within an enclosed cab.

d The commissioner is hereby authorized to approve or disapprove protective headgear and eye-protective devices required herein, and to issue and enforce regulations establishing standards and specifications for the approval thereof. The commissioner shall publish lists of all protective headgear and eye-protective devices by name and type which have been approved by him.

SUPPLEMENT II, 1976

ARTICLE V—Equipment on motorcycles and motor-driven cycles (New, 1968.)

Sec. 12-501—*Head lamps*

a Every motorcycle and every motor-driven cycle shall be equipped with at least one head lamp which shall comply with the requirements and limitations of the department. (REVISED, 1971 & 1975.)

b Deleted in 1975.

Sec. 12-502—*Tail lamps*

a Every motorcycle and motor-driven cycle shall have at least one tail lamp complying with regulations of the department. (REVISED, 1971 & 1975.)

b Either a tail lamp or a separate lamp shall be so constructed and placed as to illuminate with a white light the rear registration plate. Said lamp shall comply with regulations of the department. (REVISED, 1975.)

Sec. 12-503—*Reflectors*

Every motorcycle and motor-driven cycle shall carry on the rear either as part of the tail lamp or separately, at least one red reflector meeting the requirements of he department. (REVISED, 1975.)

Sec. 12-504—*Stop lamps*

Every motorcycle and motor-driven cycle shall be equipped with at least one stop lamp meeting the requirements of the department. (REVISED, 1975.)

Sec. 12-505—*Lamps on parked vehicles*

Section deleted in 1971.

Sec. 12-506—*Multiple-beam road-lighting equipment*

Section deleted in 1975.

Sec. 12-507—*Lighting equipment for motor-driven cycles*

Section deleted in 1975.

Sec. 12-508—*Brake equipment required*

Every motorcycle and motor-driven cycle shall comply with the provisions of § 12-301 except that motorcycles and motor-driven cycles need not be equipped with parking brakes. (REVISED, 1971 & 1975.)

b Deleted in 1975.

Sec. 12-509—*Performance ability of brakes*

Section deleted in 1975.

Sec. 12-510—*Brakes on motor-driven cycles*

(a) The commissioner is authorized to require an inspection of the braking system on any motor-driven cycle and to disapprove any such braking system on a vehicle which in his opinion is equipped with a braking system that is not designed or constructed as to insure reasonable and reliable performance in actual use. (REVISED, 1975.)

Sec. 12-511—*Other equipment*

Every motorcycle and every motor-driven cycle shall comply with the requirements and limitations of § 12-401 on horns and warning devices, § 12-402 on noise prevention and mufflers, § 12-403 on mirrors, § 12-405 on tires, and § 12-414 on emission control systems. (REVISED, 1971.)

U.S. DEPARTMENT OF TRANSPORTATION, HIGHWAY SAFETY PROGRAM STANDARD 3: MOTORCYCLE SAFETY

Purpose

To assure that motorcycles, motorcycle operators and their passengers meet standards which contribute to safe operation and protection from injuries.

Standard

For the purpose of this standard a motorcycle is defined as any motor-driven vehicle having a seat or saddle for the use of the rider and designed to travel on not more than three wheels in contact with the ground, but excluding tractors and vehicles on which the operator and passengers ride within an enclosed cab.

Each State shall have a motorcycle safety program to insure that only persons physically and mentally qualified will be licensed to operate a motorcycle; that protective safety equipment for drivers and passengers will be worn; and that the motorcycle meets standards for safety equipment.

    I. The program shall provide as a minimum that:
        A. Each person who operates a motorcycle: (1) Passes an examination or reexamination designed especially for motorcycle operation. (2) Holds a license issued specifically for motorcycle use or a regular license endorsed for each purpose.
        B. Each motorcycle operator wears an approved safety helmet and eye protection when he is operating his vehicle on streets and highways.
        C. Each motorcycle passenger wears an approved safety helmet, and is provided with a seat and footrest.
        D. Each motorcycle is equipped with a rearview mirror.
        E. Each motorcycle is inspected at the time it is initially registered and at least annually thereafter, or in accordance with the State's inspection requirements (see Periodic Motor Vehicle Inspection Standard).
    II. The program shall be periodically evaluated by the State for its effectiveness in terms of reductions in accidents and their end results, and the National Highway Traffic Safety Administration shall be provided with an evaluation summary.

MOPEDS (MOTORIZED BICYCLES)[6]

The Moped is the newest type of motor vehicle to become popular in this country. (See Figure 10-6.) The term Moped is derived from the words "motor" and "pedals." The Moped is a cross between a bicycle and a motorcycle. It can

---

[6]Much of the information in this section is from the National Safety Council's Safety Education Data Sheet No. 101, *Mopeds*.

be mounted, pedaled, steered, and stopped very much like a bicycle. Like a motorcycle, it has a motor, automatic transmission, suspension system, muffler, drum brakes, padded saddle, and a heavy frame and tires.

The Moped's chief appeal in an energy-conscious age is economy. Mopeds get 120 to 200 miles per gallon of gasoline from their small (50-cc) two-stroke engines, which are limited to about 2 horsepower. The top speed is about 30 miles per hour depending upon engine size, which is regulated in states with special Moped legislation. Exhaust emissions are so low that Mopeds are exempt from federal antipollution regulations. The noise level is also very low, lower than that of conventional motorcycles and automobiles. With gasoline prices and other automobile-related expenses rising dramatically, the Moped provides an inexpensive, attractive transportation alternative for the home-to-train commuter, the student, housewife, and retiree, the one-car family, or anyone looking for low-cost, short-range transportation. A further rise in the price of gasoline would precipitate a dramatic increase in Moped sales. At present, it is estimated that 150,000 Mopeds are in use in this country, with the industry forecasting sales of up to 200,000 annually and a goal of 4 million to 5 million annually in the early 1980s.

ACCIDENT STATISTICS

Traffic accident investigation forms do not categorize vehicles as Mopeds. Mopeds may be categorized as bicycles or motorcycles, depending on the reporting officer. European experience shows that Mopeds are safer than automobiles or motorcycles. In France, where about 10 percent of the population use Mopeds daily for transportation, the fatality rate was shown to be 6½ times lower than the rate for motorcycles, and approximately 1½ times lower than the rate for automobiles. However, a study by the European Conference of Ministers of Transport reported a death rate (fatalities per 100,000 vehicles) of approximately 8 for bicycles, 51 for Mopeds, and 171 for motorcycles (Figure 10-4).

One must use caution in making assumptions from these figures, because lifestyles in Europe are different from lifestyles in the United States. The Moped is a familiar vehicle that was a part of the transportation system in most European countries many years before the automobile. There are also special separate driving lanes for Mopeds, particularly in rural, open-road areas.

LEGISLATIVE IMPLICATIONS

There is a great deal of controversy regarding the Moped. Should it be defined as a bicycle or a motorcycle? The National Highway Traffic Safety Administration places Mopeds in the motorcycle category, and requires them to meet the same safety standards as motorcycles. The Uniform Vehicle Code also classifies Mopeds as motor vehicles.

In states without special legislation, Mopeds are usually classified as

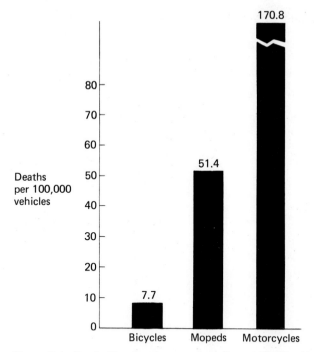

Figure 10-4 Bicycle, Moped, and motorcycle deaths per 100,000 vehicles, 1971—Germany, Belgium, Denmark, France, Netherlands, Switzerland. (Sources: European Conference of Ministers of Transport; *Report by the Committee of Deputies on Road Safety Problems concerning Two-Wheeled Vehicles*, Paris, 1974; Insurance Institute for Highway Safety. *Status Report*, Vol. 11, No. 18, November 30, 1976.

motorcycles and must meet all legal requirements for road use. Every state should require a license that would test the knowledge and skills of the operator. Some states require a special test and license, and have minimum-age requirements. Before purchasing a Moped, it is advisable to check with state or local licensing authorities to determine their legality.

OPERATION

Mopeds are fairly simple to operate. The controls can be learned while pedaling the vehicle in a parking lot or other off-street area. The engine is started by pedaling a few strokes, turning the ignition switch on the handlebar, and turning the throttle. Once the Moped is underway, the automatic transmission takes over the shifting of gears, and the operator can devote full attention to the traffic situation. Brake levers are mounted on handlebars, as on a bicycle. (Figure 10-5) Because of low power the Moped does not move out into the traffic as quickly as other vehicles, particularly on steep hills and long inclines. Pedaling a few quick strokes from a stop helps increase Moped acceleration.

Mopeds are strictly one-person vehicles, and passengers should not be carried. Mopeds have the same instability as other two-wheel vehicles on

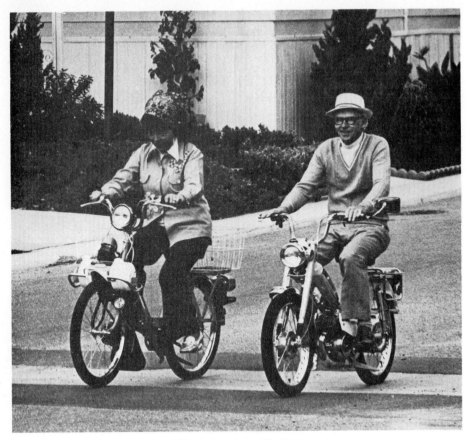

Figure 10-5 Courtesy Motorized Bicycle Association, Washington.

slippery surfaces. The same safety methods of driving a motorcycle apply to Mopeds. Driving with a headlight on, bright clothing, and a bicycle flag will help increase conspicuousness. Wearing a helmet, whether required by law or not, is good common sense.

General maintanence of a Moped can usually be accomplished by anyone who can maintain a power lawnmower or bicycle. If one is not mechanically inclined, it is best to have the servicing done where the Moped was purchased.

AREAS OF CONCERN

Safety experts predict two kinds of problems when the Moped boom arrives. First, young, unlicensed, uninsured teenagers with no background as operators of motor vehicles in traffic will move into the traffic stream on low-powered vehicles. These drivers' lack of experience or limited experience on a bicycle, plus the natural exuberance of youth, may produce a new traffic hazard. Second, although banned on expressways, Mopeds will probably be used on busy major thoroughfares and crowded secondary roads, where their low visibility and speed make them extremely vulnerable.

To minimize the dangers involved in driving a Moped, a minimum level of competency must be achieved before a Moped operator is allowed in traffic. Until education and licensing requirements are established, parents and dealers must make sure that the young driver is mature, has adequate psychophysical and physical qualifications, and has the knowledge, skills, and attitude of social responsibility needed for safe operation of a Moped.

The above information has been compiled from reliable sources but is not inclusive of all safety measures. As the use of Mopeds increases, more information will become available to help attack and study the consequent safety problems. More information can be obtained from the Motorized Bicycle Association, Washington. Information regarding state motor vehicle laws governing Mopeds can be obtained from the American Association of Motor Vehicle Administrators, Washington.

COLLEGE AND UNIVERSITY MOTORCYCLE SAFETY

Because colleges and universities have a large concentration of motorcycles, it may be desirable to develop a university motorcycle code to ensure safe operation. The following items are suggested for such a code:

   I. Definitions and designators
      A. Title of code
      B. Legislative body

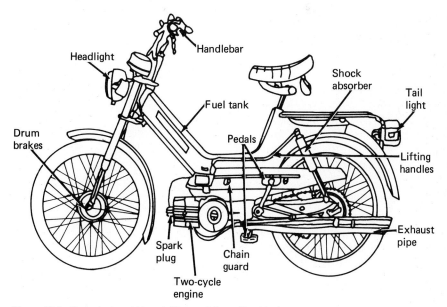

Figure 10-6 Basic design of Moped. (Source: Tribune Graphics.)

      C. Administrating agency
      D. Definitions of words and phrases
          1. Campus
          2. Minor
          3. Motor vehicle
          4. Motorcycle
          5. Operator
          6. Parental consent
          7. Park
          8. School day
          9. Sidecar
          10. Stop
          11. Store
          12. Student

II. Registration of motorcycles
      A. Procedures for registration
      B. Parental consent of minors
      C. Registration sticker
      D. Time for registration
      E. Effective period
      F. Fee
      G. Application forms
      H. State license requirements
      I. Insurance coverage

III. Equipment required
      A. Unsafe or improperly equipped motorcycles prohibited
      B. Horn
      C. Brakes
      D. Head lamps
      E. Rear lights
      F. Brake lights
      G. Rear view mirrors
      H. Handlebar height
      I. Muffler
      J. Windshield
      K. Fenders

IV. Other requirements for proper operation of motorcycles
      A. Special operator's license
      B. Required obedience to traffic laws
      C. Headgear
      D. Eye protection
      E. Adequate footwear
      F. Operator seating requirements
      G. Passenger seating and capacity
      H. Proper facility for carrying objects

  V. Rules of the road
    A. Hand signals
    B. Speed restrictions
    C. Passing on the right
    D. Passing on the left
    E. Riding the white line prohibited
    F. Weaving through traffic
    G. Approaching too closely
    H. Passing stopped vehicles
 VI. Parking
    A. Where parking is permitted
    B. Method of parking
    C. Where parking is prohibited within parking areas
    D. Storing and storage areas
    E. Special parking areas
    F. Special parking privileges for necessity
    G. Parking meters
    H. Rented spaces
    I. Meter time limits
    J. Impounding
VII. Violations
    A. Standard assessment
    B. Moving violations
    C. Payment of assessment
    D. Multiple violations
    E. Flagrant violators
    F. Revocation of driving privileges
    G. Appeals

A special motorcycle safety committee may be appointed to enlarge upon the code for specific situations. The basic objectives should be kept in mind:

1 To promote the safe operation of motorcycles and to reduce the severity and number of accidents

2 To minimize the interference of motorcycles with the educational processes of the university

3 To provide an effective and equitable program for the development of motorcycle facilities

The code suggested above was developed in detail by a special motorcycle committee at the University of Illinois at Champaign-Urbana. The committee was composed of members of the undergraduate and graduate student body, the nonacademic staff, administrative officers, and the academic faculty. The committee represented areas of competency in law, medicine, traffic engineering, driver education, law enforcement, and motorcycle dealership.

The code applies to all students who are regularly enrolled in the university, to all university staff and faculty, to all employees of the university and of related agencies located on the campus, and to all other persons who use, park, or store a motorcycle on the campus.

LEARNING EXPERIENCES

The following learning activities should provide experiences that will increase the teacher's understanding of motorcycle safety.

1 Formulate a list of acts performed by the motorcyclist and motorist that are not conducive to safe traffic.

2 Develop a motorcycle code of conduct, and have it adopted by the school, college, or university. Have it published in the school newspaper.

3 Conduct an observation survey of motorcyclists and Moped operators to determine whether they are:
  a. Wearing helmets
  b. Using eye protectors
  c. Properly clothed
  d. Driving safely
  e. Signaling their intentions

4 Teach a beginner to drive, using a prescribed step-by-step lesson plan.

5 Develop a teaching unit, which could be included in a high school driver education course, dealing with one of the following topics:
  a. The relationship between the motorcyclist and automobile driver
  b. Rules of the road that affect just the cyclist
  c. Defensive driving for the cyclist as it relates to the motor vehicle

6 Formulate a list of laws as they relate specifically to the motorcyclist.

7 Visit a motorcycle repair shop to inquire how to keep your motorcycle in good, safe condition.

8 Observe motorcyclists on your campus at a busy intersection for a 30-minute period, and report your findings to the class.

9 Take a field trip to a local traffic court where cases involving motorcycle accidents can be observed.

10 Invite a local motorcycle dealer and mechanic to describe the maintenance checks and procedures that a motorcycle owner should know.

11 Invite a local police officer to talk about motorcycle use and the major causes of motorcycle accidents.

12 Invite a member of the driver's licensing division to discuss the motorcycle driver's license examination.

13 Debate the helmet-use law.

14 Analyze the death and severity rates of states requiring the use of helmets and states with no such laws.

SELECTED REFERENCES

Aaron, James E. and Markland K. Strasser: *Driving Task Instruction, Dual-Control Simulation and Multiple-Car.* The Macmillan Company, New York, 1974, chap. 13, pp. 316–339

American Automobile Association Washington:
Guide to Safe Cycling., 1973, 47 pp.
Sportsmanlike Driving, 7th teacher's ed., chap. 11, McGraw-Hill Book Company, New York, 1975

American Driver and Traffic Safety Education Association: *Politicies and Guidelines for Motorcycle Safety Education: On-Street Riders,* 1974, 39 pp.

Bennett, Shaun: *A Trail Rider's Guide to the Environment,* The American Motorcycle Association, Westerville, Ohio, 1973

Kelley, Albert Benjamin: "Motorcycles and Public Apathy," *American Journal of Public Health,* vol. 66, no. 5, May, 1976

Metropolitan Life Insurance Co.: "Motorcycle Accident Fatalities," *Statistical Bulletin,* August, 1973

Motorcycle Industry Council, Inc.: *Reading Before Riding and Your Rithmetic Will Add Up to Motorcycle Safety, Congratulations to the Proud New Owner of a Trailbike*

Motorcycle Safety Foundation:
Safety Series Booklets:
Get Into Gear, 1974
Questions about Motorcycles and Safety? Ask a Friend, 1974
Riding Tips for the Motorcyclist, 1974
Sharing the Roadway, Motorist and Motorcyclists in Traffic, 1974
What You Should Know about Motorcycle Helmets, 1977.
Instructional materials
Guide to Motorcycle Range Design, 1977
How to Start a Motorcycle Safety Education Program in Your School and Community
Instructional Objectives in Motorcycle Safety Education, 1974
Instructor's Guide, 1976
Motorcycle Loans for Safety and Education
Motorcycle Rider Course, Motorcycle Rider Text Book, 1976
Motorcycle Safety Education Recognition Program
Research
Instructional Objectives in Motorcycle Safety Education, 1974
Motorcycle Task Analysis, 1974
References Resources
A Summary Report: Analysis of Motorcycle Accident Reports and Statistics, 1974
Licensing
Motorcycle Operator Licensing Plan, 1975
State Procedures for the Licensing of Motorcycle Operators, 1974

National Committee on Uniform Traffic Laws and Ordinances, Washington:
Model Traffic Ordinances, rev., 1968
Uniform Vehicle Code, rev., 1968
Supplement II, 1976

National Safety Council, Chicago:
Accident Facts, current ed.
Defensive Driving Course, motorcycle supplement
Motorcycles, Safety Education Data Sheet No. 98, rev.
Mo-Peds, Safety Education Data Sheet No. 101
Family Safety, Two Wheelers Are Tricky, 1975-6, Winter.

University of Wisconsin Madison: A programmed instruction series, 1972.
   Series 1: *Introduction to Motorcycles*
   Series 2: *Learning to Ride*
   Series 3: *Conditions and Procedures for Cycling*
   Series 4: *Motorcycle Maintenance and Modification*
   Series 5: *What Motorists Should Know about Cyclists*
U.S. Department of Transportation, National Highway Traffic Safety Administration, Washington: *The Development and Evaluation of a Motorcycle Skill Test, Manual, and Knowledge Test,* 1976 Available from National Technical Information Service, Springfield, Virginia
Highway Safety Program Standard 3, "Motorcycle Safety," July, 1973
Yamaha International Corporation: *Common Sense Tips for Safe Sportcycling,* Montebello, Calif., 1974, 30 pp.

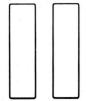

Highway Safety

OVERALL OBJECTIVE:

The student should appreciate the efforts being made by many organizations to reduce highway accidents, injuries, and fatalities.

INSTRUCTIONAL OBJECTIVES:

After completing this chapter the student will be able to:

1 Describe the nature and extent of highway accidents in the United States.
2 Discuss the programs sponsored by the National Highway Traffic Safety Administration.
3 Explain how human error can be a causative factor in highway accidents.
4 List the basic principles of the defensive driving course developed by the National Safety Council.
5 Discuss the relationship between alcohol and motor-vehicle accidents.
6 List some of the changes in the highway environment which help reduce the frequency and severity of automobile accidents.
7 Cite evidence which demonstrates a relationship between the national speed limit of 55 miles per hour and the reduction of highway fatalities.
8 Discuss the safety potential for the vehicles and equipment of the future.

THE PROBLEM OF HIGHWAY SAFETY

The United States has a highway system of nearly 4 million miles. More than 140 million vehicles are registered, with each vehicle driven approximately 10,000 miles per year. Drivers in this country clock more than 1 trillion miles annually, enough to complete more than 2 million trips to the moon. These highway figures are staggering, but even more important are the following:[1]

[1] *Accident Facts,* The National Safety Council, Chicago, 1977, p. 40.

Highway deaths in 1976	46,700
Disabling injuries in 1976	1,800,000
Cost of highway accidents in 1976	$24,700,000,000

Motor-vehicle death rates show considerable variation among the 50 states. The rates may be calculated according to the number of vehicles registered, the population of a state, or the vehicle-miles driven within the state. Owing to the mobility of our population, rates calculated on the basis of vehicle-miles driven offer the most useful information. Table 11-1 presents the number of fatalities and the mileage death rate for 1975 and 1976. A visual representation of the 1976 motor-vehicle death rates by state appears as Figure 11-1.

Highway statistics may be analyzed according to rural versus urban and day versus night fatalities. Two-thirds of the fatalities occur in rural areas. Surprisingly, half the motor-vehicle fatalities in urban areas are incurred by pedestrians. Although motor-vehicle fatalities occur more frequently in rural areas, nonfatal injuries are more frequent in cities. In both urban and rural areas most fatalities occur at night, even though fewer people walk and drive then. The nighttime death rate for both areas is more than three times the daytime rate (Figure 11-2).

Fatalities have been classified according to an hourly distribution by days of the week. In Table 11-2 the weekdays are grouped together, and their fatality

TABLE 11–1

Motor Vehicle Deaths and Mileage Death Rates by State, 1975–1976

| | Motor-Vehicle *Traffic* Deaths (Place of Accident) | | | |
| | Number | | Mileage Rate* | |
State	1976	1975	1976	1975
Total U.S.†	46,700		3.3	3.5
Alabama	1,032	975	3.9	3.9
Alaska	127	114	3.5	4.5
Arizona	737	670	4.4	4.2
Arkansas	535	566	3.7	4.1
California	4,489	4,189	3.2	3.2
Colorado	633	591	3.7	3.6
Connecticut	419	398	2.2	2.2
Delaware	121	127	3.2	3.5
Dist. of Col.	60	74	1.9	2.4
Florida	2,015	2,040	3.1	3.3
Georgia	1,290	1,391	3.1	3.5
Hawaii	149	146	3.5	3.5
Idaho	282	284	4.4	4.8
Illinois	2,073	2,084	3.2	3.4
Indiana	1,262	1,135	3.2	3.0
Iowa	785	674	3.9	3.4

TABLE 11-1 (*continued*)
Motor Vehicle Deaths and Mileage Death Rates by State, 1975–1976

	Motor-Vehicle *Traffic* Deaths (Place of Accident)			
	Number		Mileage Rate*	
State	1976	1975	1976	1975
Kansas	563	517	3.5	3.3
Kentucky	874	882	3.3	3.6
Louisiana	967	940	4.5	4.6
Maine	227	226	3.0	3.3
Maryland	677	691	2.6	2.8
Massachusetts	809	884	2.5	3.0
Michigan	1,953	1,811	3.2	3.1
Minnesota	807	777	3.0	3.0
Mississippi	677	612	4.4	4.3
Missouri	1,203	1,075	3.7	3.5
Montana	300	298	4.9	5.2
Nebraska	402	376	3.4	3.4
Nevada	224	220	4.8	4.9
New Hampshire	159	151	2.8	2.9
New Jersey	1,053	1,080	2.0	2.2
New Mexico	549	568	5.2	5.7
New York	2,359	2,458	3.5	3.8
North Carolina	1,521	1,522	3.9	4.2
North Dakota	183	169	3.9	3.8
Ohio	1,930	1,809	2.9	2.8
Oklahoma	838	763	3.4	3.4
Oregon	636	574	3.7	3.6
Pennsylvania	2,025	2,082	2.9	3.3
Rhode Island	121	112	2.1	2.0
South Carolina	820	821	3.7	4.0
South Dakota	224	198	4.1	3.9
Tennessee	1,146	1,145	3.3	3.5
Texas	3,230	3,429	3.6	4.1
Utah	254	275	3.0	3.5
Vermont	117	144	3.4	4.3
Virginia	1,020	1,030	2.8	3.0
Washington	823	771	3.2	3.2
West Virginia	497	486	4.5	4.6
Wisconsin	947	940	3.1	3.3
Wyoming	260	213	6.1	5.8
Puerto Rico‡	499	490	6.3	7.2
Guam‡	23			

*The mileage death rate is the number of deaths per 100,000,000 vehicle miles; the population death rate is the number of deaths per 100,000 population.
†Includes both traffic and nontraffic motor-vehicle deaths. See definitions of traffic and nontraffic accidents on inside of back cover.
‡Not included in Total U.S.
Source: Motor-Vehicle *Traffic* Deaths from state traffic authorities; *Total* Motor-Vehicle Deaths from National Center for Health Statistics. Reprinted in *Accident Facts,* National Safety Council, Chicago, 1977, p. 63.

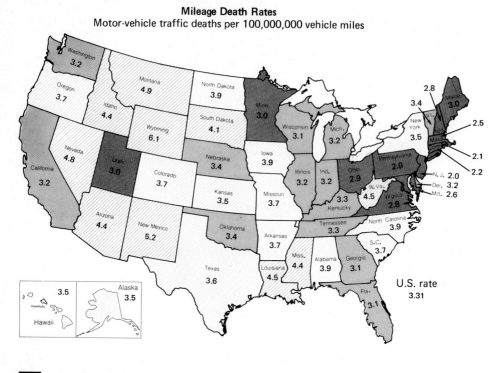

Mileage Death Rates
Motor-vehicle traffic deaths per 100,000,000 vehicle miles

■ Below 3.1—12 states
▒ 3.1 to 3.4—14 states
□ 3.5 to 3.9—14 states
▨ 4.0 and over—10 states

Figure 11-1 Motor vehicle mileage death rate by state, 1976. (Source: *Accident Facts*, 1977, p. 62, National Safety Council, Chicago.)

rates may be compared with the rates for each day of the weekend. The hours between 4 P.M. and 2 A.M. have the highest fatality rates, whereas the highest rates for all accidents occur between noon and 6 P.M. The two hours of the week when fatal accidents are most likely to occur are Friday at 11 P.M. and Sunday at 1 A.M. (Table 11-2).

Motor-vehicle death rates can also be classified according to the month of year. The first 3 months of the year have the lowest death rates. A gradually increasing rate is observed throughout the remainder of the year, except for a slight drop in December. Although these rates do not vary appreciably from month to month, it is noteworthy that the safest months are in the winter (Table 11-3).

Fatalities and death rates are demonstrably higher during holiday periods. No single holiday appears to be consistently more dangerous than the others.

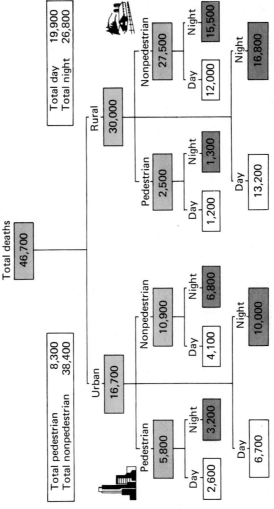

Figure 11-2 Principal classes of motor vehicle deaths. (Source: Accident Facts, 1977, p. 41, National Safety Council, Chicago.)

Over the 19 days covering the major holidays in 1976, nearly 3,700 people died in motor-vehicle accidents (Table 11-4).

There are approximately 36,000 miles in the United States interstate highway system. More than 250 billion vehicle-miles are driven on this network annually. The death rate per 100 million vehicle-miles of interstate travel is approximately 1.4. The National Safety Council estimates that if interstate-highway deaths had occurred at the same rate as deaths on all the nation's highways (3.3 per 100 million vehicle miles), there would have been 4,800 additional deaths in 1976.

Travel on turnpikes totaled 28.7 billion miles in 1976. The death rate on these highways was 1.2 per 100 million vehicle-miles. The fatality rates for interstate highways and turnpikes stand in marked contrast to the rate of 4.7 for rural roads.

TABLE 11-2
Hourly Distribution of Accidents by Day of The Week, 1976

Hour of Day*	Fatal Accidents					All Accidents				
	Total	Mon.–Thurs.	Fri.	Sat.	Sun.	Total	Mon.–Thurs.	Fri.	Sat.	Sun.
Total	100.0%	100.0%	100.0%	100.0%	100.0%	100.0%	100.0%	100.0%	100.0%	100.0%
Midnight	5.3	4.3	3.6	6.9	8.0	3.3	2.5	2.5	5.0	6.0
1:00 a.m.	5.9	4.3	3.8	8.1	10.0	2.7	1.7	1.8	4.6	6.3
2:00 a.m.	4.9	3.4	3.1	7.0	8.6	2.2	1.3	1.4	4.0	5.1
3:00 a.m.	2.8	1.8	1.8	4.5	4.7	1.3	0.7	0.8	2.3	3.3
4:00 a.m.	2.0	1.4	1.2	2.9	3.4	0.9	0.6	0.5	1.5	2.0
5:00 a.m.	1.7	1.5	1.2	2.1	2.3	0.7	0.6	0.5	1.0	1.3
6:00 a.m.	2.3	2.6	2.4	1.7	1.7	1.5	1.9	1.4	1.0	1.1
7:00 a.m.	2.2	3.0	2.3	1.3	1.3	4.0	5.4	3.8	1.4	1.2
8:00 a.m.	2.3	2.9	2.5	1.8	1.2	4.3	5.6	4.2	2.0	1.4
9:00 a.m.	2.4	2.8	2.4	1.8	1.9	3.5	4.0	3.2	2.9	2.5
10:00 a.m.	2.8	3.4	2.5	2.2	2.1	4.1	4.3	3.7	4.2	3.2
11:00 a.m.	2.9	3.5	2.3	2.5	2.3	5.0	5.2	4.7	5.4	3.9
Noon	3.9	4.1	3.0	4.2	3.8	5.5	5.6	5.2	5.7	5.4
1:00 p.m.	3.8	4.5	3.6	2.7	3.3	5.7	5.7	5.5	5.9	5.6
2:00 p.m.	4.4	5.0	4.4	3.3	3.8	6.3	6.4	6.3	6.0	6.0
3:00 p.m.	4.9	5.8	5.0	3.4	3.9	7.8	8.5	8.1	6.3	6.4
4:00 p.m.	5.3	6.0	5.9	4.3	4.3	8.4	9.2	9.1	6.3	6.6
5:00 p.m.	5.7	6.3	5.9	5.1	4.3	7.8	8.4	8.3	5.8	6.5
6:00 p.m.	5.9	6.1	6.0	5.5	5.6	5.5	5.3	5.8	5.5	5.9
7:00 p.m.	6.1	6.1	6.3	5.9	5.8	4.7	4.4	5.1	5.2	5.1
8:00 p.m.	5.2	5.2	5.9	5.1	4.6	3.9	3.5	4.2	4.5	4.4
9:00 p.m.	5.9	5.7	8.2	5.6	4.9	3.8	3.5	4.3	4.3	4.1
10:00 p.m.	5.3	5.0	7.5	5.3	4.0	3.6	3.0	4.6	4.4	3.6
11:00 p.m.	6.1	5.3	9.2	6.8	4.2	3.5	2.7	5.0	4.8	3.1

*Hour beginning.
Source: *Accident Facts*, National Safety Council, Chicago, 1977, p. 50.

TABLE 11–3
Motor-Vehicle Deaths, Mileage and Rates by Month

| Month | Deaths | | | | | | 1974–1976 Average | | |
| | Year | | | | Percent Changes | | % of Deaths | % of Miles | Death Rate* |
	1973	1974	1975	1976	1973–1976	1975–1976			
Total	55,511	46,402	45,853	46,700	−16%	+2%	100.0%	100.0%	3.4
January	3,932	3,020	3,191	3,200	−17	+†	6.8	7.4	3.1
February	3,559	2,699	2,949	3,090	−13	+5	6.3	6.9	3.1
March	4,429	3,311	3,405	3,330	−29	−2	7.2	8.0	3.1
April	4,492	3,425	3,412	3,700	−18	+8	7.6	8.1	3.2
May	4,963	3,678	4,145	4,320	−13	+4	8.7	8.7	3.5
June	5,150	4,243	4,190	4,120	−20	−2	9.0	8.8	3.5
July	5,228	4,401	4,437	4,770	− 9	+8	9.8	9.3	3.6
August	5,260	4,718	4,460	4,450	−15	−†	9.8	9.5	3.6
September	4,960	4,256	4,059	4,150	−16	+2	9.0	8.4	3.7
October	5,167	4,465	4,016	4,360	−16	+9	9.3	8.6	3.7
November	4,453	4,273	3,896	3,650	−18	−6	8.5	8.1	3.6
December	3,918	3,913	3,693	3,560	− 9	−4	8.0	8.2	3.4

*Deaths per 100,000,000 vehicle miles.
†Less than 0.5 percent.
Source: 1973–1975 deaths from National Center for Health Statistics. 1976 deaths are NSC estimates. Reported in *Accident Facts*, National Safety Council, Chicago, 1977, p. 51.

THE NATIONAL HIGHWAY TRAFFIC ADMINISTRATION

In 1966, Congress passed the Highway Safety Act (see Chapter 6) and created a National Safety Agency located in the Department of Commerce. The agency was mandated to coordinate a national highway safety program. Federal funds were made available, which encouraged states to comply with national highway safety standards.

A companion bill, the National Traffic and Motor Vehicle Safety Act, created the National Traffic Safety Agency, also located in the Department of Commerce. The purpose of this agency is the reduction of traffic accidents, injuries, and deaths. Authority was granted to establish federal motor-vehicle safety standards. The agency was empowered to determine whether vehicles were in compliance with these standards. If a vehicle failed to meet the standards or had safety defects, the agency could require the manufacturer to repair or replace the defective parts or the entire vehicle.

Later that year (1966) both agencies were redesignated as bureaus and assigned to the newly created Department of Transportation (DOT). By executive order, the bureaus were combined to form the National Highway Safety Bureau. In 1970 the bureau was made an operating administration and given its current title, the National Highway Traffic Safety Administration (NHTSA).

The NHTSA has directed its efforts toward areas that have the greatest

TABLE 11–4
Motor-Vehicle Deaths on Major Holidays, 1961–1976

Year	Memorial Day		Fourth of July		Labor Day		Thanksgiving		Christmas		New Year's	
	Immed. Deaths*	Total Deaths†	Immed. Deaths	Total Deaths	Immed. Deaths	Total Deaths	Immed. Deaths	Total Deaths	Immed. Deaths	Total Deaths	Immed. Deaths	Total Deaths
1961	462 (4)	580	509 (4)	635	386 (3)	515			523 (3)	700	337 (3)	450
1964	431 (3)	575	510 (3)	680	535 (3)	715			596 (3)	800	474 (3)	630
1965	490 (3)	655	557 (3)	740	574 (3)	765			720 (3)	960	562 (3)	750
1966	542 (3)	720	577 (3)	770	636 (3)	850			600 (3)	800	468 (3)	620
1967	608 (4)	760	732 (4)	915	606 (3)	810	764 (4)	960	684 (3)	910	372 (3)	500
1968	628 (4)	790	616 (4)	770	688 (3)	915	696 (4)	870	231 (1)	355	170 (1)	260
1969	597 (3)	800	609 (3)	810	612 (3)	815	651 (4)	815	603 (4)	755	481 (4)	600
1970	391 (2)	560	540 (3)	720	612 (3)	815	600 (4)	750	504 (3)	670	454 (3)	610
1971	557 (3)	740	635 (3)	850	616 (3)	820	679 (4)	850	645 (3)	860	456 (3)	610
1972	585 (3)	780	760 (4)	950	602 (3)	800	542 (4)	680	595 (3)	790	451 (3)	600
1973	539 (3)	720	192 (1)	295	559 (3)	750	496 (4)	620	520 (4)	650	446 (4)	560
1974	392 (3)	520	549 (4)	690	516 (3)	690	394 (4)	490	204 (1)	310	194 (1)	300
1975	425 (3)	570	508 (3)	680	407 (3)	540	508 (4)	630	412 (4)	515	402 (4)	502
1976	455 (3)	610	523 (3)	700	526 (3)	700			441 (3)	590	339 (3)	450

*"Immediate" deaths include only those which occurred by midnight of the last day of the holiday period. "Total" deaths include immediate deaths plus an estimate of delayed deaths—those which occur within twelve months after the day of accident (they are charged back to the day of the accident).

†Figures in parentheses show number of full days in each holiday period. Deaths are for these days plus the last six hours of the preceding day.

Source: Immediate deaths, press associations; total deaths, NSC estimates. Reported in *Accident Facts*, National Safety Council, Chicago, 1977, p. 57.

potential for the reduction of highway accidents: alcohol, police traffic services, emergency medical services, driver licensing, and driver education. Some of the agency's activities include:

1 The development of an accurate, portable breath-testing device

2 The development of a systematic approach to the arrest, prosecution, and referral to remedial programs of drunk drivers

3 The development of alcohol safety action projects (ASAPs), which utilize enforcement techniques, court referrals to rehabilitation programs, and close follow-ups on subsequent driving records. These projects are 100 percent federally funded. They demonstrate the effectiveness of alcohol counter-measures.

4 Support of research to determine whether drugs, both legal and illegal, contribute to a disproportionate share of highway accidents

5 The development of design specifications for ambulances

6 Assumption of responsibility for promoting the 911 emergency tele-phone system

7 Support of research projects to examine vehicle crashworthiness, restraint systems, and experimental safety vehicles

8 Implementation of safety programs on 11 Indian reservations, where motor-vehicle fatality rates are several times higher than the national average

9 Sponsorship of research on school-bus safety (in the 1973–1974 school year there were 42,000 school bus accidents, resulting in 6,000 injuries and 210 fatalities)[2]

10 Research and development activities in support of motorcycle safety

11 Development of curricula and supportive materials for driver education

Since 1966 there has been a steady reduction in the highway death rate. In 1966 the fatality rate per 100 million miles driven was 5.58. In 1972 the rate was 4.35, and by 1976 it was 3.31. Today, fewer people are killed because of poorly designed guardrails and other roadside hazards. Law-enforcement techniques and equipment are more effective. Most automobiles now on the road were built in accordance with established motor-vehicle safety standards. As a result, fewer people are being fatally injured by unyielding steering columns, shat-tered glass, or ejection from the passenger compartment.

Although the reduction in death rate cannot be attributed solely to the efforts of the National Highway Traffic Safety Administration, the cumulative positive effect of NHTSA activities cannot be denied.

As discussed in Chapter 2, accidents are usually the result of multiple causes. Highway accidents involve three major factors: human error, environ-mental hazards, and unsafe equipment. Of the three, human error is probably the most important. The National Highway Traffic Safety Administration reports

---

[2]U.S. Department of Transportation, *A Digest of Activities of the National Highway Traffic Safety Administra-tion,* 1976, p. 18.

that it is a definite factor in 77 percent and a probable factor in 95.3 percent of all motor-vehicle accidents. In descending order of frequency, the errors which most often result in highway accidents are improper lookout, excessive speed, inattention, improper evasive action, and false assumptions.[3]

REDUCTION OF HUMAN ERROR

Driving is a responsibility that demands concentration. But some motorists consider driving to be so "easy" that they do not devote complete attention to the task. This false sense of security is reinforced by the fact that passenger cars have become so automatic that they seem nearly capable of driving themselves. However, to operate a vehicle weighing over 1,000 pounds at speeds of up to 55 miles per hour is to be at the controls of a tremendous amount of force. Human morality should dictate that anything less than full concentration is unacceptable.

DEFENSIVE DRIVING

One way to improve your driving skills is to enroll in a defensive-driving course. Developed by the National Safety Council, these 8-hour programs teach people how to avoid accidents. The programs help their graduates achieve a sustained level of accident-free driving. The stress is on "preventability." The course, which is taught in more than twenty countries, emphasizes that driving is a mental task which involves planned movement in harmony with other units of traffic. A study of 8,000 defensive-driving graduates found that the group had 32.8 percent fewer accidents per year after completion of the course. Recently, Governor Rubin Askew of Florida signed a bill that requires all drivers who have had their licenses suspended to successfully complete a defensive-driving course before their licenses are reissued.

Among the more than 7 million graduates of defensive-driving courses are professional race-car drivers such as Wally Dallenbach, Tom Sneva, and Bill Vukovich. In an interview with Hayden Lynch, Mr. Dallenbach said, "When you're on the race course there's a great deal more courtesy than you find on the highways." Mr. Sneva noted that "on the track we don't have to worry about pedestrians, intersections, or drunk drivers."[4]

Some of the basic principles of defensive driving have been detailed by the American Automobile Association in a pamphlet entitled *Defensive Driving—Managing Time and Space*. Among the AAA's principles are:

1 The greatest danger is in front of you. Therefore, maintain an adequate distance between yourself and the vehicles in front of you.

2 Your position in traffic should be determined by the availability of

---

[3]Ibid., p. 41.

[4]Hayden Lynch, "Champion's Highway Safety Team Takes Defensive Driving Course," *Traffic Safety*, pp. 8–9, March, 1977.

escape routes. *Lateral positioning* means that you maintain as much space as possible between your vehicle and potential hazards such as other vehicles, pedestrians, animals, and roadside obstacles.

3 Adequate *lead time* is an important factor in planning a path of travel. At 30 miles per hour, the recommended 12 seconds of lead time means that you have planned a path of travel for 528 feet, approximately one city block.

4 Your speed and location must be adjusted to avoid having to contend with too many hazards at the same time.

5 At times, it is necessary to compromise to avoid collision.

6 Although drivers are expected to behave appropriately, we cannot depend on them to always drive as expected.

THE NATIONAL DRIVER REGISTER

The National Driver Register was established in 1960. It contains more than 5 million records of driver's-license denial, suspension, or revocation. Its purpose is to assist states in the identification of potentially dangerous drivers. The system makes traffic violations and accident records available to all jurisdictions. The register is a computerized index of state reports. Applications for a driver's license can be checked with the records of the register. In a recent year there were more than 21 million inquiries into the system, and this resulted in the identification of 176,000 motorists whose names were on the index.

ALCOHOL AND DRIVING

Drivers with a blood-alcohol concentration (BAC) of 0.10 percent or more have been involved in 50 to 60 percent of single-vehicle and 45 percent of the multiple-vehicle collisions in which the driver was fatally injured. In the United States, alcohol is a factor in at least half of all fatal traffic accidents, which occur every 20 minutes. A survey taken by the Department of Transportation discovered that among drivers who died in accidents which were judged not to be their fault, only about 12 percent had a BAC high enough to indicate intoxication. Among deceased drivers judged to be at fault, 53 percent were found to be intoxicated.[5]

The risk of having a motor-vehicle accident increases dramatically when the BAC is over 0.06 percent (Figure 11-3). When a motorist's BAC reaches 0.10 percent, the risk of having an accident is six times greater than if the individual had not been drinking. When the BAC reaches a level of 0.15 percent, the driver is twenty-five times more likely to have an accident. A high BAC also corresponds with an increase in the severity of accidents. Despite these findings, one of every fifty drivers on the highway at any given time, day or night, is legally intoxicated.[6]

[5]International Association of Chiefs of Police, *Alcohol Enforcement Countermeasures*, United States Department of Transportation, p. 32, 1976.
[6]Barent F. Landstreet, *The Drinking Driver*, Charles C Thomas, Publisher, Springfield, Ill., 1977, p. 4.

PROBABILITY OF ACCIDENTS

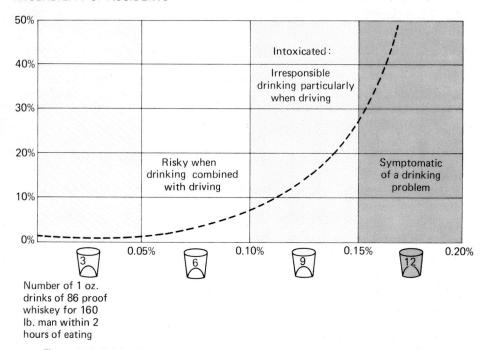

Figure 11-3 Relationship between the probability of motor vehicle accidents and the blood alcohol concentration of the driver.

The driver who represents the biggest threat to highway safety is the problem drinker. The social drinker may be intoxicated at the time of an accident, but he or she operates a motor vehicle far less frequently in this condition than does the problem drinker. Of the drivers arrested for driving while intoxicated (DWI), approximately 80 percent are problem drinkers. Studies indicate that among the drivers responsible for alcohol-related fatalities, two-thirds have had previous difficulty with alcohol. The National Highway Traffic Safety Administration estimates that fewer than 10 percent of the drivers in the United States are problem drinkers. Among our nearly 134 million licensed drivers, however, there are about 13 million problem drinkers who are also problem drivers.

Social drinkers are often capable of changing their driving habits as a result of a bad experience with alcohol. They are receptive to educational programs. Unfortunately, the problem drinker is neither receptive nor willing to change. Therefore, the problem extends beyond the mere suspension or revocation of an operator's license. A problem drinker will continue to drive with or without a license.

The Department of Transportation has developed a program known as the Alcohol Safety Action Project (ASAP). These projects began in 1970 at 9 locations. Two years later there were 35 projects in operation. These multifaceted projects attempt to deal with the problem through countermeasures of enforcement, adjudication, rehabilitation, and public information. The combined countermeasures have the potential to save 13,000 lives annually.[7]

IMPLIED CONSENT

The concept of implied consent is fairly simple. In theory, no person is deprived of his or her constitutional rights by a consent law. Driving is considered to be a privilege granted by the state; therefore, it is reasonable to expect that the licensee will obey the laws and abide by the restrictions imposed by the license. By refusing to take a chemical test for intoxication, a driver "implies" that the BAC is at such a high level that it does not warrant investigation. By this refusal, the individual "consents" to relinquish the license and the privilege of driving.[8]

Maryland was the first state to pass an "expressed consent" law. Under this type of law, the applicant for a license exhanges the right to refuse a chemical test in return for the privilege of driving. Upon initial application or renewal of the license, the individual affirms under oath that he or she will submit to a chemical test when requested to by an officer of the law. All jurisdictions in the United States operate under either implied or express consent statutes.

In most jurisdictions with implied consent laws, there are no provisions for administering a chemical test until after the person has been arrested for a DWI offense. However, police are reluctant to arrest drivers who have been drinking but may not be legally intoxicated. For this reason, many areas have enacted prearrest breath-testing laws. When an officer has reason to believe that a motorist may be in violation of the DWI statute, the officer may require the driver to give a breath sample for analysis. Ordinarily, these results can only be used to guide the officer. Results of the breath test cannot be used as evidence in court.

REDUCTION OF ENVIRONMENTAL HAZARDS

HIGHWAY SIGNS

Highway signs are an important part of the transportation system. They provide directions to motorists, warn of potential dangers, and govern the flow of traffic by providing regulatory information. To help drivers recognize and react more quickly to these signs, the U.S. Department of Transportation has developed a system of colors, symbols, and shapes which are uniform across the nation. Research has indicated that people respond more quickly to symbols than to words, and these signs communicate their messages through symbols (Figure 11-4).

[7]United States Department of Transportation, *National Transportation Trends and Choices to the Year 2,000,* p. 102, 1977.
[8]International Association of Chiefs of Police, *Alcohol Enforcement Countermeasures,* p. 92, 1976.

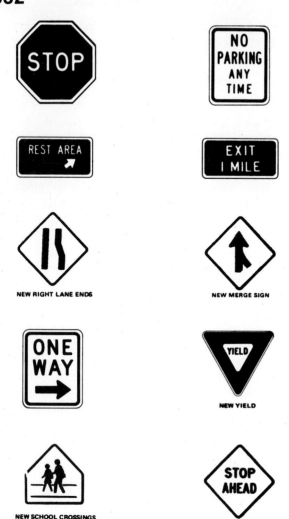

Figure 11-4 Department of Transportation highway signs.

PAVEMENT MARKINGS

Like highway signs, pavement markings are used to warn and direct motorists, and to regulate traffic. Pavement markings have been standardized by the Department of Transportation. Yellow center lines separate traffic moving in opposite directions. When there are two or more lanes of traffic moving in each direction, two solid yellow lines mark the center of the roadway. Solid yellow lines prohibit passing, whereas broken lines indicate that passing is permitted. White lines are used along the right side of the roadway to mark the end of the pavement or the separation between the roadway and the shoulder of the road. White lines also delineate lanes for traffic moving in the same direction. Solid lines prohibit crossing into another lane of traffic, but white dashes permit movement from one lane to another.

THE UNIFORM VEHICLE CODE

Laws which change from state to state or community to community can cause confusion, indecision, and motor-vehicle accidents. In an effort to establish consistency,the Uniform Vehicle Code was created to provide guidance for state governments. Similarly, the Model Traffic Ordinance was developed to guide municipalities. Both of these documents are reviewed periodically and revised when necessary. State and local governments may use the recommended codes or adopt their own standards. There is a growing trend toward acceptance of these documents, and growing recognition that standardization can help minimize the potential for traffic accidents.

THE 55 MILE PER HOUR SPEED LIMIT

In January 1974, Congress established the national 55 mile per hour speed limit. Studies show that as a result of the law the average speed on main and rural highways dropped from 60.3 to 55.3 miles per hour. Speeds on the interstate system were reduced from 65 to 57.6 miles per hour. The smallest change was recorded on secondary rural roads, where the average speed went from 52.6 to 49.5 miles per hour. From 1973 to 1975, the fatality rate dropped by 17 percent. States with the most active information and enforcement programs experienced the greatest reductions. It is estimated that over the next 10 years, enforcement of the 55 mile per hour speed limit will prevent nearly 31,400 fatalities, 415,000 injury-producing accidents, and 1.6 million property-damage accidents.[9]

The 55 mile per hour speed limit helps reduce the accident rate in several ways. It gives a motorist better control of the vehicle and more time to react to emergency situations. It creates a narrower range of highway speeds, thereby reducing the number of rear-end collisions and accidents that occur in passing situations. Collisions which occur at lower speeds cause less injury and property damage.

The legislation which created the national 55 mile per hour speed limit requires each state to certify annually that it is enforcing the law. Failure to do so may result in the withholding of federal highway funds by the Secretary of Transportation. An additional provision requires each state to submit to the NHTSA relevant laws, enforcement regulations, the number of citations issued for exceeding 55 miles per hour, and the actual speeds at which vehicles are traveling in the state. In his energy message to Congress, President Carter urged that the national 55 mile per hour speed limit be vigorously enforced.

[9]United States Department of Transportation, *National Transportation Trends and Choices to the Year 2,000,* p. 100, 1977.

It appears that this law is not unpopular among the public. A survey taken by the Kansas Highway Patrol demonstrated that 80 percent of that state's drivers believe that the limit is justified and is capable of saving lives. The survey also reported that most drivers do not feel inconvenienced by the law. Surveys conducted in other states generally report the same findings. Kansas Governor Robert Bennett launched a statewide campaign to illustrate the beneficial effects of the 55 mile per hour law. The program was a success. Both the number of accidents and the number of highway deaths were reduced. This was especially true on state and federal highways, where enforcement was vigorous.

Another demonstration program took place as a joint effort by the states of Illinois, Michigan, Indiana, and Ohio. The project was called the Combined Accident Reduction Effort (CARE). Public information media warned motorists of increased police activity on 600 miles of interstate highways during the Labor Day weekend. State police maintained high visibility and enforced the speed limit with radar, helicopter, and vascar, as well as marked and unmarked vehicles. A survey before the program clocked the average vehicle at 61.6 miles per hour, with 24 percent of the vehicles traveling at more than 65 miles per hour. During the project the average speed was reduced to 56.6 miles per hour, with only 2 percent of the vehicles exceeding 65 miles per hour. There were *no* fatalities in Illinois, Ohio, or Indiana. Michigan had 1 accident, which produced 3 fatalities.[10]

Not only has the national speed limit saved lives, it has conserved energy. A study by Continental Trailways showed that if the speed limit in 1976 had remained at 70 miles per hour, the company would have used 87 percent more fuel. The reduced speed limit saved the company 1.2 million gallons of fuel. Nationally, the 55 mile per hour speed limit provides an annual savings of 1½ billion gallons of fuel.

DEVELOPMENT OF SAFER VEHICLES AND EQUIPMENT

By reducing human error and environmental hazards, we can reduce the number of accidents. The development of safer equipment would protect drivers in collisions. The three basic elements are biomechanics, occupant-restraint systems, and vehicle structure.

BIOMECHANICS

Biomechanical research has been conducted to identify the protective capabilities and shortcomings of motor vehicles. This is done by placing anthropomorphic test dummies in a car during simulated crashes at various speeds. The test dummies are attached to instruments that identify the areas of stress and the causes of injury. Motion pictures are also used for this purpose. To date, emphasis has been placed on injuries to the head, chest, neck, and spine.

[10]Glenn B. Webber, "Four States Cooperate to Cut Holiday Toll," *Traffic Safety*, p. 21, November, 1977.

OCCUPANT-RESTRAINT SYSTEMS

The NHTSA advocates use of lap and shoulder belts by passengers and drivers. Such belts represent the single most effective safety device in the event of a crash. Seat belts currently save more than 3,000 lives per year. If the 20 percent rate of usage were increased to 80 percent, an additional 7,000 to 9,000 lives might be saved each year.

The National Highway Traffic Safety Administration has published the following information to dispel some of the misconceptions about seat belts:[11]

1 The probability of death is nearly five times greater when a motorist is thrown from a car.

2 Low speeds and short trips are as hazardous as high speeds and long trips. More than one-half of the accidents causing injury or death occur at speeds lower than 40 miles per hour. Fatalities involving nonbelted occupants have been recorded at speeds as low as 12 miles per hour. Three out of four fatal accidents occur within 25 miles of home.

3 The time and energy required to put on a seat belt are inconveniences we can live with, if we want to live.

4 A lap belt protects you from serious injury. A shoulder belt protects your head and chest. Together, lap and shoulder belts offer the best possible protection.

5 Correctly adjusted seat belts can help relieve fatigue and maintain proper riding posture. Most people find that the initial "discomfort" soon disappears, so that eventually they feel uncomfortable unless they are wearing seat belts.

6 Fewer than 0.005 percent of all injury-producing collisions involve fire or submersion. Even in those cases, the motorist is less likely to be stunned or knocked unconscious. This greatly improves the chances of escaping from the vehicle after a fire or a crash into water.

MANDATORY SEAT-BELT USE

In 1973, France became the first European country to *require* use of seat belts. As a result, automobile occupant deaths dropped 25 percent from 1972 to 1974. Several French insurance companies now offer a policy which provides a 50 percent increase in compensation for permanent disability or death when it has been verified by public authorities that the victim was wearing a seat belt. Some judges have gone so far as to rule that motorists who do not fasten their seat belts are legally responsible for up to one-third of the cost of their injuries.[12]

Among the 21 countries which have mandatory seat-belt laws are Norway, Finland, West Germany, Switzerland, Denmark, Australia, and four Canadian provinces. Seat-belt laws have been seriously discussed in this country, but the

---

[11]United States Department of Transportation, *There Are Lots of Safety Belt Myths—Why not Consider the Truths?*, 1972.

[12]Charles H. Pulley, "Buckle up Laws Save Lives in Europe," *Traffic Safety*, p. 19, September, 1977.

issue of personal liberty will probably prohibit passage. This is unfortunate because the mandatory use of seat belts could save 11,500 lives per year, reduce the number of injuries by 641,000 and yield a total savings of $84.5 billion.[13]

PASSIVE RESTRAINT SYSTEMS

An essential aspect of occupant restraint systems is usage. Lap and shoulder belts are referred to as active systems because the individual is responsible for putting on the belt. Only 20 percent of the population use this protection, and much attention has been focused on passive systems such as the air-cushion restraint system (ACRS). Activated within an instant after the crash, the system absorbs the kinetic energy of the occupants. The National Safety Council estimates that if air-cusion restraint systems were installed in all front-seat positions, the number of lives saved annually would be between 6,000 and 9,000.

The ACRS has not been without controversy. The Motor Vehicle Manufacturers Association is opposed to such a system, partly because it believes the safety of the system has not been proved. The association argues that the ACRS would not be effective in side crashes or rear-end collisions. Another major argument is that the public would be unwilling to pay the price of installation and maintenance.

Proponents of the ACRS include the Insurance Institute for Highway Safety, the United Auto Worker's Union, Ralph Nader, the Alliance of American Insurers, and the National Committee for Automobile Crash Protection. They feel that the system has been adequately tested and has been demonstrated to be safe even for people not properly seated. It is further argued that the public needs to become as concerned with safety devices as it is with optional equipment such as stereo systems and electric windows.

Late in 1977, Secretary of Transportation Brock Adams announced that passive restraints such as air bags or passive safety belts must be installed in all front-seat positions beginning in 1982. Safety programs that reduce the highway death rate by 1 per 100 million vehicle-miles would create a social benefit of approximately $5.3 billion annually. The use of occupant restraints would reduce the 1978 death rate from 3.5 to 2.8, and would save about one life in five.[14]

MOTOR-VEHICLE INSPECTIONS

A total of 34 jurisdictions now have laws requiring periodic inspection of motor vehicles. In the National Traffic and Motor Vehicle Safety Act of 1966, Congress specifically endorsed mandatory inspections. The purpose of these laws is to

---

[13]United States Department of Transportation, *National Transportation Trends and Choices to the Year 2,000,* p. 106, 1977.
[14]Ibid., p. 104.

ensure that only mechanically safe vehicles are permitted to operate, thereby minimizing the frequency of crashes resulting from vehicle defect. To be effective, the inspection must occur at least once per year, and must be performed by certified and competent personnel. In some states the vehicle rejection rate is as high as 50 percent, with such important safety factors as headlights, brakes, and suspension systems accounting for many of the rejections. The Automotive Safety Foundation reports that studies have suggested a relationship between compulsory inspection and reduction of the fatality rate.

DEFECTS INVESTIGATION

The purpose of this program is to influence manufacturers to build products free of safety-related defects. In some cases, manufacturers discover the defects and voluntarily seek to correct them by notifying purchasers who may be exposed to the risk. When defects are reported by the public, the NHTSA investigates the validity of the complaints before taking action. When an immediate threat to traffic safety is identified, a consumer protection bulletin or public advisory is issued to warn the public. From 1966 to 1975, approximately 49 million vehicles were recalled. Between 1968 and 1969, NHTSA testing of vehicles and equipment produced a failure rate of 10.1 percent. By 1975 the rate dropped to 4.1 percent.[15]

THE RESEARCH SAFETY VEHICLE PROGRAM

The primary purpose of the Research Safety Vehicle Program is to demonstrate the technical feasibility of crashworthy vehicles. Cars of the future will have a stronger occupant compartment surrounded by structures to absorb the energy of a collision. There will be fewer fires as the result of fuel-system improvements which have been mandated by Congress.

The Research Safety Vehicle Program is based on a concept known as the S3E approach: safety with energy conservation, environmental benefits, and economy. Two contracts have been awarded by the NHTSA for research and development. Minicars, Inc., and Calspan Corp. have received more than $3 million to develop a family automobile on the S3E concept by the mid 1980s. The subcompact versions will have interior comfort and size resembling present-day compact cars such as the Nova, Maverick, and Dart. The vehicle will weigh slightly more than the Chevette or Honda, yet it will be able to withstand collisions at 45 miles per hour and over. A soft front end will provide greater pedestrian protection and will reduce damage in low-speed collisions. In addition to passive-restraint systems, the energy-absorbing vehicle design will protect occupants in high-speed impacts, rollovers, and rear-end collisions. The vehicles of the future will get about 35 miles per gallon on the highway and

---

[15] *A Digest of Activities of the National Highway Traffic Safety Administration,* Department of Transportation, p. 25, 1976.

27 miles per gallon in the city. These automobiles will be constructed from materials capable of being recycled for additional use.

Table 11-5 presents the countermeasures for highway accidents and ranks them according to their potential for saving lives and reducing injuries.[16]

LEARNING EXPERIENCES

The following activities are designed to supplement the study of this chapter.

1 Develop a comprehensive "rules of the road" written test. Select a stratified random sample within the community and administer the test. Evaluate the frequency of wrong answers. Discuss how an educational program could give the general public better driving knowledge.

2 Brainstorm the skills necessary for effective driving. Create a model driving range in one of the school parking lots. Solicit volunteers among the student population and test their driving skills. After each test, explain his or her deficiencies to the volunteer.

3 Write to the National Safety Council for additional information on defensive driving. Select a safe location at a heavily traveled highway and record driver errors. Discuss your findings in class.

4 Select a panel to speak to the class on the problem of alcohol and driving. Speakers might include an officer of the state police, a lawyer, a social worker, an insurance agent, and a judge or legislator. Discuss the ASAP project, the legal issues involved in implied consent, and possible solutions to the driving hazards created by the problem drinker.

5 Create a series of slides that reproduce the standardized highway traffic symbols. Flash a sign onto the screen for a predetermined length of time to see how long a glimpse is needed for recognition of the sign. Compare the results with slides using the old written messages. Experiment with different signs by changing the color, size, shape, or the symbol itself.

6 Secure a copy of the Uniform Vehicle Code and the Model Traffic Ordinance. Discuss the provisions of each document.

7 Debate the issue of a law which would require motorists to wear safety belts. Discuss the pros and cons of a regulation which would place passive restraint systems in all vehicles by the middle 1980s.

8 In class, discuss the S3E concept. Brainstorm additional ideas for safety, energy conservation, environmental pollution, and economy. Why have the government and the automobile manufacturers waited so long to initiate S3E?

9 At a controlled intersection, observe the drivers and passengers of vehicles for usage of seat belts. Prepare a survey questionnaire of highway safety issues and distribute it to a sample population. Analyze the results.

---

[16]U.S. Department of Transportation, *National Transportation Trends and Choices to the Year 2,000,* p. 100, 1977.

TABLE 11–5

Ranking of Countermeasures by Decreasing Potential to Forestall Fatalities and Injury Accidents, Ten-Year Total

Countermeasure	Fatalities Forestalled	Injury Accidents Forestalled
Mandatory safety belt usage	89,000*	3,220,000
Nationwide 55-mph speed limit	31,900	415,000
Combined alcohol safety action countermeasures	13,000	153,000
Combined emergency medical countermeasures	8,000	146,000
Selective traffic enforcement	7,560	296,000
Impact-absorbing roadside safety devices	6,780	158,000
Tire and braking system safety critical inspection— selective	4,590	180,000
Citizen assistance of crash victims	3,750	0
Skid resistance	3,740	195,000
Regulatory and warning signs	3,670	143,000
Upgrade traffic signals and systems	3,400	133,000
Breakaway sign and lighting supports	3,250	127,000
Guardrail	3,160	52,800
Upgrade education and training for beginning drivers	3,050	131,000
Driver improvement schools	2,470	113,000
Periodic motor vehicle inspection—current practice	1,840	71,900
Bridge rails and parapets	1,520	15,300
Pedestrian and bicycle visibility enhancement	1,440	24,200
Bridge widening	1,330	51,000
Selective access control for safety	1,300	50,300
Motorcycle rider safety helmets	1,150	14,400
Paved or stabilized shoulders	928	35,800
Wrong-way entry avoidance techniques	779	3,290
Roadway lighting	759	29,600
Driver improvement schools for young offenders	692	27,000
Upgrade bicycle and pedestrian safety curriculum offerings	649	11,200
Traffic channelization	645	31,500
Roadway alignment and gradient	590	23,000
Clear roadside recovery areas	533	20,700
Median barriers	529	2,740
Pedestrian safety information and education	490	19,200
Intersection sight distance	468	18,300
Highway construction and maintenance practices	459	18,000
Railroad-highway grade crossing protection (automatic gates excluded)	276	1,080
Pavement markings and delineators	237	9,210
Warning letters to problem drivers	192	3,760
Motorcycle lights-on practice	65	1,680

*All figures have been rounded to three significant digits after internal computations were completed. All figures are subject to the caveats concerning precision of the data.
Source: *National Transportation Trends and Choices to the Year 2,000,* United States Department of Transportation, January, 1977, p.100.

SELECTED REFERENCES

Addiction Research Foundation of Ontario: *Alcohol, Drugs, and Traffic Safety,* S. Israelstam and S. Lambert (eds.), Alcoholism and Drug Addiction Research Foundation of Ontario, 1975

American Automobile Association: *You . . . Alcohol and Driving,* 1975. Copies of this pamphlet may be obtained from your local AAA or from the AAA Traffic Engineering and Safety Department, Falls Church, Va.

Automotive Safety Foundation: *Highway Safety Program Management,* Washington, 1968

Baker, Robert F.: *The Highway Risk Problem—Policy Issues in Highway Safety,* John Wiley & Sons, Inc., New York, 1971

International Association of Chiefs of Police: *Alcohol Enforcement Countermeasures,* U.S. Department of Transportation, Washington, 1976

Landstreet, Barent F.: *The Drinking Driver,* Charles C Thomas, Publisher, Springfield, 1977

National Safety Council, Chicago
    Accident Facts, 1977
    Guide to Traffic Safety Literature, 1977
    Traffic Safety Magazine, monthly

U.S. Department of Transportation, Washington:
A Digest of Activities of the National Highway Traffic Safety Administration, 1976
National Transportation Trends and Choices to the Year 2000, 1977

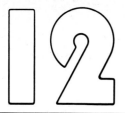

Community Safety

OVERALL OBJECTIVE:

The student should recognize the comprehensive nature of community efforts directed toward the safety and well-being of citizens.

INSTRUCTIONAL OBJECTIVES:

After completing this chapter the student will be able to:

1 Describe the activities which are necessary for civil preparedness.
2 Develop a comprehensive disaster plan which utilizes the resources of every available community agency.
3 Justify the existence of emergency-care systems.
4 Explain the components of a comprehensive emergency-care system.
5 List the responsibilities of an emergency medical council.
6 Discuss the purposes and mandates of the Emergency Medical Services Systems Act of 1973.
7 Describe how the American Red Cross helps care for disaster victims.

The community protects its citizens from danger and harm in many ways. Perhaps the most obvious illustration is the protection offered by police and fire departments. But even in small communities, safety is a principal reason for the existence of other public agencies supported by the local government. The zoning board prohibits unplanned and unsafe development. The building inspection department regulates construction and enforces fire codes. The traffic engineering division ensures safe and efficient mobility. Vital city services are maintained by the department of public works. The environmental protection agency monitors the levels of air, water, and noise pollution. The public health department inspects restaurants, grocery stores, and swimming pools.

Most communities are safe most of the time. Local governments have established the capability to protect their citizens from the hazards of everyday living. But what about extraordinary events which effect dozens of people and sometimes occur without warning? Has your community considered the possibility of a disaster? Have government officials taken appropriate steps to protect lives and property during a widespread emergency?

CIVIL PREPAREDNESS

The word "disaster" has a variety of connotations. Certainly, whenever a person suffers injury or loss of property, the event could be considered a disaster. For this chapter, a disaster is defined as an occurrence which results in loss of life, serious injury, or property damage to more than twenty-five people. The criterion for disaster is not the consequences of an event but its magnitude.

Every year American communities are struck by disaster. In each year of this century approximately 1,300 Americans have died in disasters and another 10,000 have been injured.[1] When a disaster occurs the entire community is affected. Governmental, religious, educational, industrial, and commercial institutions all suffer from the tragedy. In 1947, the S.S. *Grandchamp* was loading ammonium nitrate in Texas City, Texas. A fire broke out, which led to subsequent explosions that caused the complete destruction of everything within one-half mile of the site. In this town of 18,000 people, 570 were killed and 3,000 injured, 2,500 were left homeless, and property damage exceeeded $50 million.[2]

Preparation for disaster in this country began in the form of civil defense for protection against enemy attack. In 1916 Congress established the Council for National Defense, which consisted of the Secretaries of War, Navy, Interior, Agriculture, Commerce, and Labor. The Office of Civilian Defense was created in 1941. Ten years later President Truman signed into law the Federal Civil Defense Act, which established a national civil defense program. In May 1972, Secretary of Defense Melvin R. Laird created the Defense Civil Preparedness Agency (DCPA) as part of the Department of Defense.

The Defense Civil Preparedness Agency works with the Federal Preparedness Agency, the General Services Administration, the Federal Disaster Assistance Administration, and the Department of Housing and Urban Development. In addition, the agency works with state and local governments to achieve overall readiness to handle major emergencies. This concern for readiness covers all significant hazards from localized peacetime emergencies to the threat of nationwide nuclear attack. For the fiscal year 1977, the federal government appropriated $82.5 million to DCPA, with nearly $30 million in matching funds for state and local governments.

---

[1]Solomon Garb, and Evelyn Eng, *Disaster Handbook,* 2d ed., Springer Publishing Co., Inc., New York, 1969, p. 1.
[2]Richard J. Healy, *Emergency and Disaster Planning,* John Wiley & Sons, Inc., New York, 1969, p. 131.

DISASTER PLANNING

No community is immune from disaster. The Atlantic and Gulf Coast areas are especially susceptible to hurricanes. Explosions are most frequent in the densely populated industrial cities of our nation. Floods occur most often in areas where rivers overflow, but can also result from melting snow, notably in the mountain states of the West. The Plains are subject to tornadoes. The Pacific Coast is continuously threatened by earthquakes. High winds, transportation wreckages, riots, escape of toxic or radioactive substances, and epidemics can occur in every geographic region. Table 1-8 presents the largest United States disasters by category.

Fortunately, the effects of disaster can be minimized by cooperative planning and by appropriate action taken before, during, and after the event. In some instances the disaster can be prevented. Techniques of aviation safety, properly constructed dams, and careful use of explosives illustrate this point. Natural disasters such as tornadoes and hurricanes cannot be prevented, but much of the potential damage can. Within a 4-year period two hurricanes struck the same area. The first, Hurricane Audrey, killed 430 people. Hurricane Carla, which was designated as the greatest hurricane in recorded coastal history, killed only 40.[3] The disaster plans established as a result of the first storm helped reduce the consequences of the second.

Civil preparedness means that a jurisdiction is ready to make coordinated efforts to save lives and protect property. Community readiness requires a partnership of public and private efforts. The local government is responsible for emergency planning and must provide the necessary legal, fiscal, and administrative structure. Federal and state governments may supplement these resources at the local level, but community agencies must form the nucleus of the emergency-preparedness organization. The private sector is composed of business, industry, labor, social, civic, and health and welfare groups. As illustrated in Figure 12-1, disaster preparation is a highly complex matter which requires a vast amount of cooperation.

Disasters are characterized by large-scale destruction and injury. At a time when human needs are substantially increased, the ability to provide for these needs is diminished. Food, clothing, shelter, water, and medical supplies may be available only in limited quantities. Disaster planning can make the most effective use of the available resources. Time, equipment, personnel, and materials can be used effectively to protect property and promote human well-being. This is especially true when the disaster is unpredictable, the onset is rapid, and the impact is felt by a large number of people.

Disaster management depends upon preestablished operating procedures. Roles and responsibilities must be delineated. Lines of authority must be clarified. Communications systems must be operative. The secondary effects of

[3]Garb and Eng, op. cit., p. 2.

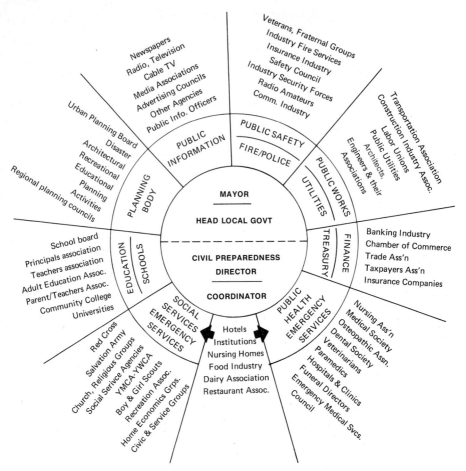

Figure 12-1 Civil preparedness organization. (Source: *Community Action for Civil Preparedness*, Defense Civil Preparedness Agency, December 1976.)

the disaster must be predicted in order to develop contingency plans. The keynote of disaster management is cooperation among agencies and individuals before the disaster occurs. This is best illustrated by one large-scale fire during which the office of emergency preparedness was asking people not to use water while the fire department was urging people to wet down the roofs of their houses.

One of the important goals of disaster management is the restoration of equilibrium after a disaster. When exposed to disaster, few people respond in a productive way. Only a small proportion of the population is capable of grasping the significance of a disaster. People have been observed sweeping dirt from the floors of their homes while the walls lay in a heap around the foundation. Disaster victims need leadership, especially during the first few hours after the disaster. If plans have not been made in advance, leadership will not be available.

Panic is a sudden, emotional state of fear which leads to irrational behavior for the purpose of self-preservation. Surprisingly, it is an uncommon occurrence during disasters. It is, however, a contagious phenomenon. The greatest potential for panic exists when people believe that the danger is severe and the onset imminent. The feeling is heightened when a person believes that there are limited escape routes, which may be closing, thereby preventing escape. Panic is not a common aspect of the postdisaster situation. The most common emotional responses in the aftermath of disaster are shock, disbelief, apathy, and nonresponsiveness.

EMERGENCY-CARE SYSTEMS

A medical emergency may be defined as a condition which requires immediate medical attention. The emergency status continues until it is determined by a health-care professional that the well-being of the patient is no longer threatened. An emergency-care system is a community or regional network of services. Currently, there is a nationwide effort to make emergency-care systems more efficient, standardized, and responsive to the needs of the community.[4]

Appreciation of the need for improved emergency medical systems was stimulated around 1966 with a report by the National Research Council entitled *Trauma, the Neglected Disease of Modern Society.* The shortcomings of the health-care delivery system had been well publicized, with one of the major problems being lack of accessibility. In 1972, Marlin K. DuVal, Assistant Secretary for Health and Scientific Affairs of the United States Department of Health, Education, and Welfare, said that "nowhere is this lack of accessibility more crucial and yet more widespread and profound than in the area of emergency care."[5]

As early as 1961 it had been convincingly demonstrated that people injured in rural counties were nearly four times more likely to die of their accidental injuries than people injured in urban areas. The states with the highest accidental automobile fatality rates are in the sparsely populated Rocky Mountain region. Rural accident victims die more often at the scene of the accident, and die sooner after the accident. These facts might lead one to conclude that the disproportionately high death rates are a function of vehicle speeds and consequent severity of injuries. To the contrary, it has been demonstrated that automobile accidents in rural areas are more often single-vehicle crashes that result in less severe injuries. The important factors which account for the differences are the accessibility and quality of the emergency

---

[4]American Hospital Association, *Emergency Services,* Chicago, 1972, p. 1.
[5]Marlin K. DuVal, "The Hidden Crisis in Health Care," in *Proceedings of the Second National Conference on Emergency Health Services,* December 2–4, Bethesda, Md., p. 3, 1971.

medical system. It is now known that up to 25 percent of the trauma fatalities can be prevented through an effective emergency system.[6]

An emergency system involves far more than the rapid transportation of a victim to a hospital. Many components must be organized to benefit the victims of serious accidents or sudden illness. An effective system can mean the difference between life and death, partial or total disability, and short or prolonged hospital stays. Unnecessary death, disability, and human suffering can be eliminated through a systematic approach to emergency care.

A modern emergency medical system must include at least the following:

1 An extensive communication network
2 Highly trained personnel
3 Efficient means of transportation
4 Sophisticated medical equipment
5 Adequate facilities
6 Adequate funding
7 Consumer knowledge of the system and willingness to use it
8 High degrees of organization and cooperation

EXTENSIVE COMMUNICATION NETWORK

Of central importance to a good emergency system is an efficient communication network. Emergencies require immediate assistance. Ideally, arrival of the ambulance at the site of an accident should not take longer than 5 minutes after notification. The public must have a means of quick entry into the system. More than 500 areas have established a 911 telephone number which connects the caller to a central dispatcher who is trained to handle emergency calls.

By using a central dispatch system, the police department, ambulance squads, and fire-rescue or emergency medical technicians can begin to respond simultaneously. Upon arrival at the accident scene, the ambulance must communicate with the hospital to indicate the nature of the emergency, the number of victims and their condition, and the estimated time of arrival at the emergency room. If emergency medical technicians are present, communication may involve the transmission of vital signs by telemetry.

Communication needs are not limited to the scene of the emergency. Hospitals may need to locate and contact physicians with special skills. If the hospital cannot handle the emergency, arrangements must be made to transport the victims to another facility. If the victim is a child, the parents need to be notified so that treatment will not be delayed. In certain situations, public health, civil defense, state police, or military agencies may be needed.

---

[6]Henry C. Huntley, "National Status of Emergency Health Services," in *Proceedings of the Second National Conference on Emergency Health Services,* December 2–4, Bethesda, Md., p. 12, 1971.

HIGHLY TRAINED PERSONNEL

A central figure in this system is the emergency medical technician (EMT), who is trained to provide basic life support. Ordinarily, training exceeds 80 hours of intensive study and clinical experience in a curriculum which is known as the Dunlap course. The essential mission of the EMT is to stabilize the victim so that the victim's condition does not deteriorate during transportation. These technicians are taught to assess the condition of the victim, determine the functioning of vital organs, extricate the victim if necessary, and provide appropriate medical management until arrival at the emergency room. Only recently have the prestige, salaries, fringe benefits, and authority been commensurate with the responsibility of the job. Since 1967, more than 145,000 people have been trained to the Department of Transportation/National Highway Traffic Safety Administration basic EMT level.

A more highly trained and skilled individual is the paramedic. Training for this specialty requires almost 500 hours. Although paramedics often have experience as military medics, some systems prefer to use fire personnel. Upon voice command from a physician, paramedics are capable of performing tasks such as intravenous infusion, administration of drugs, telemetry of electrocardiograms, and ventricular defibrillation. Paramedics truly serve as the eyes and hands of the physician.

A good system depends on many trained professionals. Police often arrive at the scene before the ambulance. For this reason, police officers must be trained in basic first aid, including cardiopulmonary resuscitation (CPR). Dispatchers must know the capabilities and limitations of the system because they serve as managers of the resources available within the system. Ambulance drivers must be totally familiar with the area and its traffic patterns. Telephone operators must remain calm, obtain necessary information, and accurately relay messages to the appropriate agencies.

With more than 43 million patients to treat annually, hospital personnel in emergency rooms need to be exceptionally competent. In the past, emergency rooms had to cope as well as they could with available personnel. In 1968, a new medical specialty was chartered as the American College of Emergency Physicians. This specialty requires a residency in emergency medicine, where the emphasis is on the diagnosis and management of trauma and critical illness. Nurses are also being encouraged to specialize in emergency medicine. In a modern emergency room, staffed with such specialists, the victim's chances of survival are excellent.

EFFICIENT MEANS OF TRANSPORTATION

In some parts of the country an ambulance ride still entails transportation without medical management. Fortunately, standards which ensure that ambulance personnel are capable of providing first aid are gradually being established. Ambulances are being designed for a smooth ride and efficient treatment. They are outfitted with life-support equipment so sophisticated that the ambulance of today serves as a mobile intensive-care unit. Since one-eighth of the beds in general hospitals are occupied by trauma victims, many of whom arrive by ambulance, it is surprising that standards were not developed much earlier.

A recent development is the use of helicopters to transport seriously injured or critically ill persons to emergency rooms. The military has used this technique for years and has successfully demonstrated the life-saving capability of air transport. In some cities helicopters are used when ground vehicles are unable to reach the emergency scene. During a freeway accident, for example, traffic may back up so far that the only way to effectively provide first aid and transportation is through the air. The cost of such a project presents an obvious hurdle. However, the helicopter has unique capabilities for law enforcement. When helicopters are used for traffic control and other special assignments, the cost efficiency can be proved. In at least 13 states emergency medical systems are assisted by helicopters operated by the state police.

Air transport can also be used in rural areas. People who live hundreds of miles from adequate hospital care sometimes need immediate medical help. In wilderness areas which are used for recreation by campers and backpackers, helicopters have been used for search and rescue missions. Congress has authorized the Secretary of Defense to provide helicopter transportation to civilians so long as the missions do not interfere with military operations. This project is known as Military Assistance to Safety and Traffic (MAST). The 23 MAST cities serve portions of 28 states. In a recent year, MAST completed 2,471 missions. From 1970 to 1975 more than 6,000 people were transported by this system.

SOPHISTICATED MEDICAL EQUIPMENT

Modern medicine is spectacular in its "space-age gadgetry." Electronic monitoring devices fill the emergency room. Coronary-care and intensive-care units immeasurably enhance one's probability of survival. Even before the victim reaches the hospital, important cardiac information can be transmitted by way of telemetry. Medical hardware is an important part of the total system.

ADEQUATE FACILITIES

Administrators and planners have been looking toward cooperation as a means of handling rapidly rising medical costs and the increased demand for medical and hospital services. Within certain geographic regions, hospitals are beginning to specialize to avoid unnecessary duplication of services, equipment, and personnel. One facility may be designated as a trauma center. Another institution may specialize in neonatal care, cardiac care, or the needs of burn victims.

In large cities, hospitals may cooperatively agree to specialize. However, in rural areas one hospital may be designated as a regional trauma facility, receiving all emergency cases in its region. Once the patient's condition is stabilized, the patient may be transferred to a specialized facility located in one of the major cities. In this way, maximum utilization of services provides cost efficiency and personnel efficiency. Highly skilled physicians and nurses can maintain peak levels of performance by practicing their skills on a daily basis.

ADEQUATE FUNDING

The establishment of an emergency medical system is expensive, but it represents a good investment. Premature deaths cost the nation billions of dollars annually. It was calculated that in one year, the 3,000 premature deaths of people under twenty-one that were caused by traffic accidents cost the nation more than ½ billion dollars. Every year there are between 7,500 and 8,500 spinal-cord injuries. The lifetime costs are calculated at between $400,000 and $600,000.[7]

Americans spend an average of $500 per person per year for health care. It has been estimated that if 2.5 percent of the health dollar were spent on emergency care, 60,000 lives would be saved each year. This figure includes approximately 15,000 fatalities related to accidents, especially motor-vehicle accidents.[8]

CONSUMER KNOWLEDGE

An efficient emergency system entails public understanding of the system and recognition of its capabilities and limitations. When an emergency occurs, the average citizen must know how to get in touch with the system. More people must be trained in first aid and medical self-help so that treatment can be rendered even before the ambulance arrives. The more a community knows about emergencies and the emergency system, the more likely that it will support the system.

ORGANIZATION AND COOPERATION

A system which depends on the services of so many people must be fully organized. Roles must be carefully defined, record-keeping standardized, policies established, and funds managed. Individuals must work together. The police officer must know the functions of the emergency medical technician. The EMT must respect the knowledge and skill of the emergency-room staff. The ambulance driver must understand the problems of the dispatcher.

[7]Paul R. Meyer, Jr., "Specialized Trauma Center Spinal Cord Injury," in *Selected Bibliography of Scientific Publications and Programmatic Reports for the U.S.A. Bicentennial Emergency Medical Services and Traumatology Conference,* May 10–12, Baltimore, Md., 1976.
[8]Huntley, loc. cit.

LEGISLATION

Even a few years ago a fully efficient emergency system would have been impossible to establish. Recent legal changes have enabled the system to become operational. Emergency medical technicians and paramedics have been given the authority to serve as physician extenders. They are protected from liability, as are other health professionals, through an extension of the Good Samaritan law.

EMERGENCY MEDICAL COUNCIL

Providing emergency care is a public responsibility. The most effective mechanism for organizing the various components of the system is an emergency medical council, whose purpose is to plan, implement, coordinate, and evaluate the system. The council must consider each of the following:[9]

1 Distribution of the population as it relates to services
2 Accessibility of transportation, and the time it takes to get from an emergency scene to the hospital
3 The capabilities of the emergency room
4 Utilization patterns of the community
5 Available communications
6 The need for first aid and safety education
7 Demographic characteristics, such as age of the population, socioeconomic status, population trends, etc.
8 Specific hazards such as recreational activities (there are 46 mountain rescue units and more than 25,000 members of the ski patrol trained in search-and-rescue and first aid)
9 Legal and regulatory barriers to an efficient system

The council should represent a broad spectrum of the community. An assessment of the current system will provide information about how the system can be improved. The council works to promote the system by offering public information and education. The council also:

1 Establishes personnel-selection criteria
2 Outlines day-to-day operational procedures
3 Develops a personnel manual which covers job descriptions, standards, salaries, rights, responsibilities, etc.
4 Facilitates agreement among various components of the system

[9]American Hospital Association, *Emergency Services,* Chicago, 1972, p. 13.

5 Establishes cooperative agreements with other towns, regions, hospitals, etc., in case of mass casualties

6 Develops comprehensive disaster plans

7 Supports education in safety and first aid to help prevent accidents and relieve the strain on the system

EMERGENCY MEDICAL SERVICES SYSTEMS ACT

In 1973 Congress enacted the Emergency Medical Services Systems Act (P.L. 93-154). The stated purpose of the act was to assist and encourage the development of comprehensive emergency medical systems. To accomplish this task, $160 million was appropriated during the fiscal years 1974–1976. The act defined such a system as one which provides the personnel, facilities, and equipment needed for the effective delivery of emergency health care within an appropriate geographic area.

Grant money was made available for the establishment of these systems, with special consideration going to applications which coordinated the new system with statewide systems. Where operations were already in existence, money was provided to expand and improve the system. Up to 40 percent of the development or improvement costs could be received from the federal government. When applicants could demonstrate exceptional need, the government could provide up to 75 percent of the funding. Special consideration was given to rural areas.

The law mandated that emergency medical systems must include the following components:

1 An adequate number of health professionals who have received appropriate training

2 Training and in-service continuing-education programs

3 Personnel, facilities, and equipment that can be connected to a central communication system (the law encouraged the use of the universal emergency telephone number, 911)

4 An adequate number of ground, air, and water vehicles appropriate to the characteristics of the service area

5 An adequate number of easily accessible emergency medical services which are collectively capable of providing services on a continuous basis, in coordination with the other health-care facilities of the system

6 Access to specialized critical medical-care units

7 An opportunity for people who reside in the service area to participate in policy making for the system

8 Provision of services to all patients without prior inquiry about their ability to pay

9 Transfer of patients to facilities which offer follow-up care and rehabilitation

10 A standardized system of record keeping which covers the treatment of the patient from initial entry into the system through discharge

11 Provision of public information and education programs which stress appropriate methods of self-help and first aid

12 Provision for periodic, comprehensive, and independent evaluation of the services of the system

13 A plan which ensures that the system will be capable of providing emergency medical services during mass casualties, natural disasters, or national emergencies

14 Arrangements with systems serving neighboring areas for the provision of emergency medical services on a reciprocal basis

ILLUSTRATIVE SYSTEMS

Many communities across the nation have been developing model emergency medical systems. In Albuquerque, New Mexico, when a caller dials 911, police, fire-rescue and emergency medical technicians, and ambulance crews are immediately dispatched. Police officers ordinarily arrive on the scene within 2½ minutes. Fire-rescue units are strategically located so that an emergency medical technician can usually provide aid within 4 minutes. Ambulances are centrally located and therefore take longer to reach the scene, but victims are transported only after their conditions have been stabilized by the EMT. Hospitals are situated near the exit ramps of two interstate highways for easy access to the emergency room.

The Seattle fire department has implemented a citizen cardiopulmonary resuscitation (CPR) training program known as Medic II. The goal of the program is to provide basic life-support education to 100,000 people. More than 25 percent of all resuscitations are initiated by private citizens who happen to be at the scene. Because irreparable brain damage begins after 3 minutes without oxygen, and a victim's chances for survival drop markedly after 5 minutes, the program will undoubtedly pay large dividends.

In 1973, Maryland mandated the development of a comprehensive emergency medical system. The purpose was to provide all citizens with quality emergency medical care regardless of their geographic location. The statewide system is linked to specialty-referral centers through a coordinated communication and transportation network. One aspect includes a med-evac helicopter transport system for the victims of serious trauma or critical illness. More than 1,200 missions are flown annually. Each crew has a medic aboard to provide professional care en route to the appropriate specialty-referral center. The Maryland Institute for Emergency Medicine receives about 75 percent of the patients. The survival rate for admissions to this facility is a phenomenal 80 percent.

Some areas are using telephone location devices. One purpose of the devices is to identify the location of callers who are so unfamiliar with the area that they cannot provide directions. The devices can be used to locate the source of a telephone call when communication has been interrupted, for example, when the victim has lost consciousness.

THE AMERICAN NATIONAL RED CROSS

The red cross is recognized worldwide as a symbol of compassion and humanitarian action. In 1862 a young Swiss businessman named Henri Dunant wrote an essay which recounted the horrors of a battle he had witnessed. His efforts eventually led to the formation of the organization known as the Red Cross.

In this country, the Red Cross grew out of the work of the U.S. Sanitary Commission and the individual efforts of Clara Barton. Ms. Barton provided nursing care for soldiers of both the Union and the Confederacy. After the Civil War she visited Europe and participated in relief efforts during the Franco-Prussian War of 1870–1871. On the basis of her experiences and her study of Dunant's writings, Clara Barton returned home to form a Red Cross Society of the United States. In 1881 she established the American Association of the Red Cross in Dansville, New York. Congress ratified the Geneva Convention in 1882, giving the Red Cross official sanction.

The original purpose of the Red Cross was the provision of services to soldiers. The unique contribution of Clara Barton to the worldwide movement of the Red Cross was the idea of an organized program of voluntary relief for disaster victims. The first disaster efforts occurred during the forest fires of 1881 in Michigan and the floods along the Ohio and Mississippi rivers in 1882. Disaster operations under her direction reached a peak during the flood in Johnstown, Pennsylvania, in 1889. At the age of seventy-six, Ms. Barton provided medical care to soldiers and civilians during the Spanish-American War.

In 1914 there were 123 chapters of the American Red Cross. By 1917, with the impact of World War I, the Red Cross network had grown to 3,287 chapters, with volunteer membership in the millions. During the war, the Red Cross operated 47 ambulance companies to bring the wounded from the battlefield to the hospital. The Red Cross assigned 20,000 nurses for wartime services. During the Depression the Red Cross was asked by the government to help distribute food and clothing. During this period the Red Cross began its blood-donor program.

During World War II the Red Cross recruited more than 71,000 registered nurses for military duty. It supplied nearly 13½ million units of blood for plasma for injured soldiers. From 1941 to 1946 the American Red Cross worked with Red Cross societies in other countries, the International Committee of the Red Cross, and the League of Red Cross Societies to provide extensive relief and rehabilitation programs for civilian victims of the war. After the war, Red Cross services were continued for the men and women of the armed forces. During the military conflicts in Korea and Southeast Asia, social-welfare and recreational programs for armed forces personnel were intensified.

In 1905 Congress granted the American National Red Cross the authority to

Local Government Authority

Disaster Coordinator

Responsibilities of government	Responsibilities of Red Cross
Protection of life and property, public health and welfare, repair or replacement of public property, and help to disaster victims (Financed by public agencies from tax funds)	The relief of persons in need as a result of disaster (Financed by Red Cross from voluntary contributions)

When disaster threatens

Government	Red Cross
Issues official warnings and designates hazardous zones Enforces evacuation from threatened areas Provides means of rescue and evacuation and directs these means Organizes and coordinates all government departments and agencies	Assists government agencies in disseminating official warnings Coordinates Red Cross resources for voluntary evacuation Mobilizes trained volunteers to assist in rescue Transports and temporarily stores household goods Assists in coordination of voluntary agencies' relief efforts

Figure 12-2 Responsibilities in natural disasters.

help meet human needs that result from disaster. Through the years, the role of the Red Cross disaster program has been reaffirmed in federal disaster legislation, most recently in the Disaster Relief Act of 1974. The Red Cross is the nation's primary voluntary agency for the relief of human suffering arising from disaster.

The Red Cross does not assume responsibility for governmental functions (see Figures 12-1 and 12-2). Red Cross disaster assistance constitutes an outright grant to needy families. Repayment is never requested, although voluntary financial donations may be accepted. Red Cross services include food, clothing, shelter, first aid, medical care, and other basic elements for comfort and survival, including blood and blood products. The primary responsibility in a disaster rests with local public-health authorities and medical resources. If no other resources are available, the Red Cross may provide direct assistance to enable victims to resume living with acceptable standards of health, safety, and human dignity. The American National Red Cross helps the disaster victims of other countries through the International Committee of the

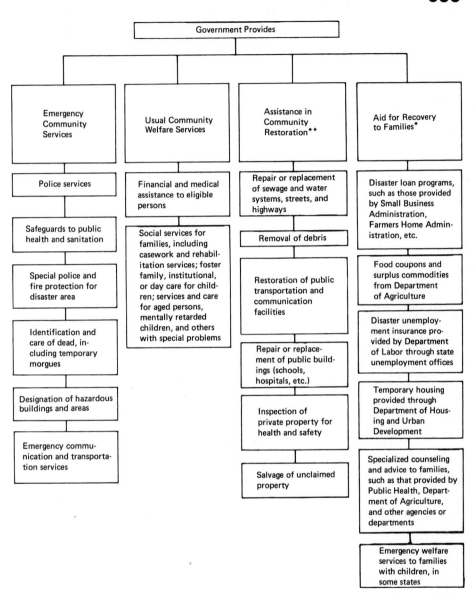

```
                          Government Provides
```

| Emergency Community Services | Usual Community Welfare Services | Assistance in Community Restoration** | Aid for Recovery to Families* |

| Police services | Financial and medical assistance to eligible persons | Repair or replacement of sewage and water systems, streets, and highways | Disaster loan programs, such as those provided by Small Business Administration, Farmers Home Administration, etc. |

| Safeguards to public health and sanitation | Social services for families, including casework and rehabilitation services; foster family, institutional, or day care for children; services and care for aged persons, mentally retarded children, and others with special problems | Removal of debris | |

| Special police and fire protection for disaster area | | Restoration of public transportation and communication facilities | Food coupons and surplus commodities from Department of Agriculture |

| Identification and care of dead, including temporary morgues | | Repair or replacement of public buildings (schools, hospitals, etc.) | Disaster unemployment insurance provided by Department of Labor through state unemployment offices |

| Designation of hazardous buildings and areas | | Inspection of private property for health and safety | Temporary housing provided through Department of Housing and Urban Development |

| Emergency communication and transportation services | | Salvage of unclaimed property | Specialized counseling and advice to families, such as that provided by Public Health, Department of Agriculture, and other agencies or departments |

| | | | Emergency welfare services to families with children, in some states |

*The chart shows how distinct and yet how closely related are the responsibilities of Red Cross and of government in natural disasters.

**Some of these programs are activated only after a Presidential Declaration of a major disaster. Federal disaster assistance is coordinated by the Federal Disaster Assistance Administration of the Department of Housing and Urban Development.

Figure 12-2 *(Continued)*

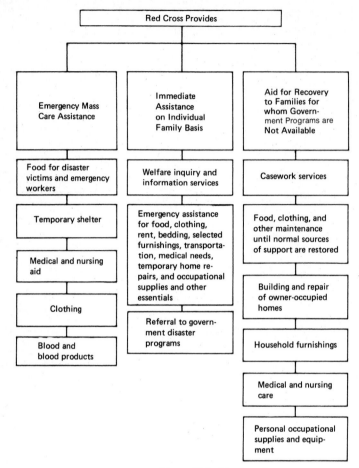

Figure 12-2 (*Continued*)

Red Cross, the League of Red Cross Societies, and the Red Cross society of the affected country.

Red Cross disaster action teams are organized to place trained volunteers at the scene of a disaster within minutes of its occurrence. The disaster action team establishes contact with public officers and appropriate authorities so that Red Cross actions are coordinated with the actions of the police, fire department, civil defense bureau, and other agencies. A determination is made of the need for Red Cross services and support which cannot be handled by the disaster action team.

Each person on the three- to six-member disaster action team must have completed the required training in order to serve. To qualify, the individual must have the following training:

1 Introduction to the Red Cross

2 Introduction to disaster services

3 Instruction in disaster-action-team responsibilities and functions

4 Instruction in damage assessment

5 Instruction in shelter management, mass feeding, and communications

6 Instruction in family service (emergency assistance to families)

7 Completion of the Red Cross standard first aid and personal safety course, or standard first aid–multi-media course

The successful efforts of the Red Cross are demonstrated every year in this country. The blood program, supported by nearly 3 million donors, helps meet a large share of the blood needs of the nation. Every year millions of Americans receive training in first aid, boating safety, home nursing, swimming, lifesaving, and other skills related to safety and health. All these activities are supported by an organization of nearly 2 million volunteers.

LEARNING EXPERIENCES

The following activities are designed to supplement the study of this chapter.

1 Identify the potential sources of disaster in your community or proximate geographic area. Analyze the community needs in a potential disaster. Develop a comprehensive plan for meeting these needs.

2 Invite the local emergency preparedness coordinator to class. Discuss the efforts of the community and the efficiency of the planned system. Compare the comprehensive plan developed by the class with the plans of the local government.

3 Prepare a list of community agencies involved in safety and identify their functions during a disaster. How do these agencies work together to provide a network of services during an emergency?

4 List the components of a comprehensive emergency medical care system. Identify the existing resources in your community. Develop a comprehensive emergency care system. What needs are not being met by the current system?

5 Invite a local or regional health-care planner, or the director of emergency care, to class. Ask him or her to describe the capabilities of the current system. Discuss ways to improve the system and to deal with unmet needs.

6 Develop a comprehensive emergency medical system, and make arrangements to present the plan to the local emergency medical council or the local governing authority.

7 Invite an EMT or paramedic to class and discuss the responsibilities, difficulties, and rewards of the job. Ask the guest to explain how some of the equipment is used, especially the devices used to communicate with hospitals.

8 Develop a plan for community education about the emergency care system. Explain how the media could be used. Write several public-service announcements which could be broadcast to inform the public of the system. What additional promotional activities could be used to gain support for the emergency-care system?

9 Invite a staff person from the American Red Cross to class. Discuss the Red Cross's local, national, and international activities. Discuss the activities of the disaster action team. Discuss the educational programs being offered locally, and the requirements for certification in each of these courses.

SELECTED REFERENCES

American Red Cross, Washington: guidelines and procedures
 No. 3001, *Authority and Legal Status of Red Cross Disaster Services,* October, 1974
 No. 3003, *Administrative Regulations,* November, 1974
 No. 3004, *Policy Position in Situations Caused by Civil Disorder,* March, 1974
 No. 3028, *Emergency Services—Disaster Action Teams,* 1975
 No. 3050, *Disaster Health Services,* February, 1976
 No. 3058, *Human Relations Team,* August, 1974
Your Community Could Have a Disaster, October, 1973
American Hospital Assocation: *Emergency Services,* Chicago, 1972
Dacy, Douglas C., and Howard Kunreuther: *The Economics of Natural Disasters,* The Free Press, New York, 1969
Defense Civil Preparedness Agency, Washington:
 Community Action for Civil Preparedness, December, 1976
 Introduction to Civil Preparedness, July, 1975
 Standards for Civil Preparedness, December, 1972
Dynes, Russell R.: *Organized Behavior in Disaster,* D. C. Heath & Company, Lexington, Mass., 1970
Garb, Solomon, and Evelyn Eng: *Disaster Handbook,* 2d ed., Springer Publishing Co., Inc., New York, 1969
Healy, Richard J.: *Emergency and Disaster Planning,* John Wiley & Sons, Inc., New York, 1969
National Safety Council, Chicago: *Accident Facts,* 1977
Noble, John H., et. al.: *Emergency Medical Services—Behavioral and Planning Perspective,* Behavioral Publications, New York, 1973
U.S. Department of Health, Education and Welfare: *Proceedings of the Second National Conference on Emergency Health Services,* December 2–4, Bethesda, Md., 1971
 Selected Bibliography of Scientific Publications and Programmatic Reports for the U.S.A. Bicentennial Emergency Medical Services and Traumatology Conference, May 10–12, Baltimore, Md., 1976

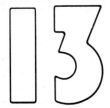

Home Safety and Protection from Fires & Disasters

OVERALL OBJECTIVE:

The student should understand that the home exposes a person to accident-producing situations, and that disaster wears many faces. The student should also know preventive and protective actions to minimize the consequences of accidents.

INSTRUCTIONAL OBJECTIVES:

After completion of this chapter the student will be able to:

1 Analyze the home-accident problem, including specific trends.
2 Describe the functions of the U.S. Consumer Product Safety Commission and its relationship to home safety.
3 List and discuss the different types of home accidents.
4 Formulate an integrated teaching unit to reduce or remove the hazards and conditions responsible for home accidents.
5 List the methods of poisonproofing a home.
6 List the miscellaneous dangers that are found in and around the home.
7 List the eight major causes of nonindustrial fires, and prescribe preventive measures for each.
8 Give five examples of how fire safety can be integrated with other school subjects.
9 Identify the emergency procedures to follow in case of fire in the home.
10 List the most frequent types of natural disasters and the preventive actions to be taken for each.
11 List the major components of a civil defense protection system.

359

HOME SAFETY

Although there has been a 61 percent decline since 1912 (see Figure 13-1), home fatalities still account for about 25 percent of all accidental deaths annually.[1] Lacking the dramatic impact of such disasters as industrial explosions, highway collisions, airplane crashes and train wrecks, accidents in the home receive relatively little publicity. Preventive efforts in this field have been neglected. Most people tend to think of the home as a haven of security, a refuge from danger. Yet more than two-thirds of the accidental injuries annually reported in this country occur in the home, and there are probably many millions of less serious injuries that never get into the official records. Home fatalities average about 27,500 each year, and home injuries over 4 million. The financial loss resulting from these accidents amounts to over $6 billion in diminished income, medical expenses, and insurance overhead. An additional loss of $1.5 billion in property damage results from home fires.[2]

Far from being a refuge, the home exposes people to more hazards in a routine day than they are likely to encounter anywhere else. It takes only a moment's thought to list many potential danger areas within the home that may cause falls, burns, poisoning, suffocation, and various other accidents—loose throw rugs, poorly lighted stairways, defective or improperly used electrical and gas appliances, leaky furnaces, kitchen knives, power tools and do-it-yourself appliances, carelessly stored poisons, plastic bags, discarded refrigerators, and flammable cleaning fluids. On the surrounding grounds, low clotheslines, upturned hoes or rakes, power mowers, and littered walks represent a few of the many hazards. There can be no doubt that education in home safety should be an important part of any accident-prevention program.

ANALYZING DATA AND FORMULATING OBJECTIVES

To organize an effective program in home safety, the appropriate school, safety council, public health agency, or farm bureau must understand the procedures that can prevent deaths and injuries within the home. Then, primary attention can be focused where it is most needed. Some of the information that should be considered in planning is supplied in Figures 13-1 and 13-2, which provide a breakdown of home-accident statistics by type of accident, age of victim, area in which the accident occurred, and activity in which the victim was engaged at the time of the accident.

Home accidents are caused sometimes by environmental hazards and sometimes by human failings but usually by a combination of both. The hazards that are most often responsible for accidents in the home—slippery surfaces; unsuitable, defective or improperly used equipment; disorder; and poor light-

[1] *Accident Facts*, National Safety Council, Chicago, 1977, p. 79.
[2] Ibid., pp. 80–81.

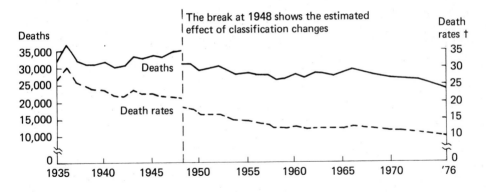

Figure 13-1 Trends in home accidental deaths and death rates. (Source: National Safety Council estimates.)

ing—are usually indicative of the family's neglect, ignorance, or faulty behavior. The other human failings to which home accidents are commonly attributed are poor judgment, inadequate supervision of children, haste, intoxication, and physical handicaps.

Home accidents, like all other accidents, are fundamentally the result of inadequate knowledge, insufficient skill, and faulty attitudes. The objectives of a home safety program should be:

1 To instruct individuals to recognize and understand the many hazards in the home
2 To help them develop a sense of responsibility toward protecting themselves and others against the possibility of home accidents
3 To teach them the knowledge and skills required to perform household tasks safely
4 To help them acquire safe, orderly habits in all their activities in the home
5 To teach them to apply self-control and self-discipline

ACHIEVING THE OBJECTIVES

The great number and variety of hazards in the home make it particularly difficult for any safety program to achieve its objectives. The dangers in our environment and our way of life are changing constantly. We have numerous conveniences, but as we have multiplied our conveniences we have multiplied our dangers. These conveniences must be used intelligently and safely. A brief comparison of the accident-prevention problems in industry and in the home will indicate some of the special conditions that make the task of promoting safe living at home especially challenging (see Chapter 14).

Type of accident and age of victim

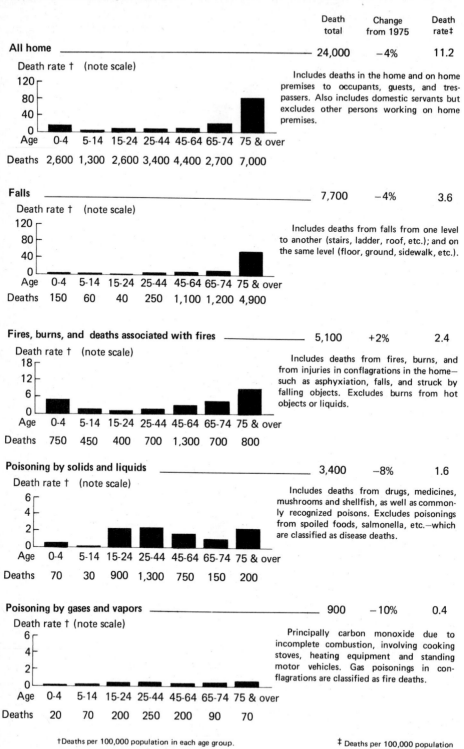

	Death total	Change from 1975	Death rate‡

All home — 24,000   −4%   11.2

Death rate † (note scale)

120
80
40
0

Age   0-4   5-14   15-24   25-44   45-64   65-74   75 & over

Deaths   2,600   1,300   2,600   3,400   4,400   2,700   7,000

Includes deaths in the home and on home premises to occupants, guests, and trespassers. Also includes domestic servants but excludes other persons working on home premises.

Falls — 7,700   −4%   3.6

Death rate † (note scale)

120
80
40
0

Age   0-4   5-14   15-24   25-44   45-64   65-74   75 & over

Deaths   150   60   40   250   1,100   1,200   4,900

Includes deaths from falls from one level to another (stairs, ladder, roof, etc.); and on the same level (floor, ground, sidewalk, etc.).

Fires, burns, and deaths associated with fires — 5,100   +2%   2.4

Death rate † (note scale)

18
12
6
0

Age   0-4   5-14   15-24   25-44   45-64   65-74   75 & over

Deaths   750   450   400   700   1,300   700   800

Includes deaths from fires, burns, and from injuries in conflagrations in the home— such as asphyxiation, falls, and struck by falling objects. Excludes burns from hot objects or liquids.

Poisoning by solids and liquids — 3,400   −8%   1.6

Death rate † (note scale)

6
4
2
0

Age   0-4   5-14   15-24   25-44   45-64   65-74   75 & over

Deaths   70   30   900   1,300   750   150   200

Includes deaths from drugs, medicines, mushrooms and shellfish, as well as commonly recognized poisons. Excludes poisonings from spoiled foods, salmonella, etc.—which are classified as disease deaths.

Poisoning by gases and vapors — 900   −10%   0.4

Death rate † (note scale)

6
4
2
0

Age   0-4   5-14   15-24   25-44   45-64   65-74   75 & over

Deaths   20   70   200   250   200   90   70

Principally carbon monoxide due to incomplete combustion, involving cooking stoves, heating equipment and standing motor vehicles. Gas poisonings in conflagrations are classified as fire deaths.

†Deaths per 100,000 population in each age group.   ‡ Deaths per 100,000 population

Figure 13-2 How people died in home accidents, 1976. (Source: Accident Facts, 1977, National Safety Council, Chicago, Ill.)

Type of accident and age of victim

	Death total	Change from 1975	Death rate‡

Suffocation-ingested object _____ 1,600   −11%   0.7

Death rate † (note scale)

Age	0-4	5-14	15-24	25-44	45-64	65-74	75 & over
Deaths	400	50	130	170	350	200	300

Includes deaths from accidental ingestion or inhalation of objects or food resulting in the obstruction of respiratory passages.

Suffocation-mechanical _____ 700   −13%   0.3

Death rate † (note scale)

Age	0-4	5-14	15-24	25-44	45-64	65-74	75 & over
Deaths	350	160	60	40	30	30	30

Includes deaths from smothering by bed clothes, thin plastic materials, etc., suffocation by cave-ins or confinement in closed spaces, and mechanical strangulation.

Firearms _____ 1,200   −8%   0.6

Death rate † (note scale)

Age	0-4	5-14	15-24	25-44	45-64	65-74	75 & over
Deaths	60	250	350	250	180	80	30

Includes firearms accidents in or on home premises. Many occur while cleaning or playing with guns. Excludes deaths from explosive materials.

All other home _____ 3,400   0%   1.6

Death rate † (note scale)

Age	0-4	5-14	15-24	25-44	45-64	65-74	75 & over
Deaths	800	250	500	400	500	250	700

Most important types included are: drowning, electric current, explosive materials, and blow by falling object.

†Deaths per 100,000 population in each age group.   ‡ Deaths per 100,000 population

Principal type in each age group:

		Population death rate†
Under 1 year	Suffocation—ingested object _____	9.6
1 to 4 years	Fires, burns _____	5.0
5 to 14 years	Fires, burns _____	1.2
15 to 24 years	Poisoning by solids and liquids _____	2.2
25 to 44 years	Poisoning by solids and liquids_____	2.4
45 to 64 years	Fires, burns _____	3.0
65 to 74 years	Falls_____	8.5
75 years and over	Falls_____	56.1

†Deaths per 100,000 population in each age group, 1976.

SPECIAL PROBLEMS

Industry employs safety engineers to make sure that all workers have safe equipment and use it properly. In the home the housekeeper is the safety engineer, and also the cook, cleaning person, launderer, seamster, nurse, chauffeur, and educator. Since the homemaker has so many roles to play, the necessity of doing the various jobs in the shortest time possible may often conflict with accident-prevention duties, and the person's safety rules will probably be somewhat flexible. The homemaker is more likely to stand on the rickety kitchen chair to reach the top shelf in the cupboard than to go down to the cellar for the stepladder. Also, unlike the safety engineer in industry, who usually deals only with able-bodied adults, the housekeeper may have to cope with irresponsible young children, aged and handicapped relatives, and a multitude of other distractions (see Figure 13-3).

The American home today is a vast machine shop containing over a billion appliances, and Americans are expected to buy millions more each year. The U.S. Consumer Product Safety Commission has awakened manufacturers to the need for safer products. Today, "many pieces of wearing apparel, carpets and rugs, mattresses and mattress pads, blankets, tents, sleeping bags and a wide range of other articles are manufactured according to the Federal Standards for Fabric Flammability."[3] Further information on the CPSC appears in the following section and in the list of references.

THE CONSUMER PRODUCT SAFETY COMMISSION[4]

The Consumer Product Safety Act established a new independent federal regulatory agency, the Consumer Product Safety Commission. The Commission's primary goal is to substantially reduce injuries associated with consumer products. On May 14, 1973, the Consumer Product Safety Commission was activated.

Congress directed the Commission to

- Protect the public against unreasonable risks of injury associated with consumer products;
- Assist consumers to evaluate the comparative safety of consumer products;
- Develop uniform safety standards for consumer products and minimize conflicting state and local regulations; and
- Promote research and investigation into the causes and prevention of product-related deaths, illnesses and injuries.

In order for the commission to be most effective, the schools and community must accept responsibility for orienting the citizenry to the functions and objectives of the commission and the procedures for using the commission.

[3]U.S. Consumer Product Fact Sheet No. 25, *Federal and State Standards for Fabric Flammability,* Washington, 1974.
[4]U.S. Consumer P.F.S. No. 52, *Some Federal Consumer-Oriented Agencies,* Washington, 1975. Also see U.S.C.P. SC-Fact Sheet.

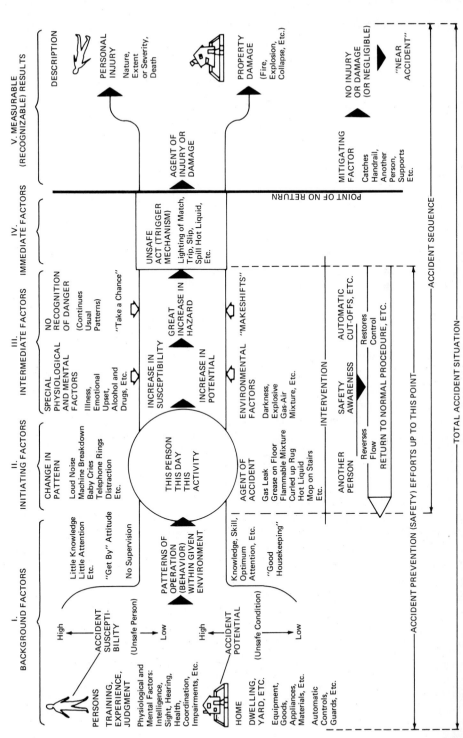

Figure 13-3 The dynamics of home accidents. (Source: Journal of Safety Research, June 1973.)

Our failure to recognize or regard the inherent dangers in and around the house and our false feeling of security while at home tend to make the establishment of safe routine procedures difficult.

The industrial employee must learn to perform only one job or to operate only one machine safely, but the housekeeper is responsible for the operation of many different machines. So many tasks compete for the housekeeper's attention that he or she may neglect the essential maintenance work necessary to keep the various machines in safe running order. It is doubtful, in fact, that housekeepers understand the mechanism of all the equipment they use.

Because of the high cost of accidents, as well as for more humane reasons, industry has given considerable attention to eliminating noise, poor lighting, excessive heat and humidity, and other conditions that contribute to fatigue and carelessness, and increase vulnerability to accidents. Although these factors also endanger homemakers, homemakers rarely initiate a systematic campaign for better working conditions. Even if they did, they could achieve only limited results. Noisy children cannot be muffled as easily as a motor, and heat must be endured if the family cannot afford air conditioning.

THE BASIC APPROACH

POSITIVE INSTRUCTION. The first objective of instruction in home safety is to help individuals recognize specific hazards around the house. It is assumed that recognition of dangerous conditions will result in their removal, and that knowledge of the risk involved in performing a task improperly will lead to the formation of safe habits. Such an approach is essentially negative, and it cannot be wholly effective unless it is combined with positive instruction.

Instructors, whether they are teachers, Scout or 4-H leaders, or parents, should point out the harmful consequences of neglect and carelessness. They must emphasize the benefits of proper behavior, and give individuals as many opportunities as possible to practice the correct procedure. Students should be taught to light the oven the right way, by striking the match before turning on the gas, and not merely told that the wrong way—turning on the gas before lighting the match—may cause an explosion when the accumulated gas ignites. This procedure is of great importance today, since more families consider turning off automatic pilot lights to save energy. In all probability, more conservative use of energy in the home will also decrease the possibility of accidents.

INTEGRATION AND CORRELATION. Instruction in home safety may be accomplished in many ways, but it is especially effective in a formal school setting, where it can be integrated or correlated with other disciplines. Since there are so many different hazards around the house, home safety can probably be taught most effectively when its several aspects are discussed in connection with related subjects. A unit dealing with household poisons such as disinfectants, insecticides, and various medicines can be included in a chemistry course; the correct use of knives and other kitchen utensils can be taught in a home economics class; and the safe use of electricity can be covered in a shop course. In this type of program, the time factor would not be restrictive, and positive learning experiences could be utilized. When time is limited, all too often a list of dos and don'ts becomes the procedure.

The integration approach gives the teacher an excellent chance to relate training in home safety to goals that are meaningful to the students. Students who enroll in home economics courses are eager to become good homemakers and will want to acquire safe cooking and sewing habits if the teacher presents them as a means to that end. Students in an electrical shop course, who are interested, for example, in making lamps for their own rooms, will be motivated to learn how to handle wiring without endangering themselves. Such courses give students a chance to gain actual experience in using safe procedures.

All students should have the chance to practice safe homemaking in their own homes, but too often parents fail to cooperate or to qualify as good supervisors. Perhaps school personnel should consider the possibility of offering a course in home management designed to attract both boys and girls. Students would then have an ideal laboratory situation in which to learn safe methods of performing essential household tasks.

REACHING ADULTS.   It is obvious that no program in home safety can be wholly successful unless it reaches the adults of the community as well as the school-age children. Maintaining a safe home environment is primarily, though by no means entirely, the responsibility of parents, and improvements are not likely to be effected without their support. It is they, not their children, who determine whether carelessness or order is to characterize the family's way of life. Children are proverbial imitators. Adults must exemplify safe behavior if they want to create an atmosphere conducive to the development of desirable safety attitudes. A home safety program can most effectively benefit the very young and the aged, the two groups among whom home accidents take the heaviest toll, by helping to make physically fit adults fully aware of their duty to protect weaker members of their family from needless risks. Most of the accidents incurred in the home by children under five years old can be avoided if the adults responsible for these youngsters exercise proper care.

It is essential to educate the present generation of adults in home safety, not only for their own welfare and the welfare of those in their care, but for the successful training of their children. If the school, despite the poor examples set by many parents, could effectively prepare all young people to maintain safe households when they come of age, hazard-free homes might be anticipated for the future. Unfortunately, the school's program in home safety is not likely to accomplish this objective without the cooperation of the older members of the community.

Education in home safety can best be provided not at school but in the home, where there are ample opportunities for young people to develop good habits by repeatedly practicing the correct procedures. If the school is to succeed in training students to establish accident-free homes, a major part of its effort should be directed toward inducing parents to give children adequate instruction in safety. It is easy for the school to teach young people to recognize and cope with specific hazards if the students' home environment fosters a respect for order and the development of responsible, considerate habits. An orderly household is likely to be a safe household. But when disorder prevails, the training students receive in a safety program may be negated by contrary influences at home.

Although older members of the family are responsible for protecting children during the first few years of their lives, their training in safe living should begin early. They must learn that knives are sharp and useful for cutting food; they must learn that matches produce fire and that fire keeps them warm and cooks their meals. They must learn the safe use of the growing number of electrical appliances, power lawn mowers, and workshop tools which are making our homes unsafe. By the time they are ready for school they should be assuming considerable responsibility for their own protection and showing some concern for the safety of others. Children will be encouraged to respect the rights of others if they associate such altruistic behavior with their parents' approval and affection. They will enjoy feeling that they have done something satisfactory, and adults can help them develop a good attitude toward safety by commending their careful, considerate acts. As they grow older, they can be shown that their helpfulness and concern for others contribute to good family living.

Desirable habits can be acquired only by actually practicing the proper procedures in a learning situation. Children should be required to participate in the family's efforts to keep the home safe. When they are still very young, they should be taught not to leave their toys on the stairs or in the middle of the floor, where people are likely to trip over them, but to return them to their proper storage place. Later they should be made responsible for keeping their rooms in order.

Parents who enforce sensible precautions against injury, taking time to explain the "why" of these precautions, bring their children through the formative years with a minimum of accidents. And when these youngsters go out into the world of schools, streets, and swimming pools, they carry with them ingrained attitudes and habits of safety which carry them through new difficulties, to a future unimaginable by their parents.

Parents must set a good example for the child if their instructions are to be effective. Too often one parent takes careless chances, and sometimes the other, after a hard day at the office, resents being asked to "do something" about flickering light sockets or a loose rug. If all members of the family would assume some share of responsibility for keeping the house in order, the homemaker's duties would be lightened, and he or she could then devote more time to functioning as a safety engineer.

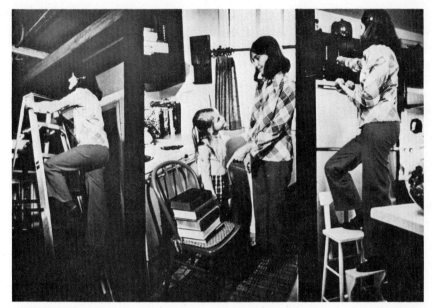

Figure 13-4 A firm step stool or stepladder will help avoid falls. (Courtesy The Country Companies, Bloomington, Ill. 61701.)

RECOGNIZING THE MAJOR HAZARDS

Comprehensive and systematic instruction must deal with all the undesirable practices and dangerous conditions that are frequently responsible for home casualties. Each of the accident categories illustrated previously should be investigated. Individuals must be taught to recognize the causes of falls, burns, poisonings, and other common accidents, and then participate in learning activities that will aid them in acquiring the knowledge, attitudes, and skills to eliminate these causes. Appropriate learning experiences may be selected from the list at the end of this chapter.

FALLS

Although statistics may not be interesting or exciting, one must remember that when they refer to fatalities and injuries, each number represents a personal loss to persons ranging from babies to senior citizens.

Over 16,000 fatalities are caused by falls. Of these fatalities, 11,500, or 71 percent, occur to individuals sixty-five or older. Of the more than 25,000 home-accident deaths that occur annually, 7,700, or approximately 25 percent, are caused by falls. The highest death rate for all home accidents, 66.8, is incurred in falls.[5]

[5]*Accident Facts*, National Safety Council, Chicago, 1977, Figure 13-1.

The following practices are among the most common causes of falls: standing on chairs or other unstable objects (Figure 13-4), including ladders that are in need of repair; skidding on small rugs or on slippery surfaces, such as improperly polished, wet, or greasy floors; tripping over objects left in the middle of the floor or on the stairs; and catching a toe on an upturned or torn carpet. Stairways that are poorly lighted or that lack a firm handrail and improper footwear or stocking feet, especially if the hose are made of slick synthetics, are factors that lead to many falls in the home. Well-fitting shoes which provide a firm base are helpful in preventing accidents. Loose-fitting shoes, high or narrow heels, untied shoelaces, sloppy cuffs, and wide or long pants and skirts all constitute tripping hazards.

The danger of falling in the home can be reduced to a minimum if a few simple precautions are taken. There would be no need for anyone in the family to stand on chairs or other unstable objects if a firm stepstool or stepladder was readily available (Figure 13-4), one large enough to enable adults to reach the highest shelves without using the top steps, where they might have difficulty in keeping their balance. From the standpoint of safety, only large rugs should be used in the house. If small rugs are preferred, they should be treated with cork or rubber to reduce the possibility of their skidding underfoot. Slippery floors are often the result of too much wax and too little polishing, but applying one of the nonslip waxes that are now on the market should virtually eliminate this hazard.

Most children love to climb. They may be expected to amuse themselves on accessible ladders, trees, garage roofs, or anything else climbable. Often this practice is dangerous because young children lack the coordination and skill to climb safely and the knowledge and experience to avoid taking foolish risks. Parental prohibitions are usually ineffectual, for young children are not likely to understand the danger involved in such a pleasurable pastime, and they realize that the parent need never discover their disobedience. Usually parents who make the dangers of climbing vivid enough to convince children of their reality succeed in preventing them from climbing only at the cost of making them excessively timid.

Ideally, parents should anticipate children's desire to climb, provide them with safe climbing apparatus such as a jungle gym or a firm ladder securely attached to the side of the garage, and instruct them in using such equipment. When this procedure is followed, children have an opportunity to participate in a valuable and enjoyable body-building exercise without endangering themselves. They may then have less desire to climb elsewhere. Even if they do climb trees and fire escapes, the skill developed in using the practice apparatus should help protect them from falls.

Since approximately 71 percent of the victims of falls are more than sixty-five years old, a program in home safety should give considerable attention to the problem of protecting the aged. As their vision grows weak and they lose their firm step, older people may need better lighting on the stairs, and a firm handrail becomes absolutely essential. Any object left in the middle of the floor or on the stairs particularly endangers older persons, for their sight may not be keen enough to detect it, and if they trip, they are less likely than a young person to recover their balance. Aged persons should be especially cautious about using the upper steps of a ladder or stepstool, for their physical frailty and poor balance make climbing dangerous. When using a ladder, make sure it is stable and sound. Always lock the spreader on a stepladder. It is a good policy not to stand higher than the third step from the top. When using a straight ladder, make sure it is long enough for the job so that it can be set at a safe angle. The "4 to 1" rule, setting the ladder base out 1 foot for every 4 feet of length, is a safe procedure (Figure 13-5). Both hands should be used when climbing, and one should not reach too far to the side. It is safer to move the ladder. A good practice is to keep your belt buckle between the rails.

Keeping an orderly home, with the furniture so arranged that it does not interfere with free passage around the room, is one of the best ways of preventing falls. The bedroom, scene of many home accidents, is often dangerous because beds, vanity benches, and other furnishings jut into the room in a way that invites people to stumble over them. Closet doors left ajar, open dresser drawers, and shoes lying in the middle of the room are other common hazards in the bedroom. When people get out of bed during the night, fumble around in the dark for robe and slippers, and grope toward the bathroom or kitchen, only half awake, they are more than likely to fall over any improperly placed object. The homemaker can eliminate this danger by seeing that the house is kept in good order and that a light switch is located within reach of the bed and at the entrance to all the principal rooms.

If one is prone to falling it may be necessary to learn how to fall without injury, as athletes, acrobats, and stunt persons do. Learning how to fall properly

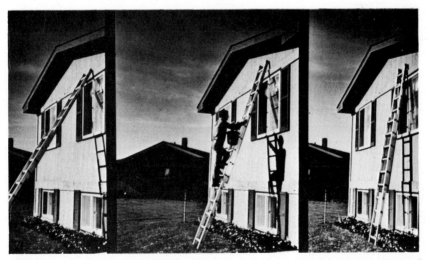

Figure 13-5 A safe angle is setting the ladder base out one foot for every 4 feet of length. (Courtesy The Country Companies, Bloomington, Ill. 61701.)

can be accomplished only by practicing on a mat under the supervision of a competent instructor. However, there are some steps one can remember to prevent injury when falling.[6]

1 Relax; do not stiffen up.

2 Turn the body to permit landing on a well padded part (one side of the buttocks, or on the thigh or shoulder)—or catch weight on a broad part of the body to take up the shock (fingers spread wide apart—arms outstretched). Dropping backward into a straight sitting position can be hard on the end of the spine. Turning only slightly to the side puts the contact on the large muscles.

3 When falling from one level to another, it is probably best to touch ground on the balls of the feet. As the feet touch the ground, bend the knees and ankles and curl the body. Attempt to put spring in parts of body by gently bending legs, hips and arms. Either stop on all fours or allow the body to roll sideward.

4 If the drop is not too great, after the legs have been bent on contact, then straighten the legs and stand or walk forward to slow down body momentum.

5 If falling forward or falling on hands and knees, reach out only moderately with the arms, have the fingers spread to distribute the area of contact, and let the arms give and fold in toward the body. Then fall to the side onto padded thigh or shoulder and roll if there is sufficient momentum to make you do so.

Practicing the above skills under the supervision of a physical education instructor would assure a person's competency in avoiding injuries.

BURNS

Severe burns are serious not only because of the immediate wound but because of the accompanying shock and the possibility of toxic poisoning, which may affect the kidneys, liver, and blood. Over one-fifth of the fatalities caused by home accidents are the result of burns, and about 45 percent of the persons who die from burns are either under five years of age or over sixty-four.

Burns occur under a variety of circumstances, but usually some personal fault is responsible. A pack of matches ignites in a person's hand because the person has failed to close the cover before striking a match. Fires start because an ash tray containing a still smoldering cigarette has been emptied into a waste-basket, or because oily rags have been carelessly stored. The flame from a gas burner may ignite a curtain that has not been securely fastened away from the stove, and rubbish fires sometimes get out of control because the refuse has not been burned in a proper container.

The improper use of flammable liquids is another common cause of burns. Many people are only vaguely aware that the fumes from gasoline, benzine, naphtha, and similar cleaning fluids are very dangerous if used near an open flame. If volatile liquids are allowed to vaporize, even switching on an electric light can cause a terrific explosion, as at least one homemaker discovered after attempting to clean the floors with gasoline. Also, few people recognize the

[6]Safety Education Data Sheet No. 5, *Falls*, rev., National Safety Council, Chicago.

danger of static electricity, which may be generated by rubbing a garment saturated with a flammable cleaning or stain-removing fluid. To avoid these dangers, the homemaker should purchase and use exclusively one of the nonflammable, nonexplosive, safe cleaning fluids now on the market.

Newspaper accounts of children burned while playing with matches are fairly frequent. Many of these incidents occur because adults have been negligent about keeping matches out of the reach of very young children. Sometimes even a careful parent cannot prevent a child from gaining access to matches. Small children who see an adult light a match may want to try the trick themselves, and if forbidden may seize the first opportunity to climb on a chair and take the matches from their "safe" storage place. If children are permitted, under adult supervision, to strike a match for an express purpose, such as lighting birthday candles or igniting the refuse in a wire basket, where it may be safely burned, they may not feel the need to "snitch" a match to perform the magic when no one is around. Rather than deny the child's request to light a match, the wise parent will teach him or her to handle matches properly, explaining that they are to be used only with the help of an adult and only in prescribed ways.

Consideration for their own safety should motivate homemakers to place pots containing liquids on the rear burners of the stove, with the handles pointing away from the edges; to take precautions against spilling or splattering hot grease; and to observe various other safety measures to minimize the possibility of burns. Often, however, adults feel that they have sufficient knowledge and skill to live safely despite hazards, and that there is therefore no need to eliminate such hazards. Perhaps the homemaker will be sure to avoid brushing against pot handles that extend beyond the front of the stove, but small children may be able to reach the handle, and their natural curiosity may induce them to investigate. If adults cannot attach sufficient reality to the possibility that they themselves may be injured as a result of their unsafe practices, they should at least recognize the danger to which their thoughtlessness subjects other members of the family. They must realize that setting the children a good example is an important part of training them to protect themselves.

In teaching students to protect themselves from the danger of burns, the instructor should stress the usefulness of controlled fires and the procedures by which they can be controlled. To supplement this positive approach, the instructor should also point out that severe burns may result if, through carelessness and disorder, fires are allowed to get out of control. Such unsafe practices as smoking in bed should be explained in terms of a dangerous combination. Since the bed is associated with sleeping, the person who smokes in bed may find the stimulus to sleep stronger than the stimulus to smoke. If the person should fall asleep, the still burning cigarette represents a "fire" that is no longer in that person's control. Numerous projects can be planned to show that when order is present and the environment is under human control, safety prevails.

In a recent hospital survey of burns it was found that hot water was the leading cause, followed by clothing, hot beverages, gasoline, chemicals, cooking grease, range ovens, conflagrations, wires, cords, and automobiles. To avoid serious hot-water burns, keep the water temperature between 135°F and 140°F. This, along with the cleaning action of the soap, should kill any bacteria. Excessively hot water may cause painful burns and can lead to more serious consequences. The very young and the very old have the greatest frequency of burn accidents; they should not be left alone or unattended when there is any danger of scalding.

TREATMENT OF BURNS When a serious burn occurs, a doctor should be called immediately, or the victim should be taken directly to a hospital. If the burn is not too serious it may be treated in the following manner.

1 Cool the burn by plunging it in ice water, or hold it under cold water; this reduces the pain and stops thermal destruction of the skin.

2 Cover the burn with a piece of clean, dry sheet or handkerchief.

3 Do not try to clean the burn, and do not put greasy ointment, grease, or butter on the affected part.

Most first-aid manuals describe in detail how to care for the various degrees of burns. If there is any question as to the seriousness of a burn, a doctor should be called, or the victim should be taken to a hospital.

GAS POISONING

Approximately 1,000 of the fatalities annually attributed to home accidents are due to gas poisoning. Many of these deaths occurred because the homemaker allowed liquids to boil over on the gas burner and extinguish the flame. When fuel gas is inhaled, the carbon monoxide combines with the red corpuscles, displacing the oxygen in the blood and causing death. The fumes expelled from an improperly banked coal furnace and the sulfur dioxide that escapes from a broken pipe in a mechanical refrigerator are responsible for many gas-poisoning fatalities. In other cases, a gas space heater used in a small closed room has consumed the oxygen in the air and caused suffocation.

The majority of gas poisoning fatalities are caused by incomplete combustion of carbon monoxide. This can involve heating equipment, stoves, or motor vehicles standing in a tightly enclosed area, usually the family garage. One of the hazardous characteristics of this deadly gas is that it is colorless, odorless, and tasteless, thus giving no warning of its presence. Despite the publicity given to the dangers of running a car motor in a closed garage, that practice continues to be responsible for a number of fatalities each year. It seems likely that carelessness rather than ignorance is responsible for these accidents.

The following precautions are suggested.[7]

[7]James E. Aaron, Frank Bridges, and Dale Ritzel, *First Aid and Emergency Care*, The Macmillan Company, New York, 1972, p. 111.

1 Gas stoves and refrigerators should be serviced carefully and regularly; an annual check or oftener.

2 No one should sleep in a poorly ventilated room where a coal or gas stove is the source of heat.

3 All gas- and oil-burning devices should be vented correctly.

4 Furnaces should be checked annually, and certainly the chimney and flue should be free of leaks.

5 Fireplaces should have sufficient drafts.

6 Indoor grills should have suitable venting; they may be placed in a fireplace.

7 A car's exhaust system should be in good repair; it should be inspected annually.

8 No one should sit in a parked car with the motor running.

9 A gasoline-burning engine should not be indoors without sufficient venting and circulation of fresh air.

10 The tailpipe on a car should be checked to make certain it does not clog when backing into snow, sand, dirt, water, or any other substance. If the car stalls in water, the ignition should be turned off.

11 No one should breathe gas, not even for a short period of time.

Common symptoms of carbon monoxide poisoning are headaches, dizziness, sleepiness, nausea, vomiting, and muscular weakness which render the victim helpless. The victim's skin frequently turns to a cherry red.

Should such an accident occur, the victim should be moved from the area immediately. The rescuer should call a physician at once, give mouth-to-mouth resuscitation, and keep the victim warm.

Other dangerous fumes may come from chemicals such as carbon tetrachloride, commonly used in the home for cleaning garments, and petroleum distillates such as gasoline, benzine, and kerosene. All these chemicals can cause asphyxiation and death.

Householders must assume responsibility for selecting and maintaining properly any equipment in and around the home that has the potential to cause gas poisoning. Such equipment should be regularly inspected, and repaired as necessary. People seem to forget that such mechanisms get old and wear out after a certain length of time. Too often, defective equipment is replaced only after it has caused serious damage.

OTHER TYPES OF POISONING

Although the death rate from poisoning by solids and liquids has declined in this century, there has been an increase from 0.8 in 1957 to 1.9 in recent years. The rate may appear to be small, but over 4,000 people die each year from this type of poisoning (Table 13-1).

Contrary to popular impressions, the majority of these fatalities occur to individuals who are over fifteen years of age rather than to young children. In a recent federal study by the National Institute of Drug Abuse, it was estimated that sleeping pills alone are associated with nearly 5,000 deaths each year, and that the users of these pills make about 25,000 trips to hospital emergency wards annually. The director of the study stated that having sleeping pills in the family medicine chest "is like having a loaded gun in the house."

TABLE 13–1

Poisoning by Type and Age, Accidental Deaths, 1975

Deaths by Type of Poisoning	All Ages	Under 5 Years	5–14 Years	15–24 Years	25–44 Years	45–64 Years	65 Years and Over
Total Poisoning by Solids and Liquids	4,694	114	49	1,332	1,853	926	420
Rate (deaths per 100,000 population)	2.2	0.7	0.1	3.3	3.5	2.1	1.9
Male	*3,147*	*66*	*36*	*1,048*	*1,318*	*476*	*203*
Female	*1,547*	*48*	*13*	*284*	*535*	*450*	*217*
Drugs and medicaments	3,132	65	19	1,056	1,282	428	282
Male	*2,038*	*36*	*11*	*818*	*894*	*165*	*114*
Female	*1,094*	*29*	*8*	*238*	*388*	*263*	*168*
Antibiotics, anti-infectives (includes penicillin)	27	3	0	2	2	8	12
Hormones, synthetic substitutes (incl. insulin)	32	0	0	4	7	8	13
Systemic, hematologic agents (includes vitamins)	61	6	3	11	12	13	16
Analgesics, antipyretics (incl. aspirin)	1,275	24	6	516	611	90	28
Other sedatives, hypnotics (includes barbiturates)	557	3	3	187	218	104	42
Autonomic nervous system, psycho-therapeutic drugs (incl. tranquilizers)	178	11	0	36	76	41	14
Other central nervous system depressants, stimulants (incl. amphetamines)	37	0	1	16	15	4	1
Cardiovascular drugs	158	4	1	1	4	28	120
Gastrointestinal drugs	3	3	0	0	0	0	0
Other, unspecified (incl. local anesthetics)	804	11	5	283	337	132	36
Other solid and liquid substances	1,562	49	30	276	571	498	138
Male	*1,109*	*30*	*25*	*230*	*424*	*311*	*89*
Female	*453*	*19*	*5*	*46*	*147*	*187*	*49*
Alcohol	391	1	1	26	124	210	29
Cleansing, polishing agents	12	7	0	2	0	2	1
Disinfectants	6	0	0	0	1	1	4
Paints, varnishes	5	0	2	2	0	1	0
Petroleum products, other solvents	54	21	5	11	5	8	4
Pesticides, fertilizers, plant foods	30	6	1	4	5	10	4

TABLE 13-1 *(continued)*
Poisoning by Type and Age, Accidental Deaths, 1975

Deaths by Type of Poisoning	All Ages	Under 5 Years	5–14 Years	15–24 Years	25–44 Years	45–64 Years	65 Years and Over
Heavy metals and their fumes	13	2	1	0	3	7	0
Other corrosives, caustics	16	4	0	1	1	4	6
Noxious foodstuffs, poisonous plants	6	0	0	1	1	1	3
Other, unspecified	1,029	8	20	229	431	254	87
Total Poisoning by Gases and Vapors	1,577	38	81	357	471	392	238
Rate	0.7	0.2	0.2	0.9	0.9	0.9	1.1
Male	*1,165*	*22*	*55*	*260*	*379*	*298*	*151*
Female	*412*	*16*	*26*	*97*	*92*	*94*	*87*
Gas distributed by pipeline	166	0	2	20	23	34	37
Liquefied petroleum gas distributed in mobile containers	51	2	2	9	14	9	15
Other utility gases	8	2	0	2	2	0	2
Motor vehicle exhaust gas	736	10	23	188	262	196	57
Carbon monoxide from incomplete combustion of domestic fuels	159	7	10	40	30	38	34
Other carbon monoxide	239	6	7	38	80	61	47
Other gases and vapors	236	11	35	57	48	49	36
Unspecified gases and vapors	32	0	2	3	12	5	10

Source: National Center for Health Statistics. Reported in *Accident Facts,* National Safety Council, Chicago, 1977.

Except for the increasing number of deaths attributed to an overdose of sleeping pills, there is little variation from year to year in the causes of accidental poisonings. As might be expected, more than four-fifths of all fatal poisonings occur in the home. Many of them are the result of the homemaker's failure to keep poisons out of the reach of small children. Although some parents are merely careless in this regard, others fail to realize the number of substances around the house that can poison a child, or an adult. There are cases on record of adults who have arisen in the middle of the night to take a dose of cough medicine but who, still half asleep, have taken instead a swig of Lysol or some other poisonous liquid. Poisons have also been mistaken for food: children have been known to eat rat poison, and strychnine has been used instead of baking powder. Botulism, a form of poisoning that results from eating improperly canned or preserved foods, also claims a number of lives every year. See Table 13-1 for other types of poisoning.

Each year thousands of children are accidently poisoned. Many are injured and many die from ingesting medicines, drain cleaners, bleaches, and other household chemicals. These chemicals are important aids in maintaining a home. They are safe and effective when used intelligently, as directed, and with caution. When they are swallowed by a child, tragedy can result.

When poisonous household chemicals and medicines enter the home, it is the responsibility of the parent to make sure that they are not swallowed by young children, who will eat and drink almost anything. The following suggestions will help "poisonproof" your home:[8]

1 Use safety packaging when available.

2 Learn how to re-secure correctly the safety feature after use, so that the product will always be packaged safely.

3 Keep household products and medicines out of reach and out of sight of your child. Lock them up when possible.

4 Store internal medicines away from other household substances. Properly re-secure the cap and keep the product in the original container. Never put any medicine or chemical in a cup or soft drink bottle.

5 Read the label on all products and heed warnings and caution.

6 Always turn on the light when giving medicines. Never take medicines in the dark.

7 Avoid taking medicines in your child's presence. The child may learn to imitate your action.

8 If you have a crawling infant, keep household products stored above the floor level, not beneath the kitchen sink.

9 If you are using a product when called to the door or telephone, take it with you; otherwise your child could get into it.

10 Have handy the phone number of your nearest doctor, poison control center, hospital, and police.

If a medicine has been prescribed for a specific illness, it should be used only as long as needed and then promptly discarded, for age may change its composition so that it becomes lethal. Discarding the bottle removes the temptation for other members of the family to use a compound that has been prepared for a particular individual in a particular state of health. One person's cure may be another person's poison, and special prescriptions should be taken only as the doctor orders. Liquids such as iodine should also be discarded after a reasonable length of time, since they become stronger as evaporation takes place.[9]

POISON FIRST-AID CHART[10]

Call your doctor immediately. If he can't be reached, call one of the following: local poison control center if available, hospital, pharmacist, police or fire department. If possible, begin first-aid treatment while another person calls for help. The nature of the poison or overdose will determine the first-aid measure to use—as shown below—*until medical help is obtained.*

---

[8]*Preventing Childhood Poisoning*, U.S. Department of Health, Education, and Welfare, Public Health Service, Food and Drug Afmin022istration, Publication No. (FDA) 75-7001, 1974.

[9]For further information on poisoning, see Consumer Product Safety Commission Fact Sheet No. 14, *Lead Paint Poisoning*, and No. 21, *Poisonous Household Substances*.

[10]*Family Safety*, National Safety Council, Summer, 1974, p. 11.

If the patient is unconscious or in convulsions:
- Do NOT force liquids on him and do NOT induce vomiting.
- Provide artificial respiration if necessary, keep him warm and take him to the hospital immediately.
- Take along the poison container, label, remaining contents or any vomited material to help identify the poison.

If the patient swallowed a corrosive or petroleum product:
- Do NOT induce vomiting.
- Dilute the poison with water or milk. *Dosage:* 1 to 2 cups for patients under 5 years of age—up to 1 quart for patients 5 years and older.
- Get him to the hospital immediately—along with the poison container, label or remaining contents to help identify the poison.

If the patient swallowed an overdose or poison that is *not* a corrosive or petroleum product:
- Dilute with water or milk. *Dosage:* 1 to 2 cups for patients under 5 years of age—up to 1 quart for patients 5 years and older.
- Induce vomiting. *To induce vomiting:* 1 tablespoon (½ ounce) of syrup of ipecac, plus at least 1 cup of water. (If no vomiting occurs within 20 minutes, dose may be repeated *only once.*) If syrup of ipecac is unavailable, induce vomiting by placing the blunt end of a spoon or your finger at the back of the victim's throat. *Do not give salt water.* When vomiting begins, keep patient face down with head lower than hips to prevent choking; place a small child across your knees in a "spanking" position.
- If no vomiting occurs within 20 minutes, repeat syrup of ipecac dose only *once* as already described—but don't waste time waiting any longer. Call doctor or hospital again for further instructions. If you can't get those instructions, take patient to hospital immediately. Bring along the container, label or remaining contents to help identify the poison—or, if vomiting occurs, a sample of the vomited material.

Examples of corrosives: sodium acid sulfate (toilet bowl cleaners), sulfuric acid, nitric acid, oxalic acid, hydrofluoric acid (rust removers), iodine, silver nitrate (caustic pencil), sodium hydroxide or lye (drain cleaners), sodium carbonate (washing soda), ammonia water, sodium hypochlorite (household bleach). *Examples of petroleum products:* gasoline, kerosene, lighter fluid, naphtha, mineral seal oil (furniture polishes), petroleum solvents and cleaners.

SUFFOCATION

Each year close to 3,000 people die from suffocation accidents. Such accidents are classified under two categories.

1 Ingested objects, which includes deaths from accidental ingestion or inhalation of objects or food, resulting in the obstruction of the respiratory passage.
2 Mechanical, which includes deaths from smothering by bed clothing, thin plastic material, and cave-ins or confinement in closed spaces.

In an average year close to 1,000 youngsters under four years old die of suffocation. Many of these deaths could have been avoided if adults had been more aware of the dangers surrounding infants. According to doctors' reports, the following items have been removed from children's lungs or windpipes: peanuts, pieces of vegetables, bacon, watermelon seeds, dried beans from a bean blower, pieces of plastic toys, pins, buttons, etc. Until children have mastered the fine art of mastication, edibles such as nuts, raw carrots, crisp bacon, and corn should be kept out of their reach and off their menu. In one instance, an ice cube lodged in an infant's throat caused some anxious moments. An ice cube lodged in the throat may not melt quickly enough to prevent suffocation. Toy balloons can be hazardous. A child who breathes in instead of out while blowing up a balloon can easily inhale the rubber and choke to death. Young children should never be allowed to play with deflated balloons. Parents should be aware of toys that shatter or have small, detachable parts such as eyes and wheels, that can be easily swallowed.

Infections of the respiratory system are the primary cause of many of these fatalities. Reports also show that babies are sometimes smothered by becoming entangled in the bed covering or their clothing, that others are strangled by gagging after vomiting, and that still others are suffocated by smoke. In a few cases, adults have rolled over onto sleeping infants and smothered them. Discarded refrigerators claim the lives of small children who explore the interior and then find that the door has snapped shut and imprisoned them. Removing the door or the latch stop on discarded refrigerators will eliminate this danger, and adequate care on the part of parents should prevent suffocation from the various other causes.

Deaths by polyethylene plastic garment, trash, and food bags continue to occur among babies and young children. Because of the extreme thinness of the material, static electricity is generated through friction, which causes the bag to adhere tightly to the skin when brought in contact with it. If the mouth and nose of a child are covered with one of these bags, the air is cut off and suffocation ensues. The material will not tear when the suffocating child fights it, and the child is unable to cry for help. These bags can become lethal instruments. They should be destroyed by burning with other trash or combustible material.

Fatalities can be avoided if parents and older members of the family take proper precautions and learn what to do in suffocation situations. Most first-aid manuals can prescribe the proper steps to take. Above all, remain calm and have a physician's phone number handy.

FIREARMS

The safe handling of firearms is discussed in Chapter 5. But misuse of firearms is a leading cause of accidental deaths in the home. Approximately two-thirds of all firearm fatalities occur in and around the home.[11] Many occur while people are cleaning or playing with guns they thought were not loaded.

Most accidental firearm fatalities occur to males, especially those between

[11] *Accident Facts*, National Safety Council, Chicago, 1977, pp. 7, 15, 80.

the ages of five and thirty-four. Over 500 fatalities per year are incurred by young men under fifteen years of age. There are several countermeasures that can reduce the number of home gun accidents.

1 Prohibit guns in the home. This is a controversial measure, but it would reduce accidents to children.

2 Take the National Rifle Association's home firearm safety course.

3 Store guns under lock and key, out of the reach of children and others not qualified to handle them.

4 Lock up all ammunition, preferably away from firearms.

5 Before bringing guns into the home, inspect them carefully to make sure the magazine and chamber are not loaded.

If all guns were treated with the respect due to loaded guns, many home gun accidents could be prevented.

MISCELLANEOUS DANGERS

In addition to casualties from the major types of accidents already discussed, approximately 4,000 accidental deaths occur in the home every year as the result of various miscellaneous causes. Individuals concerned with home safety must orient students, parents, and others to recognize and guard against some of the relatively newer hazards, such as:

1 Homemade rockets and other "space gadgets," which demand thorough understanding and close supervision

2 Backyard swimming pools, which number over 1 million and present problems of sanitation and safety

3 Many of the newer fibers which are used for clothing and which are highly flammable

4 Glass doors separating the house from the patio. Without some decorative decals on the glass, these doors can cause severe face and head injuries to youngsters as they hurry through the house.

HOME WORKSHOPS

Home workshops are becoming increasingly prevalent as the do-it-yourself movement gains in popularity. Although they promote worthwhile leisure-time activities and call prompt attention to needed repairs, they also increase the possibility of accidents. Many home workshops contain lathes, bench saws, drill presses, sanders, planers, shapers, and other power tools that are dangerous if not properly used. Amateur carpenters must learn to apply the same safety measures that industry prescribes for the protection of workers who use such tools (see Chapter 14). Volatile liquids, paints, and cleansing fluids should be stored in a safe place—away from flames, sparks, or heat. Shop teachers are in the best position to furnish the necessary instruction for the safe operation of a home workshop.

GARDENING

The principal dangers in gardening, another creative leisure-time activity, are careless handling of rakes and hoes and inefficient operation of power equipment such as mowers, hedge cutters, and trimmers. Gardeners have frequently been injured by stepping on the upturned teeth of a rake or the edge of a hoe, causing the handle to come up sharply and inflict a severe blow. This danger can be easily eliminated by storing such tools properly when they are not in use and by turning them downward when they are momentarily laid aside.

POWER MOWERS

Today, the power lawnmower is a common household device. There are approximately 25 million in use with an additional million sold each year. Despite its protective devices, a mower is only as safe as its operator. As with any power tool or power equipment, carelessness or error on the part of the operator can cause serious injury and death. It is estimated that there are close to 150,000 mower injuries each year, with the majority caused by the whirling blades. Each year 3,500 careless users have fingers, toes, hands, feet, arms, or legs mutilated in power-mower accidents.[12]

The following safety rules should be observed when using a power mower:

1 Know how to control your machine, and how to stop it quickly.

2 Don't allow youngsters, or adults who have not had proper instruction, to operate the machine.

3 Be sure the area to be mowed is clear of objects which might be picked up and thrown.

4 Disengage the clutch and put the gearshift in neutral before starting the engine.

5 Keep bystanders away from the material being discharged.

6 Stop the motor when you leave the machine.

7 Never run the engine in a closed garage or shed. Exhaust gases are dangerous, and carbon monoxide gives no warning.

8 Don't move too close to a ditch or creek, stay alert for holes and other hidden hazards, and watch out for traffic when near roadways.

9 Watch where you are driving. Beware of steep slopes and sharp turns, which can cause tipping or loss of control.

10 Don't carry passengers, and keep children and pets at a safe distance.

11 Using a checklist, conduct periodic inspections.

---

[12]"Know Before You Mow," *Family Safety*, National Safety Council, Summer, 1976, p. 12, Chicago.

Many of the precautions for the riding mower also apply to the walk-behind power mower, with the addition of the following:

1 When selecting a mower, be sure the discharge chute has a deflector plate to direct the discharge downward. The plate should be used when there is no grass-catching bag attached.

2 The mower should have a footguard in the rear to keep the operator's foot away from the blade.

3 Know the controls well enough to act quickly in case of an emergency.

4 Never adjust or leave the machine without first stopping the mower and disconnecting the spark-plug wire.

5 Avoid wet grass, as you may slip and come in contact with the blade. Clogging can also be caused by wet grass.

6 Watch your footing on steep slopes. Steer the mower across the slope, never up and down it.

7 Keep the mower flat on the ground. Never lift the mower, tilt it, or pull it toward yourself.

8 Check your fuel before starting. Avoid refueling a hot machine.

9 Store gasoline in a well-ventilated area, in a tightly capped, approved safety can. Keep gasoline away from children, living quarters, and any flame or heat sources.

10 When using an electric mower, be careful not to run over the cord or entangle it in the blades.

Caution should be taken when using a gasoline-powered rotary tiller. Before attempting to use one, make sure you know how to operate it. Most rotary tillers used around the home are rented; get adequate instruction from the rental agent.

CHRISTMAS TREE FIRES

Christmas tree fires are not so common as they were when candles were used for decorations, but, defective wiring can ignite dry needles and branches. If the following precautions are taken, there should be little danger of fires or other accidents. If a natural tree is purchased, make sure it is fresh. The higher the moisture content, the less likely the tree is to dry out and become a serious fire hazard. Fill the holder with water until the cut line is covered, and keep the water at that level. Keep the tree away from any heat source. Dispose of the tree when the needles start to drop off.

With metal trees, be careful that sharp edges don't cut the cord insulation. Metal trees should be illuminated by colored floodlights, but when the lights get hot, keep them away from little children. Plastic trees that are made of fire-resistant material should also be kept away from heat sources.

LIGHTING. Check cords. Look for frayed wires, loose connections, broken sockets, and bare spots. Lights should be fastened securely, and no bulb should come in contact with needles or branches. Don't overload extension cords. There should be no more than three sets of lights on a single cord. Keep connection joints away from the water supply for live trees.

When leaving the house or retiring for the evening, be sure all lights are turned off by unplugging them from the wall outlet. Never use wax candles on or near a tree; they are serious fire hazards. Keep decorative candles and flammable materials away from children. If trees are placed on tables, they should be kept out of reach of small children.

Before using a set of tree lights, place them on a nonflammable surface and plug them in for 10 or 15 minutes. Check for smoking and melting.

HIRING A BABY SITTER

Baby sitting is an occupation that now engages many adults and more than half the young people in America over twelve years of age. It enables them to earn millions of dollars each year. Many courses in home economics, family life, etc., offer these youngsters some training in child care, and in some schools special units have been set up for training "junior child-care aides." Unless baby sitters are properly prepared to take over the routine care of small children, the growing practice of hiring a sitter may increase the number of accidents incurred by small children. If the following precautions are observed in hiring a baby sitter, the danger in this situation should be reduced to a minimum:

1 The baby sitter should be in good health and free of any illness, even a slight cold.

2 The child should have an opportunity to become acquainted with the sitter before the parents leave so that if the child awakens during the night, he or she will be spared the frightening experience of being greeted by a stranger.

3 The sitter should be given written instructions covering the routine duties and including information on feeding the baby, stories to be read, play routine, bathing and toilet procedures, sleeping garments, and any medication to be given.

4 The sitter should receive written instructions on the procedure to be followed in case of emergency. The instructions should include the address and phone number at which the parents can be reached; the name, address, and phone number of the physician to be called, and the phone number of the doctor's exchange; the name, address, and phone number of the neighbor to be summoned if immediate help is needed; and the phone numbers of the fire and police departments.

5 The sitter should be acquainted with the special features of the home and any particular precautions that should be taken to avoid cuts, burns, and falls. Parents should point out the safe play areas and the danger spots within the house, and should show the sitter how to turn the stove on and off and where to locate light switches. The sitter should also be warned of any dangerous habits the child may have—such as a tendency to go too close to the portable fan or heater or to play with electric cords and sockets—and of the possible risk the child may incur by playing with pets or eating popcorn, nuts, candy, or suckers.

6 Parents should tell the sitter when they will return home, and should explain that no one is allowed to enter the house in their absence (except the person the sitter is authorized to summon in an emergency). If a friend is to share part of the evening with the sitter, the friend should arrive with the sitter and be introduced to the parents. All private phone calls should be discouraged in order to allow parents to call home if they feel it necessary—and also to prevent the sitter from being distracted from his or her work.

The National Safety Council's revised Data Sheet No. 66, *Baby Sitting,* has detailed information on the following:

   1 The problem
   2 Advice to the sitter
   3 Before you take charge
   4 Evening sitting
   5 Mealtime sitting
   6 Bath time
   7 Supervising play
   8 Putting charges to bed
   9 Emergency care
  10 When the parents return
  11 Parents employing a baby sitter
  12 If you are a parent of a sitter

BURGLARPROOFING YOUR HOME

The first rule when a family moves into a house or apartment is to have all the outside locks changed. If you don't know a reputable locksmith, ask the police department to recommend one.

Always install two locks, a new one and a lock with a sturdy bolt system. A vertical ring-and-bar pin-tumbler lock is superior to the common wedge-shaped or square-tongued varieties.

Install a peephole on the door with a light over it so you can see clearly. Use it! Never admit someone you don't know or who has no apparent business knocking on the door. Insist on seeing credentials of unfamiliar meter readers, delivery people, etc. If you are still suspicious, phone their company while they wait outside. Once you let an unknown person inside, you may find yourself confronted by a rapist or terrorist robber with waiting confederates.

If you must rely on a chain lock as a secondary door-security measure, be certain it will not admit a hand.

In a recent survey on how burglars enter homes, it was revealed that 48 percent force inadequate front or back door locks, 25 percent break through glass door panels to unlock front or back doors, 10 percent enter open doors and windows, 15 percent break windows, and 2 percent use a key. The use of double locks would reduce forced entries.

When all doors, including back and basement doors, have been made secure, turn to the windows. All windows should be kept locked, and screens should be sturdy enough to discourage potential cat burglars. Adequate window bolts are available at low cost. Don't ignore basement windows.

Don't leave ladders or scaffolds in place during an exterior paint job or at any other time.

At some point you will be away from your home or apartment for some length of time. A few simple precautions will help keep the premises safe.

• Temporarily stop milk, newspaper, and mail deliveries, or ask a neighbor you trust to take them in. Have someone mow the grass or shovel snow so that your home will appear occupied.

• Don't have the telephone disconnected. It could be a tipoff that the house is vacant.

• Tell the police department, landlord, or a trusted neighbor that you are going away, where you will be, and how long you expect to be gone. If you arrange to have a neighbor enter the house for any reason, arm the neighbor with a written notice that his or her presence is permitted, and tell the landlord.

• Buy an inexpensive automatic switch to turn on a few lights, and perhaps a radio, at dusk and off again later. Try to create a normal lighting pattern. A light left on all night in the living room or bedroom might tip off a burglar. Leave curtains and blinds partially open, as if you were home.

• Inventory your major valuables, appliances, etc., and put as many as possible in a safety deposit box. Note serial numbers or distinctive features (it is a good idea to mark items with your social security number) so that you will be able to identify them if they are stolen and recovered. It is also a good policy to photograph valuable possessions. Don't multiply your loss potential by leaving the house loaded with "goodies."

You think the house is secure, and you go on vacation. When you come back, you notice that something is wrong: door ajar, wrong lights on, window broken. Don't burst inside to investigate. You could surprise a burglar into violent action. Call the police and let them handle the situation. They are better prepared to take this kind of risk.

Remember that an intruder's two enemies are noise and time. A good lock system will prevent intruders from picking open a door, and a back-up bolt will mean that the intruder has to crash the door open. That requires noise and time.

Don't give out duplicate keys to casual friends, domestics, or delivery persons. If you must hide a key outside, don't put it in a mailbox or under the welcome mat. Think—where would be the last place a burglar would look?

One defense on which the experts concur is a "security room." This is a centrally located room, perhaps a bedroom, intended to be a last-ditch haven against intruders. It should be equipped with a telephone and a set of door locks similar to those on exterior entrances. If you are in the security room and a burglar is trying to get in, don't hesitate to tell the burglar that you've called the police.

TREATMENT OF CUTS, SCRATCHES, AND BRUISES

Many home fatalities are due to infections that result when so-called "minor" wounds are not properly treated. Knowledge of first aid, which is a necessity for every parent, has often saved a life; even slight injuries should receive immediate care. If safe procedures were observed at all times, all cuts and bruises would be avoided. Although homemakers may not be able to achieve this ideal state of affairs, an orderly housekeeper can prevent many small injuries. Used razor blades should be placed in a container for disposal, knives and other dangerous kitchen implements should be kept out of the reach of children, and needles and pins should be placed in a pincushion or other safe place and not left in the material being sewn.

ELECTRICAL FIXTURES AND APPLIANCES

Electricity is an extremely valuable servant when properly controlled, but when misused it becomes a powerful destructive force. Few people realize that there is ample power in an ordinary 110-volt house current to kill a human being. If people come into contact with an electric current while their hands are wet or while they are standing on a damp floor, they can receive a shock severe enough to cause death. Unless the washing machine is grounded to a water pipe and unless the pull chain used to light the bulb over the washing machine has an insulating link, the homemaker risks this possibility whenever he or she does the laundry.

People frequently become complacent about their many appliances, and allow electricity to get out of control. A busy homemaker presses a blouse to wear to the meeting which begins in an hour, dresses hurriedly, and leaves the house forgetting to disconnect the iron. The result is a fire. A parent leaves the washing machine running while talking on the phone, and a curious child, perhaps attempting to take over the homemaker's duties, suffers a mangled arm. Electrical outlets are sometimes so overloaded that the wire becomes hot enough to burn off the insulation and start a fire. Usually a fuse blows before this occurs, but too often this warning is ignored, and the fuse is "temporarily" replaced with a penny. Once the electricity is working again, the housekeeper may forget the penny and the danger until he or she is reminded by the smell of smoke. Fortunately, modern homes are equipped with circuit breakers that eliminate the use of pennies or improper fuses.

Many people fail to realize the amount of current necessary to operate all the modern home appliances: deep freeze, electric refrigerator, vacuum cleaner, several radios, television set, iron, bathroom heater and fan, toaster, furnace and air conditioners. Since many of these appliances are in use at the same time, overloading is a real danger in many homes, especially in older houses that have not been wired to accomodate all this new equipment.

When appliances are slow to heat, when a television picture fades or shrinks, and when fuses blow frequently, it is time to call a qualified electrician to handle the problem. An electrician should also be consulted before new appliances are installed; the electrician's advice is less expensive than the possible cost of overloading electrical circuits.

Only scientifically tested electrical devices should be used, but it must be understood that the approval stamp of the Underwriters' Laboratories is not a guarantee against wear. Electrical appliances should be installed, regularly inspected, and repaired as necessary by a competent electrician. Too often the head of the family, although he or she has probably had no electrical training, is expected to perform these duties. Given a similar assignment, an industrial worker would receive intensive instruction and a full set of safety equipment, including goggles. Considering the number of unqualified electricians employed in American homes, it is surprising that there are not even more accidents.

FIREWORKS

Most states forbid the sale of fireworks except to licensed pyrotechnists. Yet every Fourth of July a few deaths, some severe burns, and sometimes loss of sight result from the unauthorized use of explosives which unscrupulous merchants still sell to children and thoughtless parents. Such accidents cannot be entirely eliminated until adults fully understand the dangers of explosives and the absolute necessity of preventing children from playing with them. Many people now celebrate the Fourth by attending controlled firework displays managed by specialists and sponsored by the community. Certainly this practice is more in keeping with the spirit of the occasion and the requirements of safety than are the dangerous practices formerly associated with the holiday.

STUDENT LEARNING EXPERIENCES

Students can increase their understanding of common home hazards and the proper methods of coping with them by carrying out as many of the following assignments as available time and facilities permit:

1 List the various areas in your home—stairways, living room, kitchen, bedrooms, bathroom, basement, closets and attic, porches and balcony, and yard and garage—and note the hazards you discover in each area.

2 Develop a home safety checklist based on the hazards noted in your own home. The first question concerning the living room might be, "Are all rugs secured to prevent slipping on polished floors?"

3 List a few of the hazards noted in each area of your home. State what you have done or will do to remove them, or, if they cannot be removed, to prevent them from causing accidents.

4 List five frequently observed situations that cause falls in the home, and discuss the procedures that should be followed to avoid these situations.

5 Explain the procedure used in your home to prevent people from slipping on rugs laid on polished floors.

6 Discuss the dangers of running up and down stairs.

7 List the unsafe practices of various members of your family, including yourself. Discuss the best ways of overcoming these practices.

8 List the poisons kept in your medicine chest and the precautions taken to prevent their misuse. If possible, suggest more effective precautions.

9 List the potential dangers involved in the improper use of electricity in the home.

10 Visit an electrical-equipment store and secure information about the electrical adjustments that you may safely make in your home. Demonstrate or explain to the class some of the techniques that you have learned.

11 Collect newspaper accounts of home accidents reported during a 1-week period, and analyze their causes. Suggest procedures that might have prevented these accidents.

12 Arrange for local radio or television publicity as part of a community drive to prevent home accidents.

EVALUATION

Even though most people recognize some of the potential dangers in their homes, they are often slow to take effective remedial action. Home safety has been a relatively neglected field, and the effect of a full-scale education program has yet to be tested. Perhaps as increasing emphasis is placed on all phases of accident prevention, people will develop a generally better attitude toward safety that will stimulate the formation of orderly habits in all areas of living, including the home.

The following checklist is designed to help identify the hazards in the home, and could be used in evaluation efforts to promote safety in the home. A high percentage of affirmative answers to the following questions will indicate relatively safe homes. The negative answers will reveal the areas in which more intensive work is needed. A lowered accident rate, however, is the only real proof of the effectiveness of safety education. Teachers should analyze local data on home accidents from year to year to see whether their particular program has had any effect in their community.

A SAFE-HOME CHECKLIST

Yes No

____ ____ 1. Is the area around your driveway free from shrubs, trees, and other obstructions that would prevent a clear view by a person driving a car in or out of your driveway?

____ ____ 2. Are handrails provided for every stairway of three or more steps that leads to an entrance to your house?

Yes   No

___   ___   3. Are entrances to the house adequately lighted?

___   ___   4. Is the porch or terrace, if it is more than 10 inches above the ground, protected by a firm railing?

___   ___   5. Are clotheslines higher than head level and located away from normal paths of travel across the yard?

___   ___   6. Is the child's outdoor play area located within clear view of the kitchen window?

___   ___   7. Is the child's indoor play area located away from the normal path of traffic through the house?

___   ___   8. Do inside stairs have a firm and continuous handrail?

___   ___   9. Are stairs well lighted, with a light switch located at both the top and the bottom of the stairway?

___   ___   10. Is the bottom basement step painted white?

___   ___   11. Is there sufficient headroom (6 feet 8 inches) on all stairs?

___   ___   12. Is the stair covering firmly tacked down?

___   ___   13. Are the top and bottom of the staircase free of small rugs?

___   ___   14. Are all small rugs in the house laid on nonskid material?

___   ___   15. Are floors thinly waxed and thoroughly polished to prevent slipping?

___   ___   16. If small children live in the house, are bar gates installed at the top and bottom of the stairs?

___   ___   17. Is furniture so placed that it does not hinder free movement around the room?

___   ___   18. Do doors swing into rooms and not into halls or other normal traffic lanes?

___   ___   19. Is there a tight-fitting screen before the open fireplace?

___   ___   20. Are all cords run along the wall, instead of under rugs or furniture?

___   ___   21. Are light cords short (not more than 7 feet) and firmly connected to the wall to preclude the possibility of tripping over them?

     ___   22. Are all wall sockets fitted with guards to prevent children from inserting a finger or a piece of metal into a socket?

___   ___   23. Has all electric wiring been properly installed by a reputable electrician?

___   ___   24. Is all electrical equipment of the type recommended by the National Electrical Code and Underwriters' Laboratories, Inc.?

___   ___   25. Is all electrical equipment regularly inspected, and is any part that is found defective promptly replaced?

___   ___   26. Are there sufficient outlets for all appliances to prevent overloading the wires?

___   ___   27. Are all fuses of proper amperage (usually 15 amperes)?

___   ___   28. Are master switches or multiple-control switches placed at the entrance to each of the principal rooms?

___   ___   29. Are all portable electrical appliances, such as the washing machine, grounded to the nearest water (not gas) pipe?

___   ___   30. Are all electrical fixtures or controls in the bathroom located beyond arm's reach of the sink, tub or shower, and any metal objects?

___   ___   31. Are all electrical appliances, such as pressing or curling irons, fans, heaters, etc., disconnected when not in use?

___   ___   32. Is there an insulating link in the chain of all pull-type electric sockets?

___   ___   33. Are the locations of the various shutoffs for electricity, gas, and water known to all adult members of the family?

___   ___   34. Are all low-silled bedroom windows barred or screened to protect children from falling out?

___   ___   35. Are bunk beds equipped with a bar to prevent children from falling out?

___   ___   36. Is the rule "No smoking in bed" always obeyed?

___   ___   37. Are all kitchen shelves within easy reach? If not, is a safe and sturdy stepladder kept handy?

___   ___   38. Are all curtains located near a gas stove of nonflammable material? If not, are they securely fastened to prevent them from blowing over the flame?

Yes   No

39. Are all knives and other sharp tools kept in a special drawer, out of the reach of children?
40. Is the kitchen can opener of the kind that leaves no rough edges?
41. If grease or water is spilled on the floor, is it promptly wiped up to remove the danger of slipping?
42. Are all stove-burner controls out of the reach of young children?
43. Is the gas stove equipped with a gas pilot in good working order?
44. Is there a recently inspected fire extinguisher in the kitchen?
45. Are safety matches used, and are all matches kept out of the reach of children?
46. Is there adequate storage space for all kitchen equipment?
47. Is there adequate storage space for tools, toys, bicycles, the lawn mower, screens, storm windows, sewing equipment, etc.?
48. Is the bathtub or shower equipped with a strong grip rail?
49. Is a nonskid rubber bath mat used in the tub or shower?
50. Do all members of the household know where the nearest fire alarm is or how to telephone the fire department is case of fire?
51. Are all poisons kept in a special cabinet, properly marked, and out of the reach of children?
52. Is an approved first-aid kit readily available?
53. Are flammable materials, such as oily rags, kept in a closed metal container?
54. Are such flammable materials as tissue paper, excelsior, and old paper boxes properly stacked in the basement, away from the furnace while awaiting disposal?
55. Is the attic free of such flammable materials as wrappings and newspapers that might be subject to spontaneous combustion?
56. Are ashes collected in a metal container?
57. Are the furnace, chimney, and flues cleaned regularly?
58. Is home dry cleaning done outdoors with a nonflammable fluid?
59. Are all flammable fluids, such as kerosene and gasoline, kept outside and stored in properly marked containers?
60. Is there a special storage place for toys, and do children return them to that place when they are through using them?
61. Are guns unloaded, dismantled, and stored in a locked cabinet?
62. Are chimneys inspected above and below the roof at regular intervals, and is any loose mortar or cement properly restored?
63. Are all minor injuries incurred around the house given prompt first-aid treatment?

LEARNING EXPERIENCES

To supplement the study of this chapter, students should complete the following learning assignments, which are designed to increase their understanding of the subject matter of home safety.

1 Arrange with your parent-teacher association for the use of two homes. Set up one home to illustrate many common hazards and the other to represent a safe environment. Have your students inspect each home and report their findings.

2 Compare the costs arising from a fracture of the large bone of the upper arm, hypothetically caused by a fall from a rickety chair, with the cost of a stepladder. In estimating the cost of the injury, include the doctor's bill, the hospital bill, and the wage loss.

3 Ask the physical education teacher to explain how one can fall without being injured. Demonstrate this method before the class.

4 List some of the procedures that are recommended to protect the aged from the danger of falls.

5 Explain how a furnace may cause gas poisoning.

6 List five principles concerned with the prevention of gas poisoning.

7 List at least five common poisons frequently responsible for accidental deaths, and give the antidote for each.

8 Discuss appropriate ways of observing the Fourth of July.

9 Consult the chemistry teacher about the advisability of using ammonium sulfate or some other fire-resistant solution to fireproof Christmas trees.

10 Be prepared to debate the following resolution: "Negative teaching of home safety, utilizing such means as vivid, frightening pictures of accidents, is as effective as positive instruction."

11 Have a physician discuss with the class the dangers of barbiturates, amphetamines, and LSD (lysergic acid diethylamide).

12 Use the safe-home checklist to inspect your own home, apartment, dormitory, fraternity house, sorority house, or rooming house.

PROTECTION FROM FIRE AND DISASTER

FIRE

Fire in its many useful forms is unquestionably essential to the enjoyment of life, but danger is one of its inescapable by-products. It takes only a moment of carelessness to transform the smallest fire into a conflagration. Potential sources of destruction are found in gas burners, trash fires, furnaces, matches, cigarettes, campfires, sparks from running machinery, birthday candles, fireworks, etc. If people understand and respect the risks inherent in the routine use of fire, they need not fear them, for they can effectively guard against them by taking the proper precautions.

Analysis reveals that destructive fires, which claim approximately 6,200 lives every year and cause property damage estimated at over $4.3 billion,[13] (see Table 13-2 and Figure 13-6) are fundamentally the result either of carelessness or of failure to recognize hazards, including those represented by faulty building construction. To eliminate these causes, and to minimize the loss of life and property if a fire should break out, schools and communities must organize safety programs to achieve the following objectives.

1 To guide individuals in recognition of the most common causes of fire, and to teach them how to remove or counteract these hazards

2 To urge individuals to cooperate in the program of building properly constructed[14] fire-resistant homes, schools, and other buildings and to exercise their best efforts to bring about repairs of existing structures

[13] *Accident Facts*, National Safety Council, Chicago, 1977.
[14] Properly constructed according to the National Building Code of the National Board of Fire Underwriters.

TABLE 13-2
Estimated Building Fires* and Losses, 1975

Cause or Occupancy	Fires		Loss	
	Number	%	$ millions	%
Totals by Cause	1,264,400	100.0	3,436.6	100.0
Incendiary and suspicious	114,100	11.4	633.9	18.5
Electrical	150,500	11.9	358.1	10.4
Fixed wiring and distribution equipment	*78,400*	*6.2*	*193.4*	*5.6*
Power-consuming appliances	*72,100*	*5.7*	*164.7*	*4.8*
Heating and cooking equipment	165,600	13.1	222.8	6.5
Defective or misused equipment	*91,000*	*7.2*	*144.7*	*4.2*
Combustibles near heaters and stoves	*46,700*	*3.7*	*52.9*	*1.5*
Chimneys and flues	*15,600*	*1.2*	*23.2*	*0.7*
Hot ashes and coals	*12,300*	*1.0*	*2.0*	*0.1*
Open flames and sparks (ex. heating, cooking equip.	85,500	6.8	175.9	5.1
Welding and cutting	*14,600*	*1.2*	*56.4*	*1.6*
Sparks from machinery	*15,100*	*1.2*	*26.1*	*0.8*
Thawing pipes	*7,900*	*0.6*	*22.5*	*0.6*
Sparks and embers	*17,400*	*1.4*	*10.2*	*0.3*
Other open flames	*30,500*	*2.4*	*60.7*	*1.8*
Smoking-related	137,800	10.9	166.8	4.9
Children and fire	64,200	5.1	116.9	3.4
Flammable and combustible liquids	61,900	4.9	63.4	1.8
Fireworks and explosives	3,900	0.3	41.1	1.2
Lightning	14,200	1.1	36.1	1.1
Gas fires and explosions (ex. heating, cooking equip.)	9,500	0.7	34.9	1.0
Spontaneous ignition	11,000	0.9	21.9	0.6
Exposure	34,100	2.7	21.8	0.6
Trash burning	155,500	12.3	5.0	0.1
Miscellaneous known causes	89,300	7.1	288.7	8.4
Unknown causes	137,300	10.8	1,249.3	36.4
Totals by Occupancy	1,264,400	100.0	3,436.6	100.0
Residential	916,000	72.5	1,389.0	40.4
One- and two-family dwellings	*677,100*	*53.6*	*853.5*	*24.9*
Apartments	*158,500*	*12.6*	*337.9*	*9.8*
Mobile homes	*28,100*	*2.2*	*72.9*	*2.1*
Hotels and motels	*28,200*	*2.2*	*68.9*	*2.0*
Other residential	*24,100*	*1.9*	*55.8*	*1.6*
Industrial	58,200	4.6	745.1	21.7
Drugs, chemicals, paints, petroleum	*5,300*	*0.4*	*182.0*	*5.3*
Metal, metal products	*5,700*	*0.4*	*89.3*	*2.6*
Food products	*4,800*	*0.4*	*68.0*	*2.0*
Wood, wood products	*3,200*	*0.3*	*57.4*	*1.7*
Mines, mineral products	*1,300*	*0.1*	*43.4*	*1.2*
Other industrial	*37,900*	*3.0*	*305.0*	*8.9*
Mercantile	82,600	6.5	444.6	12.9
Stores	*25,100*	*2.0*	*169.5*	*4.9*
Motor-vehicle sales, repair, service stations	*17,700*	*1.4*	*63.4*	*1.8*
Offices and banks	*17,500*	*1.4*	*57.8*	*1.7*
Other mercantile	*22,300*	*1.7*	*153.9*	*4.5*

TABLE 13–2 *(continued)*
Estimated Building Fires* and Losses, 1975

Cause or Occupancy	Fires		Loss	
	Number	%	$ millions	%
Storage	64,500	5.1	442.4	12.9
Barns and other farm structures	*30,100*	*2.4*	*143.1*	*4.2*
Grain elevators	*2,200*	*0.2*	*55.4*	*1.6*
Garages, residential parkins	*21,700*	*1.7*	*34.1*	*1.0*
Lumber, building materials	*1,200*	*0.1*	*27.7*	*0.8*
Other storage	*9,300*	*0.7*	*182.1*	*5.3*
Public assembly and educational	75,800	6.0	303.0	8.8
Schools and colleges	*34,300*	*2.7*	*130.0*	*3.8*
Restaurants, taverns, nightclubs	23,700	1.9	62.4	1.8
Churches	*4,700*	*0.4*	*32.1*	*0.9*
Theatres, auditoriums, exhibition halls, etc.	*4,700*	*0.4*	*31.2*	*0.9*
Other public	*8,400*	*0.6*	*47.3*	*1.4*
Institutional (hospitals, homes for the aged, etc.)	30,200	2.4	40.1	1.2
Miscellaneous	37,100	2.9	72.4	2.1

*Additional nonbuilding fires include: 634,000 transportation equipment fires with $494,500,000 loss, 128,000 forest fires with $180,100,000 loss, 22,800 standing crop fires with $38,400,000 loss, and 1,056,000 grass, brush and rubbish fires with $21,000,000 loss. Totals for building and nonbuilding fires were 3,105,200 fires with $4,170,600,000 loss.
Source: Estimates of National Fire Protection Association. Reported in *Accident Facts,* National Safety Council, Chicago, 1977, p. 20.

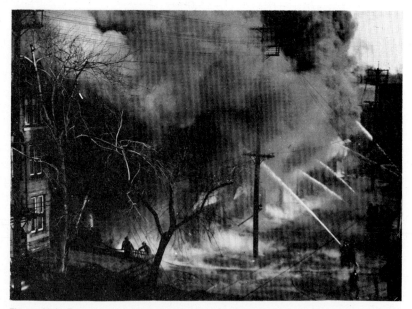

Figure 13-6 Destructive fires claim approximately 6,200 lives every year and cause property damage estimated at over $4.3 billion. (Source: Black Star.)

3 To help individuals develop safe habits in handling fires and flammable materials

4 To teach individuals what to do in case of fire

Although the material in this section is oriented primarily to an academic situation, it may easily be adapted to fire safety programs for the school, community, 4-H group, safety or public health council, Girl or Boy Scouts, PTA, etc.

ACHIEVING THE OBJECTIVES

Unlike vocational safety, which should be taught in shop classes, and highway safety, which is an intrinsic part of the driver education course, fire safety has no single, clearly defined place in the school curriculum. This chapter merely suggests the content of the fire safety program without prescribing a specific method of presentation. Each school must cover the necessary material in the way best suited to its own curriculum, the facilities available, and the needs of the community it serves.

THE BASIC APPROACH

A unit on fire safety should be included in any health and/or safety course. Whether or not the school offers such a course, various aspects of fire safety can and should be taught in connection with related fields. Precautions in using stoves should be explained in homemaking classes; the fire hazard of defective wiring and the chemistry of fire should be covered in general science courses; and protection against lightning (most dangerous in rural areas) should be integrated with instruction in farm management. If a camping or hiking trip is planned, the safety rules pertinent to the campfire should be taught as part of the students' preliminary training. Fire hazards in the home would naturally be included in the students' home safety checklist, and procedures to be followed in case of fire should be explained in connection with the school's fire drills.

Certain aspects of fire prevention, especially those not directly related to other subject areas, can easily be correlated with such courses as English and social studies. The prevention of forest fires can be covered by assigning a research project on the national conservation program. As part of their training in democratic procedures, civics students can be asked to plan a citizens' campaign for a safer school building. In studying insurance practices, an economics class might investigate the safety features a building must have to qualify for low fire insurance rates. English students can be given an essay topic such as "Fire Prevention in My Home," and a dramatics group can be encouraged to write and present a series of skits dealing with fire prevention.

Children learn best by doing; they should be given every chance to utilize the fire-prevention knowledge they have acquired. Most effective learning experiences in this area can best be provided in the home, where young people should have ample opportunity to practice the correct way to strike a match, light the gas oven, burn rubbish, and perform various other household tasks involving fire and flammable materials. Due emphasis should be given to the importance of notifying an adult in the event of a fire.

Parents are in an excellent position to help children develop safe habits by setting a good example and supervising them in the practice of proper procedures. Conversely, careless parents greatly endanger their children, not only by failing to remove fire hazards in the home but by indirectly fostering the formation of faulty behavior patterns. Adults may recognize and compensate for their own dangerous habits, but children merely imitate their parents' actions without understanding the risks that such conduct entails. The school must do all it can to extend its fire-prevention program to the entire community, utilizing newspaper articles, parent-teacher meetings, and the other media commonly employed for adult education.

In teaching people how to keep useful fires under control and how to avoid starting unnecessary fires, the instructor must constantly try to develop desirable behavior patterns while giving evidence of the possibly disastrous effects of incorrect practices. It should be made clear that fires are relatively safe as long as the proper procedures are observed. Otherwise, students become unduly fearful and react so emotionally to any possibility of fire that they increase rather than minimize the danger. Above all, students must recognize the logical relationship between careful actions and desirable consequences, and between negligence and destruction. They should be reminded constantly of the importance of conserving our natural resources.

To help individuals develop respect for safety regulations, the instructor should repeatedly stress the fact that adherence to proper procedures is a patriotic duty and a moral obligation. All students must fully understand that their carelessness in handling fire or flammable materials endangers not only themselves but many others, and may also result in extensive property damage. A still-burning cigarette flung from a car window into a forest may destroy thousands of acres of timber, which are valuable not only in themselves but as a shelter for wildlife and as protection for springs and streams. Those who tend to be careless of their own safety must be made to realize that they have no right to jeopardize others.

CAUSES OF FIRES AND PREVENTIVE MEASURES

The material to be covered in a fire safety program should include the major causes of destructive fires, particularly in homes and schools, and the most important preventive measures. This section is not offered as a comprehensive treatment of the pertinent subject matter, but merely as a guide.

SMOKING AND MATCHES

Careless smoking habits and the improper use of matches are jointly responsible for more than 25 percent of the fires reported to the National Board of Fire Underwriters. More and more department stores dealing in textiles and other combustible materials are instituting the no-smoking rule, despite the possible loss of business from inconvenienced customers. Over the years such stores have suffered enormous losses in burned merchandise, as the frequency of fire sales attests. Stores are not the only victims of careless smokers. Newspaper stories such as the following are all too common:

Cigaret Blamed for Fatal Apartment Fire

Oakland, Calif., Sept. 25, (AP). A smoldering cigaret was blamed today for a fire that raced through a six-story frame apartment house yesterday killing one woman and injuring a dozen occupants.

Fire Marshal James J. Sweeney said a cigaret apparently had been left burning in upholstered furniture in the lobby. Damage was estimated at $100,000.

Many smokers have flagrantly dangerous habits. They light cigarettes even when handling gasoline and other highly flammable materials. They flick live ashes on the carpet, or forget to flick them at all, so that the ashes fall on clothes or furniture. They leave a cigarette smoldering on the edge of an ash tray, or even on the edge of a desk or table if an ash tray is not handy, become distracted, and leave the room. The cigarette falls where it will, possibly going out but just as possibly igniting a rug or a slip cover.

If there are smokers in the home, clean ash trays should be conveniently placed in every room but kept away from curtains and other materials that burn easily. An ash tray should never be emptied into a wastebasket. Everyone should make it an inflexible rule never to smoke in bed. Too often smokers feel that this practice is not dangerous for them, since *they* would never be careless enough to fall asleep while smoking. Despite their best intentions, the inclination to sleep may be overpowering. Even if they remain awake, a hot ash can easily drop from a cigarette unnoticed and smolder down to the highly flammable mattress stuffing. If one is going to smoke in the bedroom, it is safer to do so while sitting in an upright chair.

Although safety matches are preferable to the old-style kitchen matches, users must make it a habit to close the cover on the book of matches before striking the match, and to discard the used match in a nonflammable receptacle since it may continue to smolder even after the flame is out. When matches are used outdoors near any sort of vegetation, they should be broken into two before they are thrown on the ground. Failure to observe this practice can easily cause a forest fire.

A flashlight, *not* a match, should be used when one needs to find something in a dark closet. Since a match is often more readily accessible than a flashlight, many people tend to ignore this rule. The best procedure is to have an electrician install a light in all storage areas. Although some accidents occur because of deficiencies in the match itself, a more serious problem is the use of matches by young children. Children are fascinated by matches, and their natural curiosity about fire constitutes a hazardous situation. All too often, children become frightened when lighting a match and may drop it on their clothing or some other flammable material. The International Association of Fire

Chiefs strongly urges parents to plan a definite course of instruction for their children on the proper use of matches.

Matches should be stored in a metal container and, like poison, kept out of the reach of children. Youngsters should be allowed to use matches for worthwhile purposes, however, if an adult is present to supervise. Such opportunities help children learn the proper use of matches and tend to curtail their desire to play with matches on their own.

ELECTRICITY

The wiring in many older homes and schools cannot accommodate modern electrical appliances. Some homes are festooned with a hodgepodge of poorly insulated wires and lamp cords, hung on nails or tacked against wood without any regard for safety requirements. Fires attributed to such practices cause an estimated loss of $365 million every year; it is obvious that many people lack even a rudimentary understanding of electricity.

If a circuit, protected by a 15-ampere fuse and intended for lamps and small appliances, is used for large appliances that need a heavier wire, the fuse will blow, indicating that something is wrong. If this warning is ignored and the 15-ampere fuse merely replaced with a 20- or 30-ampere fuse, or with a copper penny, the wire may become hot enough to ignite the lath at the baseboard outlet. Individuals must recognize this hazard; they must understand the necessity of entrusting the matter of wiring to a competent electrician, who will know the type of circuit needed to service the number of appliances in use.

Leaving appliances such as irons, toasters, hot plates, and heaters unattended while the current is on is the second-ranking cause of fires that are due to misuse of electricity. Individuals should be trained to remove the plug or at least to switch off the current before leaving an appliance even "for a minute." Such distractions as a telephone call or a visitor at the door can easily extend the minute indefinitely. Most modern irons are equipped with a pilot light to indicate that the current is on and an automatic control switch to minimize the danger of overheating. In addition, a strong metal stand should be provided for the iron to protect the board in case the user, despite the best intentions, forgets to turn off the iron before leaving the house.

Cheap electric toys are sometimes poorly insulated reproductions of such household appliances as stoves and irons. They are extremely dangerous if unattended. Children should be permitted to operate electric toys only in the presence of watchful adults, who must see that the toys are not used near faucets or grounded metal fixtures and that the toys are disconnected as soon as youngsters stop playing with them. Children should be permitted to operate electric toys only if the toys carry the Underwriters' Laboratories mark on the cord and toy itself. Electric toys that use house current should be operated through a transformer that reduces the voltage. Toys that become as hot as regular kitchen equipment should not be used by children. They may cause serious burns or start a fire. Although toys sometimes specify the age group that should use a toy, not all youngsters in that age group have the ability to use the toy safely.

HEATING UNITS

Furnaces are not dangerous when properly installed, maintained, and operated. Good insulation and adequate clearance above the furnace and around it will prevent wooden joists and other flammable material from igniting. In older homes, which lack the fire-resistant features of modern buildings, the heating unit should be surrounded by noncombustible material. Asbestos millboard may be used to protect adjacent structures, or sheet metal may be installed over wooden partitions, with a 1-inch space allowed between the metal and the partition. Coal- and wood-burning stoves are again becoming the vogue as other fuels become scarce and expensive. Caution should be used when igniting the fuel. Kerosene or other volitile liquids should never be used; their vapors can cause an explosion.

The common hot-air furnace is relatively safe if it is correctly operated. Improper firing may cause dangerous overheating and send explosive and poisonous fumes through the house. The gas furnace usually gives little trouble, except when it is necessary to have the gas turned off for a time and then turned on again. It is best to have the local power company handle this matter. A properly installed oil furnace is ordinarily dangerous only if the burners become clogged. This hazard can be avoided by having accumulated soot periodically removed and having the burners regularly oiled and adjusted by a competent service person. Portable space heaters used in a closed room often consume all the available oxygen and can produce carbon monoxide. They should be properly vented to allow oxygen to enter the room. Other hazards associated with space heaters are: contact with the flame or hot surface area, explosion of accumulated gas while attempting to light the burner, electric shock, and explosion of flammable liquids. Space heaters have their place when used properly, but they can cause fires, injury, and death if they are not properly installed and operated.

The principal hazard represented by the kitchen stove is the possibility that some flammable substance will come into contact with the burners. Spilled grease should be promptly wiped up, flimsy kitchen curtains should be securely fastened so that they cannot blow over the flame, and clothes should not be placed near the stove for quick drying. In those few homes that still have coal- or wood-burning kitchen stoves, the same precaution must be taken when starting the fire. Precautions must also be taken to see that hot coals do not fall out on the kitchen floor and that adequate insulation is provided for surrounding structures.

An open fireplace should be protected by a securely fitted screen to prevent sparks from falling on the floor or carpet. But even when this precaution is taken, the fireplace must never be used as an incinerator for Christmas wrappings, corrugated paper boxes, and other refuse that can easily blow out into the room. The hearth should not be left until the fire has settled down and there is no danger of burning material spilling onto the floor. Many fires have been caused by burning logs that have slid under the screen and rolled out of the fireplace when no one was watching.

The use of improper fuel—such as coal, charcoal, and styrofoam packaging—and improper ventilation can cause carbon monoxide poisoning. One should also make sure that the fire is completely out when leaving the house and before retiring for the evening.

Chimney fires are becoming more frequent as more fireplaces are being used because of the energy crisis. Chimney fires are usually the result of soot building up in the flue. All chimneys, flues, and stovepipes should be inspected, cleaned, and if necessary repaired before fires are started in the fall. Removing the accumulated soot saves fuel, increases heat, and minimizes the danger of fire. If cracks or loose bricks are detected in the chimney, under or above the roof, a reliable brick mason should be employed to "point" the chimney and remove the hazard. Proper attention to these matters costs considerably less than a fire that might result from neglecting them.

EXPLOSIVE MATERIALS

The improper use of flammable liquids is responsible for a large proportion of the deaths attributed to fires in the home. Such use is more often the result of ignorance than of carelessness. Not every person who uses a hair spray is aware of the fire hazard presented by this flammable fluid. Most people realize that gasoline, benzine, naphtha, and other dry-cleaning fluids are flammable and should not be used near an open flame, but few people understand that the vapor or fumes released from these highly volatile liquids can flow as far as 200 feet from the point of evaporation and can explode even without contact with a flame. A spark caused by switching on a light or the static electricity generated by rubbing a garment saturated with a flammable cleaning fluid may be enough to touch off an explosion, especially on a dry day when little air is stirring. Even one pint of gasoline, when vaporized, can produce 300 cubic feet of explosive force. All household members must be made to understand that gasoline is more dangerous than TNT or dynamite and must be handled accordingly. If flammable liquids must be used, they should be stored in an appropriate metal container, preferably away from the house and in a well-ventilated area.

Paint spraying, like dry cleaning, can be extremely hazardous unless the proper precautions are observed. Paint removers, synthetic thinners, and many quick-drying paints containing the highly flammable plastic, pyroxylin, evaporate easily and give off explosive vapors. Therefore, paint spraying should be done out of doors, and the no-smoking rule should be strictly observed. Highly flammable material should not be stored in the house.

Liquids having a flash point[15] at or below 200°F are considered flammable.

[15]The temperature at which the liquid vaporizes sufficiently to produce a flammable or explosive mixture near the surface of the liquid.

Gasoline has a flash point below 25°F; lacquer, ethyl alcohol, and varnish above 25°F but below 75°F; and kerosene and turpentine above 70°F but below 200°F.

Any natural or artificial gas escaping from defective pipes, stoves, or refrigerators represents an extremely serious hazard. Many people who know that such fumes are lethal when inhaled in sufficient quantity do not realize that they are also explosive. A gas leak was considered responsible for a school explosion in New London, Texas, that killed 294 persons. To prevent such disasters, there must be more widespread knowledge of the danger of gas and the procedures to be followed if a leak is detected. The windows should be opened immediately. If the leak cannot be promptly found and stopped, the gas company should be called to take care of the matter.

Failure to follow the correct procedure in lighting the gas oven is a common cause of explosions in the home. Homemakers who turn on the gas before striking a match apparently do not understand how rapidly the gas flows from the open jet. By the time they strike a match they may be surrounded by gas fumes, and the resultant explosion is likely to cause a severe burn. When lighting an appliance that does not have an automatic pilot light, apply the lighted match to the burner while turning on the gas. Oven doors should be opened before lighting so that any accumulated gas will be dissipated.

Any odor of unburned gas should receive immediate attention. If the odor is not strong, look for extinguished pilot lights or partially opened valves on the range, heater, or other gas appliance. If the odor is strong, open all windows and doors, leave the building, and call the gas company from an outside phone. If a light is needed, use a flashlight and do not turn on the electricity; a spark from the switch could cause an explosion.

Among the various causes of explosions in the home, probably the one least often recognized is a concentration of dust particles, mixed with air and exposed to an open flame. Such a combination has often resulted in serious explosions in grain elevators, coal mines, and in factories where there is sugar, starch, or flour dust. On a smaller scale, explosions may be caused in the home by dumping the contents of the vacuum cleaner into the fire in the fireplace, incinerator, or coal- or wood-burning stove. Dust should always be wrapped securely in newspaper before it is burned.

RUBBISH AND OTHER FLAMMABLE MATERIAL

Half of all fires in the home start in the basement. Many are due, at least in part, to the stacks of newspapers, paper boxes, excelsior-filled packing cases, and other highly combustible materials all too frequently stored there. A hot ash from a cigarette or the cinders from a coal furnace or fireplace can easily ignite such material. Any fire that gets started in this way is likely to be serious, for it will grow rapidly, fed by the accumulation of trash. Fire is almost certain to break out if the rubbish includes oily rags, paints, or other materials subject to spontaneous ignition.

The garage and attic are also favorite storage places for trash. The garage is particularly dangerous because of oil drippings from the car, but the attic is not much safer. The boxes, trunks, books, and old clothes stored there are likely to become thoroughly dried out by the summer heat and thus particularly susceptible to fire. Ideally, trash should be promptly disposed of and not allowed to accumulate. Since it is unrealistic to expect that this practice will be generally adopted, cellars, garages, and attics should be cleaned out regularly, not just once a year during Fire Prevention Week in October. All oily rags and similar material must be placed in a closed metal container and stored in a cool, open place.

Various plastic materials commonly found in the home have a low ignition point and rapid burning rate, particularly celluloid and other synthetics made of pyroxylin, a highly flammable compound containing nitrocellulose and camphor. Such materials, because of their low kindling point, can easily catch fire from a spark or the tip of a cigarette. They should be kept away from open flames, electric wiring, and lighted cigarettes.

Some Christmas tree ornaments—icicles, tinsel, etc.—are made of flammable plastics and may be easily ignited by poorly insulated or otherwise defective wiring, which may also ignite the tree itself. Despite the children's protests, the tree should be disposed of as soon as it becomes dry, usually 3 or 4 days after Christmas. Such precautions as inspecting tree lights carefully, disconnecting them when an adult is not in the room, and treating the tree with a fire-resistant spray can also do much to prevent fires during the holiday season.

OUTDOOR FIRES

When you are building a fire outdoors to burn leaves or rubbish, to cook a meal, or to provide warmth at a campsite, every precaution must be taken to keep the fire under control. If carelessly tended, it can easily spread to nearby underbrush, causing the destruction of acres of forest land or doing other extensive damage.

To remove the rubbish and litter hazards discussed previously, trash should be burned at least once a week. A small accumulation of rubbish can usually be safely burned outdoors in a wire basket or other metal container, but disposing of the trash collected over several months in one big bonfire is dangerous. Such a conflagration may be difficult to control, especially during the windy fall months when cleanup campaigns are most common. A trash fire should not be left until it has burned out completely and a pail of water has been thrown over the ashes to make sure that the last spark has been extinguished.

Fully one-third of the forest fires in this country are attributed to campers and other sportspersons. Although careless smoking habits and careless use of matches are undoubtedly responsible for many of these fires, improperly tended campfires are also a major cause. A picnic fire or campfire should be built in an outdoor fireplace provided for this purpose or on a bare spot of ground, free of leaves and other flammable underbrush. Roaring fires should be avoided. Using a small bed of coals for cooking purposes will result in a better meal and greater safety. Even after the fire has settled down, it should never be left while the campers go off to swim or explore the surrounding area. Before the fire is abandoned, it should be spread out and thoroughly soaked with water.

LIGHTNING

Ninety percent of all lightning fires occur in rural areas, and 20 percent of destructive farm fires and 90 percent of live stock deaths are caused by lightning. This subject is discussed more fully in connection with farm safety (see Chapter 14). The city dweller faces relatively little danger from lightning, but should nevertheless take the precaution of staying away from windows, fireplaces, porches, doorways, television sets, electric appliances, telephones, and grounded metal objects during an electrical storm. Outside television antennas and lead-in wires should be well grounded and have an approved lightning arrester installed by a competent serviceperson. If a person is outside when the storm hits, the person should, if possible, take shelter in a steel skyscraper or an automobile with a metal top. When a lightning storm starts, avoid high places and seek low spots. It is also wise to get off the golf course and stay away from wire fences. Any lightning casualties that occur despite these precautions must be considered inevitable. Such accidents are among the few that can be attributed to an uncontrollable natural force rather than to human ignorance and carelessness.

The Lightning Protection Institute of Chicago, a nonprofit organization, provides the latest information dealing with lightning protection. The main work of the institute is educational. It works to promote the science and improvement of lightning protection, and to establish proper safeguards against the dangers of lightning.

CONSTRUCTION FAULTS

In pioneer times lumber was plentiful and cheap. Frame dwellings, which are particularly susceptible to fire, became the prevailing type of construction. For more than a century, the building code published and constantly revised by the National Board of Fire Underwriters has exerted an increasing influence upon construction practices. Fire-resistant walls, interior partitions, floors, and roofs represent the current building trend. Much present-day building material is noncombustible, such as metal lath, light-steel protected framing, reinforced concrete, and heavy-steel studs. Fire-retarding materials inserted between walls and partitions to prevent the spread of fire from floor to floor are now commonly used.

Even with our modern building codes, many construction faults still exist. Many new homes have been found to have no fire barriers. False ceilings, unstopped walls, non-fire-resistant wood paneling, flammable plastic tiles, and some of the newly developed insulation materials are suspect. All are materials that can trigger a fire. A prudent potential homeowner should thoroughly examine the construction of a house before purchasing it.

Many homes built more than 20 or 30 years ago, before the building code was modernized and generally observed, show evidence of poor construction and improper care. Defective heating plants, open stairways, halls, and laundry chutes, wooden shingles, and other hazards characteristic of older houses have been at least partially responsible for many serious fires. Without efficient fire-protection service in most communities, many of these homes would have burned to the ground years ago.

Owners do not always realize that even an old house can be made relatively safe, and that they need not trust solely to luck and the fire department to protect their lives and property. Wooden shingles can be replaced with asbestos or slate, open spaces between walls and under floors can be filled with fire-resistant material, and fire stops can be built in strategic places. The cost of these alterations is negligible when compared with the damage that can be done by a fire. Homeowners who fully understand the danger represented by poor construction will recognize the practicality and necessity of making improvements.

Many older school buildings, like older homes, can only be labeled fire-traps. Today in many of our elementary and secondary schools students are enrolled in buildings that do not meet proper fire safety standards. Schools which have many floors, furnish only inferior or poorly located fire escapes, and fail to equip all doors with panic bolts are particularly dangerous. Folding wooden chairs used in the auditorium, which doubles as a gymnasium in some schools, represent another all too common fire hazard.

Fortunately, many school fires occur after students have gone home. But a daytime fire, such as the Our Lady of the Angels fire of December 1, 1958, which cost 94 lives, will long be remembered. The nation was shocked by that catastrophe. But open stairways, improper storage of waste material, lack of automatic fire detectors, lack of fire-barrier doors, inadequate fire-alarm systems which fail to alert the local fire department immediately, and careless fire drills have not always been dealt with adequately. These hazards are still present in too many schools.

Notorious school-fire disasters have demonstrated the necessity for safe schools, and present-day building and maintenance practices are a great improvement over those of 25 years ago. In many states the construction of "fireproof" schools is required by law. Although the standards for schools are often included in the statute governing the construction and maintenance of all public buildings, some states have studied the problem of school fires deeply enough to formulate a special school-building code that requires safe design features and fire-retardant construction.

Design is fully as important as construction. Even if a building is made almost entirely of "fireproof" material, there is still danger if its combustible contents are not properly protected or if its stairways are open to permit the rapid spread of smoke and flames. The building itself may not burn, but more fire fatalities are due to the effects of inhaling smoke than to actual burns. Even a small amount of smoke from a fire inside the building may be enough to cause a disastrous panic unless students have been thoroughly trained in efficient fire-drill procedures. In addition to construction and maintenance codes, statutes have been enacted in many states to govern fire-drill procedures and other matters relating to fire prevention. Requirements are usually revised periodically to meet new conditions.

PROCEDURES TO BE FOLLOWED IN CASE OF FIRE

Although people who understand fire hazards and conscientiously attempt to remove or compensate for them can minimize the possibility of fire, they cannot entirely eliminate it. They cannot personally prevent fires caused by lightning, arson, or the carelessness of others, and a useful fire can get out of control despite all precautions. A fire safety program must cover not only preventive measures but the procedures to be followed in a fire.

ESCAPING FROM A FIRE

If a fire should break out, the first and most important rule is to keep calm. The death toll in many major fire disasters would have been considerably lower if the victims had "kept their heads." Planning and rehearsing a rational procedure to be followed in case of fire, however remote the possibility may seem, should enable people to carry out that procedure when an emergency actually occurs, instead of endangering themselves further by making a frantic, ill-considered attempt to escape.

An escape plan involves:

1 A meeting of all members of the family to figure out two possible escape routes in case of fire. The plan should include every room, especially the bedrooms. The procedure is to be rehearsed frequently. (See Figures 13-7 and 13-8.)

2 Definite instructions as to what individuals should do if they are awakened and smell smoke. They should be cautioned against opening a door before feeling it to determine whether it is hot; told how to brace the door with their feet, if the door is not hot; advised to open the door a few inches to find out whether the hall area is hot and/or smoky; and reminded that they may have to use a window if they want to secure fresh air or call for help, or lower themselves to the porch roof, or even drop (not jump) to the ground if an escape ladder is not available (Figure 13-9).

3 A previously arranged place for gathering outside, to make sure that all occupants are out of the house and to prevent anyone from going back to rescue a person who has already left the building.

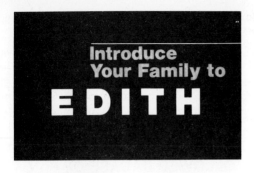

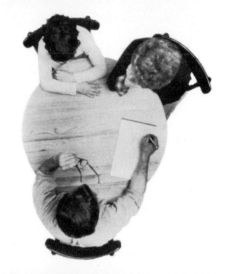

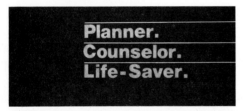

Figure 13-7 Introduce your family to EDITH (Exit Drills In The Home). (Source: National Fire Protection Association, Boston, Mass.)

Fires in schools where well-planned fire drills (see Chapter 4) have been conducted frequently enough to establish orderly exit procedures have rarely resulted in many fatalities. There have been serious school fires in which not a single life was lost because students had been trained to perform fire drills quickly and carefully. In other, potentially less dangerous fires many deaths have been caused by panic—the result of little or no practice in evacuating a building.

EDITH (Exit Drills In The Home) is a plan to save your life in case of fire.

EDITH

Don't wait for smoke and fire to surprise you. Plan your home fire escape now. If you live in an apartment, ask the management to schedule drills. Practice during Fire Prevention Week and once or twice more during the year. If you move, make a new plan right away!

Discuss and Plan Ahead

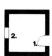

Sit down with your family today and make step by step plans for emergency fire escape.

Diagram two routes to the outside from all rooms, but especially from bedrooms. Locate the enclosed exit stairs in an apartment building.

Put the fire department number on your phone.

Choose a place outdoors for everyone to meet for roll call; locate the call box or neighbor's telephone for calling the fire department.

Discuss why you shouldn't go back inside once you're out. (People have died returning to a burning building.)

You May Need To Make a Purchase

Buy a smoke detector for each level of your home. If the bedrooms are not all in the same area, you need a smoke detector outside each sleeping area, too.

Each person should have a whistle (for warning others) to keep by the bed. Some family members may need a special escape ladder.

Practice

• Start now sleeping with the door closed, unless you have a good system of smoke detectors. The door holds back smoke and fire while you escape.

• Practice testing the door for fire. If it's warm, you'll have to use your alternate escape route. If not, brace your shoulder against the door and open it cautiously. Be ready to slam it if smoke or heat rush in.

• Make sure children can operate the windows, descend a ladder, or lower themselves to the ground. (Slide out on the stomach, feet first. Hang on with both hands. Bend the knees while landing.) Lower children to the ground before you exit from the window. They may panic and not follow if you go first.

• Practice what to do if you become trapped. Since doors hold back smoke and fire fighters are adept at rescue, your chances of survival are excellent if you do the right thing. Put closed doors between you and smoke. Stuff the cracks and cover vents to keep smoke out. If there's a phone, call in your exact location to the fire department even if they are on the scene. Tell children not to hide. Wait at the window and signal with a sheet or flashlight.

• Practice crawling in smoke.

• Have children practice saying the fire department number, the family name, street address, and town into the phone.

Figure 13-8   EDITH is a plan to save your life in case of fire. (Source: National Fire Protection Association, Boston, Mass.)

Even if people have a plan of action to be followed in case of fire in their schools, homes, places of business, or other familiar locations, they may still be subject to panic if fire breaks out in their hotel or in some other strange place. In this event, knowledge of the following rules, applicable to nearly all situations, may prevent serious consequences.

1 Always be prepared for fire. Check your nearest exit before going to your room.

2 If aroused by fire, check to see whether the door to your room is hot. If it is not, place your foot behind it and pull it just enough to feel whether there is any pressure from the hall. If you open the door without taking these precautions, you may allow flames, smoke, and superheated air to rush in upon you.

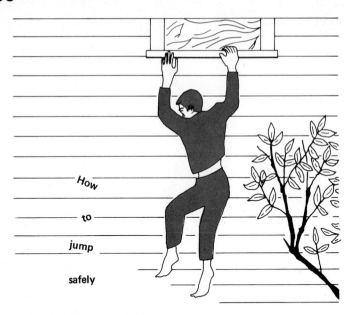

(but *don't* if you can avoid it)

From a window:

- Slide across sill on your stomach, feet first.
- Hang by your hands—it'll cut distance to ground by a third or more.
- Push away from house—then drop.
- Roll when you land.

From a porch roof:

- Never hang and drop from eaves—you might swing in and break your back on porch railing or floor.
- Jump to soft ground or into bushes—or yell for a ladder.

Figure 13-9 How to jump safely. (Source: Seconds Save Lives, pp. 8 and 9, The Country Companies, Bloomington, Ill.)

Air at a temperature between 300°F and 500°F seriously endangers life, and at 500°F it sears the lungs. In many major fire disasters, at least 50 percent of the deaths are caused by inhaling smoke and superheated air.

3 If it seems safe to leave the room, cover your mouth and nose with a wet towel and crawl on the floor, where the smoke is least dense. (Fig. 13-10.) Close the door behind you to prevent a draft from feeding the fire. If there is a panic rush for the main exit of the building, keep away from the crowd and attempt to find another exit.

4 If you plan to escape by a window, make a rope from bed sheets and clothing and fasten it securely to the radiator or bed. Do not jump, except as a last resort. More people have been saved by waiting for the fire department to come and rescue them than by leaping from burning buildings.

5 Do not enter a burning building to recover property. Only an attempt to save a life justifies taking this personal risk.

6 If burned, report for medical treatment as soon as possible.

RESIDENTIAL SMOKE ALARMS

In one recent year, an estimated 8 million householders purchased residential smoke alarms, a piece of equipment they hope they will never need.

Fires kill about 6,500 people in their homes each year, often during their sleeping hours. Fire officials are enthusiastically endorsing this new tool for early detection of fire. It has been estimated that 50 percent of fire-related deaths would be eliminated if every home had at least one smoke alarm.

The detector is concealed within a small container that fastens to the ceiling, usually in a hallway near the bedroom area. The alarm cannot prevent a fire, but its loud signal can arouse heavy sleepers before blinding smoke and deadly fumes prevent their escape. An analysis of fire deaths showed that four of five people killed in residential fires died not from burns but from toxic fumes. Besides strong demands for the smoke detectors from homeowners, laws have been enacted in several states to require smoke alarms in all new dwellings. The federal government requires alarms in all new, federally financed housing. A recent survey showed that 13 states mandate this protective device in all new residential construction, and 23 states require smoke alarms in specified types of residences.

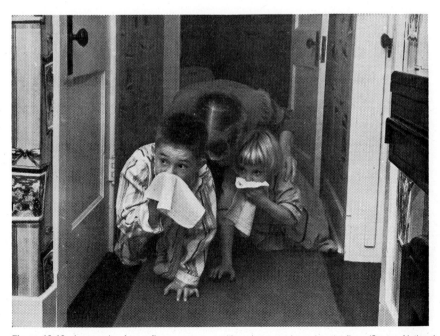

Figure 13-10 In escaping from a fire, cover your mouth and nose and crawl on the floor. (Source: National Safety Council, Chicago, Ill.)

Although smoke-alarm legislation has not yet been enacted in many states, many people believe that most states will eventually enact such legislation.

The following section, reprinted from *Family Safety* magazine, deals in detail with the various aspects of smoke detectors and alarms.

WHAT YOU SHOULD KNOW ABOUT SMOKE DETECTORS[16]

Smoke detectors for home fire protection have become big business almost overnight. If you are considering purchasing one to guard your family, you may be bewildered by the large selection of devices on the market today. Here are the answers to a few of the questions that might puzzle you as you shop.

Five years ago, no one had ever heard about smoke detectors. Why do I need one now?

The United States has more fire deaths and damage than any other nation in the world. Last year, more than 5,000 people died in home fires—roughly 15 every 24 hours.

Fire authorities believe that more than half of those lives could have been saved if the victims had been warned of impending disaster. Most home fires occur at night while the household is asleep. A smoke detector will rouse you and give you and your family from three to forty minutes to escape.

"Most people don't really believe it could happen to them," says David Lucht of the National Fire Prevention and Control Administration, part of the Department of Commerce. "But if I could take members of the average American family into a burning house and let them see what could happen to them and their home, they'd run right out and buy a smoke alarm."

You may be interested in smoke detectors because a local ordinance requires you to have one. A Federal law requires detectors in all new mobile homes. All homes purchased with loans guaranteed by the Federal Housing Authority or the Veterans Administration must have detectors. According to the Fire Equipment Manufacturers' Association, state codes in Massachusetts and Connecticut specify that a detector be installed in all new single-family dwellings. Similar legislation on a county or city level is proliferating all over the country. Some municipal codes require placement of a detector in existing homes when the property changes hands or when major repairs are made.

What are the major types of smoke detectors and how do they work?

Two types of units are on the market today: photoelectric and ionization detectors.

A photoelectric detector contains a lamp that directs a light beam into a central chamber. In the chamber is a light-sensitive photocell ("electric eye"), angled so that the light beam can't ordinarily reach it. But when smoke enters the chamber, the smoke particles scatter the light beam and some of the light enters the photocell. The photocell "sees" the light and sets off an alarm.

An ionization detector contains a radioactive source that allows some electricity to flow within the chamber. When smoke particles enter the unit, they impede the flow of current. Electronic monitoring devices measure the current reduction and set off an alarm.

How do I decide which type is best for my home?

A photoelectric detector provides early warning of smoldering fires with or without heat. Conversely, some ionization detectors respond more slowly to certain types of smoldering-only fires, but will probably respond faster than photoelectrics in a fire that gives off relatively little visible smoke.

[16] *Family Safety*, National Safety Council, Chicago, Winter, 1976–1977, pp. 26–27.

Photoelectric detectors must be connected to the house current. Ionization detectors may be powered by house current or batteries. Some house current models can be plugged directly into an outlet. Other "wired-in" types will probably have to be installed by an electrician. Wired-in models have this advantage: if your home has more than one detector, you can have the system wired so that all alarms will sound when any one unit detects smoke. But if a fire knocks out the electrical wiring of a home, a fairly rare occurrence in the early stages of a home fire, a house current unit without battery back-up will be useless.

Of course, a battery model requires you to change the batteries periodically. All Underwriters Laboratories (UL)-approved units feature an audible trouble signal that tells you when the batteries are nearing the end of their useful lives. Some manufacturers recommend changing the batteries every 12 months whether or not the unit signals.

Either type of unit will do a good job. Be sure that the model you select carries the UL label.

How many detectors should I have and where do I put them?

The number of detectors you need for complete protection depends on the size and arrangement of your house. Any detector should be placed on the ceiling or, if on a sidewall, about six or twelve inches from the ceiling. Locating a smoke detector to guard the sleeping area of a home is usually simple—mount the unit in the hall immediately outside the bedrooms.

Placement of units in other areas of the home can be a complex matter, and you may need expert help. The important thing is to locate the units between the bedrooms and other areas of the house so that the detector can intercept smoke as it approaches the bedroom area.

How much will an adequate protection system cost me?

Smoke detectors generally range in price from about $40 to $140, depending on type and installation requirements. You can find models priced as low as $19.95. Battery models are usually more costly than plug-in types. Those that are permanently connected to the house current are probably most expensive because of installation costs.

In addition to the initial cost, you will assume the minimal costs of batteries or bulbs and electricity. Smoke detectors are usually guaranteed by the manufacturer for one to five years.

You can keep your detector in working order by doing the light maintenance chores recommended by the manufacturer. Both ionization and photoelectric detectors need a yearly vacuuming. Some models require cleaning with alcohol. You should check occasionally for insects in the unit. Any detector should be tested periodically by blowing cigarette or candle smoke into the chamber.

Won't my smoking friends set off a false alarm?

Late-model detectors are factory-adjusted so they will protect you without sounding off every time you light a cigarette or burn a piece of toast. Sometimes a combination of circumstances will result in an alarm. But a false alarm should be a rare, minor problem. If it does occur, you can look upon it as an assurance that your protection system is working for you.

Do ionization detectors give off dangerous amounts of radiation?

Ralph Nader's Health Research Group recently warned that some ionization detectors have the potential for emitting dangerous amounts of radiation. Not so, says the Nuclear Regulatory Commission, pointing out that even a damaged or faulty detector would leak only a "negligible" amount of radiation. A smoke detector emits so little radiation that one authority says, "If you sat 24 inches from your detector for 497 years, you'd receive a dosage of radiation equivalent to one tooth X-ray." A far greater danger is death by fire if your home is not protected by a smoke detector.

FIGHTING A FIRE

Fire-fighting efforts during the first 5 minutes of a fire are worth more than the work of the next 5 hours. Quick action prevents a small fire from becoming a conflagration. It is essential that people know exactly what to do if they detect a fire so that they will be able to keep their heads, size up the situation, and take appropriate action immediately.

If clothing catches fire, it should be torn off away from the face. Above all, the victim should be kept from running, since that would merely fan the flames. If a rug or woolen blanket is readily accessible, it should be wrapped around the victim's neck to keep the fire from the face, or thrown on the victim and brushed down toward the feet. In some circumstances, it may be possible to smother the flames by placing the victim on the floor and rolling the victim in a rug.

One must understand that fire burns because three elements are present: (1) a substance that will burn—fuel, (2) sufficient heat to cause ignition, and (3) oxygen. Remove any one of these and the fire is extinguished. The fuel may be removed; the heat may be quenched by water; and the oxygen supply may be shut off by smothering.

If the person detecting a fire has any doubt about his or her ability to extinguish it, the fire department should be summoned immediately. A fire in a wastebasket can probably be put out promptly by dropping a book on the flames, but the fire department should be called at once if the fire has already ignited the curtains.

Everyone should know how to summon the fire department so that in an emergency valuable time will not be wasted looking up the number in the phone book or hunting for a fire signal box. People should know the location of the fire-signal box nearest their homes, schools, or places of business. If a box is not close to the scene of the fire, one should use the nearest phone. People need merely tell the operator that they want to report a fire; the operator will know what to do. When a signal box is used, the person reporting the fire must stay at the box until the fire apparatus arrives in order to direct the firemen. Obviously, if two or more people detect the fire, at least one should stay behind to fight the flames with a rug or fire extinguisher while the other reports the fire.

When using a fire extinguisher, stay as near as possible to the door and aim directly at whatever is burning. If the fire is spread out over the floor, aim at the nearest part of the fire and sweep it out completely in front of you as you move forward. If flames are traveling up the wall, put out the fire at the bottom first and then follow it up.

Today, fire extinguishers are relatively inexpensive, and in a fire they may be worth many times their purchase price. Everyone should give serious thought to providing at least one for the home, car, and place of business. The most commonly used fire extinguishers are described in Figure 13-11.

Because fire safety education can be easily implemented in school programs, the following student learning experiences are suggested.

Class "A" fires occur in ordinary combustible materials such as wood, cloth and paper. The most commonly used extinguishing agent is water which cools and quenches. Fires in these materials are also extinguished by special dry chemicals for use on Class A, B & C fires. These provide a rapid knock down of flame and form a fire retardant coating which prevents reflash.

Class "B" fires occur in the vapor-air mixture over the surface of flammable liquids such as greases, gasoline and lubricating oils. A smothering or combustion-inhibiting effect is necessary to extinguish Class "B" fires. Dry chemical, foam, vaporizing liquids, carbon dioxide, and water fog all can be used as extinguishing agents depending on the circumstances of the fire.

Class "C" fires occur in electrical equipment where non-conducting extinguishing agents must be used. Dry chemical, carbon dioxide, and vaporizing liquids are suitable. Because foam, water (except as a spray), and water-type extinguishing agents conduct electricity, their use can kill or injure the person operating the extinguisher, and severe damage to electrical equipment can result.

Class "D" fires occur in combustible metals such as magnesium, titanium, zirconium and sodium. Specialized techniques, extinguishing agents and extinguishing equipment have been developed to control and extinguish fires of this type. Normal extinguishing agents generally should not be used on metal fires as there is danger in most cases of increasing the intensity of the fire because of a chemical reaction between some extinguishing agents and the burning metal.

Figure 13-11 Classification of fires. (Source: The Fundamentals of Fire Extinguishment, The Ansul Company, Mainette, Wis.)

STUDENT LEARNING EXPERIENCES

The following assignments are designed to give students an opportunity to apply and extend their knowledge of fire prevention, and give the teacher an opportunity to estimate the extent of their learning.

1 With the assistance of the local fire department, arrange a demonstration of spontaneous ignition. Tell the class what you have done in your home to remove this danger.

2 Collect newspaper, radio, and television accounts of home fires reported during a 1-week period. List the causes and consequences of these fires and the steps that might have been effective in preventing them. Discuss your findings before the class.

3 With the assistance of your dramatics teacher, present a play or skit dealing with fire safety. Copies of The Rehearsal or The Intruder may be obtained from the National Board of Fire Underwriters.

4 With the aid of your general science teacher, set up a demonstration to show the correct wire size for electric outlets and the effect of overloading these outlets.

5 Late in September, arrange for the local fire chief or fire marshal to speak to an assembly on "Fire Prevention in October—and Other Months Too!"

6 Use the following checklist, adapted to suit your particular situation, to survey your home for common fire hazards. Enlist the assistance and cooperation of your family in making this survey. List some of the hazards detected in each area of your home and describe what can be done to remove them or prevent them from causing fires.

7 Have a member of the fire department demonstrate the use of extinguishers for the various classes of fires.

HOME FIRE SAFETY CHECKLIST

Yes   No

Yard and garage hazards

____   ____ Have you removed all combustible rubbish, leaves , and debris from your yard?

____   ____ Have you removed all waste, debris, and litter from your garage?

____   ____ Is an adult always present during the entire time trash, leaves, etc., are being burned out of doors?

____   ____ Is trash and refuse burned in a suitable outdoor incinerator?

____   ____ Have weeds, dried leaves, and rubbish been removed from vacant property adjacent to yours?

____   ____ Does your garage have a concrete, brick, or earthen floor?

____   ____ If your garage is in the basement or attached to the house, have cutoffs or barriers been provided to prevent passage of gases, smoke, or odors into the house?

Housekeeping hazards

____   ____ Do you keep your basement, storerooms, and attic free of rubbish, oily rags, old papers, mattresses, broken furniture, etc.?

____   ____ If you use an oil mop, do you keep it in a metal container or other safe, well-ventilated place, where it will not catch fire by spontaneous ignition?

____   ____ Do you destroy or dispose of oily polishing rags or waste after use?

____   ____ If you store paint, varnish, etc., are the containers always kept tightly closed?

____   ____ Do you deposit ashes in metal containers used for that purpose only, and dispose of them at frequent, regular intervals?

____   ____ Has your family been forbidden to use gasoline, benzine, or other similar flammable fluids for cleaning clothing or floors in your home?

Heating and cooking hazards

____   ____ Is your gas- or oil-heating equipment of a type which has been examined and listed by the Underwriters' Laboratories, Inc. or the American Gas Association Laboratories?

____   ____ Is your central heating equipment inspected and serviced by a reliable serviceman before the heating season?

____   ____ Are all flue pipes, vent connectors, gas vents, and chimneys inspected each fall, and cleaned and repaired when necessary?

____   ____ Are walls, ceilings, and partitions near boilers, stoves, furnaces, and heating pipes protected by noncombustible insulation or is adequate separation provided?

____   ____ Have you eliminated all vent connectors and flue pipes which pass through attics, floors, or ceilings?

____   ____ Are wood floors under stoves and heaters protected by insulation or ventilated air space?

____   ____ Is the cooking equipment kept clean and free of grease?

____   ____ Are curtains near stoves and other heating equipment arranged to prevent their accidentally blowing over the burners or flames and igniting?

____   ____ Are rooms in which room heaters are used properly ventilated for life safety during operation?

____   ____ Is your portable oil heater always set so that it is level to ensure proper operation?

Yes   No

_____ _____ Do you always refill the fuel tank or compartment of your oil heaters and oil stoves outdoors and in the daylight?

_____ _____ Do you regulate the flame and properly maintain your oil heater or stove to keep it from smoking?

_____ _____ If you use a wick-type oil heater, do you trim the wick and clean it regularly?

_____ _____ Do you always turn out your portable oil or gas heater upon retiring at night?

_____ _____ Do you always make sure that your portable heater is placed well away from curtains, drapes, furniture, etc.?

_____ _____ Are the gas connections for portable gas heaters or appliances made of metal?

_____ _____ Is your inside basement door at the head of the stairs properly fitted and kept closed at night?

_____ _____ Are members of your family forbidden to start fires in stoves, fireplaces, etc., with kerosene or other flammable liquids?

_____ _____ Is the fireplace equipped with a metal fire screen?

Electrical hazards

_____ _____ Do you allow only reliable electricians to install or extend your wiring?

_____ _____ Are all of your electrical appliances—including irons, waffle irons, mixers, heaters, lamps, fans, radios, television sets, etc.—listed by Underwriters' Laboratories, Inc.?

_____ _____ Do all rooms have an adequate number of outlets to avoid need for multiple attach-ment plugs and long extension cords?

_____ _____ Are your electric irons and all electrical appliances used for cooking equipped with heat-limit controls?

_____ _____ Have you provided special circuits for heavy-duty appliances such as washing machines, refrigerators, ranges, ironers, etc.?

_____ _____ Do you use only 15-ampere fuses for your household lighting circuits?

_____ _____ Are all flexible electric extension and lamp cords in your house in the open—none placed under rugs, over hooks, through partitions or door openings?

Matches and careless-smoking hazards

_____ _____ Do you keep matches in metal containers away from heat and away from children?

_____ _____ Do you extinguish all matches and cigarette and cigar butts carefully before disposing of them?

_____ _____ Do you see to it that there are plenty of noncombustible ash trays in all rooms?

_____ _____ Are all members of your family instructed not to smoke in bed?

Preparation in case of fire

_____ _____ Do you know the location of the fire-alarm box nearest your residence?

_____ _____ Do you know how to turn in a fire alarm?

_____ _____ Do you know the telephone number of the fire department?

_____ _____ Do you have a plan of escape from your home in case of fire?

_____ _____ Do you hold fire drills in your home?

_____ _____ When you employ "sitters," do you instruct them carefully on what to do in case of fire?

_____ _____ Did your entire family take part in completing this checklist?[17]

EVALUATION

Any evidence that students recognize and understand fire hazards and preven-tive measures indicates that their training in fire safety has been effective. Knowledge of these matters must be more than superficial if it is to lead to

---

[17]National Board of Fire Underwriters, New York.

proper behavior. To discover how much students have really learned, the teacher must attempt to judge their awareness of the close cause-and-effect relationship between the various hazards and destructive fires, and between preventive measures and safety. Students should be able to explain why turning on an electric switch can cause flammable vapors to ignite, why oily rags should be enclosed in a metal container, and why a match should be broken in two before it is thrown on the ground.

Objective tests, especially those given both before and after students have received instruction in fire safety, are one means of measuring how much knowledge has been absorbed.

In the final analysis, the effectiveness of fire safety education must be measured not by how much students know about hazards and precautions, but by how much they apply that knowledge. Teachers must have evidence that hazards are being eliminated and that the proper procedures are being voluntarily observed before they can be sure that any real learning has taken place. If safety education is successful in this area, the ultimate result will be the control of fire. We must realize that evaluation is not a means to an end, but should be considered as a continuous process.

EMERGENCY SERVICES AND DISASTER PROTECTION

A major emergency affecting a large number of people can occur at any time and anywhere. It can be a peacetime disaster such as a flood, tornado, earthquake, fire, hurricane, blizzard, or forest fire, or it can be nuclear attack. In any type of general disaster, lives can be saved if people are prepared for the emergency and know what actions to take.

"Although seemingly unprepared, we have always been able to rally our forces and gain an ultimate victory." This has been our stand since our country first won its independence from Great Britain. But atomic bombs, atomic energy, radiation, germ warfare, and radioactive fallout place us in a position where an aggressor can directly attack our civilian population without first overcoming our armed forces.

Aggression as an instrument of national policy has not been ruled out by all countries of the world. Common prudence demands that we make every effort to protect our people. Because of the many possible disasters aside from war, prevention must be the first step in a disaster-protection program. The lightning rod lessens the danger of disaster from lightning; fires can be curbed by fire-resistant construction, fire control, and the elimination of combustibles. But the general public remains apathetic to the need for a program of protection against disaster.

The most destructive disaster would be the unleashing of an all-out war. The devastation of two Japanese cities was caused by two *small* nuclear bombs. Since then, the power of nuclear weapons capable of being used against home-front targets has increased more than a thousandfold. All that is needed is for someone to press the panic button, or start turning the keys to the destructive mechanism.

An all-out attack on this country would involve our cities as well as our military installations. The people would be a target. Planning for disaster prevention and protection is vital if we are to meet such circumstances, but the planning cannot be left only to emergency services and disaster-protection agencies; they are helpless without the understanding and cooperation of the people. A workable plan, which will ensure at least partial recovery from any initial enemy attack, is imperative. We must realize the seriousness of the situation. We must not use civil defense warning signals to welcome home a victorious baseball team. We must not forget Hiroshima and Nagasaki.

Lethal radioactivity can be blown hundreds of miles from an atomic explosion. The mushroom-shaped cloud that rises when a thermonuclear weapon is exploded sucks up tons of dust and dirt and carries it into the upper atmosphere to a height of 20,000 to 80,000 feet. As the cloud rises and brings the dust with it, the radioactive particles of the exploded bomb attach themselves to the dust. When the wind blows downward, these heavier-than-air particles of dust with radioactive particles sticking to them fall to earth. This "fallout" can be lethal. The dangers just described, plus the blast and the subsequent fires, burns, contaminations, and poisons from primary radiation, should impel the population to give heed to some form of prevention program.

Our defensive weapons are being constantly improved, but an unready home front increases our vulnerability. With a good emergency-services—disaster-prevention program, and a protection program to speed postdisaster recovery, we can reduce our vulnerability. Our investment in disaster protection can pay dividends in diminished apprehension and a stronger sense of security.

DISASTER PROTECTION

Our nationwide emergency-services and disaster-protection system is constantly being improved and enlarged. The heart of the system is fallout shelter protection against the radioactive materials from a nuclear attack. The system includes warning and communication networks, methods of measuring fallout radiation, lifesaving and recovery procedures, emergency broadcasting stations, local governmental organization for emergency operations, citizen training in emergency skills, and military forces for times of emergency.

Schools also have an important part to play in disaster-protection programs. The federal Office of Emergency Services and Disaster Protection and many individual states have prepared disaster-preparedness guides for school administrators. Some of the subjects covered are.[18]

1. A Realistic Approach to Civil Defense
2. Identifying a need
3. The New Approach to Protection
4. The school, a vital Link in Civil Defense

[18]*A Realistic Approach to Civil Defense, A Handbook for School Administrators,* Office of Emergency Services and Disaster Protection, Department of Defense, Washington, 33 pp.

5. Civil defense, a Study in Science
   a. The Weapon
   b. Fallout
   c. Fallout Radiation
   d. Radioactive Decay
   e. Exposure
   f. Shielding
6. The School Plant
   a. The Safest Place
   b. Improvising
7. Building for Tomorrow
8. Developing a Shelter System
9. The Community Shelter Planning Program
10. Warning and Communication Systems
11. In the Shelter
12. Interschool System Organization for Civil Defense
    a. Staff Utilization
    b. In-Service Civil Defense Education of Staff
13. The Shelter Drill
14. Civil Defense in the Curriculum
15. Civil Defense Adult Education
16. The School as a Community Agency

The Office of Emergency Services and Disaster Protection has prepared a self-teaching course that provides an orientation to civil defense. The units deal with protection, nuclear weapons effects, shelters, warning emergency operations, and program support and governmental responsibilities for civil defense.[19]

With the aid of federal and state governments, cities and counties throughout the United States are developing local civil defense systems. Although these local systems have been set up primarily as a protection against nuclear attack, they have done a remarkable job in major peacetime disasters. They have warned people of impending storms, tornadoes, hurricanes, floods, and earthquakes.

In most communities a citizens handbook that describes what should be done in times of emergency is available through the local office of civil defense.

A dynamic civil defense organization can keep all citizens alert to the dangers presented by a nuclear attack, and can prepare citizens for natural disasters. Confidence in local and state programs will go a long way toward avoiding panic, which can kill and injure more people than the disaster itself.

NATURAL DISASTERS

TORNADOES

Tornadoes are small but deadly stoms that skip across the land, cutting a swath of destruction. They are characterized by winds that whirl at great speeds and usually by thunderstorms. A tornado can be described as a rotating, funnel-

[19]*Civil Defense, U.S.A., a Programmed Orientation to Civil Defense*, Office of Emergency Services and Disaster Protection, Department of Defense, Washington.

shaped cloud that usually moves from a southwest direction. Tornadoes occur almost everywhere, but they are most frequent in the central section of the United States. They usually occur in the spring.

If one lives in a tornado area or belt, it is particularly important to know the procedures to follow to protect oneself. The U.S. Weather Bureau issues forecasts for areas most likely to experience tornadoes several hours before the tornadoes are expected to occur. If a tornado is sighted, the bureau issues a public tornado warning. When this occurs, people should keep their radios or televisions tuned in for further weather information.

When a tornado watch is announced, it means that a tornado is expected in or near your area. When this occurs, tune in your local radio or television station and watch the sky for a funnel-shaped cloud.

After the warning is issued you should take shelter immediately. You must take quick action to protect yourself from flying debris and from falling or blowing away. The best protection is an underground shelter or a steel-framed or reinforced-concrete building. If you are at home, head for the basement and go to the corner nearest the storm. If no basement is available, take refuge under a heavy table or bench, and stay away from the windows. If you are outdoors, you should go to a nearby ditch or ravine. Do not remain in a trailer or mobile home. If you are driving in open country, drive away from the tornado's path at a right angle.

If you are in school in a city area, seek shelter near an inside wall on a lower floor. Avoid large rooms such as the gymnasium or auditorium, especially if the roof is not well supported. In rural school areas, the tornado cellar or a nearby ravine or ditch is the safest place to go.

If you are in a factory or industrial plant, follow safety officials' instructions as to where workers are to move for their greatest protection.

FLOODS AND HURRICANES

There are certain emergency actions associated with major floods, hurricanes, and storm tides. People living in areas where these disasters are likely to occur are usually given a long period of warning before they are asked to move to safer locations. There are certain procedures to follow when asked to evacuate. They are:

1 Follow the instructions, advice, and specific directions given by your local government.

2 Secure your home before leaving. If there is time, bring out your possessions from the house or tie them down securely. Bring in anything that might be blown or washed away. Board up the windows, disconnect electrical appliances, turn off the gas, and move other objects to an upper floor. If you are trapped at home by a flash flood, go to the second floor or the roof, where there is a better chance of being spotted and rescued.

3 If you are directed to leave the area, leave before the roads become blocked, make sure you have a full tank of gasoline, follow recommended routes, and watch for wash-outs, fallen electric lines, slides, and falling or fallen objects.

, **4** When reaching a body of water, make sure it is safe to cross. Put your car in low gear, and drive slowly to avoid splashing water into your engine, which can cause it to stall. Test your brakes after reaching the other side.

EARTHQUAKES

If you live in an earthquake area, the following procedures are recommended.

1 Keep calm and don't panic.

2 Remain where you are. If outdoors, stay there and keep clear of anything that might collapse or fall. If indoors, stay there. Many people are injured by falling walls, electric wires, etc., when entering or leaving buildings.

3 When indoors take cover under a desk, table, or sturdy bench. Stand or sit against an inside wall, preferably in the basement. Stay away from windows and outside doors.

4 If you are driving an automobile, pull off the road and stop as soon as possible. Remain in the car. When you resume driving, watch for hazards created by the earthquake.

After a natural disaster, certain precautions should be taken before one attempts to resume normal activities.

1 Use extreme caution when reentering a building that may have been weakened by the storm.

2 Check for electrical shortages, and keep away from fallen wires.

3 Keep lanterns, torches, or lighted cigarettes out of buildings because gas lines may have ruptured.

4 Use extreme caution when checking for gas leaks in your home. Do not use matches or candles. If gas is present, open all doors and windows, turn off the main gas valve, leave the house, and then call the gas company.

5 If electrical appliances are wet, turn off the main power switch, unplug the appliances, dry them out, reconnect them, and then turn on the main power switch. If fuses blow when the power is restored, turn off the main power again and inspect for short circuits. If in doubt call a qualified electrician.[20]

The best way to meet all disasters is to remain calm and avoid panic. If individuals follow directions and take instructions provided by their local, state, and federal governments, they can feel relatively secure if a disaster should strike.

[20]Much of the information in this section has been obtained from the *Citizen's Handbook—In Time of Emergency*, Office of Emergency Services and Disaster Protection, Washington.

LEARNING EXPERIENCES

The following activities are designed to supplement the study of this chapter.

1 Arrange for a home clean-up campaign *before* Fire Prevention Week in October, making special provisions for the removal and proper disposal of rubbish from attics, basements, and other common repositories for trash.

2 List the particular precautions that can prevent fires in the various areas of the home and school—the kitchen, attic, basement, furnace room, etc. Pay particular attention to such potential danger spots as chimneys and hot pipes, electrical equipment, and fireplaces.

3 Interview someone who has been in a serious fire, and explain the correct and incorrect procedures that the person followed at the time.

4 Visit a local store or factory equipped with automatic sprinklers. Discuss the value of this system, and of any other devices used to protect the buildings from fire, with the owner or the person in charge of fire prevention.

5 Check your neighborhood to determine where there is a fire-alarm box and where it is located.

6 Secure from the school or local library any of the better books describing the bombing of Hiroshima and/or Nagasaki or the bombing of London, with a view to discovering what happens when disaster strikes. Report your findings to your class.

7 As a class project, set up a disaster-prevention program for your school.

8 Invite your local emergency services and disaster agency director to address a student assembly on the subject "An adequate emergency services and disaster program can save lives."

9 Have a member of the fire department demonstrate the proper use of fire extinguishers.

10 Using the checklist below, survey your school for common fire hazards. List the most serious hazards you find and plan ways to remove or compensate for them. Discuss your suggestions at an assembly or a PTA meeting.

SELF-INSPECTION BLANK FOR SCHOOLS

If precautions are taken to minimize the danger of fire and to provide for safety in case fire occurs, real progress will be made in protecting life and property. Intelligent thought and care put into practice can eliminate practically all fires within schools.

Instructions

Inspection is to be made each month by the custodian and a member of the faculty, at which inspection only Items 1 to 20 need be reported. At the quarterly inspection, a member of the fire department should accompany the above inspectors, and the complete blank should be filled out. The report of each inspection (monthly and quarterly) is to be filed with the Board of Education or School Commissions.

Questions are so worded that a negative answer will indicate an unsatisfactory condition.

Date_____

Name of School_____City_____

Class: Elementary_____Junior High_____Senior High _____

Capacity of School?_____Number now enrolled _____

(1) Are all exit doors equipped with panic locks?_____Are these locks tested each week to ensure ease of operation? _____ Do these lock securely so that additional locks, bolts, or chains are not necessary?_____Are such additional locks open whenever building is in use?_____

(2) Are all outside fire escapes free from obstructions and in good working order?_____Are they used for fire drills? _____

(3) Is all heating equipment, including flues, pipes, and steam lines:
(a) In good, serviceable condition and well maintained? _____
(b) Properly insulated and separated from all combustible material by a safe distance?_____

(4) Is coal pile inspected periodically for evidences of heating? _____

(5) Are ashes placed in *metal* containers used for that purpose only?
_____

(6) Is remote control provided whereby oil supply line may be shut off in emergency?_____

(7) Where is outside shut-off valve on gas supply line? _____
_____

(8) Check any of the following locations where there are accumulations of waste paper, rubbish, old furniture, stage scenery, etc., and explain under remarks:—attic, basement, furnace room, stage, dressing rooms in connection with stage, other locations_____

(9) Is the space beneath stairs free from accumulation or storage of any materials? _____

(10) What material or preparation is used for cleaning or polishing floors?
_____
Quantity on hand?_____Where stored? _____

(11) Are approved metal cans, with self-closing covers or lids, used for the storage of *all* oily waste, polishing cloths, etc.? _____

(12) Are approved metal containers with vapor-tight covers used for all kerosene, gasoline, etc., on the premises?_____
Why are such hazardous materials kept on the premises? _____

(13) Are premises free from electrical wiring or equipment which is defective? _____
_____
(If answer is *No,* explain under *Remarks.*)

(14) Are only approved extension or portable cords used? _____

(15) Are all fuses on lighting or small-appliance circuits of 15 amperes or less capacity? _____

(16) Are electric pressing irons equipped with automatic heat control or signal and provided with metal stand?_____

(17) Are sufficient fire extinguishers provided on each floor so that not over 100 feet of travel is required to reach the nearest unit? _____
In manual training shops and on stage, 50 feet? _____

(18) Have chemical extinguishers been recharged within a year? _____
Is date of recharge shown on tag attached to extinguisher?_____

(19) Is building equipped with standpipe and hose having nozzle attached?
_____
Is hose in good, serviceable condition?_____

(20) Is a large woolen blanket available in the domestic science laboratory for use in case clothing is ignited?_____

Remarks (Note any changes since last inspection)
The following items to be included in each quarterly inspection:—

(21) Building construction: Walls_____Floors_____Roof _____
No. stories_____No. classrooms _____

(22) Which sections of buildings are equipped with automatic sprinklers?
_____

(23) Are there at least two means of egress from each floor of the building? _____
   Are these so located that the distance measured along the line of travel does not exceed
     From the door of any classroom, 125 feet? _____
     From any point in auditorium, assembly hall, or gymnasium, 100 feet? _____
(24) Are all windows free from heavy screens or bars? _____
(25) Do all exit doors open outward? _____
(26) Are all interior stairways enclosed? _____
   Are doors to these enclosures of self-closing type? _____
(27) Are windows within 10 feet of fire escapes glazed with wire glass?
   _____

(28) Are manual training, domestic science, other laboratories, and the cafeteria so located that a
   fire in one will not cut off any exit from the building? _____
   _____

(29) Is a smoke-tight projection booth, built of incombustible materials, and vented to the outside,
   provided for the motion-picture machine?
   _____

(30) Are heating plant and fuel supply rooms cut off from the main corridor by fire-resistant walls,
   ceiling, and doors? _____
(31) Do all ventilating ducts terminate outside of building? _____
(32) State type of construction of any temporary buildings in school yard.
   _____

(33) Is nearest temporary building at least 50 feet from main building?
   _____

(34) How often are fire drills held? _____ Average time of exit? _____
   _____

(35) Are provisions made for sounding alarm of fire from any floor of building? _____
   _____
   Is sounding device accessible? _____ Plainly marked? _____
(36) Give location of nearest city fire-alarm box. _____
   _____

   How far distant from the premises? _____
Remarks

                Inspector _____ Title _____
                Inspector _____ Title _____ [2]

SELECTED REFERENCES

Aaron, James E., A. Frank Bridges, and Dale O. Ritzel: *First Aid and Emergency Care,*
   The Macmillan Company, New York, 1972
Allstate Insurance Company, Skokie, Ill.: *What You Should Know about Tornadoes*
Country Companies, Bloomington, Ill.: *The Fireproof Mind. Seconds Save Lives*
Department of Defense, Office of Emergency Services and Disaster Protection,
   Washington:
   A Realistic Approach to Civil Defense
     Civil Defense, U.S.A., 1968
   Federal Civil Defense Guide
   Introduction to Civil Defense, 1972
   Personal and Family Survival, rev.
   Publication Index, MP-20, latest ed.
   Unit 1. Civil Defense Protection Against What?
   Unit 2. Nuclear Weapons Effect

---

[2] The National Board of Fire Underwriters. Chicago. Approved and adopted by the National Association of
   Public School Business Officials. Endorsed by the International Association of Fire Chiefs.

Unit 3. Shelters
Unit 4. Warning, Emergency, Operations and Support Programs
Unit 5. Governmental Responsibilities for Civil Defense
Emmons Howard: "Fire and Fire Protection." *Scientific American,* p. 21, July, 1974
Lighting Protection Institute: *Lightning Protection Guide,* Chicago, 15 pp.
Metropolitan Life Insurance Company: *Statistical Bulletin,* p. 6, January, 1975
National Fire Protection Association, Boston:
  Baby Sitters Handbook
  Clothing Can Burn
  Don't Let Your Family Burn
  Escape from Fire Wherever You Are
  Fire, Electricity and Your Home
  Fire Safety in Your Home
  High Rise Fire Safety
  Home Fire Detection, 1975
  In Case of Fire—Have You Made Your Escape Plan?
  Introduce Your Family to EDITH (Exit Drills in The Home)
  Know Your ABC and D of Portable Fire Extinguishers
  Sparky's Fire Department Inspectors Handbook
  What's Cooking
  Your Guide for Home Fire Fighting
National Safety Council, Chicago:
  Accident Facts, published annually
  Safety Education Data Sheets:
  No. 2, rev., *Matches*
  No. 5, rev., *Falls*
  No. 6, rev., *Cutting Implements*
  No. 7, rev., *Lifting, Carrying, Lowering Inanimate Objects*
  No. 8, rev., *Poisonous Plants*
  No. 9, rev., *Electric Equipment*
  No. 12, rev., *Flammable Liquid in the Home*
  No. 15, rev., *Hand Tools*
  No. 16, rev., *Non-Electric Household Equipment*
  No. 20, rev., *Utility Gas in the Home*
  No. 21, rev., *Solid and Liquid Poisons*
  No. 49, rev., *Bathroom Hazards*
  No. 58, rev., *Winter Walking*
  No. 61, rev., *Floors in the Home*
  No. 62, rev., *Ice Boxes and Refrigerators, Hazards of Discarding*
  No. 66, rev., *Baby Sitting*
  No. 68, rev., *Safety in "Do it Yourself"*
  No. 76, rev., *Safety in Bad Weather Conditions*
  No. 86, rev., *Cigarette Fire Hazards*
  No. 90, rev., *Flammability of Wearing Apparel*
  No. 91, rev., *Home Lighting*
  No. 92, rev., *Safe Use of Pesticides*
Farm Safety Review, "Home Fires," vol. 35, no. 5, September-October, 1977
                              pamphlets
  All About Fire Books, K-1, K-2-3, and K-4-6
  Did George Do It?
  Energy Crisis
  Family Emergency Almanac
  The Hazard Haunted House
  The Hazard Hunter

Home Poisons
Plug Into Electrical Safety
Winter Snow Falls
Family Magazine, selected articles:
    "Mower Use with Less Injury," Summer, 1969
    "Stairs Can Be Your Downfall," Fall, 1970
    "Slips, Scalds and Shock that Breed in the Wetlands," Fall, 1971
    "The Low Down on High Rise Fires," Winter, 1971–1972
    "Five Steps to a Fire Safe Home," Fall, 1972
    "Look Up and Live," (electrical hazards), Fall, 1972
    "In The Mouth of Babes," Spring, 1973
    "CO Means Colorless and Odorless and Danger," Fall, 1973
    "The Name of the Fire Game—GET OUT," Winter, 1973–1974
    "A New Look at Child Poisoning," Spring, 1974
    "What Do You Do Now?" (child poisoning), Summer, 1974
    "This Book is Not For Kids," (matches), Fall, 1974
    "Garden Variety Mishaps," Spring, 1975
    "When Water Won't Work," (fire extinguishing), Spring, 1975
    "Should You Do it Yourself?" Summer, 1975
    "Summer is Flu Time," Summer, 1975
    "Disaster," Summer, 1975
    "Fire Has Its Place," Fall, 1975
    "When to Fight a Fire," Winter, 1975–1976
    "What if You Smell Gas," Winter, 1975–1976
    "Know Before You Mow," Summer, 1976
    "Fight Fire with Firemen," Fall, 1976
    "Watch Out the Heat's On," Fall, 1977
Outdoor Power Equipment Institute, Inc., Washington:
    Mow in Safety
    Powermowerman
    Safety Sammy Sez (riding mower safety)
Segal, Louis: "What Price Clothing Fire Safety," *Fire Journal,* January, 1972
Strasser, Marland K., James E. Aaron, Ralph C. Bohn, and John R. Eales: *Fundamentals of Safety Education,* 2d ed., The Macmillan Company, New York, 1973, 501 pp.
The Ansul Company: *The Fundamental of Fire Extinguishment,* Marinette, Wisc.
Thygerson, Alton: *Accidents and Disasters,* Prentice-Hall, Inc., Englewood Cliffs, N.J., 1977, 411 pp.
U. S. Consumer Product Safety Commission, Washington:
    Fact Sheets
    No. 1, *Power Mowers*
    No. 2, *Hedge Trimmers*
    No. 3, *Bathtub and Shower Injuries*
    No. 4, *Tent Flammability*
    No. 5, *Non-Glass Doors*
    No. 6, *Stairs, Ramps, and Landings*
    No. 7, *Power Saws*
    No. 8, *Swimming Pools*
    No. 9, *Kitchen Ranges*
    No. 10, *Bicycles*
    No. 11, *Televisions* (fire and shock hazards)
    No. 12, *Fireworks*
    No. 13, *Carbon Monoxide*
    No. 14, *Lead Paint Poisoning*
    No. 15, *Tricycles*

No. 16, *Extension Cord/Wall Outlets*
No. 17, *Flammable Fabrics*
No. 18, *Insecticides and Pesticides*
No. 19, *Glass Doors and Windows*
No. 20, *Infant Falls*
No. 21, *Poisonous Household Substances*
No. 22, *Playground Equipment*
No. 23, *Flammable Liquids*
No. 24, *Laundering Procedures*
No. 25, *Flammable Fabrics Standards*
No. 26, *Floors*
No. 27, *Snowmobiles*
No. 28, *Matches and Lighters*
No. 29, *Skiing and Skiing Equipment*
No. 30, *Standards and Development Under CPSA*
No. 31, *Repurchase Regulations*
No. 32, *Substantial Hazards-Section 15*
No. 33, *Aerosols*
No. 34, *Space Heaters and Heating Stoves*
No. 35, *Hair Dryers*
No. 36, *Wringer Washing Machines*
No. 37, *Glass Bottles*
No. 38, *Mini-Bikes*
No. 39, *Mobile Homes*
No. 40, *Christmas Decorations*
No. 41, *Plastics*
No. 42, *Football and Football Equipment*
No. 43, *Crib Safety—Keep Them On The Safe Side*
No. 44, *Fireplaces*
No. 45, *Fondue Pots*
No. 46, *Poison Prevention Packaging*
No. 47, *Toys*
No. 48, *The Elderly and Stairway Accidents*
No. 49, *Sleds, Toboggans and Snow Disks*
No. 50. *Electric Blenders, Mixers, Choppers/Slicers, and Grinders*
No. 51, *Chain Saws*
No. 52, *Some Federal Consumer Oriented Agencies*
No. 53, *Upholstered Furniture*
No. 54, *Electric Baseboard Heaters*
No. 55, *Federal Hazardous Substances Act*
No. 56, *Ladders*
No. 57, *Smoke Detectors*
No. 58, *Vinyl Chloride*
No. 59, *Electric Home Workshop Tools*
No. 60, *Trouble Light*
No. 61, *Electrical Toys*
No. 62, *Electricity*
No. 63, *Refrigerators*
No. 64, *Pressure Cookers*
No. 65, *Gas Water Heaters*
No. 66, *Baby Walkers*
No. 67, *Oven Cleaners*
No. 68, *Misuse of Consumer Goods*
No. 69, *Counter-Top Cooking Appliances* (portable)
No. 70, *High Chairs*

No. 71, *Bunk Beds*
No. 72, *Drain Cleaners*
No. 73, *Clothes Dryers*
No. 74, *Toy Chests*
No. 75, *Hammers*
No. 76, *Electric Irons*
No. 78, *Garden Tractors*
No. 79, *Furnaces*
No. 80, *Consumer Deputies*
No. 81, *Refuse Bins*
No. 82, *Batteries*
No. 83, *Kitchen Knives*
No. 84, *Roller Skates, Ice Skates, Skateboards*
No. 85, *Trampolines*
No. 86, *Baby Rattles*
No. 87, *Airless Paint Spray Guns*
No. 88, *Antenna Electrocutions*
No. 89, *Home Canning Equipment*
U.S. Department of Health, Education and Welfare, Rockville, Md.:
Safe Toys for Your Child
We Want You to Know about Preventing Childhood Poisoning
Wilson, Rexford: "A Fire Safe House," *Farm Safety Review,* November–December, 1972
Worick, Wayne, W.: *Safety Education—Man, His Machines and Environment,* Prentice-Hall, Inc., Englewood Cliffs, N.J., 1975, 288 pp.

U.S. CONSUMER PRODUCT SAFETY COMMISSION AREA OFFICES

Atlanta Area
   1330 West Peachtree Street, N.W.
   Atlanta, Georgia 30309
   404-881-2231

Boston Area
   100 Summer Street
   Boston, Massachusetts 02110
   617-223-5576

Chicago Area
   230 South Dearborn Street
   Chicago, Illinois 60606
   312-353-8260

Dallas Area
   Rm 410C, 500 South Ervay
   Dallas, Texas 75201
   214-749-3871

Denver Area
   Suite 938, Guaranty Bank Building
   817 17th Street
   Denver, Colorado 80202
   303-837-2904

Kansas City Area
    Traders National Bank Building
    1125 Grand Avenue
    Suite 1500
    Kansas City, Missouri 64106
    816-374-2034

Los Angeles Area
    3660 Wilshire Boulevard, Suite 1100
    Los Angeles, California 90010
    213-688-7272

New Orleans Area
    Suite 414, International Trade Mart
    2 Canal Street
    New Orleans, Louisiana 70130
    504-527-2102

New York Area
    6 World Trade Center
    Vesey Street, 6th Floor
    New York, New York 10048
    212-264-1125

Philadelphia Area
    400 Market Street
    Continental Building, 10th Floor
    Philadelphia, Pennsylvania 19106
    215-597-9105

San Francisco Area
    160 Pine Street
    San Francisco, California 94111
    415-556-1816

Seattle Area
    3240 Federal Building
    915 Second Avenue
    Seattle, Washington, 98174
    206-442-5276

Cleveland Area
    Plaza Nine Bldg., Rm 520
    55 Erieview Plaza
    Cleveland, Ohio 44114
    216-522-3886

Minneapolis Area
    Federal Building, Fort Snelling, Rm 650
    Twin Cities, Minnesota 55111
    612-725-3424

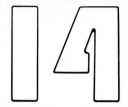

Occupational Safety

OVERALL OBJECTIVE:

The student should recognize the hazards of the workplace and be able to discuss the different efforts being made toward occupational safety.

INSTRUCTIONAL OBJECTIVES:

After completing this chapter the student will be able to:

1 Discuss the extent of injuries, illness, and fatalities in the workplace.
2 Explain the purposes and provisions of worker's compensation laws.
3 List the reasons why Congress enacted the Occupational and Safety Health Act (OSHAct).
4 Describe the responsibilities of the agencies created under OSHAct.
5 Explain the procedures that are followed during an OSHA inspection.
6 List the penalities for violations of OSHA standards.
7 Discuss employee rights and responsibilities under OSHAct.
8 Describe the functions of industrial safety administration.
9 Appreciate the losses created by occupational accidents.
10 Explain the hazards associated with farming as an occupation.
11 Explain why OSHAct will not materially change the hazards of farming.

There is ample evidence to demonstrate that good occupational safety records are a result of organized safety programs. Safety is not the exclusive responsibility of management or the safety officer. A good safety program promotes safety throughout the system. People are often the least reliable component in a system, and safety must be a meaningful part of the work experience of every worker. As in other areas of accident prevention, individuals must accept responsibility for safe living.

PERSPECTIVE ON OCCUPATIONAL SAFETY

The results of safety programs in the workplace are impressive. Between 1912 and 1976 accident fatality rates dropped by 71 percent. Since World War II accidental deaths among workers on the job have been cut by 24 percent. The

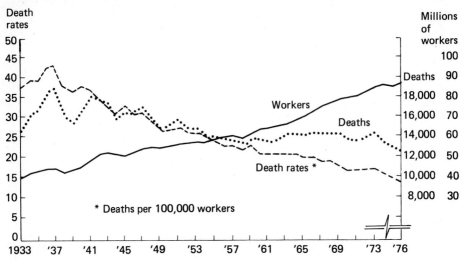

Figure 14-1 Trends in work accidents, 1933–1976. (Source: Accident Facts, The National Safety Council, Chicago, 1977, p. 23.

workplace death rate in 1945 was 33 per 100,000 workers. By 1976 the death rate was reduced by more than half, to 14 per 100,000 workers. Figure 14-1 depicts the gradually declining occupational death rate. It shows that the work force has more than doubled while the actual number of worker deaths has declined by several thousand.

Although it is true that death rates have also decreased away from the workplace, the ratio of on-job to off-job fatalities has increased from 1.82 in 1945 to 3.06 in 1976. The injury ratio has displayed a similar trend, with a growing proportion of accidental injuries occurring off the job. Three out of four deaths and more than half the injuries suffered by workers in 1976 occurred off the job (Table 14-1).

Member companies of the National Safety Council (NSC) generally have better safety programs than nonmembers. Member companies also have lower injury rates. In Table 14-2, the injury rates for National Safety Council members are compared with the rates for nonmembers. Over the years, member companies have averaged 70 percent lower frequency rates and 40 percent lower severity rates than nonmember companies.

There can be little doubt that organized safety efforts have contributed to the reduction in workplace death and injury statistics. But a great deal more remains to be done. Work accidents still kill more than 12,000 people annually. Work injuries disable another 2.2 million, 80,000 of whom become permanently impaired. A workplace death occurs every 42 minutes. There are 35 per day, or 245 per week. A workplace injury occurs every 4 seconds. There are 6,000 per day, or 34,600 per week. It has been estimated that 390,000 new cases of disabling disease occur each year from exposure to toxic materials at work.[1]

[1]Nicholas Askounas Ashford, *Crisis in The Workplace: Occupational Disease and Injury,* The M.I.T. Press, Cambridge, 1976, p. 3.

TABLE 14–1

Trends in On-Job Off-Job Deaths and Injuries

Year	Death Ratio Off Job/On Job*	Injury Ratio Off Job/On Job
1945	1.82	1.38
1950	2.03	1.28
1955	2.20	1.23
1960	2.12	1.15
1965	2.59	1.29
1970	3.17	1.48
1975	2.91	1.45
1976	3.06	1.41
Change 1945–76	68%	+2%

*Deaths per 100,000 workers.
Source: *Accident Facts,* National Safety Council, Chicago, 1977, p. 25.

Industry loses more than 245 million man-days to work injuries annually. Fatalities are considered to cause an average loss of 150 days per case. Permanent disabilities are calculated in terms of actual days lost plus an allowance for lost efficiency resulting from the impairment. It is estimated that in future years the time loss caused by current work accidents will total 120 million man-days. Of the $52.8 billion which accidents cost in 1976, work accidents accounted for $17,800,000 or one-third of the total (Table 14-3).

TABLE 14–2

A Comparison of the Injury Rates Between National Safety Council Industry Members and Nonmembers

Year	Injury Frequency Rate			Injury Severity Rate		
	NSC Members	Non-members	% NSC Rates Lower	NSC Members	Non-members	% NSC Rates Lower
	Manufacturing					
1965	4.6	16.8	−73	450	830	−46
1966	5.1	17.6	−71	470	810	−42
1967	5.1	18.0	−72	460	830	−45
1968	5.3	17.9	−70	480	790	−39
1969	5.7	18.9	−70	500	830	−40
1970	6.0	19.1	−69	500	860	−42
	Mining					
1965	23.5	37.9	−38	4,024	6,970	−42
1966	21.9	38.4	−43	4,016	6,534	−39
1967	22.4	37.5	−40	4,019	6,092	−34
1968	22.2	36.7	−40	4,494	7,983	−44
1969	21.8	37.6	−42	3,597	6,506	−45
1970	22.2	39.2	−43	3,793	6,644	−43

Source: Manufacturing nonmember–Total U.S. experience projected from BLS rates, less experience of reporters to NSC. Mining nonmember–Industrywide rates from Bureau of Mines, less reporters in U.S. Bureau of Mines safety competitions. Reported in *Accident Facts,* National Safety Council, Chicago, 1977, p. 27.

TABLE 14–3
Itemized Cost of Work Accidents in 1976

Item	Cost in $ Billions
Wage loss	3.6
Medical expense	1.9
Insurance administration	2.4
Fire losses	2.0
Indirect costs*	7.9
Total	17.8†

*Includes the money value of time lost by workers other than those with disabling injuries, who are directly or indirectly involved in accidents.
†Cost per worker amounts to approximately $185.
Source: *Accident Facts*, National Safety Council, Chicago, 1977, p. 5.

The part of the body most frequently injured in 2.2 million disabling work injuries, was the trunk. About 38 percent of all compensation for work injuries was paid to people with trunk injuries. According to the California Department of Industrial Relations, most of these injuries were sprains, strains, hernias, and dislocations. The thumb and fingers are the second most frequently injured part of the body, with the most common injuries being lacerations, punctures, and abrasions. Table 14-4 shows the number of cases and the percentage of total work injuries for each body part.

TABLE 14–4
Body Part Injured in Various Types of Industries

Industry	No. of Injuries*	All Parts	Eyes	Head, Face, Neck	Back and Spine	Trunk	Arms (incl. hands)	Legs (incl. feet)	Other and Unspec.
Total†	269,108	100%	5.2	7.0	24.0	7.9	29.4	22.6	3.9
Agriculture	14,089	100%	7.1	7.0	19.4	9.7	26.9	23.5	6.4
Mineral Extraction	2,074	100%	7.5	7.9	19.3	8.2	29.5	24.5	3.1
Construction	22,204	100%	7.2	5.7	24.0	7.1	27.0	25.1	3.9
Manufacturing	82,540	100%	7.4	5.6	21.6	6.8	36.1	19.9	2.6
Transportation and Public Utilities	22,930	100%	3.4	10.0	27.9	8.1	21.8	24.7	4.1
Trade	51,751	100%	3.5	6.4	24.7	7.2	33.6	21.6	3.0
Service	35,009	100%	4.2	8.1	26.4	8.0	24.8	23.5	5.0
State and Local Government	38,424	100%	3.1	8.9	25.7	10.8	20.3	25.6	5.6

*Injuries severe enough to cause absence from work for a full day or shift beyond the day of the accident.
†Includes 87 cases for which the industry could not be determined.
Source: California Work Injuries, 1974, State of California, Department of Industrial Relations. Reported in *Accident Facts*, National Safety Council, Chicago, 1976, p. 30.

Frequency and severity rates vary widely among different industries. In a 3-year study among reporters to the NSC, the frequency rates ranged from a high of 35.49 for underground coal mining to a low of 1.63 for automobile manufacturing. Severity rates were highest in mining and marine transportation (river craft and other craft, and stevedoring), and lowest in the aerospace industry. Some individual companies have compiled fantastic safety records. One chemical company has recorded 66,645,399 man-hours of work without a disabling injury. Table 14-5 presents a comparison of industry types among NSC reporters, listing their frequency and severity rates from 1974 to 1976.

WORKER'S COMPENSATION

Industrial injuries and fatalities were all-too-common occurrences in the American workplace before 1911. Workers and their families received little or no compensation for their losses. There was no incentive for employers to support safety programs since employers were not legally responsible for injuries to their employees. This was true because:

1 Employers claimed assumption of risk as a legal defense. They claimed that the employee, aware of the risks and agreeing to accept employment, also agreed to accept those risks as a condition of employment. Accidental injury was accepted as an inherent risk in earning a living.

2 Employers claimed contributory negligence as a defense against liability. Since most accidents involve some degree of inappropriate behavior, the employees were considered responsible for their misfortunes.

3 Employers cited the fellow-servant rule. According to this doctrine, an employer could not be held liable for an injury to an employee that was caused by another worker.

4 Salaries were pitifully low and went to pay for the basic necessities of life. Legal action was expensive, took months or years to complete, and usually resulted in such small awards that the employee was discouraged from legal action.

5 Labor unions were weak, and employees found that if they made trouble for the employer they would lose their jobs.

Several books such as *Law of the Killed and Wounded* and *Our Murderous Industrialism* helped to stimulate public concern for workplace safety. Following the lead of several European countries, our nation passed its first effective worker's compensation law in 1908. The law offered protection only to federal employees in hazardous occupations. By 1913, 21 states had enacted worker's compensation laws, and the positive effect on industrial accidents was immediately evident. Today, 87 percent of the nation's workers are covered by laws in all 50 states. Coverage and benefits vary widely from state to state.

Worker's compensation laws provide coverage for most American workers against accidental injuries arising out of and in the course of employment.

TABLE 14–5
Three-Year Frequency and Severity Rates among Reporters to the National
Safety Council, 1974–1976

Industry	Frequency Rate	Severity Rate
All industries	10.87*	668*
Aerospace	1.92	127
Air transport	30.19	586
Automobile	1.63	190
Cement	11.11	974
Chemical	4.07	371
Clay and mineral products	19.66	1037
Communications	5.56	253
Construction	14.92	1549
Electrical equipment	3.20	153
Fertilizer	7.83	723
Food	18.03	746
Foundry	15.99	990
Glass	11.46	456
Government employees	6.39†	604‡
Iron and steel products	14.22	693
Leather	18.93	636
Lumber	17.83	2102
Machinery	7.30	319
Marine transportation	15.49	3918§
Meat packing	24.67	749
Mining, surface	10.09†	1972†
Mining, underground coal	35.49†	5019†
Mining, underground except coal	26.26†	4338†
Nonferrous metals and products	8.87	809
Petroleum	7.00¶	673¶
Printing and publishing	9.74	373
Pulp, paper, and related products	9.85	690
Railroad equipment	24.42	1526
Rubber and plastics	5.43	426
Sheet metal products	6.24	402
Shipbuilding	10.82	589
Steel	3.98¶	686¶
Storage and warehousing	4.40	179
Textile	3.86	280
Tobacco	10.21	668
Transit	33.30	888
Wholesale and retail trade	7.74	229
Wood products	16.46	910
Other industries	6.05	354

*Based on Z16.1 Standard. Rates are not fully compatable from year to year due to changes in numbers
 of reporters and increased representation of service, trade, and government.
†1970–1972.
‡1967–1969.
§Includes 29 disaster deaths in 1975.
¶1971–1973.
Source: *Accident Facts,* National Safety Council, Chicago, 1977, pp. 36–37.

Employers are required to compensate the employee regardless of whether negligence can be proved. The intent of these laws is to provide basic economic security in the event of injury, without attempting to fix blame. The underlying philosophy recognizes that the employer and employee are joint participants in an enterprise which benefits both parties. In effect, the employer pays for the loss and passes the loss on to the consumer. Certain classifications of workers are excluded from coverage by worker's compensation laws. Workers in very small companies (three to four employees), domestic servants, farm laborers, executives and owners, and workers covered by other compensation laws are not eligible for worker's compensation benefits.

Worker's compensation laws require employers to prove their ability to pay for workers' compensation judgments. Insurance companies sell policies to guarantee such economic surety. Most employers purchase worker's compensation insurance rather than assume the responsibility themselves. Rates are calculated on the basis of industrial risk and previous experience with the company. The employer thus has the incentive to provide a safe workplace and to expect safe behavior from the employees. Rates are ordinarily expressed in terms of dollars per $100 of payroll (i.e., $2.70 per $100 of payroll). In an effort to reduce the amount of claims, the insurance carriers hold inspections, maintain accurate accident records, and provide recommendations for improving safety in the workplace.

As a system for the effective delivery of basic economic security against work-related injury and disease, the benefits of worker's compensation laws are many. Primarily, they provide protection against the interruption of income. The level of compensation depends on:

1 Whether the disability is total or partial
2 The employee's weekly wage level
3 Maximum duration of benefits as stated in the law
4 Maximum dollar limits established by the law
5 Waiting periods prior to collecting benefits, usually 3 to 7 days

The salary compensation represents a proportion of the wage ranging between 50 and 60 percent. Minimum and maximum limits are usually specified so that workers are guaranteed a basic level of income regardless of wage level. The maximum limit is intended to discourage people from staying out of work because their compensation checks are nearly equal to their paychecks.

Medical care and rehabilitation are provided under worker's compensation laws. Medical benefits are generally granted in all cases of injuries included under the law. There is no waiting period for this benefit, which provides medical, surgical, nursing, and hospital benefits as well as rehabilitation. Most states place no limit on the amount payable under this benefit.

It is important to note that employees with physical handicaps do not contribute to higher rates for worker's compensation premiums. In most instances, the handicapped employee who is selectively placed and properly trained will have a safety record equal to or better than that of the general working population. Worker's compensation rates are based on accident data, not on the physical limitations of employees.

THE OCCUPATIONAL SAFETY AND HEALTH ACT (OSHAct)

In recent years Congress has become keenly aware of the need for safety legislation. Safety bills pertaining to highways, motor vehicles, consumer products, the environment, and flammable fabrics are illustrations of this concern. The Williams-Steiger Act, better known as the Occupational Safety and Health Act, was signed into law on December 29, 1970. It affects more than 5 million firms as well as most state and federal agencies. More than 60 million workers are protected by the law, which President Nixon called one of the most important pieces of legislation ever passed by Congress. I. W. Abel, president of the Steelworkers Union, said it was a Magna Carta for the workers of America.

Many factors contributed to the passage of P.L. 91-596. Some of them were:

1 A steadily rising workplace injury rate from 1961 to 1970
2 A number of spectacular disasters, especially in mining
3 Mounting research evidence linking the workplace with chronic diseases such as cancer, emphysema, and pneumoconiosis (black lung disease)
4 Strenuous lobbying by worker groups, notably the AFL-CIO
5 Better educated workers, who perceive the importance of safety in the workplace
6 The national economic losses resulting from occupational illness, injury, and death.

OSHAct states that "the Congress finds that personal injuries and illnesses arising out of work situations impose a substantial burden on, and are a hindrance to, interstate commerce in terms of lost production, wage loss, medical expenses, and disability payments." The purposes of OSHAct are "to assure so far as possible for every working man and woman in the Nation safe and healthful working conditions, and to preserve our human resources." For this reason, the general duty clause requires employers to provide a workplace free from recognized hazards that are likely to cause death or serious physical harm to employees. Beyond complying with OSHAct standards, employers have a positive duty to protect their employees from recognized danger, and to provide a safe and healthful place of employment.

It is important to remember that the act was intended to improve both safety and health. Safety hazards are aspects of work which can cause burns, shock, cuts, bruises, etc. The harm is usually immediate and sometimes violent. Health hazards refer to toxic and carcinogenic chemicals and dust, and to physical and biological agents. The harm is usually not immediately known and may take years to diagnose. Respiratory disease, heart disease, cancer, and neurologic impairment result in a shortened life expectancy and a diminished quality of life.[2]

AGENCIES OF OSHAct

To accomplish its mandate OSHAct created several agencies. The Occupational Safety and Health Administration, located in the Department of Labor, sets standards, conducts inspections, issues citations, and assesses penalties for violations. The Occupational Safety and Health Review Commission is an independent, quasijudicial review board consisting of three members appointed by the President. Its purpose is to carry out the adjudicatory functions of the act. This agency rules on all enforcement actions. Employers have 15 days to challenge a violation or assessed penalty. If no challenge is brought forth within this time limit, the review commission automatically upholds the actions of the Occupational Safety and Health Administration. The outcome is final. It is not subject to review by any court or agency.

Congress established the National Institute for Occupational Safety and Health (NIOSH) to assist the Secretary of Labor in carrying out the act. NIOSH conducts research, experiments, and demonstrations that relate to occupational safety and health. Safety standards can be developed or revised as a result of these efforts. The agency conducts educational programs to ensure an adequate supply of personnel to carry out the provisions of OSHAct. NIOSH is required to publish a list of all known toxic substances and their levels of toxicity. Unlike the Occupational Safety and Health Administration, NIOSH is located in the Department of Health, Education, and Welfare.

Most Americans depend on worker's compensation benefits for basic economic security in the event of injury, illness, or death arising from employment. Serious questions have been raised with regard to the fairness and adequacy of these benefits. For this reason, Congress authorized OSHA to conduct a study to evaluate the effectiveness of state worker's compensation laws. The National Commission on State Workman's Compensation Laws was created for this purpose. The 15-member commission, appointed by the President, was given 1 year to make recommendations. After reporting in July 1972, the commission was dissolved.

A 12-member National Advisory Committee on Occupational Safety and Health (NACOSH) was also established by the act. The committee is composed of representatives of management, labor, occupational safety and health professionals, and the public. The purpose of NACOSH is to advise, consult with, and make recommendations to the Secretary of Labor and the Secretary of Health, Education and Welfare on matters relevant to OSHAct.

[2]Ashford, op. cit., pp. 8–9.

INSPECTIONS, INVESTIGATIONS, AND RECORD KEEPING

After presenting appropriate credentials, OSHA inspectors (compliance officers) are authorized "to enter without delay and at reasonable times any factory, plant, establishment, construction site, or other area, workplace or environment where work is performed by an employee of an employer." The inspection is comprehensive, including the workplace and all pertinent conditions, structures, machines, apparatus, devices, equipment, and materials. The inspector may question the employer, a reasonable number of employees, and an employee representative. Both the employer and the employee representative may accompany the compliance officer during the inspection.

Employers are required to maintain accurate records of work-related deaths, injuries, and illnesses. Excluded from this requirement are minor injuries which require only first-aid treatment and which do not involve medical treatment, loss of consciousness, restriction of work or motion, or transfer to another job. Employers must maintain accurate records of employee exposure to potentially toxic materials or harmful physical agents. Employees are entitled to observe such monitoring and to have access to these records. Any employee who has been exposed or is currently being exposed to toxic materials or harmful physical agents at dangerous levels must be informed of this fact by the employer.

If an employee believes that there is a violation which may threaten physical harm, or that an imminent danger exists, he or she may request an inspection. The request must be made in writing and must be signed by the employee. If the employee so requests, the employer's copy will not identify the person asking for the inspection. The requested inspection should occur as soon as practicable. Employees who request inspections or testify in proceedings on behalf of themselves or others may not be discharged or discriminated against in any way.

If the inspection reveals a violation, the compliance officer will issue a citation. The written citation must describe in detail the nature of the violation. The citation will also fix a reasonable amount of time in which the violation may be corrected. Each citation must be prominently posted at or near the site of the corresponding violation. If the violation has no direct or immediate relationship to safety or health, a "notice" may be issued in place of the citation.

A typical OSHAct inspection consists of several steps. The compliance officer:

1 Shows credentials and asks to see the top management officer

2 Explains the reason for the visit: random visitation, request by employee, death or multiple-injury accident, or high-priority industry

3 Describes the procedures to be followed during the inspection

4 Asks to see records relevant to accidental injuries, deaths, or illness

5 Asks to see the employee representative

6 Conducts a walk-through inspection

7 Talks with employees and asks questions pertinent to the inspection

8 Conducts a closing conference with the employer to describe the results of the inspection

9 Gives the employer copies of applicable laws and standards if a violation exists

10 Issues citations for serious violations

11 Assures the employer that any trade secrets observed during the walk-through inspection will be kept confidential

PENALTIES

Any employer who willfully or repeatedly violates the requirements or standards of the act may be assessed a civil penalty of not more than $10,000 for each violation. A citation for serious violations can result in a penalty of up to $1,000 for each violation. An employer who fails to correct a violation may be fined up to $1,000 for each day beyond the specified deadline. If an employer is convicted of willfully violating a standard, leading to the death of an employee, the penalty cannot exceed $10,000 and/or imprisonment for 6 months. The penalty for giving advance notice of an inspection is a fine of up to $1,000 and/or a 6-month prison term. Violations of posting requirements can bring a fine of up to $1,000 for each violation.

EMPLOYEE RIGHTS AND OBLIGATIONS

Under OSHAct, the employee has broad protection against harmful or dangerous working conditions. The employee has the right:

1 To observe the monitoring of harmful substances, and to have access to the records of such monitoring

2 To ask for an OSHA inspection

3 To have an employee representative accompany the compliance officer

4 To have citations posted at or near the place of violation

5 To appeal to the Occupational Safety and Health Review Commission if the time designated for correction of a violation seems excessive

6 To provide input to OSHA for the establishment or revision of safety standards

7 To exercise these rights without fear of dismissal or discrimination

OSHAct does not specifically mention employee responsibilities. Since there are no penalties for unsafe actions by employees, the effectiveness of the act depends on employee self-regulation. The safety and health procedures mandated by the employer should always be followed. Where regulations call for the use of safety materials, the employee should use such equipment in a responsible manner. If an occupational injury or illness occurs, the employee should notify the employer so that the employer may voluntarily investigate and correct the violation before receiving a citation. Whenever employees are aware of unsafe conditions they should report them to the employer. Whenever employees observe a dangerous environmental condition or unsafe human act, they should take appropriate action to remove the potential for harm.

COMMENTS ON OSHAct

Before OSHAct, safety efforts were fragmented and varied greatly from workplace to workplace and from state to state. The amount of money spent by individual states on occupational safety and health ranged from $2.20 to less than 0.01¢ per worker.[3] The accident rates demonstrated similar variability. The states with the best safety and health programs had death rates of approximately 19 per 100,000 workers. States with poorly organized programs averaged death rates of 110 per 100,000 workers. OSHAct will certainly help standardize safety efforts and foster greater efficiency in the management of safety programs. OSHAct has increased our awareness of workplace safety. The maintenance of records by employers of employee injury, illness, and death has also enhanced our awareness of the safety and health problems that face workers. Workers now feel entitled to safety as a matter of individual rights.

There can be little doubt that OSHAct will positively affect the safety and well-being of the American worker. The greatest impact will probably occur in the target industries, those with the highest injury frequency rates (stevedoring, roofing and sheetmetal, meat and meat products, miscellaneous transportation, and lumber and wood products). It remains doubtful that OSHAct will fully achieve the goal Congress had in mind, a safe and healthful workplace for every working man and woman. From April 28, 1971, through December, 1975, OSHA made 117,754 inspections, resulting in 76,533 citations alleging 386,000 violations, and penalties totaling more than $10 million. There are not enough compliance officers to effectively inspect the 5 million workplaces covered by OSHA. Even if there were, safety is not guaranteed by the enforcement of standards for environmental conditions. Safety and health require a commitment by everyone in an organization. Appropriate attitudes, a high skills level, and safe behavior should be integrated into a safe workplace environment.

ADMINISTRATION OF INDUSTRIAL SAFETY

The workplace is an ecological unit. Efforts at safety must be made with the awareness that accidents are caused by multiple factors. Some conditions which are not especially dangerous by themselves pose a definite threat when combined with other minimal dangers. Carbon monoxide is often present where heat, stress, and noise are found. Under such conditions, an employee, especially one poorly prepared for the job, may make errors of concentration or

[3]Steven Pausner and George Clark, "OSHA's Ancestors: Previous Laws of the Workplace," *Job Safety and Health,* vol. 2, pp. 16–21, April, 1974.

judgment which could lead to an accident. Any attempt to reduce the level of potential danger must be directed toward the correction of multiple factors.

Organized safety programs began more than 60 years ago with the passage of worker's compensation laws. The science of safety administration has been developed only during the last 20 years. The broadly conceived task of safety administration is to minimize the workplace danger potential, thereby reducing workplace illness, injury, severity, and fatality rates. In companies where these rates are already low, the evidence suggests that the top management is strongly involved in the safety programs. The central purpose of safety administration programs is the development of safe attitudes, behavior, and skills levels so that safety can become an integral part of the employee's approach to occupational responsibilities. Effective safety programs permeate the workplace.

In addition to controlling hazards and avoiding accidents, safety administration involves many activities which actively promote safety. Among these activities are to:

1 Screen applicants carefully and place them in suitable jobs.

2 Train employees in safe levels of knowledge and skill.

3 Make safety a part of occupational training so that safe behavior can be practiced as the job is being learned.

4 Maintain accident records, and analyze these data to determine causes, trends, dangerous areas, dangerous activities, dangerous times of the day, etc.

5 Inspect the workplace regularly for unsafe environmental conditions and unsafe acts, and correct these dangerous situations.

6 Develop or revise policies according to the findings of inspections and records. Enforce these policies consistently.

7 Develop an effective system of communication with both employees and management to stimulate cooperation throughout the organization.

8 Provide in-service education for employees so that they can maintain levels of knowledge and skill adequate to changing technology.

9 Investigate the causes of injury or illness and identify methods for their prevention.

10 Procure, distribute, and evaluate information on the effectiveness of the safety equipment used by employees.

11 Plan, implement, and evaluate safety education programs. Some companies now provide safety education on subjects not directly related to the workplace—defensive driving, home fire safety, first aid—in recognition of the fact that "safety" in one aspect of life leads to "safety" in other areas.

12 Set a good example.

Contrary to popular belief, safety is not synonymous with lost production. Research has demonstrated that the opposite is true. There is a relationship between safety effectiveness and production effectiveness. The highest levels of efficiency can be correlated with the best injury records. A poor safety record negatively affects profit in the following ways:[4]

1 Operating costs are increasd by the time lost to injuries.

2 Production costs are increased by the loss of materials, goods, and human services.

3 Disabling injuries cause the loss of trained and experienced workers, who must be replaced by untrained and inexperienced workers.

4 The cost of the employee benefit package is raised.

5 Worker's compensation premiums are raised.

6 The personnel department becomes busy filling out claims forms, insurance forms, and accident report forms; screening for a replacement; training the new employee; and filling out a set of forms for the new worker's file.

7 Human suffering causes a noticeable drop in employee morale, and often leads to a loss of good will in the community. Some people believe that a safe (good) company produces a safe (good) product. Poor management contributes to accidents and allows inferior products to be manufactured. In a very real sense, "safety control" is quality control.

CAUSES OF OFF-THE-JOB ACCIDENTS

Off-the-job accidents occur under a wide variety of circumstances. It is not easy to identify the major causes or to plan appropriate preventive action. An accident report may show that a worker has been injured while trying to hang a picture at home, but it rarely gives enough details to indicate exactly how the accident happened. The victim may have been using defective equipment, wearing inappropriate clothing, or concentrating on something other than the task at hand. But it is particularly difficult to imagine the cause of such an accident when the victim has a perfect safety record on the job, where he or she performs similar tasks every day.

There is evidently a discrepancy between workers' careful behavior on the job and their conduct at home. The obvious explanation is that many employees are too irresponsible to behave safely when they are away from warning signs and the watchful eye of the supervisor. Perhaps some vocational students and employees associate safety principles exclusively with the specific tasks that they have learned to perform in the school shop and the plant. The improper work habits acquired before this training may still govern their activities at home. Another possibility is that employees conduct themselves safely on the job because they realize that factory work is dangerous, but they fail to take precautions while performing various household chores because they underestimate the hazards.

---

[4]John V. Grimaldi and Rollin H. Simonds, *Safety Management,* 3d ed., Richard D. Irwin, Inc. Homewood, Ill., 1975, pp. 73–397.

The inferior tools used in many homes undoubtedly contribute greatly to the higher incidence of off-the-job accidents. Industry makes sure that employees have good equipment, but employees are often negligent about equipping themselves with adequate tools for their work around the house. In attending to household repairs, they are often content with tools that have been ruined by improper handling or that are otherwise unsuitable. When they need a screwdriver, they rarely bother to select one that is properly squared and of the appropriate width and thickness. All too often the ill-fitting screwdriver is held in one hand and the screw in the other, so that the hand holding the screw is in excellent position to receive a serious gash if the tool should slip. Countless unsafe practices of this sort are commonplace in many homes today.

SCHOOL INDUSTRIAL SAFETY PROGRAM

The experience students gain in the school's electrical, forging, woodworking, printing, automotive, welding, foundry, and pattern-making shops; in chemistry and physics laboratories; and in such courses as home economics and driver education undoubtedly helps prepare them for successful work in industry. The vocational safety program is patterned in part on the accident-prevention techniques employed in the modern plant, but it is considerably less intensive. In itself, the program cannot orient students to the safety requirements of their future jobs. Students must understand that factory work, which involves long hours of repetitive labor under the pressure of high production quotas, demands even greater skill and more attention to safety than are required in the school's shops and laboratories.

Adolescents tend to emulate adults, especially those with whom they identify. Vocational students are more likely to respect accident-prevention rules if they understand that the most skilled factory workers conscientiously observe safety regulations, and that cautious behavior is not associated exclusively with sissies and teacher's pets. Students' familiarity with the safety practices of industry should facilitate the adoption of similar methods in the school. If students understand the functions of the safety engineer, they should be willing to accept the appointment of a student to a corresponding position in their shop class. Teachers will find it to their advantage to acquaint students with the following features of the industrial program:

1. *Management support.* All managerial levels support the safety program. The employers' interest in accident prevention is evident in their willingness to finance protective equipment, to maintain a safety staff, and to permit time off the job for safety meetings. Through periodic conferences with the safety engineer, operating executives are acquainted with all phases of the safety program and with their responsibility for ensuring its success. Superintendents and foremen, recognizing that safety is a vital part of the operation of the plant, and that it facilitates production, devote considerable time and effort to gaining workers'

acceptance of safety regulations and to instructing new employees in the proper procedures.

2. *Safety director.* A safety director or safety engineer is appointed to take charge of the program. In addition to qualifying as an accident-prevention expert, the person selected for this position must possess such qualities as vision, initiative, persistence, good judgment, diplomacy, leadership ability, and above all, sympathy. The safety director's job is to see that adequate protective devices are provided and used and that safe operating procedures are established and faithfully practiced. In most plants the safety director is affiliated with the employee-relations department. Safety is an important consideration in the various functions of that department: hiring personnel, providing desirable working conditions, and administering health and insurance programs.

3. *Plant inspections.* The safety engineer regularly inspects the factory for hazardous conditions and unsafe procedures and initiates action to eliminate any danger spots that are discovered. The engineer makes sure that the necessary mechanical safeguards are installed on equipment in accordance with the specifications of state law and insurance-company requirements, and that all operators use the guards provided for their machines and wear any special protective apparel that is appropriate to their work. Most companies furnish work gloves, goggles, and aprons free of charge and make safety shoes available to employees at cost. When the safety engineers detect hazards that cannot be compensated for by protective devices, they determine the steps that must be taken to remedy the situation. Equipment may have to be rearranged, machinery may have to be redesigned, or new procedures may have to be developed.

Supervisors make frequent checks to ensure that the safety engineer's recommendations are faithfully carried out. They watch particularly for the following hazards:

a. *Chemical hazards.* Unlabeled acids, improper handling of caustics, etc.

b. *Electrical hazards.* Open switches, defective portable lights, etc.

c. *Fire hazards.* Improperly stored oily rags, flammable liquids used near a flame, etc.

d. *Faulty fire-protection equipment.* Unsafe fire escapes, defective fire extinguishers, etc.

e. *Machine-operation hazards.* Defective equipment, failure to use guards on saws, power presses, grinding wheels and other dangerous machines, etc.

f. *Material-handling hazards.* Defective trucks, conveyors, etc.

g. *Power-transmission hazards.* Unguarded belts, defective pulleys, etc.

h. *Poor lighting*

    i. Poor housekeeping. Improperly stored tools, scraps left on the floor or workbench, etc.

    j. Poor ventilation

    k. Yard hazards. Open pits, unguarded railroad crossing, etc.

    l. Seasonal hazards. Icicles, slippery walks, etc.

4. *Health services.* Many companies require all potential employees to undergo a thorough examination, covering general health and physical fitness, intelligence, emotional stability, and aptitude, to make sure that they are wholly suited to the job for which they are being hired. Even minor ills may lower their efficiency and drive and thus increase their vulnerability to accidents. Emotional immaturity may interfere with their ability to concentrate on a given task. High intelligence may indirectly endanger them if they are given dull, routine jobs that cannot hold their attention.

    In addition to providing medical examinations for new employees, most companies see that all on-the-job injuries receive prompt first aid and any additional care that seems necessary. As a minimum service, the factory owner maintains someone on the staff who is trained in administering first aid. Larger plants usually employ a graduate nurse, and some companies have an entire medical department. Employees are encouraged to report all injuries, no matter how slight. Every injury case is thoroughly followed up to ensure satisfactory and complete treatment.

5. *Accident reports.* Industry keeps careful accident records, which are conscientiously analyzed and used as a basis for planning the safety program. Casualties are classified by departments, equipment inflicting the injury (lathe, hammer, etc.) part of equipment causing injury (gear, pulley, etc.), activity in which the victim was participating at the time of injury (cleaning, oiling, etc.), method of contact with object causing the injury (fell, struck against, etc.), and the proximate cause of the accident (defective equipment, lack of skill, etc.). Abex Corp., a New York industrial equipment manufacturer, keeps track of minor injuries. The safety director feels that a high incidence of first-aid cases in one area eventually leads to a bad accident. The records enable the safety engineer to spot poor supervisors and accident repeaters, to identify the departments that need help in preventing accidents and the conditions that must be corrected, and to stimulate friendly rivalry among departments for the best safety record or the greatest accident reduction. To foster this sort of competition, some companies reward winning departments with trophies, special privileges, or bonuses.

6. *Color code for identifying shop hazards.* Many accidents occur because workers are either unaware or temporarily forgetful of the dangers involved in various areas around the shop. Sometimes they simply do not notice a hazard until they stumble against or over it. To

avoid this possibility, all danger spots should be painted a distinguishing color. It is also desirable to identify first-aid and fire-fighting equipment in this way. The following color code indicates how paint may be used to promote industrial, farm, and other areas of safety.[5]

- *Fire-protection Red* has for many years been used to designate fire-protection equipment such as fire-alarm boxes, fire-hose locations, sprinkler pipings, containers for flammables, etc. Other uses should be discouraged. It should not be used to designate danger areas because of its low visibility as compared to yellow or orange and because such use is confusing. Not only should the fire-protection equipment be painted red or with bands of red, but the wall against which it hangs should be painted red, and a red square should be placed on the floor below the equipment and on the wall above.
- Fire-protection red should be used on fire extinguishers, fire hose, hose connections, hydrants, apparatus, fire doors, alarm stations, and fire blankets.
- *High-visibility Yellow* should be used to mark all levers and gear handles to indicate a need for caution. In alternate stripes with black it should be used to mark strike-against, stumbling, falling, or tripping hazards. Yellow is very bright and should be restricted in use to those places where it has real meaning. Yellow paint would be desirable on aisles to direct the flow of traffic, on the gear-shift handle, brake, and clutch on a tractor, on the adjusting screws of a power saw, and on handles of power tools. Caution signs, guardrails, barricades, low beams, and pipes should be painted yellow. Yellow and black stripes should be used on such hazards. Yellow is very bright and should be restricted in use to those places next to drives, and raised sills in barn doors.
- *Alert Orange* should be used to indicate dangerous parts of machines and equipment, particularly moving parts which are uncovered or which cannot be fully covered (edges of gears). Machine guards that can be opened or removed should be painted orange on the inside as well as on the dangerous part which is exposed. If the dangerous part is large, the color will be more effective if a bar of orange is placed along the danger edge. Alert orange should be used on the interior of switch boxes, fuse boxes, power boxes, and machinery guards and on the exposed parts of pulleys, gears, cutting edges, rollers, or presses.
- *Safety Green* should be used to designate first-aid kits and cabinets for quick location. The Green Cross symbol should be placed on the wall above first-aid equipment so it can be easily seen from a distance. Safety green should not be confused with high-visibility green. Safety green should be used to identify first-aid kits, stretchers, and other first-aid equipment.
- *Purple* is the basic color for designating radiation hazards.
- *Black or White* or a combination of black and white is used for housekeeping markings. Stairways (risers), refuse cans, food-dispensing equipment are examples of the places where these basic colors are being used.
- *Precaution Blue* should be used to indicate the need of caution. Blue may be put on switch boxes and handy receptacles as a reminder to use caution and to be sure that everyone is free of danger from the equipment.
- It is well to hang a large blue tag with the words, *Do not operate,* on any machine which is being repaired, until it is all ready to go.
- Background paint of high-visibility buff on the other parts of machines and equipment, especially shop tools, will add greatly to the efficiency and safety. Dark colors tire the eyes. Soft colors, such as high-visibility buff, will add to visibility and be restful to the eyes as well as increase the effectiveness of the other colors. Severe color contrasts should be avoided to keep the brightness ratio low.

---

[5]N.J. Wardle, "Paint for Safety," *Agricultural Leaders' Digest*, June, 1952, p. 16. See also Russell DeReamer, *Modern Safety Practices*, John Wiley & Sons, Inc., New York, 1958, p. 123.

An alert shop teacher can all but eliminate the possibility of vocational accidents, which are usually attributed to environmental hazards, unsafe student behavior, or a combination of both. The instructor should take steps to remove or compensate for such common accident causes as crowded work areas, disorder, poorly arranged equipment, poor lighting and ventilation, improper floor covering, undesignated and inadequately guarded danger zones, defective equipment, and insufficient protective devices. The instructor should also establish and faithfully use an efficient accident-reporting system, set up procedures for handling emergencies, and see that even the slightest injury receives prompt first aid. A well-qualified teacher can keep unsafe student behavior at a minimum by providing the class with careful instruction, conscientious supervision, and intelligent, sympathetic guidance.

FARM SAFETY

There are currently between 3 and 4 million people in this country who work on farms and ranches. The injury and illness rates for agriculture are exceeded only by the rates for the mining and construction industries. In 1976 there were 1,900 agriculture-related work deaths. This represents a death rate of 54 per 100,000 workers, which is four times greater than the average death rate for all industries, 14 per 100,000 workers. National Safety Council data show that an estimated 190,000 disabling injuries have resulted from agricultural work. More than one-third of these injuries were characterized as severe, permanent, or fatal.

Many agencies have been working as advocates of agricultural safety and attempting to reduce the hazards associated with farming. A few of the organizations that have had a significant impact on the gradually declining accident rates are:

1 National Safety Council
2 4-H Clubs
3 Future Farmers of America
4 U.S. Department of Agriculture
5 American Society of Agricultural Engineers
6 American National Standards Institute (ANSI)
7 National Fire Protection Association
8 Occupational Safety and Health Administration
9 U.S. Consumer Product Safety Commission

The primary aim of farm safety education is to help farm residents acquire knowledge, attitudes, and behavior patterns which will protect them from the numerous hazards of agricultural work. With the guidance of the instructor, students must develop a general safety code which includes the following rules:

1 Never work when you are too tired to do so carefully.

2 Always allot enough time to a task to perform it safely and properly. Avoid rushing, for haste causes many accidents.

3 Always lift a heavy object the safe way. With your feet together, your back straight, and your knees bent, make the lift by straightening your knees and keeping the load as close as possible to your body.

4 Always keep tools and machines in good operating condition, and use them only for their intended purposes. Plan regular inspections of all equipment, and remove or correct all hazards.

5 Practice good housekeeping at all times. Observe the maxim "A place for everything, and everything in its proper place."

6 Avoid overexposure to sun to prevent heat exhaustion and skin cancer. See that even the slightest injury receives immediate first-aid treatment.

GENERAL PRECAUTIONS

Farmers should be able to use modern implements without endangering themselves. Most of these implements are furnished with adequate safety devices. The best safety device, however, is a safe operator. The teacher must make sure that students understand the danger involved in using equipment improperly. Students must also recognize the need for taking precautions so that they will voluntarily obey the following safety rules, which have been developed by the Farm Equipment Institute and the American Society of Agricultural Engineers to govern the use of farm machines (see Figure 14-2).

1 *Keep all shields in place.* Shields are intended for your protection; use them. The best designed and most expensive shield is worthless if it is not in place when the machine is operated. Yet accidents have been reported involving careless or lazy farmers who have used an implement while the safety shield provided by the manufacturer remained in the tool shed. Sometimes a shield must be removed for servicing, but a few minutes spent in replacing it may save a lifetime of regret.

2 *Stop machine to adjust and oil.* If you adjust or oil machinery while it is in motion, your wrench may slip so that your hand comes into contact with a moving part, your sleeve may get caught in a sprocket or moving part, or you may slip and fall against a moving part. Work safely by turning off your machine before oiling or adjusting it. It takes only a minute to stop and start the motor.

3 *When mechanism becomes clogged, disconnect power before cleaning.* When you are trying to relieve a clogged mechanism, the obstruction often clears unexpectedly. If the power is still on when this happens, your hand or foot may be drawn into the machinery along with the material causing the clogging.

4 *Keep hands, feet, and clothing away from power-driven parts.* Avoid reaching around or climbing over implements while the power is on. If you slip and lose your balance, your hand or foot may be drawn into the machinery, or your clothing may be caught on a moving part. (Remember that sleeves or overalls can wind around a smooth, round shaft in motion as easily as around a

Speed	**Crossing slopes**	**Uphill**
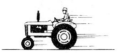	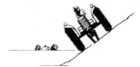	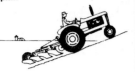
Select safe speed for each job. Slow down when turning. Cut speed when working on slopes, near ditches or on rough, uneven ground.	Cross slopes slowly. Look-out for dips, raises, rocks, gullies, etc., that could trigger upset. Set wheels wide as practical for job.	Go up slopes carefully. Use power gear if pulling heavy rolling load. On grades, engage clutch smoothly—don't jerk. Back the tractor up really steep grades.
Downhill	**Ditches**	**High hitch**
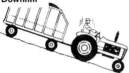	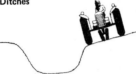	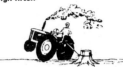
Use lower gear, especially with heavy rolling load. Keep loads within ability of tractor to control and stop them. Wagons hauling heavy loads should have brakes.	Drive slowly when crossing or working along shallow ditches or grass waterways. Stay safely clear of irrigation or large open drainage ditches.	Hitch only to drawbar or regular hitch points. Set drawbar no higher than 17 inches from ground. Engage the clutch smoothly, not suddenly.
Public roads	**Loads on front**	**Loads on drawbar**
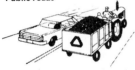	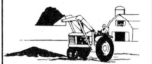	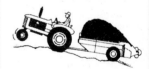
Observe traffic rules. Signal intentions. Identify rig with SMV emblem. Turn corners slowly. Shift down when going up or down grades with load.	Operate front-end loader according to instruction manual. Handle rig smoothly—avoid abrupt turns, jerky starts and stops. Don't overload. Add rear wheel weights.	Add front-end weights for balance. Handle tractor carefully on slopes, when crossing ditches, on rough ground. Avoid hitting rocks, stumps, etc., with trailing vehicle.
Hidden obstacles	**Misuse**	**Mud**
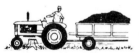	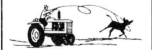	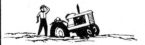
Slow down in tall weeds or grass. Watch for hidden logs, stumps, rocks, holes, etc. Keep speed moderate at night and when visibility is poor.	Use tractor for the jobs it's designed to do—not for running errands, herding cattle or just plain horseplay.	When you can't back out, get help. Don't chain blocks to drive wheels—chassis can revolve around the axle if wheels stick. Avoid muddy spots when possible.

Figure 14-2 In operating a tractor, these common pitfalls should be avoided. (Source: Farm Safety Review, September–October 1967, p. 8.)

square shaft.) Do not wear loose clothing when you are working near moving parts—better still, disconnect the power before doing any work on or around machinery.

5 *Keep off implements, and keep others off, unless a proper seat or platform is provided.* If you ride on an implement, except on a seat or platform intended for this purpose, you may be thrown off balance and flung into the machinery or out in front of it. This can easily happen if the implement stops short, drops into a hole or ditch, or goes over a bump. If you are riding on a platform, do not get down until the power is shut off. Even then, do not just jump down, for your clothing may catch on a projecting part of the machine and cause a fall. Look carefully before you dismount and use the proper footholds in descending.

HUMAN FACTORS ENGINEERING

Human factors engineering can help prevent farm accidents. This branch of engineering attempts to correct accident situations by adapting the machine to the individual's physical and mental limitations. Such engineering is directed at environmental factors which diminish the capability of workers to properly use their acquired knowledge and skills. Important gains have been made in reducing the levels of stress, noise, vibration, discomfort, fatigue, and boredom which ordinarily accompany the tasks of farming.

Some of the important causes of agricultural injury and illness are not directly influenced by human factors engineering. Contributing to these high rates are factors such as:

1. *Bad weather.* Agricultural workers must endure the outdoor elements of temperature and climate. They are frequently imperiled by windstorms, rainstorms, and tornadoes. If a person has any choice of shelter during a lightning storm, the person should choose in the following order:
   a. Buildings protected from lightning and large metal or metal framed buildings (avoid use of electrical equipment)
   b. An automobile with metal top and body
   c. Large unprotected buildings
   d. Small unprotected buildings

   It is best to stay away from open doors or windows, and from fireplaces, stoves, piping, or other metal objects. Do not go out of doors or remain out during thunderstorms unless you must.

   If remaining out of doors is unavoidable, keep away from:
   a. Small sheds and shelters in exposed locations
   b. Isolated trees
   c. Wire fences
   d. Hilltops and large open spaces where protection is not provided by taller objects

Seek shelter in a cave, a depression in the ground, a deep valley or canyon, the foot of a steep or overhanging cliff, or in a dense grove of trees. If you are caught in an open area and have no other alternative, your best bet is lying on the ground, away from isolated trees.

When a person becomes unconscious from a stroke of lightning, call a doctor and apply the same emergency treatment recommended for electric shock. The immediate application of artifical respiration is very important. In addition to causing burns, the passing of electric current through the body often paralyzes the nerves and muscles affecting the heart and breathing mechanism.

2. *Animals.* Although they are not a major cause of injury, farm animals are large and constitute a significant hazard.
3. *Agricultural chemicals and pesticides.* These poisonous substances are especially dangerous. The harmful effects are often quite subtle and produce no immediate symptoms. When a person has used such chemicals for several years, the concentration in the body builds to a toxic level that can cause severe and chronic disability. Safety measures should be taken when mixing, applying, and storing these substances.
4. *Location.* People who are injured in a rural area may have to be transported a considerable distance before they can receive proper treatment. Burns, fractures, cuts, and other injuries are likely to be particularly serious if they do not receive prompt medical attention. Therefore, accidents represent an even greater threat to farmers than to urban residents, who have ready access to doctors and hospitals. A rural accident victim may die from loss of blood en route to the hospital, although an immediate transfusion could have saved his or her life. The inconvenience involved in seeing a doctor often influences farm residents to neglect minor injuries thereby increasing the possibility of infection or serious complications.
5. *Machinery.* Farm machinery is characterized by heavy equipment designed to tear, dig, pull, compact, and shred. Machinery is not capable of distinguishing between a stock of corn and a leg. Because of the tasks they perform, agricultural machines demand adequate knowledge, a high level of skill, and extreme caution when being operated.
6. *Long working hours.* Like other businesspersons, the farmer has deadlines to meet. Weather plays an important role in setting and achieving these deadlines. The farmer cannot fully plan a work schedule and must take advantage of good weather. Fatigue and boredom lead to carelessness and an attitude which permits "taking chances."
7. *Safety administration.* In industry, specialists operate and administer the safety program. On the farm, it is the farmer alone who must take the initiative for safety. The owner of a farm must be a farmer, mechanic, chemist, electrician, plumber, carpenter, businessperson, and safety administrator. Obviously, the farmer's ability to perform these tasks is suspect.

LOSSES

Losses from agriculture accidents are especially costly. Some of the reasons for this are:

1 Agriculture equipment is intended to reduce the number of people needed to effectively farm many acres. The equipment is usually large and quite expensive, with most of it costing more than $10,000 and some of it costing as much as $30,000.

2 Agricultural equipment is quite sophisticated. Automobile replacement parts are kept in stock, and repairs usually take less than a day to complete. Farm equipment requires highly specialized mechanics. Often, the repairs must wait until parts can be shipped from the manufacturer. This delay can mean the difference between profit and loss for the year's work.

3 Agricultural injuries are particularly severe. Among all professionally treated farm injuries that require one-half day or more away from work, the average medical bill is $120.[6] Many farmers are not adequately covered by health insurance so that the cost of injury is often direct and unexpected.

4 Most farm work is completed by the farm family, an unsalaried unit of highly motivated personnel. When injury causes the loss of one or more family members, salaried workers must be employed. When money is the primary source of motivation, productivity usually suffers. If the injury produces permanent disability to the farmer, the consequences are multiplied by the number of years the individual could have otherwise continued to work.

TRAUMA

The biggest safety problem facing agricultural workers is trauma. Ironically, the varied machinery which has reduced the number of people exposed to the hazards of farming has also contributed to the high degree of risk that faces today's farmers. Since 1951 the annual number of machinery-related accidental deaths has dropped by more than 50 percent, but machinery remains the single most important contributer to the high death rate among agricultural workers (Table 14-6).

It is generally recognized that the tractor is the most dangerous piece of farm equipment. Most injuries from tractors result in crush wounds or fractures. More than half of the tractor fatalities are caused by overturns. As a result, the Occupational Safety and Health Administration has established a standard for protective roll-over equipment on tractors.

HIGHWAY USAGE

In recent years many main highways intended for fast-moving traffic have been constructed in rural areas. Previously, the average farm resident drove to town over a lightly traveled dirt road, which he or she habitually entered without

[6]National Safety Council, *Farm and Ranch Safety Guide*, Chicago, 1973, p. 6.

TABLE 14-6

Nontransport Deaths from Accidents on Farms* by Type, 1951–1974
(excluding farm home deaths)

Year	All Types†	Machinery	Drowning	Firearms	Falls	Struck by Obj.	Fires, Burns	Elec. Curr.	Animals	Poisoning	Suffocation	Lightning
1951	2,580	851	334	332	274	154	151	76	151	37	29	70
1953	2,572	895	345	319	258	141	140	69	143	38	35	53
1955	2,482	826	386	282	225	146	125	101	119	40	38	59
1957	2,420	884	404	306	198	124	98	87	99	23	25	53
1959	2,407	892	365	268	204	162	121	84	87	49	29	69
1961	2,403	913	377	253	195	126	133	102	80	45	37	56
1962	2,246	852	366	219	175	140	101	56	108	54	32	53
1963	2,309	894	361	245	165	152	124	64	70	50	31	52
1964	2,279	875	362	238	135	160	118	88	87	31	38	36
1965	2,321	943	377	226	148	133	102	86	77	43	39	44
1966	2,165	907	323	210	143	138	99	77	70	44	30	26
1967	2,183	912	350	220	153	130	96	72	72	42	36	23
1969‡	1,954	467‡	317	180‡	121	350‡	74‡	71	78	26	56‡	27
1970	1,795	444	282	155	125	310	57	83	63	39	46	29
1971	1,717	428	268	148	112	269	59	59	69	31	47	29
1972	1,712	452	262	142	120	262	40	64	70	28	54	26
1973	1,769	447	262	146	119	285	40	72	82	29	51	22
1974	1,617	377	234	109	118	292	30	86	54	41	50	21

*A place is a farm if it has 10 or more acres of land and $50 or more of agricultural products are sold each year, or if it has less than 10 acres but $250 or more of products are sold each year.
†Includes some deaths not shown separately.
‡Data for 1969 and later years not comparable with previous years due to classification changes.
Source: National Center for Health Statistics. Reported in *Accident Facts*, National Safety Council, Chicago, 1976. p. 88.

453

hesitation, knowing that any oncoming car would be moving slowly enough for its driver to avoid collision. Today, when the road to town accommodates a fast-moving traffic stream, approaching motorists may not be able to stop in time to avoid hitting a car that suddenly turns onto the highway from a secondary road or farm driveway. Rural drivers must assume their share of responsibility for their own safety and that of other motorists by coming to a *complete* stop before entering the main highway and waiting until the road is clear before turning into it. They must also be careful to give the proper signal before turning off the highway.

Although the majority of motor-vehicle accidents are caused by human factors, faulty automotive equipment is often a contributory factor in rural accidents. Periodic inspection and replacement of worn or damaged parts will prevent accidents from failure of the steering gear or brakes, or from faulty headlights. Retreading or replacement of worn tires will reduce the likelihood of skidding, help avoid blowouts, and prevent the necessity of changing tires on a busy highway.

Farmers can help reduce greatly the number of motor-vehicle accidents on rural highways by habitually treating other drivers with courtesy and consideration. When moving agricultural equipment on the main highway, the farmer must avoid any conduct that will force motorists to make a sudden change in their driving pattern. Farm vehicles being pulled by tractors at dusk are particularly hazardous, and all such vehicles should be lighted 1 hour after sunset. A high flag on slow-moving vehicles that are used on hilly roads will increase the distance at which the vehicles may be seen over hilltops. Lights and reflectors, required by highway regulations, are recommended for self-protection. In areas where livestock must cross the main road, adequate signs should be posted to warn drivers of this hazard.

Farm residents should be reminded of the special rules applying to pedestrians and cyclists in rural areas. It is particularly important that children who must use main highways to travel to and from school be taught to practice safe pedestrian habits at all times, and to exercise the necessary caution when crossing the road and getting on and off the school bus (see Chapters 4 and 8). Bicycle riders who use the highway at night must understand their obligation to motorists, and the precautions to be taken for their own safety after dark (see Chapter 9).

TOOLS

Before farms became highly mechanized, many farmers' tool kits could not pass the most superficial safety inspection. Standard equipment consisted of a good ax, a saw or two, a few hammers—usually with loose handles—one or two screwdrivers, and a pair of pliers. Even then these tools were inadequate, and today a full supply of good tools is essential for servicing modern farm equipment. Unfortunately, the old habit of neglecting tools persists. Farm residents must be influenced to observe the high standards that industry has established for the maintenance and use of machines and tools.

A study of farm casualties shows that the following practices are most often responsible for tool-related accidents:

1 Working with an inappropriate tool, for example, using a flat file to open a paint can

2 Using a defective tool such as a hammer with a loose handle

3 Using a tool incorrectly, for example, applying pressure toward the body, rather than away from the body, when working with a pointed or sharp-edged tool

4 Working in inappropriate clothing, for example, wearing a loose-sleeved shirt when working with a lathe or circular saw

To eliminate these practices, teachers must persuade farm residents to adhere to the following principles when using hand tools:

1 The tool selected should be designed for the job to be done. A screwdriver should not be used unless it fits snugly into the head of the screw. All tools should be sturdy enough to withstand a reasonable amount of pressure.

2 The tool selected should be in good working condition. Such tools as files or chisels with loose handles, dull saws with improperly set teeth that vary in height, dull axes, mallets with damaged heads, and hammers with greasy handles should never be used.

3 All tools must be correctly used. When you are handling scythes, knives, and other sharp-edged tools, pressure should be applied away from the hand and body. A wrench should be pushed with the open palm so that the fingers will not be injured if the tool slips. Stationary tools should be securely fastened down.

4 When electrical tools are used, the power switch should be within easy reach of the operator.

5 Protective apparel such as gloves or goggles should be worn when sharpening tools, repairing barbed-wire fences, or performing other tasks in which safety equipment is necessary.

6 All tools should be properly stored: securely fastened in a properly identified spot, with cutting edges protected.

When we note the high injury and illness rates for agriculture workers and recognize that machinery is involved in many of these accidents, it is surprising that OSHA has not identified agriculture as a target industry. Actually, there is little that OSHAct could do by way of enforcement. Many agricultural workers are self-employed and rely on family members to help with their work. Of the 2,100 farm work deaths in 1975, only 600 occurred to nonfarm residents. Of the 200,000 disabling agricultural injuries in 1975, 150,000 were incurred by farm residents. Since OSHAct standards apply only to employees, education rather than enforcement is the best method for reducing farm injuries and accidents.

One way to identify the needs of a farm safety education program is to analyze accident data. Another method is to develop an inspection inventory which specifies safety hazards. When a questionnaire such as the following checklist is analyzed, the need for farm safety education becomes apparent.

FARM FIRE SAFETY INSPECTION BLANK

Answer each question with "yes" or "no." Questions which receive "no" answers indicate potential danger spots which need prompt attention and correction. *Inspect* your farm yourself—*today!*

	Yes	No
Lightning		
Have lightning-protection systems of a type approved by Underwriters' Laboratories been installed on your property?	___	___
Have lightning-rod installations been checked and put in good condition within the past year?	___	___
Are lightning-rod systems grounded in moist earth?	___	___
Are wire fences that are attached to buildings properly grounded at the fence post nearest the building?	___	___
Are ground cables protected from livestock's rubbing against them, particularly at the corners of buildings?	___	___
Do radio and television antennas have approved lightning arrestors?	___	___
Electrical		
Has the wiring been checked by a qualified person since installation?	___	___
When new machinery was added to the load on a motor, was the wiring inspected and any necessary new wiring installed by a qualified electrician?	___	___
Is electricity delivered to a centrally located pole and switch box, and distributed from there to buildings?	___	___
Are the wires leading to remote buildings of sufficient size to reduce the possibility of a drop in voltage?	___	___
Do you inspect your fusebox regularly to see that approved fuses of specified capacities are being used?	___	___
Are electric-light bulbs in exposed locations in barns and outbuildings protected by glass or metal guards?	___	___
Have you removed all extension cords over hooks, nails, or beams, or stretched through doors?	___	___
Flammable liquids		
Are motor fuels stored away from all combustible materials?	___	___
Do you have approved safety cans for any necessary transportation of gasoline?	___	___
Are greases, oils, and flammable liquids stored in an oil house located away from other buildings?	___	___
Your heating system		
Have your stoves, furnace, chimney, and smoke pipes been inspected and cleaned in the past year?	___	___
Are walls adjacent to stoves protected by metal or plaster board, leaving 6 inches of air space between protection and wall?	___	___
Does your heating system provide adequate heat without "forcing" or overstoking in very cold weather? (Note: If "forcing" is necessary, you need better building insulation or more adequate heating equipment to provide sufficient heat for your house.)	___	___
If you have a shingle roof, does your chimney have a spark arrester?	___	___

	Yes	No

Has the chimney been examined for cracks lately, especially in the attic and above the roof line?

Do any smoke pipes in your house or outbuildings pass through partitions? If so, are the pipes protected by an approved metal thimble to prevent the walls from charring and igniting?

Do you prohibit the use of kerosene for starting or quickening a fire in your home?

Does your fireplace have a metal screen in front of it to prevent sparks from flying onto carpet or furniture?

Portable heaters

Are your portable oil heaters of a type which has been examined and listed by Underwriters' Laboratories?

Is your portable oil heater always placed on a level floor in order to ensure proper operation?

Do you always refill its fuel tank outdoors and in the daylight?

If you use a wick-type portable oil heater, do you trim the wick and clean it regularly?

Do you regulate the flame of your portable oil heater to keep it from smoking?

Is the latch which fastens the upper to the lower part of the heater secure?

Do you always turn your portable oil heater out upon retiring at night?

Outside the home

Do you keep grass and weeds cut short around your home, barn, and other buildings?

Are all buildings on your farm accessible to fire trucks at all times?

Do you have milk cans or other containers available to carry water to neighbors' property in the event of fire there?

Do you have cables for dragging farm equipment from burning sheds?

The barn

Are lightning rods properly installed and in good condition?

Is the hayloft well ventilated?

Do you prohibit the stacking of trash and manure against the barn?

Do you take care not to store damp hay in the barn?

If you have a blower for drying hay, has the installation been inspected by a competent electrician?

Are light fixtures, fuse boxes, and switches kept free of dirt, dust, and chaff?

Are exposed light bulbs in the barn protected by glass or metal guards from damage by animals or human carelessness, or to keep the bulbs from setting fire to hay, straw, or dust?

Is smoking in the barn prohibited?

Is the storage of tractors and other equipment in the barn prohibited?

Fire protection

Is the number of the nearest fire department posted prominently near the phone?

Have you made arrangements with the nearest fire department to assure its response at a time of fire?

Does the fire department have a map of your farm, with streams, ponds, or fire cisterns clearly marked?

Do you have an adequate emergency water supply (at least 3,000 gallons) on your farm? Is it accessible to fire trucks or portable pumps?

Do you have approved fire extinguishers placed conveniently near any area of special fire hazard?

Do you have approved fire extinguishers on your motor vehicles?

Have your fire extinguishers been inspected and recharged within the past year?

	Yes	No
Do employees and members of your family know how to use your fire extinguishers?	___	___
Do you have enough garden hose and an adequate supply of buckets for carrying water?	___	___
Do you have ladders long enough to reach to the roof for rescuing members of your family from your home in case of fire?	___	___
Have your family and employees been instructed and drilled in locating proper exits from your house and buildings, and in closing all windows and doors in case of fire?	___	___
Have you set up a definite plan of action for a fire emergency?	___	___

Equipment

	Yes	No
Do hay and corn driers have automatic controls to shut off fans and close dampers in case of overheating?	___	___

Do all of the following have Underwriters' Laboratories (U.L.) labels:

	Yes	No
Brooders	___	___
Crop driers	___	___
Electric cooking appliances	___	___
Electric fences	___	___
Electric irons	___	___
Electric refrigerators and deep freezes	___	___
Electric heaters	___	___
Electric stoves	___	___
Fire extinguishers	___	___
Fuel tanks	___	___
Gasoline pumps	___	___
Gasoline or kerosene stoves	___	___
Incubators	___	___
Liquefied-petroleum gas systems	___	___
Oil burners	___	___
Portable oil heaters	___	___
Radios	___	___
Roof covering	___	___
Television sets	___	___

Name _____

Address _____

LEARNING EXPERIENCES

The following activities are designed to supplement the study of this chapter.

1 Compare the injury, illness, and fatality rates of various industries. Identify the causes of industrial accidents and recommend ways by which the danger could be reduced.

2 Secure a copy of your state worker's compensation law. Compare the current provisions of the law with the provisions of the laws of nearby states. Analyze the benefits, and make suggestions for improving the provisions of the law.

3 Debate the pros and cons of the Occupational Safety and Health Act.

[7]National Board of Fire Underwriters, New York.

4 Invite an OSHA inspector (compliance officer) to class to discuss the act and its standards, inspection procedures, violations, and penalties.

5 Arrange a field trip to a local industrial plant. Meet the safety administrator and tour the facility. Ask the safety administrator to discuss the responsibilities of the position. Discuss the qualifications needed for this position.

6 Obtain a copy of a safety handbook published by a local industry, and analyze the regulations and procedures in the guide. What changes would you recommend?

7 Develop a safety checklist for a high school shop. Use the checklist to survey the school's vocational facilities. Make suggestions for improvement to the industrial arts teacher. Use a similar checklist to survey a home workshop.

8 Write to several manufacturers of farm equipment for pamphlets describing their machinery. Analyze the potential hazards of the equipment. Determine the adequacy of the safety information distributed by the manufacturer.

9 Imagine that you are a farmer. What safety policies would you encourage to protect yourself, your family, and your employees? Consider issues such as machinery, poisons, animals, lightning, drowning, and electrical current.

SELECTED REFERENCES

Ashford, Nicholas Askounas: *Crisis in the Workplace: Occupational Disease and Injury,* The M.I.T. Press, Cambridge, 1976

Binford, Charles M., Cecil S. Fleming, and Z. A. Prust: *Loss Control in the OSHA Era,* McGraw-Hill Book Company, New York, 1975

Gordon, Jerome B., Allan Akman, and Michael Brooks: *Industrial Safety Statistics: A Re-Examination,* Praeger Publishers, Inc., New York, 1971

Grimaldi, John V., and Rollin H. Simonds: *Safety Management,* 3rd ed., Richard D. Irwin, Inc., Homewood, Ill., 1975

International Labour Office: *Accident Prevention: A Worker's Education Manual,* Geneva, 1961

National Safety Council, Chicago:

Accident Facts, yearly

Farm and Ranch Safety Guide, 1973

Farm Safety Review, magazine

Guide to Occupational Safety Literature, 1976

Pausner, Steven, and George Clark: "OSHA's Ancestors: Previous Laws of the Workplace," *Job Safety and Health,* vol. 2, pp. 16–21, April, 1974

Petersen, Dan: *Safety Management: A Human Approach,* Aloray, Inc., Englewood Cliffs, N.J., 1975

———: *Safety Supervision,* AMACOM, New York, 1976

Samuels, Sheldon: "A Greater Voice for the Worker," *Job Safety and Health,* vol. 2, pp. 23–26, February, 1974

Appendix A

NORTH CAROLINA INITIATES A NEW PROGRAM TO PROVIDE K–9 TRAFFIC SAFETY EDUCATION

North Carolina has assigned a high priority in its comprehensive plan for highway safety to establishing a new traffic safety education program that will reach one million students in kindergarten through ninth grades annually. In the course of programming the curriculum development phase of this high priority action item, the Governor's Highway Safety Program (GHSP) has the full cooperation of the Department of Public Instruction (DPI). A research and development project has been in progress for seven months. The output of this project is a family of curriculum guides and materials for K–9 traffic safety education developed with participation of K–9 educators, tested in pilot programs, definitively evaluated, and incorporated in its completed form into a plan for statewide implementation. The GHSP is sponsoring these efforts with state and federal highway safety funds, the federal share furnished through the National Highway Traffic Safety Administration. The curriculum is intended both to meet the highway safety education needs perceived to be common in nature for any state, and in particular to serve the special needs of this state as evidenced by traffic accident profiles, demographic characteristics, transportation facilities, climate, geography, and topography of North Carolina. Three overriding concepts and principles guide the formulation of curriculum for the planned statewide program. These are:

1. Communicating facts and providing instruction to the public for the purpose of enlarging and improving knowledge and understanding of highway traffic safety calls for a program of public information and education that must be rigorously designed, not casually left to chance.

2. In the same perspective, the program must begin in an organized, formal sense, not when young people become eligible for driver education and training courses because they reach 15 years of age, but rather not later than when children first enter school at prekindergarten or kindergarten levels.

3. Additionally, a program of traffic safety education for young people must be provided in school from pre-K or K through 9th grades in a manner that grows both in coverage by units of instruction and in depth by degrees of attention through advancing grade levels so that young people are knowledgeable about traffic safety in the areas of coverage listed to the extent indicated by their participation in the highway traffic environment prior to the time when they are trained and licensed to drive: pedestrian safety; bicycle safety; passenger safety; school bus safety; mini-bike, Mo-Ped, and motorcycle safety; farm vehicle and other work or recreation vehicle safety; pre-driver education and training aspects of motor vehicle and traffic safety.

The North Carolina Governor's Highway Safety Program, together with the Department of Public Instruction, in recognition of the principles presented above, has initiated a new program to provide K–9 traffic safety education in North

National Safety Council Transactions, "School and College," Joseph E. Lema, vol. 23, National Safety Council, Chicago, 1974.

460

Carolina's school systems. To accomplish the program, the GHSP assembled a research and development study team composed of: Research Triangle Institute (prime contractor); Appalachian State University, East Carolina University, the University of North Carolina Highway Safety Research Center, and the National Safety Council (subcontractors); 100 school officials, administrators, and teachers in K–9 grades of selected pilot schools in four school systems—Asheville City, Buncombe County, Greenville City, and Pitt County Schools; and an Advisory Committee on Traffic Safety Curriculum established by the DPI.

The team outlined above was formed to provide a broad base of inputs desirable and warranted in view of the magnitude of the effort along with the serious nature of the problem and the associated degree of betterment possible, considering the high number of traffic accident involvements of young people who are not yet licensed to operate motor vehicles and are not eligible for driver training courses available only at 15 years of age. This situation is characterized by these facts: annually 3,500 pedestrians and bicyclists are killed or injured as a result of traffic accidents in the state, with 50 percent of these casualties comprised of young people under 15 years of age, a group whose individual participation in the highway traffic environment is generally limited to walking or cycling; the state has no current organized, formal traffic safety education program for young people under 15 years of age (true in most states today); and the costs of initiating a new K–9 traffic safety education program statewide are substantial to reach 1,000,000 pupils and 40,000 teachers in K–9 grades of 150 school systems.

A synopsis of a four-part Professional Guide which presents K–9 Traffic Safety Curriculum developed for North Carolina and used in pilot programs of traffic safety education in K–9 grades of 14 schools involving 8,000 pupils and 300 teachers is provided in the following paragraphs.

The K–9 Traffic Safety Curriculum is divided into four levels, addressing the special needs and abilities of the children at those levels.

Level A corresponds approximately to the K–1 grade levels. Little or no reading skill is required. Units in pedestrian, bicycle, school bus, and passenger safety are presented. Emphasis is placed on development of perceptual skills, especially in regard to pedestrian safety.

Level B is aimed at 2–3 grade levels. Pedestrian, bicycle, school bus, and passenger safety units are included. Perceptual and judgmental skills are emphasized. Bicycle safety becomes extremely important, since this is the age at which most youngsters begin driving their bicycles on the street.

Level C corresponds to the 4–5–6 grade levels. Units in pedestrian, bicycle, school bus, and passenger safety are presented. A unit on mini-cycle safety and an optional farm vehicle safety unit are introduced. The scope of all units is widened to include activities in which students can reach out into the community to investigate and express their concern for the safety of others as well as themselves. Activities include in-depth identification of hazards and opportunities for problem solving and exploration of attitudes. The natural laws which affect vehicles and pedestrians are also presented.

Level D, prepared for 7–9 grade levels, is structured differently than the K–6 elementary units. The emphasis in Level D is on preparation for the driving task. Three units are presented. The first unit in the series (grade 7) presents more sophisticated approaches to pedestrian, bicycle, school bus, and motorcycle safety, plus an optional section for farm vehicle safety. The second unit, (grade 8) deals with passenger safety, trip planning, first aid, and other activities which begin changing the student's focus of concern to the driver's responsibilities. Students explore the complexities of the traffic environment and investigate the problems and solutions our advanced technology has produced. The third unit (grade 9) deals directly with preparation for driver education. The total fabric of the highway transportation system and the relationship of the individual driver, pedestrian, and others to the system are examined. The students explore the mental and physical factors important to safe behavior behind the wheel. Attitude clarification and formation are emphasized.

The curriculum and materials prepared and acquired from various sources for K–9 traffic safety education pilot programs in North Carolina are directed towards accomplishing the goals of: reducing traffic accidents, deaths, and injuries experienced by young people under 15 years of age; increasing knowledge and understanding of safety relationships involving various highway users—drivers, passengers, cyclists, and pedestrians—as they impact on each other in the highway traffic environment and as they interact with roadway/roadside elements and vehicle design features; developing an attitude of responsibility towards identifying and assessing risks and making informed, judicious decisions for safe behavior in the traffic stream; and fostering a desire to support actions within the community that are conducive to improving highway safety.

Within the curriculum are a variety of teaching/learning experiences that address the fulfillment of certain needs of the student in learning to think for himself and to behave safely, including:

1. A sense of how the student relates to the traffic environment. This includes an understanding of how the student relates to drivers as a pedestrian, a bicyclist, and a passenger.

2. Information about the traffic environment. He needs to recognize and understand traffic signs, signals, and markings. A knowledge of what others expect of him is helpful, for example, a knowledge of the Rules of the Road.

3. The ability to identify and assess hazards. An accident is an unintended event which results in damage or injury, but most accidents are caused by a series of misjudgments. Students need to explore the causal relationships in accidents and learn to identify behaviors which are likely to result in accidents.

4. Knowledge of how to avoid or handle hazardous situations. The student needs to identify alternative actions which produce safe results, as well as to practice safe, responsible behavior. This includes practice in motor and perceptual skills.

5. A positive attitude toward safety. The student needs to develop a positive feeling about turning down unreasonable risks. Acting safely means thinking ahead and acting in one's best interest.

Material covered in each level of curriculum (A, B, C, D) is organized into units which are appropriate to particular grade levels and is published in one of four color-coded looseleaf hard-cover binders. Each unit is divided into general topics or concepts. Under each concept heading are listed objectives—broad behavioral outcomes which the lessons attempt to encourage.

Next is content for discussion, which presents facts to convey or background information. Suggested learning activities follow. Activities are listed numerically. Art work and other worksheets which may be useful to reproduce, either as transparencies or in quantity for each student, also labelled numerically to correspond with appropriate activities, are incorporated directly after the concept reference in the text. Stories, poems, songs, etc. are found in a supplemental section at the end of a unit. Resource lists for each unit also are found at the end of the unit. While the entire curriculum is organized so that it may be used for regular, independent safety lessons, the activities readily lend themselves to integration within existing subject areas for Levels A, B, and C, which cover K–6 grades.

The curriculum allows for a wide variety of activities, especially in terms of role playing, hands-on activities, and decision making by the student. Emphasis is placed on informing the student of his special place in the highway traffic environment as a driver, passenger, cyclist, or pedestrian and on engendering an understanding of his responsibilities and limitations, as well as those of others, so that the student can make intelligent decisions about his behavior. Each unit begins with an introduction which offers background information on the state-of-the-art concerning a specific topic, for instance, pedestrian safety. This is followed by statements of unit objectives and checklists for teachers preparing to instruct pupils in selected traffic safety subjects. Basic curriculum content and suggested activities are then presented for the respective units. An example of items incorporated into curriculum content and suggested activities for units in Level C, grades 4–6 is presented in the list of topics below:

Pedestrian Safety: Basic Facts About Pedestrians; Pedestrian Skills; Walking during Conditions of Limited Visibility; Identification of Pedestrian Hazards; Traffic Signs and Signals; and Pedestrian Responsibility.

Bicycle Safety: Advantages and Limitations of Bicycles; Natural Laws Limiting Drivers, Bicyclists, and Pedestrians; A Bicycle Is A Vehicle; Drive A Bike That Fits; Know Your Bicycle; Predict Possible Hazards; and Drive With Skill and Control.

School Bus and Passenger Safety: Going To and Waiting for the Bus; Entering the School Bus; The Proper Use of Safety Belts; Riding in the Car; and Trip Planning.

Vehicle Safety: Hazards Unique to Farm Vehicle Operations; and Precautions for Slow-Moving Vehicles.

Mini-Cycle Safety: Know Your Machine; Know How to Handle Different Driving Surfaces; and Drive With Skill, Control and Safety.

Masters for reproduction, activity sheets, and resource references are listed for a unit following the presentation of curriculum content for that unit as it occurs within the document containing the total curriculum for a specific level.

STUDY DESIGN FOR EVALUATION OF PILOT PROGRAMS

An evaluation is being conducted in three parts. First, knowledge tests were developed for the third, sixth, and ninth grade levels, based on the curriculum content. Forty items were developed for each grade level designated, and 20 items from each group of 40 were randomly chosen for pretests which were administered early in the semester. After students have received exposure to the curriculum in pilot-program schools, follow-up tests, including all 40 items, will be administered. These tests have been field tested in other schools prior to adoption.

The sample for the knowledge-testing encompasses 12 third-grade classes, 12 sixth-grade classes, and 12 ninth-grade classes. An equal proportion of these classes are experimental and control in the western and eastern areas of the state involved in the pilot programs.

Analysis of data thus acquired will answer a basic question: How much knowledge did the students acquire as a result of the pilot program? A statistical test will be made to indicate whether the change in amount of knowledge is great enough to be significant.

For the second part of the evaluation, a filming system will be utilized for recording behavior in the school vicinity, again early and late in the semester in both experimental and control schools. Observations of selected behavior characteristics will be recorded.

For the third part of this evaluation, a questionnaire has been developed and will be mailed late in the semester to a sample of teachers who participated in the pilot program. The questionnaire concerns their evaluation of the utility of the curriculum and materials developed for K–9 traffic safety education.

The GHSP and the DPI have scheduled major tasks in research and development of a new statewide K–9 traffic safety education program: develop curriculum and materials for pilot programs; conduct pilot programs in 14 schools—eight in Asheville/Buncombe County area and six in Greenville/Pitt County area; evaluate pilot programs; adjust and complete curriculum in form for statewide use; determine plan for accomplishing statewide implementation of the program in K–9 grades; and commence first phase of statewide implementation.

In closing, I would offer four observations that relate to experience gained in the process of curriculum development for traffic safety education, especially with respect to ensuring that such programs are designed for maximum utility and practical implementation. First, it was found to be of major value to have the direct assistance of 100 school officials, administrators, and teachers currently active in K–9 education in the determination of methods for communicating traffic safety education guidelines to teachers and instruction to pupils at varying grade levels. Secondly, it is substantially beneficial to acquire and assess curriculum currently in use in other states and communities, as well as instructional materials now available, to aid in applying the curriculum as an early step. A third point which is of major importance, in our estimation, is that pilot programs should be conducted at all grade levels in a representative group of schools prior to initiation of statewide implementation. A fourth and sometimes easily forgotten matter for consideration is that substantive evaluations of program effectiveness are essential to avoid misrepresentation of potential accomplishments due to a lack of information stemming from adequate testing of program actions. In fact, it is as critical that a definitive study design for evaluation be soundly conceived, applied both in experimental and in control group situations, and utilized objectively in making decisions governing directions for the program, as it is logical to recognize that all states and communities should have organized, formal traffic safety education programs at the early childhood levels, oriented toward the special needs of individual states and communities.

Appendix B

INSTRUCTIONAL PROGRAM FOR ILLINOIS

It is not possible to include the entire content of all twelve units. Therefore, only introductory materials and unit objectives are given. Each unit contains various episodes, episode objectives, and learning activities. Unit 4 is presented in its entirety to illustrate the format and makeup of the units.

THE HIGHWAY TRANSPORTATION SYSTEM

THE HIGHWAY TRANSPORTATION SYSTEM

The HTS is an important and complex system consisting of numerous man-machine combinations with a variety of goals that use a rather uniform communication network and operate in a variety of regulated environments. The safe operation of this system has become one of the nation's leading social and economic problems.

OFFICIAL PLAN FOR CONTROLLING HTS SAFETY PROBLEM

The National Highway Safety Act requires each state to have a comprehensive driver education program, as a part of the overall Highway Safety Program, to reduce traffic accidents.

APPROACH FOR DEVELOPMENT OF DRIVER EDUCATION PROGRAM

The program of instruction for driver education is best derived from an analysis of motor vehicle operator tasks.

DRIVING TASK MODEL

The role of the driver in the HTS is primarily that of processing information and making decisions. Driving an automobile consists of making skilled and properly timed actions under varying road and traffic conditions, based on sound judgments and decisions. These decisions are in turn dependent upon previously acquired knowledge and the gathering of accurate information pertinent to the immediate traffic situation.

Source: Driver Education for Illinois Youth, Office of Superintendent of Public Instruction (now Office of Education), State of Illinois, Springfield, Ill., 1972.

IMPLICATIONS FOR DRIVER EDUCATION

Driving requires a type of social and mental behavior that needs to be learned and acquired through formal training and supervised experience. From learning, man develops the set of expectations, correlations, and judgments upon which sound driving decisions are made. Because of the tremendous variety of traffic situations, a broad type of learning is required.

GENERAL OBJECTIVES FOR DRIVER EDUCATION

The goal of driver education is the development of traffic citizens who will be competent and responsible users of the highway transportation system.

THE HIGHWAY TRANSPORTATION SYSTEM

The operation of motor vehicles takes place in the highway transportation system (HTS). This highway transportation system, invented by man, is one of the elaborate and important systems which make our present way of life possible. The education of citizens for the safe and efficient use of such a vital system is now considered a necessary and legitimate function of the public schools.

The purpose of the highway transportation system is to move people and goods from one place to another in a relatively safe, efficient, and convenient manner. As a system, the HTS consists of an assembly of elements that carries out the desired functions by the interdependent operation of the component parts. The major components are: the people who use the system, the vehicles that carry people and goods, and the highway environment in which the vehicles are operated.

Although most of our citizens are drivers, the entire population uses the HTS either as passengers or pedestrians. Those who operate nonmotorized vehicles, principally bicycles, become a fourth category of users. The people using the HTS operate or ride in millions of vehicles of various sizes, performances, and conditions. The operation of such vehicles takes place in close proximity to other vehicles going in the same or opposite directions and on roadways crossing one another. These highways differ in design, construction, and condition which are in turn modified by various circumstances such as weather and light. Altogether, there are over four million miles of roadway in the HTS which link together all points of the country and reach the most remote hamlets.

As the number of motor vehicles increased by the thousands each year, and then by millions, the problem of providing adequate highways and regulating road traffic multiplied. Many highways have become obsolete and inadequate for the volume of high speed traffic that uses them. Traffic jams are daily occurrences at such peak hours. Traffic volumes continue to double and redouble. To compound the problem, the streets and highways are built, owned, and maintained by several thousand different political subdivisions. Bad roads, inadequate signs, crowded highways and/or low illumination make it easier for drivers to commit errors.

In a democratic and mobile society such as ours, the individual driver is entrusted with a considerable degree of responsibility for the control and maintenance of his motor vehicle. The variety of these motor vehicles with their wide range of sizes and performance capabilities make driver judgments increasingly difficult. When some piece of equipment, accessory, or load becomes defective or out of adjustment, the vehicle can become difficult, hazardous, or even impossible to control in a proper manner.

Almost everyone who reaches legal driving age may own and drive a motor vehicle. Selection and control of drivers is by separate licensing, police and court authorities in the fifty states, and thousands of local municipalities. As a result, the HTS is used by millions of drivers of varying ability, age, and temperament who must make decisions critical to proper operation of the total system.

The continuous interaction of the HTS elements generates a multitude of traffic situations and a variety of traffic environments in which the driver-vehicle units must operate. The result is a complex system consisting of numerous man-machine combinations with a variety of goals which use a rather uniform communication network and operate in a variety of regulated environments. The safe and efficient operation of the HTS then becomes dependent upon the performance of the various functions or responsibilities of the major components.

In this kind of man-machine system whose total system functioning is critically dependent upon the performance of the vehicle operator, errors and malfunctions can be expected. These errors or malfunctions can result in the breakdown of the overall operation of the system. The number and type of driver errors and the time at which they occur will determine the degree of safety for the HTS operation.

When such a vital system does not operate safely, whether because of improper use, mismanagement, or poor design, grave and serious consequences result. Not only does the system become less efficient and economical to operate, but thousands of lives are lost annually and millions of dollars in resources are destroyed. Since a vast amount of goods and numbers of people are moved on our highways, all conflicts and delays in movement are costly. It is estimated that highway traffic accidents cost the nation a minimum of 11 billion dollars annually. Highway traffic safety has become one of the nation's leading social and economic problems. The magnitude and complexity of the problem will cause it to be a major and challenging problem for years to come.

OFFICIAL PLAN FOR CONTROLLING HTS SAFETY PROBLEM

Highway traffic accidents are symptoms of some HTS malfunction. The complex nature of the solution to the traffic problem has taxed the thinking, imagination, and energies of the ablest men. To prevent motor vehicle accidents, or to significantly reduce their number, calls for the continuous application of many skills and talents.

Over the years an official, comprehensive plan for attacking the highway traffic problem has evolved. In this plan called the Highway Safety Action Program, the major program areas were identified, as shown in Figure 1. For each area a set of traffic accident prevention measures was recommended for implementation and evaluation. A comprehensive traffic safety education program, including the need to understand and support all other areas, was recognized as fundamental to the total program. This program has been modified somewhat and now serves as the basis for the present traffic safety program administered by the National Highway Traffic Safety Administration of the United States Transportation Department.

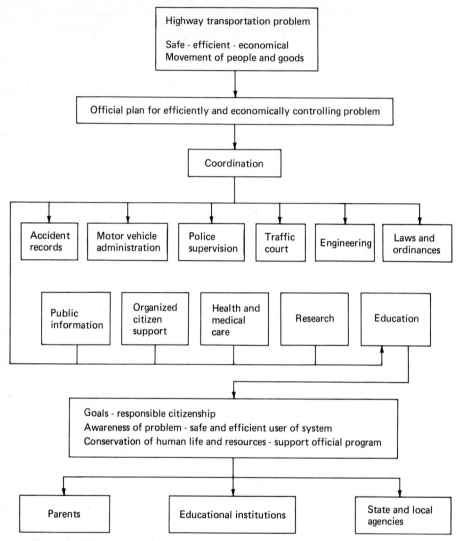

Figure 1 Highway safety action program.

The Highway Safety Act of 1966 requires each state to have a highway safety program designed to reduce traffic accidents and the deaths, injuries, and property damage resulting therefrom. For a state to be approved, it must provide a comprehensive driver education program. This act reinforces the belief held by most traffic safety specialists that driver education is a most significant part of the total traffic accident prevention program. Since the need for driver and traffic safety education has been clearly established, our concern and energies should be directed toward the development and implementation of the most effective program of instruction.

APPROACHES FOR DEVELOPMENT OF DRIVER EDUCATION PROGRAM

Since automobile driving takes place in the HTS and the various components influence each other, the entire system must be considered. This calls for the use of the systems analysis technique. Systems analysis is a kind of problem-solving technique that can be used by curriculum designers for better decision-making. A picture of the functional requirements of the system as a whole and those of the major components unfolds when using systems analysis methods. This technique also makes possible the delineation of operator interaction with system equipment and other environmental factors required during typical trips. Within this context of information, the performance requirements of the human operation can be defined. These definitions should then guide the development of an effective instructional program.

Because a system exists to facilitate man's control or modification of his environment, it is best understood in terms of its intended use. Systems analysis, then, begins with a statement of the particular system purpose. For the HTS the problem becomes one of how to provide safe and efficient movement of goods and persons from one location to another or how to prevent accidents and congestion. Accidents and congestion are malfunctions in the system and result from conflicting interaction of man, vehicle, and the roadway network. A breakdown in one or more of the components can create problems.

To solve the problem, the system is broken down into the major components, as identified in Figure 2. At this point, the systems analyst starts thinking and asking questions which can lead to at least two major approaches. These are the accident causation and task analysis approaches.

In the accident causation approach the questions relate to the various factors that cause accidents. What are traffic accidents? What causes them? What is the role of each system component in an accident? How can traffic accidents be prevented or minimized? To answer such questions requires an investigation and study of accidents and their common causes are identified, programs can then be designed to prevent or minimize them. With this approach, the goal of driver education is the prevention of traffic accidents.

The task analysis approach begins by asking such questions as, "What is the best roadway for such a system? How should the car be designed for the task it is to serve? What are the performance capabilities of the competent driver? How can the system best be managed and controlled?" The focus of this approach is on people and the tasks they are asked to perform rather than on accidents and how they happened. Investigation and research are concerned with defining the tasks that the driver or pedestrian must do to become competent and responsible when using the system. Using this approach, the goal of driver education becomes one of developing responsible users who become competent in performing specific tasks. Research is aimed at improving the product so that errors or malfunctions are reduced to a minimum.

The present instructional program for driver and traffic safety education has evolved primarily from the use of the accident causation approach. The problem in the use of this approach is that the real causes of traffic accidents have been found to be quite elusive. Auto accidents are of many types and are the result of a variety of circumstances which exist before and at the time of the accident. They occur in

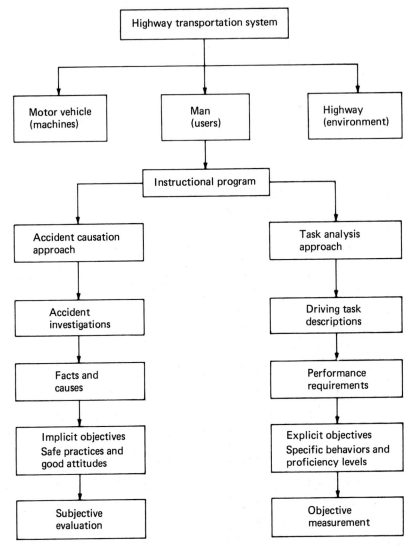

Figure 2 Approaches for curriculum development.

a rather complex system where the continuous interactions of elements can generate an infinite number of situations and conditions. In addition to these many situational factors, traffic accidents may also be a function of such factors as personal characteristics, experience and training, operating procedures, equipment, and fatigue or other temporary driver conditions. Therefore, it has been found that the exact causes cannot be accurately assigned to even a small number of antecedents.

Concepts of the meaning of the term "accident" vary so much it is difficult to determine the limits of meaning. Traditionally, accidents have been understood to be chance events developing without foresight or expectation and resulting in injury, damage, or loss. The term is often used synonymously with injury or loss. This concept has an insurance or engineering purpose. They tend to describe the immediate mechanism and consequence. Furthermore, whether or not an "accident" is considered an accident and is reportable varies in different states according to the degree of damage or injury.

The United States Public Health Service defined the accident sequence as a chain of events or series of interactions between a person and the environment or agent including the measurable or recognizable consequence. The consequence may be, for example, a slip or fall which does not result in any injury, or it may include unintended injury, death, medical expense, or property damage. This should be modified explicitly to state that the consequence is undesirable and unplanned. The accident is then defined as the event that causes the recognizable, undesirable results of the sequence which need not be injury, damage, or loss.

Not only is the accident researcher faced with difficult conceptual and methodological problems, but most of the official traffic accident records are known to be incomplete or unreliable. The fact is traffic accidents do not lend themselves readily to observation. No one knows when or where the next accident will occur. The people involved are seldom prepared to note the circumstances of complicated events compressed into a few confused seconds. The best information must, therefore, be derived from the results and such fragmentary evidence as the surprised participants or witnesses may recall. Once an analysis of the available information is made and the causes determined, there is no way to check as to whether the conclusions reached are correct.

When so little is positively known about the specific or common accident causation factors, it is difficult to plan effective accident prevention programs. As a result, the general objectives for driver education have tended to be all inclusive, thus, too broad in scope. They lack the guidelines that enable teachers to formulate a set of instructional objectives which can be defined in terms of specific behavioral outcomes. Therefore, many programs of instruction rely predominantly on the learning of facts, physical skills, and lists of dos and don'ts. These not only are incomplete, but also tend to be somewhat irrelevant.

In its broadest sense, the traffic accident should be considered an error in the overall function of the HTS. As such, accidents are only a negative malperformance index of the HTS operation to which the driver, in most cases, contributes. The real difference between an accident and any other driving error is that the accident is usually destructive and sometimes terminal. Since the safety of a system is usually defined in terms of the magnitude of the variable errors that occur, a safe HTS is, therefore, one in which the variable errors are brought under control and minimized. If this definition is valid, then the greatest achievements in highway safety can best be attained through the study of driving rather than through the study of accidents. This does not, however, mean that traffic accident research should not continue to be used for evaluation purposes.

Task analysis is the systematic study of the behavioral requirements to be performed. For such a study to be trustworthy, the analyst must keep in mind the system mission, performance specifications, operational problems, and system environment. The question that must be answered for each task is, "What must be learned and to what degree?"

It is the task analysis results that become the key to the development of a valid instructional program. To know what human beings must accomplish in systems and to express these accomplishments as human functions makes possible the accurate identification of the required capabilities. When the particular capabilities and responsibilities required by man to perform the variety of driving tasks are established, an effective program of instruction can be designed. The flow chart in

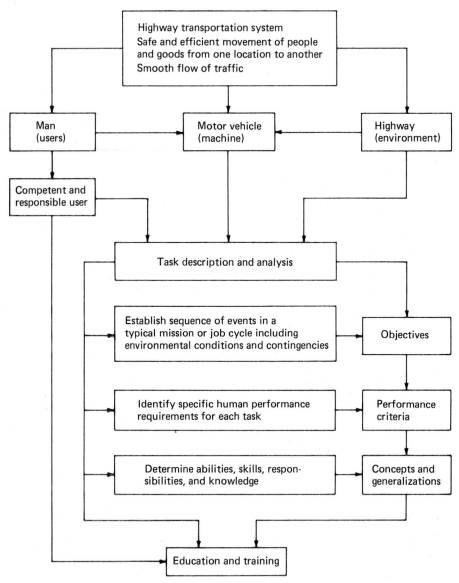

Figure 3 Task analysis approach to program development.

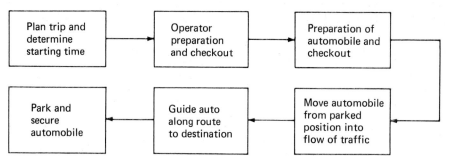

Figure 4 Typical automobile trip activities.

Figure 3 illustrates the procedures to follow in deriving the behavioral objectives necessary to the development of a relevant program of instruction are illustrated.

For our purposes the driving task is defined as the total of all related activities taking place from the inception of a trip to its termination. The inception of a trip occurs when the decision to undertake a trip is made and a destination chosen. The term "driving task," thus, has a broader scope and time dimension than the word "driving" and involves activities before as well as during the actual trip. Figure 4 shows the sequence of major events in a typical trip.

Important contingencies such as environmental conditions and machine malfunctions . . . may be critical to trip success. Tire blowout, brake failure, fog, icy roads, and human errors are examples of contingencies present during the operation of motor vehicles.

Task descriptions are statements of those events which constitute the interactions of drivers and other highway users with their vehicles and with the highway environments. These are statements which specify exactly *what* it is that the operator vehicle units are doing. They provide the kind of information to which all subsequent plans for operators in the system must constantly be referred. They evolve into statements of human performance requirements.

When properly stated, the task descriptions serve as a basis for writing instructional objectives in terms of what the students should be able to accomplish. Generally, the level of detail for specifying task activities is about the same as that used in a good manual of instruction for a beginner. In fact, a good set of task descriptions could be utilized as a procedural manual.

The term "task," as used here, is defined as a major operation to be performed by the driver or the man-vehicle unit in the system as part of a given trip. It consists of a group of activities that often occur in close proximity with the same displays and controls and that have a common purpose. Each task such as route finding, cornering, and the selection of a safe field of travel may be performed many times within a given trip. Some may be discrete while others, like tracking and speed control, are continuous.

Major tasks are broken into subtasks and task elements. Subtasks are those components of the task in which the operations performed are quite dependent upon each other and are performed sequentially as a unit. Task elements are the psychomotor activities performed by the operator. Since the driver performs a number of interrelated subtasks simultaneously, it becomes necessary to identify their interrelationships. Such subtasks can then be ordered into a hierarchy that can assist in describing the organizational content of driving.

DRIVING TASK MODEL

Using information derived from driving task descriptions and analysis, it is possible to design a suitable driving model for instructional purposes. The interaction of the major HTS components are shown in Figure 5. In man-machine systems the most important function for man is usually decision-making. Therefore, the driving task model used for curriculum development in this guide is one which has, for its major point of reference or orientation, the making of responsible decisions. Heretofore, several models of the driving task included decision-making as a significant function, but the major emphasis has been on one or more other important factors such as observing, guidance, interpretation of traffic situations, planning, foresight, identification of hazards, judgment, analysis, and attention.

In the HTS there is a driver in a vehicle, with or without passengers, on a roadway that has geometric features within a varied environmental setting. There are many other vehicle-driver units on this road. The road that the driver is using is part of an existing highway system of other roads with similar or different traffic environmental conditions. This system has a multitude of origins, destinations, geometric designs, traffic features, and facilities. The driver must have strategies and tactics which will enable him to perform the task of moving his vehicle efficiently, safely, and conveniently to his destination.

On a typical trip once the qualified driver has determined the starting time and general route, he must choose a series of specific paths along which he can safely operate his motor vehicle. In following these many paths, he will encounter a variety and multitude of traffic situations generated by the interaction of other highway users and the various traffic elements present. To make wise choices and take proper actions under these conditions, the driver must continuously make accurate sensory perceptions, estimates of spatial relationships, and predictive or value judgments. When called for, applicable stored knowledge from related experiences is integrated with incoming data. All these actions as illustrated in Figure 6, are integrated or interact in such a way as to form what may be classified as an operational cycle. Many times before such a cycle is completed, a special form of perceptual feedback occurs which is the result of the continuous sensory impressions interacting with formulative or stored experiences. Such feedback could indicate a need for further information or validation of the mental actions up to that moment. Depending on the interpretations made, the cycle in process could be interrupted, resumed, or abandoned as the circumstances may dictate. During the operation of vehicle controls, other sensory feedback is received as a result of neuromuscular performances. Finally, there is an evaluation of the direction and movement of the vehicle to determine whether or not the time-space placement is in accord with the chosen plans.

Based on this brief analysis of the driving task, it should be obvious that the role of the driver in the HTS is primarily that of processing information and making decisions. Physical skills are important, but they are easily mastered by almost everyone. Using the brake, accelerator, and steering at different times to varying extents are not particularly difficult skills. The difficult aspect of the driving task is the mental ability involved in deciding what control to use, when to use it, and to what extent. Involved also are the social responsibilities and assessments of risks. The fact that the modern high-powered automobile is relatively easy to operate

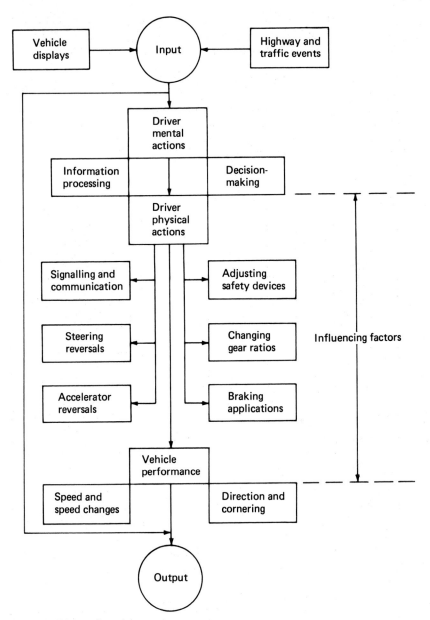

Figure 5 Driving task model.

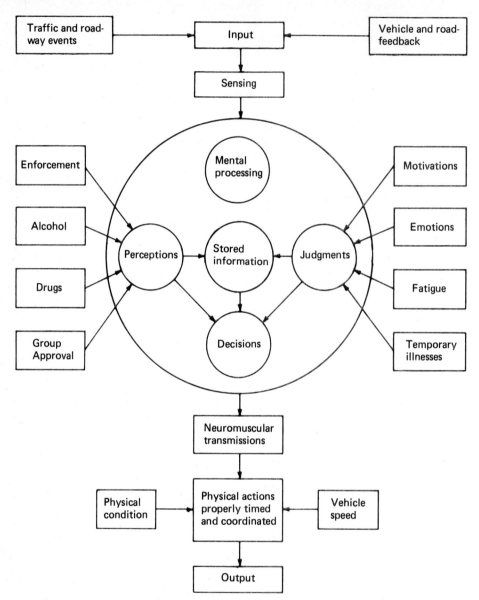

Figure 6 Human functions required for driving task.

from a physical standpoint makes the job of education and training more difficult because one first has to overcome the belief that there is nothing to it.

The various types of information processing functions are usually difficult to distinguish when they occur together in the same situation. Such processes cannot be observed directly, but may be inferred from some end results. The fact that the human being is so complex and variable makes it impossible to describe driver functions except in general terms. Until more specific research is available, we should be able to make considerable progress by assuming that human information processing and decision-making when driving is in no fundamental way different from that required for similar kinds of human activities.

HUMAN FUNCTIONS REQUIRED

Sensory Perception—In the HTS, the interaction among drivers, vehicles, and highway environment is never static in a significant sense. Rather, it is a combination of physical and perceptual factors typically changing in split seconds. Therefore, driving involves the perceptual organization of complex stimuli which must be accomplished within a given time in a given situation. This involves human sensing and identification of the pertinent traffic events or elements.

Through visual perception the driver learns of the presence of pedestrians, the presence and meaning of traffic controls, of the roadway conditions, and the number, position, movement, and speed of other vehicles. He must observe and identify many events from all directions that are related to his vehicle movement. Since the driver's senses are usually being exposed to more traffic stimuli than he can become aware of, it is necessary that he follow a process of selecting, sorting, and organizing those key events which will affect his progress. Therefore, it is important that beginning drivers be taught a process for systematic and efficient information gathering under a time constraint.

It is rather obvious that visual perception does develop significantly as a result of the various activities encountered by the human in normal life situations. However, in almost every field of endeavor the perceptions of the well-trained person are keener, more critical, and more analytical than those of the novice. In the case of automobile driving, the consequences are too great to limit the development of visual perceptions to random experiences.

An analysis and interpretation needs to be made of the traffic or elements perceived. Basically, this involves the estimation of speed-space-time factors, the evaluation of the hazards present, and the assessing of risks involved.

The driver must operate in close proximity to other vehicles of different sizes and speeds going in the same and opposite directions. He must also operate on highways and streets where there are areas of limited space due to curbs, embankments, and other obstacles. As a result, the driver must develop a good sense of lateral judgment.

Proper timing of vehicle movements or maneuvers is essential in order to avoid conflicts with other HTS users. In order to achieve proper timing, the driver must judge to some extent the performance capabilities of his own vehicle and those of other vehicles. He must be able to estimate speeds or changes in speeds, stopping distances, safe following distances, and the time or distance required for the changes in direction. For example, the passing driver will need to judge how fast the lead vehicle is traveling, how fast oncoming vehicles are traveling, and when an acceptable gap exists for the maneuver. This also assumes the driver can judge the acceleration potential of his car at the given speed before passing, and that his car is functioning properly. In any such maneuver the driver will also need to determine whether or not adequate traction can be maintained under the circumstances being encountered.

A most important class of judgments required of drivers is the prediction of other highway users' actions or behavior. In most real driving situations, there are usually other drivers and pedestrians present. Generally, the rules of the road can provide a valid set of assumptions about what the behavior of other drivers is likely to be. However, with such a large number and variety of drivers or pedestrians using the HTS, errors and deviant acts on the part of others can be and must be expected.

To be able to predict the hazardous moves other drivers might make requires the ability to interpret the behavior of these drivers. The behavior of other drivers may be based on the physical characteristics of the persons, the type of automobiles being driven, and the kind of roadway or traffic conditions being encountered.

To achieve a safe pathway for travel also requires the appraisal of the traffic events or elements for their hazard potential. To determine whether or not an event or object is hazardous requires the person to classify his perceptions into categories of "expected effects" rather than just appearances. Will the activity of the other vehicle or surface conditions possibly cause loss of traction? Will an object obstruct the view or lessen the visibility of one or more of the highway users? Some events or objects may be unpredictable and, hence, call for special attention.

Once the driver has assessed the nature of the hazards and their probability for happening, he must determine the level of risk involved. The risks to be taken are dependent to a great extent on the accuracy of the evaluation of consequences for the various hazards and the willingness of a person to gamble with certain true odds.

For each of the various hazards that are identified, it is necessary for the driver to estimate the consequences. There is a need to associate potential dangers with current spatial relationships. The probability of a serious conflict or collision must be estimated for each of the alternatives available. When a collision appears unavoidable, consideration should be given to minimize the impact.

In the present highway transportation system the individual driver is entrusted with the responsibility for making most of his own traffic decisions. In metropolitan areas it has been estimated that each driver is confronted with about 100 decisions for each mile traveled. Of these, at least 20 decisions require some action, generally of an evasive or defensive nature.

The decisions that must be made are many and varied. To begin with, the driver must select a general route to follow and a time to start in order to arrive at his destination on time. All along the selected route the driver must choose a series of specific pathways along which he can safely guide his vehicle. Then he must decide when, where, what, and how much action to take.

Many situations the driver encounters have limited alternatives, so the decisions about what action to take are simple. Other situations may call for decisions that are difficult and complex. Some may be difficult because the driver is required to hold so much information in his head at the same time or he may need to make a series of decisions in a short span of time. Some are continuous such as those related to speed or direction; some are general and long range; others are critical and specific.

Decision-making, as required in driving, generally has to do with those mental processes that lead to the selection "one" from among a known set of response alternatives. Because of the consequences, the goal for decision-making during driving becomes one of being able to select with a high degree of certainty the best alternative. This means that practice in making the various types of driving decisions is a necessity.

At times the driver may encounter traffic situations that are rather uncommon and quite complex. In these situations it may be possible that a selection will have to be made from responses and resources not already known by the driver. Such situations as these will call for mental activities that can be classified as problem-solving.

After making a decision or selecting a course of action, the driver is required to translate his solution into an appropriate physical response. First, he must translate the results of his analysis into a set of instructions. Second, he must act physically on the vehicle controls to make the vehicle conform to his course of action. He must turn the steering wheel, accelerate, decelerate, brake, change gear ratios, signal, or use various safety devices. Certain kinesthetic cues such as road feedback will enable him to make any necessary corrections or adjustments. At times a high degree of coordination is required between the feet, hands, and eyes. Many such responses will need to become semiautomatic or habitual. These control actions must be performed under static and dynamic conditions, and they may vary somewhat from vehicle to vehicle.

STORED INFORMATION—What information is needed for performance of the driving task? Certainly a driver must have a store of prior knowledge for gaining an understanding of what the traffic situations demand and upon which to base his decisions and actions related to control of his vehicle. Experience and information stored in one's memory can have a profound effect on what he perceives, how he interprets, and, therefore, what decision he makes.

There are two classes of stored or retained information that are essential to the safe operation of motor vehicles. These are the long-term and short-term retention of information.

There are two classes of stored or retained information that are essential to the safe operation of motor vehicles. These are the long-term and short-term retention of information.

Long-term retention is like a set of instructions that have been programmed into the mind and are valid over any and all cycles of the task operations. To interpret or classify inputs in terms of their effects, the driver must use rules that are stored in his long-term memory and that represent alternative courses of action.

Long-term retention includes classifications, nomenclature, and background knowledge for interpretations of perceptual information, as well as memory of procedures for maneuvers. All estimates or predictions required by the driver are based upon rules stored in memory, such as rules of the road, rules for vehicular dynamics, and rules having to do with human behavior in general. For the more complex decision-making or problem-solving situations, the driver will need to recall concepts and general rules or strategies from which inferences can be deduced. Then there are the large number of potential emergency conditions for which required procedures may be critical to the performance of infrequently practiced tasks.

Another important category of information that should be readily available to the driver is the knowledge of those factors that can impair or adversely affect his driving proficiency. The driver needs to be able to recognize those psychophysio-logical conditions or social factors which can improve or impair one's driving capabilities. Knowledge about the effects of alcohol on his driving competencies is also a prerequisite for the responsible driver. In addition, he will want to be informed about those practical control or compensatory measures that can be taken.

Short-term retention of information is peculiar to a single task or cycle of operations which must be retained for seconds, minutes, or even hours. These data are generally combined with other information and retained for use at the proper time. This type of retention has a distinctively limited capacity as compared with long-term memory.

A most important and frequent use of short-term retention for the motorist has to do with route finding and the processing of information from signs, signals, and roadway markings. The driver must also memorize temporarily the configuration of traffic around him while carrying out his own maneuvers. The range and precision of such short-term memory can be a significant factor in becoming proficient at making decisions.

Driving a modern automobile presents us with an interesting paradox. To the casual observer, the ability to drive a car safely may consist merely of acquiring a few simple psycho-motor skills in addition to learning the "Rules of the Road." From this viewpoint and with all the power assists, plus an automatic transmission, driving does appear to be becoming easier and simpler; however, driving is really a complex task. We now know that competent drivers do not just guide vehicles. They are involved in a complex and constant process of observing, evaluating, and deciding how best to control the speed and position of the car in order to achieve the safe and efficient movement of the car. An efficient and sure means of communication must be used between driver and driver, driver and pedestrian, and from the highway system to the driver. We are finally beginning to recognize that driving is not just a physical task; it is primarily a mental and social task.

Since driving requires a type of social interaction and interdependence, it involves the thinking and actions of millions of people. The maintenance and the strategic operation of motor vehicles must be accomplished by the HTS users who think, plan, and make decisions. These required behavioral patterns evolve from learning experiences. From learning, man develops the set of expectations, com-mitments, correlations, and judgments upon which sound driving decisions are made. This process is expedited through formal training and supervised practice.

Driving an automobile is a task which is learned and one that does not emerge on the basis of growth processes. As such, the individual needs a set of learning experiences that will enable him to achieve acceptable levels of performance proficiency. The all-pervasive role of the automobile in our society, the large number who drive, and the costs associated with malperformance are compelling reasons for formal programs to be included in general education programs of public schools.

If we are to accept today's challenge of highway traffic safety, a systematic analysis of the driving task should be the basis for program development. We must ask two questions. What does a safe driver really need to know? How can we teach young drivers so that their behavioral patterns can be influenced to the point they will become competent and responsible drivers? The task analysis approach can be used to define the scope and breadth that driver education must take in order to meet the challenge it faces.

From a task analysis of driving, it can be inferred that it is the errors in observation, decisions, or actions which can and do lead to hazardous situations, near collisions, collisions, injuries, and fatalities. Therefore, the content of our driver education course should be selected on the basis of the perceptions, judgments, decisions, and actions that are required in everyday traffic situations including emergencies. Furthermore, a careful study should be included of the various factors which affect man's ability to perceive, to make judgments, and to make decisions, and take actions that are involved in driving. Teachers will need to know the best methods for the development and improvement of these abilities, as well as the skills or habits involved in learning to drive.

By its very nature the analysis of the driving task contributes to the formulation of instructional objectives in terms of desired behavioral outcomes. The basis for selecting the required concepts and generalizations is also provided. In addition, the method leads to a structure for classifying and organizing knowledge that can be useful for organizing and administering the instructional program. By using this approach there should evolve a program of training and education that is comprehensive, relevant, motivating, and measurable.

GENERAL OBJECTIVES FOR DRIVER EDUCATION

The general objective of the HTS is the safe and efficient movement of people and goods from one location to another. This objective is accomplished by men who operate vehicles and communicate with other users in a network of streets and highways under a variety of contingencies. It is important that each user clearly understand this system objective and that his actions are in accord. Furthermore, they should recognize their role in achieving this system objective and the consequences of errors on their part or on the part of others.

The goal of driver education is the development of traffic citizens who will be competent and responsible users of the highway transportation system. To achieve this goal the following general objectives as derived from the driving task model are suggested:

1. The students are able to recognize and define automobile driving as primarily a mental and social task involving the interaction of men and vehicles with the highway environment in a rather complex highway transportation system whose malfunction results in serious economic and social consequences.

2. The students can apply in a variety of highway traffic situations learned information about traffic laws and regulations, vehicle capabilities and limitations, vehicle operational practices, and highway environmental features.

3. The students can demonstrate those mental and physical competencies, including appropriate strategies and tactics, for driving proficiently along safe and legal pathways in a variety of highway system environments under varying conditions and contingencies.

4. The students have information that will enable them to determine a set of strategies for preventing various psychological, physiological, social, or other factors from having an adverse effect on one's ability to perform the driving task in a proficient manner.

5. The students can define the legal and moral responsibilities of highway users necessary for the safe and efficient operation of the highway transportation system; they have those concepts and values which will predispose them to accept such responsibilities.

UNITS OF INSTRUCTION

UNIT 1.0   NATURE OF THE DRIVING TASK

Unit 1.0 attempts to give the student a general orientation and overview of the course. Such an introduction not only provides a base line or road map for future reference and the development of specific goals, but can also establish the motivational background for student learning which can continue throughout the course. In essence this first part tries to answer the questions, "Why am I here? What can I hope to accomplish? What will I be doing?"

The orientation provides a motivational background for the student by giving a description of the features of the system and the task requirements. The student gets acquainted with the purpose of the system at large and, more specifically, the functions of the operator performing the driving task. He will also get, as part of his orientation, some general information on how the system malfunctions to enable him to better appreciate and later anticipate these disturbances and failures that are a part of the operational environment whenever he is a user of the system.

Along with the establishment of goals and motivations, there needs to be initiated the development of fundamental concepts or generalizations which can serve as dominant themes and rationales throughout the course. For example, it is necessary at the outset for the student to recognize that automobile driving takes place in a system, a highway transportation system, and that this system is complex and extremely important in our way of life. As only one of several million users of the system, the student can begin to develop a sense of pride and shared responsibility for the efficient operation of this vital system. He should also begin to comprehend that automobile driving today is primarily a mental and social task.

In a complex system like the highway transportation system, it is not sufficient for the vehicle operators to be competent at their individual task. In addition, each operator of a vehicle needs to understand the relationship of his task to the functioning of the total system. At all times he driver should be able to relate his individual objectives to the goals of the system. In general the student should clearly recognize that what he learns or does is not only important to himself but to the system as well.

NATURE OF THE DRIVING TASK

EPISODE 1.1 General Nature of Our Highway Transportation System
EPISODE 1.2 Role of the Driver in the HTS
EPISODE 1.3 HTS Failures and Their Consequences

The basis for the instructional program is an analysis of the driving task. In order to define the driving task, it is necessary to have a brief description of the highway transportation system. When this transportation system is not functioning efficiently, serious traffic problems are generated. It is because of the serious nature and broad scope of the highway traffic problem that driver and traffic safety education can be justified.

UNIT OBJECTIVE   The student can describe and define the general nature of the driving task in our complex highway transportation system (HTS) and the consequences of system failures.

UNITS 2.0, 3.0, AND 4.0   BASIC KNOWLEDGE AND SKILLS FOR VEHICLE OPERATION

In order to properly develop the human functions and abilities required for the driving task, it is first necessary to build up a file of usable information as outlined in Units 2–4. Past experiences and information that have been stored in the driver's memory can have a pronounced effect on what is perceived. A body of related information is also a prerequisite for making sound judgments and formulating wise decisions. Fortunately, most students already have a rich background of experience that has provided them with a reservoir of manipulative skills and information related to motor-vehicle operation. A diagnostic testing program can help determine the extent of each pupil's entering behaviors.

The instructional materials to be selected for these units are best limited to those required for competent operation of the vehicle in the more common and less complex environments. This is in keeping with the principle that we learn and recall best that which is meaningful and has immediate application. In these beginning units, four major categories of knowledge emerge that can be utilized, expanded upon, and reinforced in the duration of the course. These categories are: rules and regulations, vehicle capabilities and limitations, vehicle operational practices, and pertinent physical environmental features.

UNIT 2   TRAFFIC LAWS AND RULES FOR DRIVER PERFORMANCE

EPISODE 2.1 Signs, Markings, and Signal Controls
EPISODE 2.2 Right-of-Way Regulations and Speed Restrictions
EPISODE 2.3 Laws for Specifying Maneuvers

A most important attribute of any complex system involving numerous man-machine units is the set of procedures or practices that need to be followed for its safe and efficient operation. These procedures and rules usually evolve with the use of the system, and in the case of HTS, are subject to change. Traffic regulations establish the specifications for conventional behavior so that all drivers have an equal chance to reach their destination with a minimum of frustration and inconvenience.

These traffic laws and rules that regulate or assist in the formulation of strategy for movement are learned and followed in a more effective manner when they are studied in the context where they are applied. This also gives an opportunity for introducing learning activities involving the various environmental conditions or events. Those traffic laws which deal with driver condition and responsibility will be introduced toward the end of the course. Once the student has a perspective of the total driving task, he can then develop a better rationale for the enactment and enforcement of this type of law.

UNIT OBJECTIVE The students are able to define traffic regulations and their requirements and recognize the various situations or conditions under which they apply.

UNIT 3.0   VEHICLE PERFORMANCE AND CONTROL CAPABILITIES

UNIT OBJECTIVE The student can define and recognize, in a manner sufficient for safe and effective operation, the capabilities and limitations of motor vehicles under the various conditions to be found in the HTS; he recognizes that a wide range of performance capabilities exists among the different vehicles used in the HTS.

EPISODE 3.1 General Performance Capabilities for Motor Vehicles
EPISODE 3.2 Vehicles with Reduced or Increased General Performance Characteristics
EPISODE 3.3 Factors and Forces That Affect Vehicle Control Systems

If the driver is to keep his motor vehicle under control, he must have a knowledge of its capabilities and limitations. The automobile is a machine that is capable of a certain range of performance. To make the necessary judgments and decisions in driving requires that the operator know what vehicles can or cannot do under various conditions. Such knowledge is also required for predicting the possible actions of other drivers. It does not seem necessary or advantageous to introduce driver actions in this unit.

UNIT 4.0   HABITS AND SKILLS FOR VEHICLE OPERATIONS AND MANEUVERS (Example of complete unit)

EPISODE 4.1 Predriving Habits
EPISODE 4.2 Operation of Vehicle Controls
EPISODE 4.3 Procedures and Skills for Routine Maneuvers

4–6 LAB AND CLASS HOURS

The actual control of the automobile is dependent upon the driver's physical ability to operate the controls for movement and guidance. Motor skills are also necessary for the operation of various devices or switches such as turn signals, lights, horn, windshield wipers, defroster, ventilators, etc. Since the timing and coordination are critical, these skills and abilities need to be developed into fixed habits before the driver can operate in traffic with any degree of safety.

For efficient and effective learning of such skills to take place, it is necessary that students have an understanding of the purpose or function of the controls and the reasons for given sequential procedures to be followed. These skills and related information are acquired from progressive experiences provided in the classroom and laboratory as needed. Therefore, learning activities in this unit are usually integrated with those of other units.

UNIT OBJECTIVE **The student is able to identify and operate skillfully the vehicle control systems, safety devices, and accessories in accordance with given safe and efficient procedures; he can define and demonstrate the proper procedures and skills for routine maneuvers.**

EPISODE 4.1 Predriving Habits

EPISODE OBJECTIVE **The student can describe and demonstrate pre-driving checks or habits.**

4.11 Outside predriving checks
4.12 Seat adjustment, seat belts, and mirrors
4.13 Safety devices, controls, and accessories

EPISODE 4.2 Operation of Vehicle Controls

EPISODE OBJECTIVE **The student can demonstrate skill in the operation of vehicle controls for moving and stopping the car**

4.21 Starting the engine, idling, and securing car
4.22 Moving the car forward and backward-tracking
4.23 Deceleration and downshifting
4.24 Braking to a stop

EPISODE 4.3 Procedures and Skills for Routine Maneuvers

EPISODE OBJECTIVE **The student can describe and demonstrate pre-driving checks or habits.**

4.31 Signaling and communication
4.32 Lane changing
4.33 Cornering and turning
4.34 Turning the car around
4.35 Passing and being overtaken
4.36 Parking
4.37 Merging with high speed traffic

SUGGESTED LEARNING ACTIVITIES UNIT 4.0

1. Identify, classify, and list in proper sequence the procedures for various actions and maneuvers; student can justify the sequences. (Safety and legal reasons or efficiency.)

2. Diagram and label the recommended steps for performing certain maneuvers.

3. Demonstrate the correct procedures, habits, and skills in laboratory lessons.

4. Name by listing each of the information instruments, regulating switches, driving control devices, and safety aid devices found in a typical automobile.

5. Describe the function and operation of each of the regulating switches.

6. Explain how the proper use of each safety aid or device increases the safety and well-being of each person using them. Describe the proper use and function of each device.

7. Describe where each of the instruments, switches, and devices of the four groups is located. You may wish to diagram (using labels) the instrument panel and driving cockpit of your family car or other vehicle. Include the driving controls in their approximate location.

8. Construct a diagram of the instrument panel and driving cockpit of a (1) bus, (2) truck, (3) sports car, (4) foreign car, or (5) vehicle of your choice.

9. Describe the proper body position for operating a motor vehicle that is (a) moving forward, (b) backing straight, and (c) making a backing turn.

10. Create a standard operating procedures (SOP) check list that a driver could use and should perform before, during, and after a trip.

UNITS 5.0, 6.0, 7.0   DRIVING STRATEGIES AND TACTICS

Basic to the development of effective driving performance is the recognition that there exists a repeated and integrated cycle of man-machine unit operations. From the driving model adopted in . . . this guide, it is clear that perception, judgment, and decision-making are considered as critical in driving as the motor skills of controlling the vehicle. Although these human functions or abilities and their related skills are integrated into observable classes of behavior, there seems to be no doubt that errors or poor performance can occur at any point in the cycle and in a combination of one or more. Therefore, it is important to set up separate training programs and evaluative criteria for each definitive ability. For each of these abilities, which must be practiced if proficiency is to be acquired, there is a body of knowledge that must be integrated for proper training to take place.

When the motor vehicle is being operated in the HTS, the driver will come upon a variety of road and traffic situations, some of which may tax his capabilities to the limit. This broad scope and range in the complexity of traffic situations that the driver faces is what makes the task of the driver educator so difficult. It becomes obvious that the broader the learning the better able the driver will be to cope with the variety of problems encountered in the HTS. Since the tremendous variety of driving situations far exceeds man's capacity to retain and utilize information, a basic goal of this part of the curriculum is " learning to learn" by the student. This is a kind of learning which enables the student, without further teaching, to continue to cope with new situations and problems. Therefore, the structure of the content is oriented toward the kinds of traffic situations to be encountered rather than the types of environmental settings.

Of critical importance is the classification of various traffic and driving situations into categories that can provide for this broader type of learning experience and effective transfer of training. Training opportunities may then be programmed into the classroom and laboratory which can provide a rich background of experience equivalent to the two or three years driving experience that the average beginning driver now picks up on a trial and error basis. Training exercises in the classroom can be presented with slides, transparencies, film strips, and on motion picture loops of the desired scenes. Learning experiences in the laboratory should be correlated closely with those in the classroom.

In the laboratory the teacher should choose routes with as many varied experiences as practical and work for general patterns of action so that transfer to similar situations will take place in the future. Attention will need to be given to the hazardous elements that may be common to many situations. This means an analysis of many local hazardous situations will be conducted to find out what these common elements are.

This is the most important part of the curriculum and should serve as the focal point for the development of learning experiences in other units. It is recommended that the units in this part be coordinated with those in other parts in such a manner as to facilitate continuous referral throughout the entire driver education course.

UNIT 5.0   PERCEPTION OF SYSTEM EVENTS

EPISODE 5.1 Nature of Sensory Perception
EPISODE 5.2 Principles for Efficient Observation and Perception
EPISODE 5.3 Identification of Significant HTS Events and Cues

Driving decisions and performance to a large extent depend on a clear, complete, and accurate picture of the immediate surroundings. Wherever a driver fails to perceive important events related to driving, there is a reasonable chance for an improper action with serious consequences. Any substantial misrepresentation of things as they really are is also a serious handicap to safe driving. A driver's habits of comprehending the driving scene show up clearly in his timing of routine action in traffic.

The critical factor for perception in traffic is the ability of the driver to use his sensory capacities in a systematic way. Under the pressure of time, the driver must develop efficient observational and identification procedures. This unit should include visual training to increase the rapidity of observation, as well as to increase the span of recognition of the individual. Such exercise can also demonstrate the need for alertness and the procedures for its development. It is recommended that the classroom training program be initiated in Unit 2.0 with the use of digit and sign slides.

In the laboratory the teacher should have the student master the basic motor skills of car operation before beginning intensive training in "reading" the traffic scene. Undue attention to motor skills will tend to interfere with training for visual perception except that which is needed to learn such skills. When these operational tasks become semiautomatic so that drivers no longer have to formulate the acts in the mind, then, attention is freed for perception of the total traffic scene.

UNIT OBJECTIVE The student is able to demonstrate the ability to observe and recognize, in an efficient and effective manner, the pertinent HTS events and conditions for vehicle guidance along selected routes.

UNIT 6.0   JUDGMENT OF SYSTEM EVENTS

UNIT OBJECTIVE   The student is able to make judgments of traffic situations, evaluate highway characteristics, traffic control and weather conditions, estimate spatial relationships, and predict the behavior of other highway users.

EPISODE 6.1 Concepts and Principles for Improvement of Judgmental Abilities
EPISODE 6.2 Evaluation of Highway Characteristics, Traffic Controls, and Weather Conditions
EPISODE 6.3 Prediction of the Probable Behavior of Other Highway Users
EPISODE 6.4 Estimation of Spatial Relationships

Once the driver perceives the traffic situation at hand, he must then interpret and evaluate the various actions and system events for their hazards and risks so he can select the best path and speed to take. This calls for the ability to make judgments.

Judgment in driving may be defined as the cognitive process of categorizing input from the traffic scene in terms of effects, rather than in terms of appearances. It is a process of relating what is perceived to the stored information and experiences pertinent to the situation being encountered. Therefore, most of the information required for making sound judgments should have been learned in previous units.

Specific judgments can be developed or improved to a high degree through proper training and structured experiences. The training program should focus on driving input, subtasks to be performed, and relevant stored information. Such a program should introduce certain regularities into sequences so the driver can better prepare and organize his responses. As a result, many of the intellectual tasks, which are rather difficult initially, may become simple procedural tasks with minor perceptual control.

UNIT 7.0   DECISION-MAKING FOR A PLAN OF ACTION

EPISODE 7.1 Principles and Procedure for Making Decisions
EPISODE 7.2 Driving Decisions for Various Traffic Situations
EPISODE 7.3 Pretrip Planning

6–10 LAB AND CLASS HOURS

In any man-machine system the men are the decision-makers; they control and are responsible for the power of the machine. For the motor vehicle operator decisions range in their complexity from those that are virtually automatic or predetermined by the situation to those that are based on a variety of complex judgments. Some traffic situations are so complex that the real meaningful information is often camouflaged to such an extent that only a trained observer can analyze it properly for the best course of action. Decision-making is further complicated because of the limited time span.

Decision-making by drivers involves mental processing that leads to the selection of a response from among a learned set of alternatives. Even in the simplest driving tasks, alternatives are usually available to the operator. This means that a training program should be required that can be applied through performance to the driving task. The training media, both simulated and actual, should include driving situations that depict uncertainty, complexity of events, limited time, and conflict among alternatives. Instruction for route selection should also be based on principles of decision-making applicable to driving.

UNIT OBJECTIVE   The student is able to determine an appropriate plan of action, including strategies and tactics required to carry out the plan, for various traffic situations that are to be encountered under varying conditions and contingencies.

UNITS 8.0, 9.0, 10.0, 11.0, and 12.0   HIGHWAY USER RESPONSIBILITIES

In the complex highway transportation system that has evolved, much more than competent vehicle operators is required. The users of the HTS need to become responsible and safe users if the system is to operate effectively. Real safety requires that self-control, insight, and a sense of responsibility be present. The last five units are concerned primarily with driver condition and responsibilities.

The program of instruction in the first seven units has been intentionally limited to those learning activities that are directly related to the development of a competent driver. Once the student has learned the role certain human functions have in driving, and the proficiency levels that must be obtained, he is then psychologically ready to study those factors which can impair or adversely affect his driving proficiency. As a responsible user of the HTS, he will be faced with decisions as how best to handle such influences either as a driver or pedestrian.

Units 8.0 and 9.0 include those factors and conditions which can adversely affect both the physical and mental abilities that are required of man when driving. Some factors, such as emotions and fatigue, are internal to man; others are external like alcohol, drugs, and social forces. A knowledge and understanding of the various influential factors present should enable the driver to realistically assess his capability to drive at any given time. He should also be able to evaluate the proficiency levels of other drivers with which he, or other members of his family, may wish to ride.

The last three units are derived from the basic requirements for responsible driving that have been enacted into law. These requirements are: (1) be a licensed and qualified driver, (2) know and obey prescribed "Rules of the Road," (3) operate the vehicle in a reasonable and prudent manner at all times, (4) have a registered and mechanically safe vehicle, (5) never operate a motor vehicle under the influence of intoxicating liquor or other drugs which render the driver incapable of safe operation, (6) perform certain duties and assume prescribed responsibilities in the event of involvement in a traffic accident, and (7) know and observe pedestrian rights and duties.

It should be assumed that these are basic or minimum requirements. A competent and responsible driver should have pride in achieving much more than the minimum standards. He should want to earn the praise of his peers and develop a self-image of always being known for performing to the best of his ability. He should continually strive for that degree of excellence of which he is capable.

These units, when properly taught, not only promote greater safety on the highways, but also provide an excellent medium for the development of self-control, accurate thinking, and personal and social responsibility. Social responsibilities are more easily taught in connection with an activity that the student feels to be vitally significant. If we are successful in doing this, our youthful drivers can become the best drivers on the highways.

UNIT 8.0   DRIVER CONDITION AND BEHAVIOR

EPISODE 8.1 Functions of the Human Brain Related to Driving
EPISODE 8.2 General Physical Conditions Which Can Affect Driving Capability
EPISODE 8.3 Emotions and Their Effect on Driving Proficiency
EPISODE 8.4 Motivations for Responsible Driving

How one performs the driving task in various traffic situations depends somewhat on his emotional state, his motivations, and his general physical health. Therefore, it is important that the beginning driver be able to recognize how certain emotional responses or actions of self-expression can affect his driving efficiency. No one is immune to emotional upsets and physical ills, so it is necessary to learn how to handle such factors in order that they do not seriously affect, temporarily, one's driving ability.

UNIT OBJECTIVE   The student can determine a set of strategies for preventing certain psychophysiological factors or social forces from having an adverse effect on his driving proficiency.

UNIT 9.0   ALCOHOL AND OTHER DRUGS

EPISODE 9.1 Nature and Scope of Drinking-Driving Problem
EPISODE 9.2 Effect of Alcohol on the Body as Related to Driving Task
EPISODE 9.3 Concepts, Definitions, and Classifications of Drugs and Their Effect on Driving Abilities
EPISODE 9.4 Legislation, Enforcement, and Controls for Drinking-Driving and Drug Abuse Problems

From a study of prevailing research and statements by respected scientists, it can be concluded that the driving ability for some persons will definitely become impaired with a blood alcohol concentration of 0.05 per cent, and that the driving ability of all persons is impaired by the time the blood alcohol level reaches 0.10 per cent. Unfortunately, many alcohol impaired persons have performed the driving task several times without adverse effects because of chance factors. Such experiences can lead to misconceptions about one's ability to drive with relatively high blood alcohol level in spite of statistics to the contrary.

Alcohol and other drugs have a serious effect on the driving task because of the fact that only slight amounts are necessary to affect those mental functions that we use to control our driving acts. Small amounts of alcohol and many other drugs first affect a person's restraints or inhibitions. Then a person's self-control is further weakened because his emotional drives are no longer held in check by judgment and reason. Without normal inhibitions, a driver will take risks that are both needless and dangerous.

UNIT OBJECTIVE **The student can demonstrate a knowledge of the concepts and generalizations which will enable him to make wise decisions in regard to the use of alcoholic beverages or other drugs anytime he will be using HTS as a driver, passenger, or pedestrian.**

UNIT 10.0   OBEDIENCE TO AND ENFORCEMENT OF TRAFFIC LAWS

EPISODE 10.1 The Nature and Scope of Traffic Laws
EPISODE 10.2 Enforcement of Traffic Laws
EPISODE 10.3 Interpretation of Traffic Laws Regulating HTS User Behavior or Conditions
EPISODE 10.4 Enactment and Administration of Effective Legislation and Enforcement

In a democratic and mobile society, the control and responsibility for the operation of motor vehicles rests almost completely with the individual. Traffic laws and regulations not only establish specifications for conventional behavior, but they furnish a social device for the control of those drivers who prove by their actions that they are not willing to assume the responsibilities inherent in driving.

The problem is one in which individual action is necessary, but extremely difficult to secure. The best way to influence the behavior of the driver is not by preaching slogans, using the scare technique, or bombarding him with messages which make no change in his thinking. The behavioral patterns that exhibit social respect evolve from properly chosen and guided learning experiences. From learning, man develops the set of expectations, commitments, correlations, and judgments upon which sound driving decisions are made. The more effective education, the less need for a penalizing type of enforcement.

UNIT OBJECTIVE **The student is able to determine a person's shared legal and moral responsibilities when using the HTS; he recognizes the need for a system of just traffic law enforcement.**

UNIT 11.0 POST CRASH PROCEDURES AND RESPONSIBILITIES

EPISODE 11.1 Legal and Moral Responsibilities of a Reasonable and Prudent Person
EPISODE 11.2 Insurance Protection Against Economic Consequences of Traffic Accidents

Even the most proficient and responsible drivers are subject to traffic accidents. Therefore, HTS users should know what steps to take before and afterwards in order to best protect the life, limb, property, and legal rights of those involved. Doing the right thing in the proper way at the appropriate time may save a life or minimize injuries; it will always minimize, and often avoid, legal problems.

UNIT OBJECTIVE The Students can describe and define the legal and moral responsibilities of persons involved in or driving into a traffic accident situation.

UNIT 12.0 SELECTION, INSPECTION, AND MAINTENANCE OF SAFE VEHICLES

EPISODE 12.1 Selection of Safe and Economical Equipment
EPISODE 12.2 Observation and Interpretation of Vehicle Subsystems for Proper Performance
EPISODE 12.3 Preventive Maintenance

Each individual vehicle driver or owner shares with the automobile manufacturers and service agencies the responsibility for equipping and maintaining a safe operating vehicle. Improperly equipped or maintained vehicles can, and do, lead to serious malfunctions which result in vehicle and HTS failure. To discharge this responsibility effectively requires that each driver have the knowledge and observational skill to determine whether or not his vehicle is functioning properly and is in need of maintenance or repairs. As an intelligent consumer of an expensive and complicated machine with many equipment options, the automobile driver can have a decided effect on whether or not safety is given the highest priority in production and sales of motor vehicles. The kind of vehicle and monthly installment payments may also influence the degree to which the owner can afford required maintenance or repair costs.

UNIT OBJECTIVE For the various vehicles used, the students can contrast the performance characteristics and optional equipment available in terms of safety, economy, and convenience; they can evaluate the performance or functioning of the various vehicle subsystems to determine the need for corrective maintenance or repairs.

Appendix C

HIGHWAY SAFETY PROGRAM STANDARD 4.4.3.

Each state shall have a motorcycle safety program to ensure that only persons physically and mentally qualified will be licensed to operate a motorcycle: that prospective safety equipment for drivers and passengers will be worn: and that the motorcycle meets standards for safety equipment.

A statewide motorcycle education program which provides for both classroom and laboratory instruction is a pressing need under present-day traffic conditions. It is obvious that the primary purpose of such a program should be to qualify young people for the proper and safe operation of motorcycles on streets and highways. The state should ensure that operators are properly tested and licensed, encouraged to operate in compliance with applicable traffic laws, make sure that operators and passengers wear approved protective clothing and that safety equipment is installed on all registered motorcycles, provide for inspection on a regular basis, and establish and maintain adequate records on crashes, injuries, deaths and traffic law violations.

A motorcycle, according to experienced operators, is a responsive and safe machine until it is operated by the unskilled user. It is not inherently dangerous, but it cannot be handled casually. Two things make a high level of performance necessary in cycling: first, the stability of the machine is not built-in but is provided by the operator; and second, the operator is exposed rather than protected, as is any passenger riding behind him. In the final analysis, motor vehicle safety lies in the hands and good judgment of all drivers. There is a growing need for instruction about motorcycles, not just for the cyclists but for all users of the public highways.

As people living in a highly mobile and traffic-oriented society, we must of necessity possess a foundation of traffic knowledge which will enable us as operators of motor vehicles to make the right decisions under street and highway traffic conditions. The school can be the best source for acquiring this knowledge. The need for education to respond is more and more apparent.

RESPONSIBILITY FOR MOTORCYCLE EDUCATION

Motorcycles are here to stay and registrations will continue to grow in the foreseeable future. Thus, it is incumbent upon the states and local school districts to assume responsibility for motor cycle education. New instructional programs, consisting of both classroom and controlled off-street operation, should be expanded to include motorcycle education; and curriculum objectives in traffic safety should be examined and revised, as needed, to meet the demands of the time.

Source: Office of the Superintendant of Public Instruction, Safety Education Division, *Driver Education for Illinois Youth*, 1972, pp. 133–159.

More teachers of motorcycle education will be needed during the next decade. Thus, state colleges and universities with teacher preparation programs should provide courses in motorcycle education, both theory and practice, to meet the needs of the states which they serve.

Business and industry should support motorcycle education programs as a part of traffic safety. This could take various forms, but one way would be to provide scholarships for students preparing to teach in this area.

A new dimension in traffic safety, the motorcycle, cannot be ignored by the states and local school districts without severe consequences to youth. Properly conceived and implemented, school programs in motorcycle education can be an important factor in helping to assure that those who operate or ride on motorcycles do so safely.

6.02   STATE REQUIREMENTS—SECTION 27-23, UNIFORM TRAFFIC ACT STATES THAT THE COURSE OF INSTRUCTION GIVEN IN GRADES 10 THROUGH 12 SHALL INCLUDE AN EMPHASIS ON THE DEVELOPMENT OF KNOWLEDGE, ATTITUDES, HABITS AND SKILLS NECESSARY FOR THE SAFE OPERATION OF MOTOR VEHICLES INCLUDING MOTORCYCLES INSOFAR AS THEY CAN BE TAUGHT IN THE CLASSROOM. (AMENDED BY ACT APPROVED AUGUST 11, 1967.)

An educational program, regardless of its organizational pattern, must impress youthful operators of motor vehicles that there are many things to be learned and much information to be acquired about traffic problems if they are to become proficient and safe users of public streets and highways. In nine out of ten accidents, human behavior is prominent among the contributing factors.

The following plan is recommended for incorporating motorcycle educational curricular materials in the present high school driver education program:

Incorporate into the present required thirty clock-hours of classroom Driver Education instruction an additional unit of work which would require the addition of two or three hours of instruction concerning the integration of motorcycle materials into the Driver Education Program. Also, emphasis should be placed on special legal requirements of the rider, registration of the rider, registration of the motorcycle, licensing of the motorcycle driver and special regulations applying only to the motorcycle. This was legally required of all operators of motor vehicles and motorcycle riders after January 1, 1969.

The following curriculum material is provided so that motorists might more intelligently share the highway transportation system with motorcyclists. Inasmuch as over 90 percent of the auto-cycle collisions find the former to be held legally at fault, it would appear that there is a need for educating motorists.

The numerical references interface with Section II–Curriculum, thereby making it more complete. Incorporation of this material should not be limited to the classroom instruction, but should also be used in the laboratory experiences, particularly on-street and simulation. (Italicized numerical entries were inserted for clarity. These numbers do not appear in the original curriculum.)

UNIT 1.0—NATURE OF THE DRIVING TASK

EPISODE 1.3 Highway Transportation System Failures and Their Sub-sequences

1.32 Social and economic consequences of system failure
    1.321 Number of types of accidents and trends
        –Motorcycle accidents occur during the same days of the week and hours of the day as motor vehicle accidents
        –Motorcycle accidents are more likely to occur on a clear, dry day
        –Personal injuries to the rider usually are to the head and appendages
        –In over 90 percent of car-cycle accidents, a vehicle operator cut off a cyclist
          —Driver turning left cut off approaching cyclist
          —Driver cut off riding path of cyclist when turning right
          —Other car-cycle accidents happen on the straight-away when a driver cuts off a cyclist when attempting to pass
    1.322 Accident causation factors
        –Driver did not see cycle
        –Driver saw cycle and believed he could still perform the maneuver
        –Driver saw cycle too late
        –Driver failed to yield
        –Driver was speeding
        –Driver following too closely
        –Inexperience of cyclist
        –Cyclist was distracted
        –Cyclist's emotional mood
    1.323 Costs of traffic accidents and congestion
        –Car-cycle accidents cost approximately $750 on average

SUGGESTED LEARNING ACTIVITIES   **UNIT 1.0**

1. Survey five to ten experienced automobile drivers and ask them how easy (or difficult) it is for them to distinguish motorcycles in the traffic stream.
2. Ask these drivers what percentage of car-cycle accidents are probably the fault of the auto driver; what percent are probably the fault of the cyclist?

UNIT 2.0—TRAFFIC LAWS AND RULES FOR DRIVER PERFORMANCE

EPISODE 2.2 Right-of-way Regulations and Speed Restrictions

2.25 Emergency vehicles, school buses, motorcycles and bicycles
   2.251 Cyclists must obey the same laws as other vehicle operators; therefore, they should receive the same consideration extended to others

UNIT 3.0—VEHICLE PERFORMANCE AND CONTROL CAPABILITIES

EPISODE 3.2 Vehicles with Reduced or Increased General Performance Characteristics

3.26 Motor-driven cycles and motorcycles
   3.261 Various kinds and uses—street, trail, street/trail, multi-purpose
   3.262 Acceleration capability is related to and is dependent upon the cycle's horsepower and the weight of the cyclist and his passenger and the weight of the cycle
   3.263 Acceleration capability also is reduced on an upgrade
   3.264 Directional stability and handling capability can seriously be affected by road surface
   —"Traction reducers" include: water, frost and ice, dew, gravel, sand, leaves, oil, paint strips, paper, bumps, bridge gratings, sewer covers, tree sap, grain, water from autos' air conditioners, mud and other objects on the road (Also listed under 3.316)
   3.265 A cyclist will try to maintain directional stability and handling capability by varying his lane position (Also listed under 5.332)
   3.266 Handling capability also is affected by cyclist's hand signals. Since most of his controls are hand-operated, the cyclist must temporarily take his hand off the controls to signal his intention if the vehicle is not equipped with directional signals
   —He often may supplement electric directional signals with hand signals (Also see 5.334)
   3.267 Complex handling of controls upon a variety of road surfaces, traffic and leaning attitudes of the machine make demands upon the cyclist for which he may be ill prepared due to inexperience
   3.268 Stability in turns and curves is dependent upon the road surface just before, into and just after the turn or

curve. It also is dependent upon body and machine lean (especially in crosswinds), and on passenger's weight and actions

    —Nervous or unknowledgeable passengers may not lean with the rider, thereby adversely affecting the travel path

3.269 Braking and decleration

    —Downshifting and throttling back can slow the cycle

    —Cycles are equipped with front and rear brakes which supply 70–75 percent and 25–30 percent braking power, respectively

    —Since controls are easy and close for the cyclist to operate, his reaction time may be reduced below that of an automobile driver (Also see 6.4221)

    —Under normal conditions, and up to approximately 30 mph, some cycles may be stopped in a shorter distance than other vehicles; therefore, vehicle operators should allow a greater than normal following distance when behind a cycle traveling 30 mph or below. (Also see 6.4222, 6.423, 6.4243, 7.2215)

    —Above 30 mph, many vehicles can be stopped in a shorter distance than most cycles. Above 30 mph, road surface conditions and/or the lateral slope of the road may make it difficult or impossible for the cyclist to employ 100 percent braking effort and remain upright. This is even more true in a turn or curve where the cycle is in a leaning attitude (Also see 6.4222)

EPISODE 3.3 Factors and Forces that Affect Vehicle Control Systems

3.31 Role of traction in vehicle movement and control

    3.316 Factors and conditions which affect coefficient of friction

        —Factors affecting traction include: water, frost and dew, gravel, sand, leaves, oil, paint strips, paper, bumps, bridge gratings, sewer covers, tree sap, grain, water from autos' air conditioners and other objects on the road.

3.36 Loading and load distribution

    —Passengers and luggage adversely affect a cycle's center of gravity by moving it higher and to the rear, thereby reducing the ease of handling. Passenger's space needs may cause the operator to move forward on the saddle, thereby crowding him and making it difficult to shift, brake and turn

SUGGESTED LEARNING ACTIVITIES   **UNIT 3.0**

1. Describe at least three situations in which a motorcyclist could lose control of his cycle. Explain how you, as a vehicle operator, would follow the cyclist in each of the situations you have described.
2. Discuss how you would operate a motor vehicle if you were following a cyclist carrying a passenger.

UNIT 5.0—PERCEPTION OF SYSTEM EVENTS

EPISODE 5.2 Principles for Efficient Observation and Perception

5.23 Organization and identification of data
    5.232 Concepts or laws of proximity, similarity, size, continuity and closure
        —Because of cycle size, it is difficult to estimate cycle speed (Also see 6.363)

EPISODE 5.3 Identification of Significant Highway Transportation System Events and Cues

5.33 Actions and informational cues supplied by other users
    5.331 Vehicle lights—turn signals, brake lights, etc.
        —Location of electric signals on cycles
        —Since electric signals do not cancel automatically, it is possible that the signals would remain on after the intent of their use has passed. Audible sound of signals is drowned out by engine noise
        —In order to be seen, cyclists may flash the headlight from high to low beam at intersections
        —In order to be seen, cyclists ride with the headlight on (legal requirement in Illinois) (Also see 12.111)
    5.332 Movement of cycle—speed change, direction of front wheels, exhaust fumes, weaving
        —Cyclists vary position in lane to see what is happening on the road ahead and to be seen by other drivers
        —To maintain control, cyclists usually will slow considerably before riding onto a gravel road or a road that is sprinkled with gravel
        —When approaching a sharply angled railroad crossing, a cyclist will slow and maneuver in such a way that he may cross it at nearly a right angle
        —A cyclist may modify his path of travel slightly in order to avoid road surface objects or conditions which may reduce his control
    5.334 Driver actions—hand signals, movement of head,

adjusting safety devices, talking with passengers *and other operator movements*
  —Some older cycle models are not equipped with electrical signals. Operators probably will give an interrupted hand signal to stop, slow or turn because they must simultaneously operate the clutch lever when shifting
  —Cyclists usually will lean their cycle and body when negotiating a turn (Also see 6.364)
5.34 Developing of efficient visual habits
  5.343 Scanning and search techniques
    —Because of varied lane positions, cyclists may hold on the road and check from side to side, especially at intersections, for the presence of cyclists
  5.344 Check mirrors and over shoulders regularly
    —Look for cyclists, especially in the two rear blind spots

SUGGESTED LEARNING ACTIVITIES UNIT 5.0

1. Describe what a cyclist would do if he were approaching railroad tracks. What would you, as a driver, do to allow the cyclist to cross the tracks safely?
2. Observe two unmarked intersections for fifteen minutes apiece. Note the number of cycles which travel through or turn at the intersection. Note the direction in which they travel through the intersection. List what the automobile operators are doing; i.e., tell whether the driver allows the cyclist to turn, tell whether the drivers are aware of the cyclist's presence, etc. Report your findings to class.
3. Explain how you would know that a cyclist ahead of you intends to turn right.
4. Discuss ways of detecting cyclists, especially at intersections. What clues should you look for which would help you to know the intended travel path of a cyclist? How could you avoid cutting off a cyclist if you are making a right turn?

UNIT 6.0—JUDGMENT OF SYSTEM EVENTS

EPISODE 6.3 Prediction of the Probable Behavior of Other Highway Users

6.31 Human limitations and capabilities for tasks
  —Vehicle operators and cyclists vary in their experience and ability to control their vehicles—with many being relatively inexperienced, especially early in the riding season (March–June)
6.36 Ranking of probable actions of other users based on conditions and cues given
  6.361 Common errors that can be expected for similar situations
    —Vehicle cuts off cycle
    —Left turns

   —Right turns
   –Vehicle overtaking cycle does not allow enough space for cycle after passing
   —Vehicle overtaking cycle uses part of cycle's lane
   –Vehicle tailgating cyclist

6.362 Quality of communication given and received
   –Cyclist's inability to give continuous hand signals

6.363 Prediction of speed
   –Because of cycle size, it is difficult to estimate cycle speed (assume cyclist is traveling at posted speed)
   –Noise and small size make cycles appear to be fast-moving

6.364 Prediction of direction
   –Hand or electrical signals
   —Leaving signal on after intended use—must be manually canceled
   –Body lean and lean of machine
   –Lane position
   –Varies with road surface ahead

EPISODE 6.4 Estimation of Spatial Relationships

6.41 Estimation of speeds and time intervals
  6.413 Speed and rate of closure of other traffic units
   –Cycle speed may vary in accordance with road and weather conditions, and cycle power capabilities

6.42 Judgment of distance and changing spatial relationships
  6.422 Estimation of distance for vehicle to stop or change direction
   6.4221 Mental and physical reaction time
    –Cyclist's reaction time may be faster than motorists due to location of cycle controls
   6.4222 Braking distances for various vehicles and types of brake applications under given conditions
    –At 30 mph and below, some cycles may be stopped faster than an automobile
    –At speeds over 30 mph, most cycles need a longer stopping distance than automobiles
    –To warn motorists of their intent to slow/stop, cyclists may apply the foot (rear) brake first and thus cause the taillight to glow (1969 to present—stoplight activated by either hand or foot brake)
    –When adverse road and/or weather conditions exist, cyclists will travel more slowly and brake sooner than under normal conditions

6.423 Optimum following distances for conditions and types of vehicles
  –Cyclists should be given a three-second following distance under normal conditions due to their machine's ability to stop quickly at low speeds. Under adverse road/weather conditions, follow cycles at a four-second distance (Also see 3.269)
6.424 Estimation of space required for maneuvers
  6.4243 Lane changes, intersections, interchanges, passing, parking
    –When changing lanes or passing a cyclist, allow the cyclist as much space in his lane as you would allow a motor vehicle; i.e., start change/pass far in back of cycle and do not use part of the right lane to negotiate the maneuver (Also see 7.224)
    –When returning to the right lane after passing a cycle, give the cycle an adequate "space cushion" by returning only when you can see that the cycle is behind you
    –Avoid tailgating at intersections. Also, at slow, intersection speeds, cycles may be stopped more quickly than motor vehicles

SUGGESTED LEARNING ACTIVITIES   UNIT 6.0

1. Explain how it is possible for the reaction time of a cyclist to be less than that of an automobile driver. Describe how you would interact with a cyclist on a roadway whose speed was 25 mph, 35 mph.
2. Make a chart of suggested following distances for various motor vehicles. Explain why you should follow each vehicle in the time—distance you have charted.

UNIT 7.0—DECISION MAKING FOR A PLAN OF ACTION

EPISODE 7.2 Driving Decisions for Various Traffic Situations

7.22 Decisions for common traffic situations
  7.221 Movement within traffic flow
    7.2211 Types of roadways
      –Follow cyclists at a greater distance when roadway surface is sprinkled with gravel, sand or other "traction reducers" such as chuckholes
      –Follow cyclists at a greater distance when roadway is mountainous

 7.2212 Lane selection and usage
—Allow cycle the same amount of "road space" that you would allow any other vehicle
 7.2213 Lane changing *and passing*
—Look for a cycle *ahead* of a vehicle you may be passing
—Allow cyclist to "own" his whole (legal) portion of a travel lane
 7.2215 Following and being followed
—Allow more space ahead of your vehicle if cyclist ahead of you must cross railroad tracks
—Use a three-second following distance
—At speeds under 30 mph, allow a four-second following distance
—When being followed, signal early
 7.222 Intersections
 7.2221 Uncontrolled and controlled ·
—Signal intentions early
—Look for cyclists entering your right or left turning paths and yield to them
—Allow a cyclist the same courtesy you would an automobile operator
 7.224 Passing and being passed (Also see 6.4243)

SUGGESTED LEARNING ACTIVITIES UNIT 7.0

1. Diagram and explain what actions you would take as a vehicle operator in the following situations: (a) vehicle turning left in front of cycle, (b) vehicle turning right in front of cycle, (c) vehicle pulling in front of a cycle from a crossroad, driveway or alley, (d) vehicle tailgating a cyclist, (e) vehicle overtaking cycle, (f) cycle overtaking a vehicle, (g) cycle overtaking a vehicle on right, (h) vehicle following cyclist, (i) cycle following a truck or large vehicle, (j) cycle riding at a corner where vehicles are parked, (k) cyclist carrying a passenger.

UNIT 8.0—DRIVER CONDITION AND BEHAVIOR

EPISODE 8.2 General Physical Conditions Which Can Affect Driving Capability

 8.21 Effects of fatigue on driving performance
 8.211 Sources and nature of fatigue
 8.212 Effect upon driving efficiency
—Riding in the open wind creates wind buffeting and noise. Wind effect can camouflage fatigue
—Engine noise, vibration and road shock

            –Monitoring traffic and the roadway overtaxes a rider
                 more quickly than a driver

    8.213 Measures used to delay the onset of fatigue and
            control its effects on driving
            –Cyclists should take breaks often and limit their
                 daily riding to fewer hours than when driving an
                 auto—but some do not

EPISODE 8.4 Motivations for Responsible Driving

    8.44 Role of beliefs, attitudes and values
            –Overassess ability and take unnecessary chances
            –Disobey some traffic laws
            –While they feel they can control their machine, cyclists may
                 not possess the capabilities necessary in some situations
                 where others' responses are important to cyclists' safety
            –Most cyclists do obey traffic laws and cooperate with other
                 drivers in the highway transportation system, but when
                 riding some tend to display various attitudes and emotions
                 more than automobile operators

    8.46 Development of self-concept or self-understanding profile as
            related to driving
            –A few cyclists may display a daring image; evidence:
            —Failure to share roadway
            —Lack of, or failure to use, safety gear
            —Taking unnecessary risks
            —Punish themselves or cycles to prove superiority

UNIT 9.0—ALCOHOL AND OTHER DRUGS

Because of the importance of balance in cycle riding, the heavy demands of riding cycles and the lack of protection for their bodies, the results of cyclists' errors (even slight errors) due to being under the influence of alcohol and other drugs are magnified.

UNIT 10.0—OBEDIENCE AND ENFORCEMENT OF TRAFFIC LAWS

EPISODE 10.1 The Nature and Scope of Traffic Laws

    10.12 Classification of laws
          10.1243 Traffic laws and laws pertaining to motorcycles
               –Headlight on at all times cycle is operated
               –Helmets, compulsory wearing of (in some
                 states)
               –Eye protection (mandatory in Illinois)
               –Miscellaneous laws vary from state to state
                 making compliance sometimes difficult

EPISODE 10.3 Interpretation of Traffic Laws Regulating Highway Transportation System User Behavior or Condition

10.32 Conditions for earning and maintaining a legal operator's license
–Special cycle licenses and tests
–All operators in the highway transportation system must obey traffic laws

SUGGESTED LEARNING ACTIVITIES   **UNIT 10.0**

1. State which motor vehicle laws pertain to cyclists. Name any laws which cyclists must obey, but automobile drivers need not obey.

UNIT 11.0—POST CRASH PROCEDURES AND RESPONSIBILITIES

When involved in an accident (due to the nonprotective nature of his man-vehicle traffic unit), a cyclist usually will need immediate and more extensive medical attention than the average driver involved in an accident.

UNIT 12.0—SELECTION, INSPECTION AND MAINTENANCE OF SAFE VEHICLES

EPISODE 12.1 Selection of Safe and Economical Equipment

12.11 Legal and illegal equipment regulations
12.111 Lamps and other lighting regulations
–In order to be seen, cyclists usually will ride with

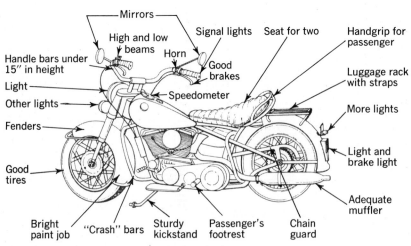

Figure 1 The well-equipped motorcycle–for safety!

This information is provided by the Motorcycle Industry Council Government Relations office. As State Assemblies continue to pass and/or amend motorcycle equipment requirements, subsequent charts with current dates will be issued. Phone, telex, or write to the

Motorcycle Industry Council offices listed below for additional information concerning motorcycle equipment requirements or for additional copies of this chart.

STATE	SAFETY HELMET	EYE PROTECTION	REARVIEW MIRROR	BRAKES	HANDLEBAR HEIGHT	PASSENGER SEAT	PASSENGER FOOTRESTS	PASSENGER HANDHOLD	SAFETY BARS	PROTECTIVE CLOTHING	TURN SIGNALS	SPEEDOMETER/ODOMETER	HEADLIGHT DAYTIME USE	PERIODIC INSPECTION
Alabama	●	●	●	●-7		●	●			●				
Alaska	■-22	●	●-6	●-8	●-13	●	●	●						
Arizona	■-3	●	●	●-7	●-13	●	●	●						●-19
Arkansas	●	●	●	●-7		●	●	●	●				●	●
California	●		●	●-8	●-14	●	●	●			●			●-21
Colorado	●-1	●	●	●-7		●	●							●
Connecticut	*	●	●	●-8h	●-13	●								●-21
Delaware	●-1	●	●	●-7	●-13	●					●			
Dist. of Col.	●	●	●	●-8	●-13	●	●	●				●-17		
Florida	●	●	●	●-8	●-13	●	●						●	●
Georgia	●	●	●-5	●-7		●	●			●-16				
Hawaii	●-1	●	●	●-7	●-13	●	●							
Idaho	●			●-7		●								
Illinois		●	●	●-7	●-13	●	●	●					●	
Indiana	●	●	●-5	●-8	●-13	●	●						●	●
Iowa	*	●	●	●-7	●-13	●	●						●	●-20
Kansas	●-4f	●	●	●-9	●-13	●	●				●			●-21
Kentucky	●-1	●	●	●-7		●	●				●	●-17		
Louisiana	■-3	●	●	●-8	●-13	●	●				●			
Maine	●-1	●	●	●-7	●-13	●	●						●	
Maryland	●-1	●	●-6	●-7	●-13	●	●							●-20
Massachusetts	●	●	●	●-7	●-13	●	●							●
Michigan	●	●-2	●	●-8	●-13	●	●							●-21
Minnesota	●	●	●	●-7	●-14	●	●						●	●-21
Mississippi	●		●	●-8	●-10	●	●					●-17		
Missouri	●		●	●-7	●-13	●	●							
Montana	●		●	●-8		●	●						●	
Nebraska	●-g		●	●-7	●-12	●	●							●
Nevada	●	●	●-6	●-8	●-13	●	●				●			●
New Hampshire	●	●	●	●-7	●-13	●	●				●	●		●
New Jersey	●-1	●	●-6	●-7	●-13	●	●	●						●
New Mexico	●-1	●	●	●-7	●-13	●	●							●
New York	●-1	●	●	●-8	●-13	●	●					■-23c	●	●
No. Carolina	●		●	●-7		●	●						●	●
No. Dakota	●-1	●	●	●-8	●-13	●	●					●		●-21
Ohio	●	●	●	●-7	●-13	●	●							●-21
Oklahoma	●-3	●	●-6	●-8	●-11	●	●					●-17		●
Oregon	●	●	●	●-7	●-14	●	●							●-21
Pennsylvania	●	●	●	●-8	■-14d	●	●	●						
Rhode Island	*	●	●	●-9	●-13	●	●	●				●-17a		
So. Carolina	●-1	●	●	●-7	●-13	●	●							●
So. Dakota	●-3d	●	●	●-9	●-13	●	●							
Tennessee	●	●	●	●-7	■-13	●	●		●-15				■-d	
Texas	●-1	●	●	●-7	●-13	●	●							●
Utah	●-2	●-2	●	●-7	●-14	●	●					●-18		●
Vermont	●-1	●	●	●-7	●-13	●	●							●
Virginia	●	●	●	●-8b	●-13	●	●							●
Washington	●	●	●-5	●-8	●-13	●	●						●	●-21
W. Virginia	●-1	●	●	●-7	●-13	●	●						●	●
Wisconsin	●	●	●	●-7	●-13	●	●					●-h	●	●-21
Wyoming	●	*	●	●-8	●-13	●	●						●	

● Requirement in law
1 Reflectorization
2 Where speeds exceed 35 mph
3 Under 18 years
4 Under 16 years
5 Left side
6 Left and right side
7 One wheel
8 Both wheels
9 Must meet performance standard
10 10" above fasten point
11 12" above fasten point
12 15" above fasten point
13 15" above seat
14 Handgrips below shoulder height
15 Over 750 cc if operator under 18 years

16 Foot wear
17 Speedometer
18 Odometer
19 Annual emissions inspection
20 Upon transfer of title
21 Random
22 Under 19 years
23 Speedometer with both mile and kilometer calibrations

a If originally equipped by manufacturer
b For motorcycle manufactured after 7/1/74
c For motorcycle manufactured after 9/1/80
d Effective 7/1/77

e Effective 1/1/78
f Effective when Federal funds are no longer withheld for failure to comply with Federal law
g Not enforced
h Newer models

Many state inspection regulations require that any equipment installed on a motorcycle must function properly even though the equipment is not required by law.

* Denotes removal of requirement since March, 1976 list was distributed.
■ Denotes change in status since March, 1976 list was distributed.

Although this chart represents information from the most authoritative sources available as of the date shown above, the Motorcycle Industry Council is not responsible for accuracy or completeness.

MOTORCYCLE INDUSTRY COUNCIL, INC.
4100 Birch St. Suite 101 • Newport Beach, Calif. 92660
(714) 752-7833 • Telex 67-8302
1001 Connecticut Ave. N.W. Suite 522 • Washington, D.C. 20036
(202) 872-1381 • Telex 89-508

Figure 2 State motorcycle equipment requirements.

the headlight on. Legal requirement in some states (including Illinois)

—Wearing a safety helmet is required in most states

6.03 LICENSE REQUIREMENT—A LICENSE TO OPERATE A MOTORCY-CLE MAY BE ISSUED TO PERSONS UNDER 18 YEARS OF AGE IF THEY CAN QUALIFY BY EXAMINATION.

The implementation of an effective state motorcycle safety program requires the participation and support of the local governments. It is at the local level where motorcycle safety can be most effectively fostered by campaigns which seek to develop well-informed, well-trained and safety-motivated motorcycle operators.

There are certain actions which are instituted by the state to promote safe motorcycle operation and eliminate unsafe practices of motorcycle operators. . . .

REGISTRATION—A motor-driven cycle is now defined as every *motorcycle* or every bicycle with motor attached with less than 150 cubic centimeter piston displacement. A special distinguishing plate will be issued to motorcycles having less than 150 cubic centimeter piston displacement.

DRIVER'S LICENSE—A driver's license to operate a motor vehicle, including motorcycles, cannot be issued to anyone under 18 years of age unless he has successfully completed an approved Driver Education course. The Driver Education course must include instruction in the classroom part which orients automobile and motorcycle drivers to the problem of sharing the road together safely.

A driver's license must be classified to indicate the type of vehicle and operation for which the applicant has qualified by examination or such other means which the Secretary of State has prescribed. Therefore, no person may obtain a motorcycle license until he has successfully completed a motorcycle examination.

MOTORCYCLE LICENSE CLASSIFICATIONS—A class L license restricts an operator to driving a cycle with 150 cubic centimeters or less. Anyone under 18 years of age or who has taken his examination on a motor-driven cycle is restricted to the L classification.

An M classification requires the operator to be 18 years of age or older and permits him to drive any cycle.

Instruction Permits—An instruction permit for a motor-driven cycle is restricted to the operation of such cycle during daylight hours only, and it is not valid unless the holder thereof is practicing under the direct supervision of a licensed motor-driven cycle operator or motorcycle operator who is at least 21 years of age. A motorcycle instruction permit is valid for practice driving only when the holder thereof is under the direct supervision of a licensed motorcycle operator who is at least 21 years of age.

In order to obtain a motor-driven cycle instruction permit, a person under 18 years of age must successfully complete an approved Driver Education course. He must have the Illinois Driver Education Certificate to obtain this permit.

An examination for a motorcycle or motor-driven cycle driver's license requires the applicant to demonstrate his ability to exercise ordinary and reasonable control in the operation of a motorcycle.

MOTORCYCLE PROGRAM—THE MOTORCYCLE EDUCATION AND TRAINING COURSE SHOULD CONSIST OF BOTH CLASSROOM INSTRUCTION AND CONTROLLED OFF-STREET OPERATION.

An individual completing a motorcycle instructional program should understand and appreciate each essential facet involved in safe operation of a motorcycle under all traffic conditions, classes of roads and highways, and climatological conditions.

After successful operation of an approved Driver Education course, a school district may offer a special motorcycle instructional program consisting of 10 to 12 hours of classroom instruction and six hours of motorcycle driving instruction. The program is not required by law, and if schools elect to incorporate motorcycle instruction, it must be approved by the Superintendent of Public Instruction.

ADMINISTRATIVE PROCEDURES

In order that your motorcycle rider education course be successful, several administrative factors must be considered. Naturally you will begin by obtaining the consent of the administration and school board. A thorough proposal will have been developed supported by a sound budget to better assure your obtaining their consent.

PERSONS ELIGIBLE TO TEACH—The instructor shall be certified to teach driver education and have additional training and experience with motor-driven cycles and motorcycles.

PERSONS ELIGIBLE TO ENROLL—Any resident of the local school district who has reached his sixteenth but not his twenty-first birthday, or has completed the driver education course, is eligible to be enrolled (in) and attend the elective course in motor-driven cycle driver education.

WHO MAY OFFER THE COURSE—Those schools which have met the qualifications set forth by the Safety Education Section of the Office of the Superintendent of Public Instruction.

WHEN TO OFFER THE COURSE—Classes may be offered before school, after school, during regular school hours, Saturdays and evenings. The course should be conducted during the early fall, late spring and the summer months to insure better weather conditions.

HOURS OF INSTRUCTION—With a growing emphasis upon riding strategies, and new audio-visual media to interestingly portray strategies, a class of novice riders could benefit from 12–16 hours of classroom instruction; some of the time might be of an independent study nature using new media. If a practice riding area has no auxiliary "trail" area, most novices will be able to master the suggested off-street riding program in 4–5 hours exclusive of on-cycle, on-center-stand preliminaries.

WHERE THE COURSE MAY BE HELD—The course should be offered at the school and the laboratory sections must be conducted on an off-street area where traffic is not present.

CYCLE IDENTIFICATION—Cycles may have the dealer stickers on them for the purpose of identification.

Cost—This depends upon how many students you will instruct, of course, and what facilities you have. Assume you have seven motorcycles (six for instruction, one for a stand-by); use this formula:

Administrative and planning hours × teacher salary +

Class hours × teacher salary +

$\dfrac{\text{Number of students}}{\text{Number of cycles (6)}}$ × range hours × teacher salary +

Insurance +

Miscellaneous expenses (oil, gas, extra spark plugs, fair wear and tear) $5/cycle.

Insurance—You ought to obtain insurance locally, if possible. If the insurance carrier of the driver education vehicles or other local agent is not disposed to serve you at a reasonable rate, contact the Office of the Superintendent of Public Instruction, Safety Section in Springfield for other sources.

EQUIPMENT AND FACILITIES

Motorcycles—They may be obtained from dealers on a free-loan basis. As with automobiles, the factory reimburses them for rider education vehicles. Have a loan agreement signed just as with automobiles. (See Appendix A) It is recommended that motorcycles in the 100cc–150cc engine size be used. They should have a center stand so that on-stand simulation sessions might be conducted. Be prepared to do minor adjustments (engine idle, chain adjustment, adding oil, changing bulbs and spark plugs) yourself.

Helmets—Because of the personal nature of a helmet, dealers may be reluctant to lend these. The Office of the Superintendent of Public Instruction will assist you in this matter, if need be; but try approaching dealers for a donation of one to two helmets each, or approach service clubs for donations for helmets and have their name printed on the helmet. Maintain helmets' inside cleanliness with a spray disinfectant between usage.

Traffic Cones—If you do not have some, borrow 40–50, six-inch cones from the city public works department.

Traffic Signs—These may be obtained from the city and mounted on poles welded to old auto wheels. Small signs that are mounted in traffic cones can be obtained from driver education supply houses. Include stop, yield, RR, one-way and do not enter signs.

First Aid Kits—If students wear gloves and have long sleeves, you rarely need one; but have a good one available. The school nurse should be able to select one.

Fire Extinguisher—A dry-chemical extinguisher should be kept on hand. Care in refueling cycles before the day's use will avert gasoline spills on hot engines.

Gasoline—A five-gallon container should be stored according to accepted regulations. Many motorcycles require premium fuel.

Storage—Motorcycles should be stored in an approved area with ignition and fuel turned off. Keep the ignition keys and helmets in a secure location.

Miscellaneous—A motorcycle manual, tool kit, extra bulbs, fuses, engine oil, pre-gapped spark plugs and two-cycle oil (if required) should be on hand.

Situation "simulators"—Railroad tracks may be simulated by fastening two 6-foot-long 2 × 4's approximately three feet apart; it may be placed at various angles on the range. A pail full of gravel or sand should be spread at a couple of turns during advanced lessons. Newly painted lines in a parking lot or range will provide a built-in reducer.

Students' attire—Students should furnish all attire with the exception of a helmet, unless they have an approved (Z90.1) helmet they wish to bring. They should have leather gloves, long pants (bell-bottoms must be fastened), long sleeves, shoes with heels high enough to cover their ankles, and glasses or goggles with safety lenses.

TEACHING SUGGESTIONS

Classroom and practice riding sessions should be integrated. Riding should start after the second or third hour of class instruction. Students want to learn to ride and they should not be delayed long.

In order to teach the integrated course, it would be desirable to teach the first four units in this order: 1, 3, 4, 2. Unit 5 activities should begin concurrently with Unit 1 or 3. It will be noted that portions of Units 3 and 4 are more properly taught during the practice-riding sessions.

You may find it necessary to omit certain items from your course of instruction. Be certain to include data and learning experiences that will contribute significantly to the welfare of your students.

In preparing this curriculum, it was assumed that students in a motorcycle rider education course will have already successfully completed a driver education course. If some have not, then, supplementary study will be required if they are to keep pace.

Off-street practice riding area—A paved surface free of excessive amounts of loose material is needed. Minimum dimensions for such an area would be 100 × 200 feet. More desirable is 150 × 300 feet, and 200 × 400 feet will permit several intersecting streets to be incorporated in the design. An existing driving range would be ideal. It is relatively easy to lay out a design for various skill areas for motorcycles. You do not even need a tape measure. Some practice areas that may be designated by cones appear below. Entrances and exits should be determined for particular areas and enforced.

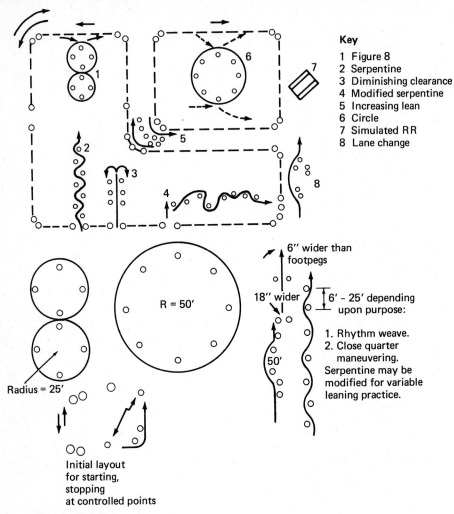

Key

1 Figure 8
2 Serpentine
3 Diminishing clearance
4 Modified serpentine
5 Increasing lean
6 Circle
7 Simulated RR
8 Lane change

R = 50'

6" wider than footpegs

18" wider

6' – 25' depending upon purpose:

50'

1. Rhythm weave.
2. Close quarter maneuvering. Serpentine may be modified for variable leaning practice.

Radius = 25'

Initial layout for starting, stopping at controlled points

Figure 3 Mini-range.

CURRICULUM GUIDE

This curriculum guide lists the topics under each unit that you will want to teach; however, it is not a subject matter text. In a few instances additional inclusions are made to clarify topics found to be lacking in several sources. From the sources you will find subject matter and audio-visual materials that treat the topics listed. Each unit has behavioral objectives, content references and learning activities that you may find helpful in planning lessons for your students. An off-street lesson guide provides a suggested chronology of riding experiences.

Index